T0177496

Integrative Sleep Medicine

Weil Integrative Medicine Library

Published and Forthcoming Volumes

SERIES EDITOR

Andrew Weil, MD

Integrative Sleep Medicine

EDITED BY

Valerie Cacho
Integrative Sleep Physician
Sleep Life Med
Honolulu, HI, USA

Esther Lum
Pulmonary and Sleep Physician
Board Certified in Pulmonary, Sleep, and Integrative Medicine
Denver, Colorado, USA

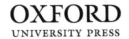

OXFORD
UNIVERSITY PRESS

Oxford University Press is a department of the University of Oxford. It furthers
the University's objective of excellence in research, scholarship, and education
by publishing worldwide. Oxford is a registered trade mark of Oxford University
Press in the UK and certain other countries.

Published in the United States of America by Oxford University Press
198 Madison Avenue, New York, NY 10016, United States of America.

© Oxford University Press 2021

Library of Congress Cataloging-in-Publication Data
Names: Cacho, Valerie, editor. | Lum, Esther, editor.
Title: Integrative sleep medicine / [edited by] Valerie Cacho and Esther Lum.
Other titles: Weil Integrative medicine library.
Description: New York, NY : Oxford University Press, [2021] |
Series: Weil integrative medicine library | Includes bibliographical references and index.
Identifiers: LCCN 2021008537 (print) | LCCN 2021008538 (ebook) |
ISBN 9780190885403 (paperback) | ISBN 9780190885427 (epub) |
ISBN 9780190885434 (online)
Subjects: MESH: Sleep Wake Disorders—therapy | Integrative Medicine—methods | Sleep
Classification: LCC RC547 (print) | LCC RC547 (ebook) | NLM WL 108 |
DDC 616.8/498—dc23
LC record available at https://lccn.loc.gov/2021008537
LC ebook record available at https://lccn.loc.gov/2021008538

DOI: 10.1093/med/9780190885403.001.0001

1 3 5 7 9 8 6 4 2
Printed by Marquis, Canada

To my loving husband, Danny, thank you for your support, without it this book wouldn't have been possible.
To my kids, Ava and Jacob, follow your dreams.
—Valerie

To my mom and dad, who always believed in me;
To my husband, who always encouraged and supported me;
To my son, whom I will always believe in.

This book was made possible by all of them.

With love and gratitude,
—Esther

CONTENTS

FOREWORD

ANDREW WEIL, MD

Series Editor

Good sleep is a key component of healthy lifestyle—good both in terms of quality and amount. Most people need seven hours of sleep at night; some do well on less, a few on more. Good sleep has a normal "architecture" with distinct phases characterized by brain wave frequency. An initial plunge into deep (non-rapid-eye-movement or NREM) sleep is followed by a phase of rapid eye movement (REM) sleep in which dreaming occurs. These two phases alternate cyclically until waking. Smoking, sleep apnea, stress, and various medications distort sleep architecture, depriving many people of restorative sleep.

Judging just by the brisk sales of sleep aids, both prescription and over-the-counter products, I think it is clear that many people in our society do not sleep well and are not getting the health benefits from it they should. Many have trouble falling asleep; others are unable to stay asleep. Many become dependent on pharmaceutical sleep aids, none of which reproduce natural sleep architecture, most of which suppress dreaming.

Inquiry into the sleeping habits of patients should be part of any medical history, whether or not insomnia is the reason for seeing a doctor. If a problem with sleep is suspected, referral to a sleep medicine specialist might be indicated. Sleep medicine is a new field, rapidly developing to address a growing need.

So many factors can interfere with sleep that identifying them is often challenging, addressing them even more so. Integrative medicine practitioners are trained to assess lifestyles of patients and recommend changes to improve health and manage common problems. This volume on *Integrative Sleep Medicine* will help all health professionals better understand the complexity of sleep disorders and the diversity of treatment approaches for them.

Drs. Cacho and Lum have compiled an impressive amount of information on their subject and present a great array of evidence-based therapies to manage the problems with sleep affecting so many people today. I thank them for their work and welcome this addition to the expanding Weil Integrative Medicine Library Series published by Oxford University Press.

PREFACE

It is an honor and a privilege to present this new addition to the Weil Integrative Medicine Library.

Sleep is an inherently integrative process, playing crucial roles in memory consolidation, mood, and health. It naturally follows, then, that an integrative approach would work best for maintaining healthy sleep and addressing sleep disorders.

Sleep medicine is a relatively new field that has experienced explosive growth in the past few decades, and clinicians are still learning how to best apply the wealth of scientific discoveries. While it is often easier to view and treat sleep as an isolated process, sleep and wake are a true yin/yang phenomenon. Because of this, sleep cannot be compartmentalized without sacrificing a greater understanding of it. Notably, a recurrent theme that appears throughout the book is the bidirectional nature of sleep and its impact on our lives. In fact, one would be hard pressed to describe any aspect of our lives that sleep does not influence in some way.

Just as we speak of cardiovascular health, we can also speak of sleep health. Too often sleep is seen as the first thing to be sacrificed rather than regarded as the foundation of a healthy lifestyle. Yet sleep health is an essential part of overall health and disease prevention. Integrative sleep medicine recognizes the pivotal role that sleep plays in our lives, places equal emphasis on maintaining sleep health as treating sleep disorders, and utilizes an evidence-based, holistic perspective.

This text is particularly timely. As we go to press, the country is still trying to emerge from a devastating pandemic that has left almost no one untouched. Covid-19 itself appears to have a direct impact on sleep, causing both hypersomnia and insomnia, and it has been posited that adequate sleep and melatonin play a role in fending off the disease. In addition, the stressors and disruptions created by the pandemic have wreaked havoc on the sleep of many tens if not hundreds of millions more, resulting in a worldwide increase in insomnia and sleep disturbances. This is reflected in an increase of prescriptions for both sleep and anti-anxiety medications.

Short term sleep disturbances can lead to long term sleep disorders and their attendant risks, and many are now at risk of developing chronic insomnia.

However, this progression is not inevitable, nor do we need to wait for studies of the pandemic's impact in order to take steps now. If addressed early, measures can be taken to prevent the progression, such as keeping a regular sleep/wake schedule, being physically active, and getting appropriate light exposure, to name a few.

We hope you will find this book helpful in addressing the growing need for better sleep, and we hope it contributes to improving the sleep health of many.

Sleep well,
Valerie Cacho
Esther Lum

ACKNOWLEDGMENTS

Thank you to Dr. Andrew Weil for seeing the potential in us. Andrea and her team at Oxford. Dr. Rubin Naiman for his support and pioneering work in integrative sleep medicine. And our contributors, who shared their time and expertise in the creation of this book.

ABOUT THE EDITORS

Valerie Cacho, MD, is the president and founder of Sleep Life Med, an integrative sleep medicine practice based in Ewa Beach, Hawaii. She completed her sleep fellowship at the Cedars Sinai Medical Center in Los Angeles, California. Dr. Cacho is board certified in Sleep and Internal Medicine by the American Board of Internal Medicine.

Esther Lum, MD, is a board certified pulmonary and sleep medicine physician with over two decades of experience practicing sleep medicine. She completed her fellowship training at Washington University in St. Louis, Missouri. Dr. Lum is board certified in Pulmonary Disease and Sleep Medicine by the American Board of Internal Medicine, and she is board certified in Integrative Medicine by the American Board of Physician Specialties.

CONTRIBUTORS

Hovig K. Artinian, MD, MAT
Pediatric Pulmonology and Sleep
  Medicine Physician
Helen DeVos Children's Hospital,
  Spectrum Health
Michigan State University
Grand Rapids, MI, USA

Michael Beshir, PharmD
Clinical Pharmacist
Department of Inpatient Pharmacy
Rush Oak Park Hospital Institution
Oak Park, IL, USA

Valerie Cacho, MD
Integrative Sleep Physician
Sleep Life Med
Honolulu, HI, USA

Ann Marie Chiasson, MD, MPH
Director, Fellowship in Integrative
  Medicine
Associate Professor of Clinical
  Medicine
Andrew Weil Center for Integrative
  Medicine
College of Medicine, University of
  Arizona
Tucson, AZ, USA

Chana Chin, MD
Assistant Clinical Professor
Department of Pediatrics
CHOC Children's Pulmonary and
  Sleep Medicine and the University
  of California, Irvine Department of
  Pediatrics
Orange, CA, USA

José Colón, MD, MPH, ABLM, IFMCP
Sleep Medicine Specialist and Pediatric
  Neurologist
Lee Health, The Children's Hospital of
  Southwest Florida
Fort Myers, FL, USA

Kayla Cook, PharmD
Clinical Pharmacist
Department of Pharmacy
Rush Oak Park Hospital
Chicago, IL, USA

Frederic C. Craigie, Jr, PhD
Clinical Psychologist/Medical
  Educator
Andrew Weil Center for Integrative
  Medicine
University of Arizona College of
  Medicine
Tucson, AZ, USA

Natalie D. Dautovich, PhD
Assistant Professor
Department of Psychology
Virginia Commonwealth University
Richmond, VA, USA

Param Dedhia, MD
Director of Sleep Medicine
Health and Healing
Canyon Ranch
Tucson, AZ, USA

Sutapa Dube, MD
Clinical Assistant Professor
Department of Psychiatry
University of Arizona College of
  Medicine
Tucson, AZ, USA

Stephen Paul Duntley, MD
Visiting Professor
Department of Neurology
University of Colorado School of
  Medicine
Aurora, CO, USA

Joseph M. Dzierzewski, PhD
Associate Professor
Department of Psychology
Virginia Commonwealth University
Richmond, VA, USA

Nicola Finley, MD
Physician
Medical Department
Canyon Ranch
Tucson, AZ, USA

Erin E. Flynn-Evans, PhD, MPH
Director, Fatigue Countermeasures
  Laboratory
Human Systems Integration
NASA
Moffett Field, CA, USA

Sophie von Garnier, EdM, MA
Department of Counseling Psychology
Santa Clara University
Santa Clara, CA, USA

Michael A. Grandner, PhD, MTR
Associate Professor
Department of Psychiatry
University of Arizona College of
  Medicine
Tucson, AZ, USA

Mindy Green, MS
Retired Clinical Aromatherapist
Department of Research and
  Development
Aveda Corporation (Estee Lauder)
Minneapolis, MN, USA

Diana Grigsby-Toussaint, PhD, MPH
Associate Professor
Department of Behavioral and Social
  Sciences and Department of
  Epidemiology
Brown University
Providence, RI, USA

Cassie J. Hilditch, PhD
Research Associate
Department of Psychology
San Jose State University
San Jose, CA, USA

Alex Holland, MAc
Vice President of Strategic Initiatives
Arizona School of Acupuncture and
    Oriental Medicine
Tucson, AZ, USA

Janna L. Imel, PhD
Graduate Student
Department of Psychology
Virginia Commonwealth University
Richmond, VA, USA

David Kiefer, MD
Clinical Assistant Professor
Department of Family Medicine and
    Community Health
University of Wisconsin-Madison
Madison, WI, USA

Elizabeth B. Klerman, MD, PhD
Professor
Department of Neurology, Harvard
    Medical School
Massachusetts General Hospital
Boston, MA, USA

Alison Kole, MD, MPH, FCCP
Pulmonary Medicine
Summit Medical Group City MD
Berkeley Heights, NJ, USA

Michael Kurisu, DO
Director
Center for Integrative Medicine
University of California at San Diego
San Diego, CA, USA

Jaclyn L. Lewis-Croswell, PsyD
Psychologist
Department of Psychology
Psychology Center of Tampa Bay
Tampa, FL, USA

Esther Lum, MD
Pulmonary and Sleep Physician
Board Certified in Pulmonary, Sleep,
    and Integrative Medicine
Denver, Colorado, USA

Caroline Maness, MD
Neurology Resident, Chief Resident
Department of Neurology
Atlanta, GA, USA

Jennifer L. Martin, PhD
Professor of Medicine
Department of Medicine
University of California
Los Angeles, CA, USA

Joanne S. Martires, MD
Assistant Professor
Pulmonary, Critical Care, and Sleep
    Medicine
Rush University Medical Center
Chicago, IL, USA

Robert Maurer, PhD
Clinical Psychologist, Faculty
Family Medicine Spokane
Spokane Teaching Health Center
Spokane, WA, USA

Ashwin Mehta, MD, MPH
Integrative Medicine
Memorial Healthcare System
Hollywood, FL, USA

Rubin Naiman, PhD
Clinical Assistant Professor of
    Medicine
Andrew Weil Center for Integrative
    Medicine
University of Arizona
Tucson, AZ, USA

Patrick J. O'Connor, PhD
Professor
Department of Kinesiology
University of Georgia
Athens, GA, USA

Jason C. Ong, PhD
Associate Professor
Department of Neurology
Northwestern University Feinberg
  School of Medicine
Chicago, IL, USA

Kaustubh Vijay Parab, MBBS, MPH
Doctoral Student & Research Assistant
Department of Community Health
University of Illinois at
  Urbana-Champaign
Champaign, IL, USA

Smita Patel, DO, FAASM
Integrative Neurologist and Sleep
  Specialist
iNeuro Institute
Des Plaines, IL, USA

Iris A. Perez, MD
Attending Physician, Associate
  Professor of Clinical Pediatrics
Department of Pediatrics
Keck School of Medicine of USC/
  Children's Hospital Los Angeles
Los Angeles, CA, USA

Valencia Porter, MD, MPH
Founder
Resilient Health
San Diego, CA, USA

Shadab A. Rahman, PhD, MPH
Instructor in Medicine; Associate
  Neuroscientist
Division of Sleep Medicine; Division
  of Sleep and Circadian Disorders,
  Department of Medicine
Harvard Medical School; Brigham and
  Women's Hospital
Boston, MA, USA

Tarah Raldiris, PhD
Assistant Professor
Department of Psychology
Flagler College
St. Augustine, FL, USA

Reuben Ram, MD
Physician
Department of Family and Sleep
  Medicine
David Geffen School of Medicine
  at UCLA
Los Angeles, CA, USA

Noshene Ranjbar, MD
Assistant Professor
Department of Psychiatry
University of Arizona
Tucson, AZ, USA

Scott Ravyts, MS
Clinical Psychology Doctoral
  Candidate
Department of Psychology
Virginia Commonwealth University
Richmond, VA, USA

Morgan P. Reid, MS
Doctoral Student
Department of Psychology
Virginia Commonwealth University
Richmond, VA, USA

Kaddy Revolorio, PsyD
Psychology Postdoctoral Resident
Department of Mental Health
Veterans Affairs Greater Los Angeles
    Healthcare System
North Hills, CA, USA

Shauna L. Shapiro, PhD
Professor
Department of Counseling Psychology
Santa Clara University
Santa Clara, CA, USA

Jong Cheol Shin, PhD
Postdoctoral Research Associates
Department of Behavioral and Social
    Science
School of Public Health, Brown
    University
Providence, RI, USA

Mary Anne Tablizo, MD
Pediatric Pulmonary and Sleep
    Medicine Specialist
Lucile Packard Children's Hospital
    Pulmonary and Sleep Medicine
    Center and Valley Children's
    Hospital Pediatric Pulmonary
    and Sleep
Palo Alto, CA, USA

Lynn Marie Trotti, MD, MSc
Associate Professor
Sleep Center and Department of
    Neurology
Emory University School of Medicine
Atlanta, GA, USA

Andrew S. Tubbs, BSc
Graduate Research Associate
Department of Psychiatry
University of Arizona College of
    Medicine—Tucson
Tucson, AZ, USA

Jeanne Wallace, MD, MPH
Professor of Medicine
Olive View-UCLA Medical Center
Sylmar, CA, USA

Carly L. A. Wender, PhD
Postdoctoral Research Fellow
Center for Traumatic Brain Injury
    Research
Kessler Foundation
East Hanover, NJ, USA

Claire E. Wheeler, MD, PhD
Assistant Professor
Health Promotion
OHSU-PSU School of Public Health
Portland, OR, USA

Emerson M. Wickwire, PhD
Associate Professor
Departments of Psychiatry and
    Medicine
University of Maryland School of
    Medicine
Baltimore, MD, USA

Manisha Witmans, MD, FRCPC, FAASM
Associate Clinical Professor
Department of Pediatrics
University of Alberta
Edmonton, Alberta, Canada

1

Perspectives on Integrative Sleep Medicine

ESTHER LUM

Feeling rested and refreshed after a peaceful night of sleep is a universal desire, as there is simply no equivalent to a good night's rest. Sleep, like nutrition and physical activity, is one of the key underpinnings of human health and well-being. Though the relative importance of each may be debated, survival is shortest without sleep.

Despite its importance, sleep deprivation and impaired sleep are pervasive in modern life. As a whole, Americans have lost touch with the innate ability to sleep along with the natural circadian rhythms that help drive the sleep–wake cycle. Add to that the stressors of daily living, and the result is a society that has forgotten how to sleep, leaving a multitude of individuals struggling to find remedies.

A growing body of knowledge points to a myriad of health conditions associated with sleep disorders, including cancer, depression, and cardiovascular disease. While this heightened awareness has led to more articles and features in the general press, the wealth of information is often confusing and misinterpreted by both patients and clinicians alike. Furthermore, fundamental questions remain, beginning with why we even sleep at all.

Over the past couple of decades, there has been increasing concern over Americans getting enough sleep. An analysis by the US Centers for Disease Control and Prevention (CDC) of a 2014 survey concluded that more than one-third of Americans do not get enough sleep on a regular basis,[1] and the CDC has called insufficient sleep a public health epidemic. A study from 2015 suggests that adolescents may be among the hardest hit, with decreasing sleep duration noted in this group during the study period of 1991–2012.[2] While the effects of sleep deprivation are serious for adults, the consequences in adolescents may be even more severe during this key period of their development, adversely impacting mental health, school performance, weight gain, and substance abuse.

Although some studies have argued against a recent significant decline in the average sleep duration of Americans, surveys suggest that whether the decrease is real or not, more than 40% of Americans do not feel they get enough sleep on a regular basis,[3] and the consequences of this lack of sleep are very significant. Drowsy driving alone is thought to be the cause of more than 800 fatalities annually,[4] and a Rand study from 2017 estimates that the United States loses up to 9.9 million working hours and $411 billion annually due to insufficient sleep.[5]

As society has become increasingly 24-hour over the past few decades, night shift and alternative work schedules more frequently encroach on time traditionally used for sleep. Healthy practices that promote quality sleep, including good nutrition and physical activity, have become more difficult to integrate into busy yet increasingly sedentary lifestyles. The original iPhone was released in 2007, and since then, smartphones and electronic media have become ubiquitous in daily life. Often present in the bedroom, electronics are distractions that have been clearly shown to disrupt sleep quality, in part due to the light emitted by these devices, which affects the circadian rhythm. On a more global scale, light pollution, which is excessive artificial light outside at night, negatively impacts the circadian rhythms of humans and wildlife alike. More than 80% of the world's population is thought to live under light-polluted skies.[6]

Lack of sleep and poor quality of sleep have become recognized as important public health issues, and sleep became a metric for the first time in the Healthy People 2020 objectives. Healthy People provides science-based, 10-year national objectives for improving the health of all Americans.[7]

Despite this growing awareness, sleep deprivation and sleep disturbances remain prevalent in the population. While the use of electronics, the presence of light, and a 24-hour society are not likely to change at any time in the foreseeable future, measures can be taken to improve sleep if the importance of sleep is recognized and prioritized by both individuals and society alike.

Historical Views of Sleep

To sleep, perchance to dream.

This famous line from Shakespeare's *Hamlet* is often quoted to describe the desirability of sleep. However, the actual meaning of "sleep" in the quote refers to death, and it reflects a view of sleep as a time of passivity akin to death. This view was commonly held even in recent history, until the electroencephalogram (EEG) was invented and brain activity was noted during sleep. Prior to this discovery, sleep was often defined by what it was not: wake.

Yet in other times and societies, different views of sleep existed. In Greek mythology, the gods Hypnos (sleep) and Thanatos (death) were brothers, but, despite this, sleep was viewed as a healing process. The ancient Greeks created healing temples or *asclepeions* that were dedicated to the healing god Asclepias.[8] Visitors to the temples sought spiritual and physical healing, and the temples promoted a holistic approach that included purification through diet and exercise. An important part of the healing process was temple sleep, which occurred when patients slept in the temple with the hope that Asclepias would appear in their dreams and tell them how to be healed. Patients also reported their dreams to priests who would assist in dream interpretation to find a cure. Asclepeions were the forerunners of our modern-day hospitals, and many physicians such as Hippocrates received their training there.

Other societies have revered dreams and the insights that they bring. Native Americans such as the Iroquois took dream interpretation very seriously and used dreams to guide their actions. Children were encouraged from a young age to recall their dreams and interpret their meaning.[9] Dreams were used to make important decisions, such as going to war or choosing spouses. Practices such as fasting and sweat lodge ceremonies were undertaken to promote dreaming, and dreams were often shared among tribe members to determine their underlying meaning and appropriate actions to take in response. A shaman often used dreams in his or her role as a healer.

Native Americans as a whole believed that dreams were an extension of reality, allowing communication with other realms and spirits. This view of the dream world as a form of alternate reality is not unique to Native Americans. Other ancient cultures including Egyptians, Hebrews, and Australian Aborigines recognized dreams as prophetic communications from ancestors or spirits.[10] The Old Testament describes God speaking to leaders through dreams numerous times.

Although science and medicine long relegated sleep to be a physical state of little interest, many cultures throughout history have recognized sleep as an important experience in people's lives, one that provided spiritual connection, insight into their own lives, and a foundation for healing. Modern medicine has yet to fully recognize or study many of these potential benefits of sleep and dreaming.

ALTERNATIVE SLEEP PATTERNS

The evolution of human sleep patterns must have been heavily influenced by the environment and circumstances of ancient humans. Humans evolved in concert with the day–night cycle and were exposed to the elements and predators during sleep, with the most obvious result being the preference to sleep at night. With modernization and industrialization came the development of easily controlled climate and lighting, severing the connection between sleep and the outside environment.

Moreover, sleep is impacted by physical activity and other occurrences during the day, and, as a result, sleep in industrialized societies is far removed from how it originally evolved.

Most Americans consider the ideal sleep pattern to be one consolidated sleep period at night. Epidemiologic studies suggest that 7–9 hours is the optimum for most people, with exceptions for both short and long sleepers. However, modern sleep patterns are heavily influenced by various timing constraints, such as jobs, children, and school start times. Social preferences, such as meals and gatherings, also influence sleep timing. Furthermore, the ubiquitous presence of light in various forms from indoor lighting, electronic media, and night lights influence sleep patterns as well.

The data are clear that sufficient sleep is foundational for optimum health, but the best way of obtaining that sleep remains undefined. Humans are very adaptable to different situations, and, like diet, there may be many healthy patterns of sleep. Other sleep patterns that differ from the current "ideal" have been described. While there is limited concrete information on how humans used to sleep in earlier eras, written documentation suggests that a bimodal pattern was common in pre-industrial Europe, and the mid-day siesta continues to exist today in some countries. An examination of some different sleep patterns may yield insights regarding other sleep practices, which include varying timing and duration of sleep.

The Spanish Siesta

Most people have heard of the word *siesta*, a Spanish term describing an early afternoon nap or rest. The Spanish siesta occurs during the hottest part of the day, when it is often too hot to work outside. It also coincides with a natural circadian decline in alertness that occurs in the early afternoon. Although the prevalence of the afternoon siesta has declined over the years as more people have moved to the cities, the afternoon break during the day continues to be practiced in parts of Spain. Traditionally, a typical Spaniard worked in the morning, had an afternoon siesta period, then worked later into the evening, with dinner and bedtime subsequently delayed as well.

Although the term "siesta" is Spanish, the practice of a siesta has not been limited to Spain or Europe. Siestas are commonly practiced in Asia, especially by the elderly, and considered to be a healthy practice. Other countries with a siesta habit include the Philippines, Nigeria, and Italy, countries with warm climates like Spain. Even in the United States, where siestas are not considered a standard practice, it is not uncommon for the elderly to take a nap during the day. The siesta is also not a recent phenomenon. Ancient Islam had a siesta, as did the Romans.

Are these bimodal sleep patterns healthy? There are data suggesting that a regular siesta habit may be beneficial,[11] and the Spanish Society of Primary Care

Physicians (SEMERGEN) released a statement recommending the daily siesta based on a review of research.[12] The Spanish have one of the longer life expectancies in the world,[13] and while numerous factors play into that, it suggests that the siesta itself does not negatively impact health and potentially could support it.

First and Second Sleep

In another bimodal sleep pattern, one quite different from the siesta, a first and second sleep period at night have been described, dating back to times before the Industrial Revolution.

In a descriptive book of nighttime in pre-industrial Europe, the historian Ekirch[14] details this pattern of sleep. People slept a couple hours after sunset (referred to as the first sleep), woke for 1–2 hours, and then slept again (the second sleep) until dawn. During the wake time between the first and second sleep, various activities took place, such as reading and relaxing, as well as less sedentary ones like chopping wood or sewing. Ekirch found references to the first and second sleep in various types of writings and documents from that time period, though these references diminished around the seventeenth century.

Traditional Societies

The sleep patterns of more traditional societies are thought to reflect that of ancient humans, which has prompted scientific interest. People in such societies are much more exposed to the elements and lack the electricity and artificial lighting that may impact their circadian rhythms.

While these societies are now few and far between, some still exist and have become subjects of interest. In a study of three preindustrial human societies, the Hadza, Kalahari San, and the Tsimané, Yetish et al. examined sleep duration, timing, relation to natural light, ambient temperatures, and seasons.[15] These societies do not use electricity or artificial light, and they are exposed to variations in day length, season, and daily temperature. Using actigraphy, their patterns of sleep were assessed and, perhaps not surprisingly, were found to correlate with their natural environment.

Sleep time among the three groups was similar, between 5.7 to 7.1 hours. Sleep times of the Tsimané and San in the winter were longer than in the summer by 56 minutes and 53 minutes respectively, and sleep onset was on average about 3.3 hours after sunset. There was also a strong correlation between the initiation of sleep and a fall in ambient temperature and between wake onset and the nadir of daily temperature. Both naps and nocturnal wake periods were infrequent.

Interestingly, interviews of the Tsimané and San found that neither group had a word for insomnia. Five percent of these populations had sleep onset problems and 9% had sleep maintenance problems, but fewer than one-third of these had them more than once a year.

In another study of a rural population without electricity in Madagascar, segmented sleep was noted, with a peak of activity observed after midnight.[16] Frequent napping was also present, and the population slept 6.5 hours per night. This nighttime pattern appeared to be similar to the first and second sleep noted by Ekirch.

In these studies of non-electrified populations, it was noted that sleep quality, as measured by sleep efficiency, was generally fairly poor, lower than that of most post-industrial populations. Sleep duration was also shorter, but circadian rhythms were more stable.

The siesta, first and second sleep, and unimodal sleep pattern all represent different accommodations for the need to sleep. It is hard to draw broad conclusions from limited data of alternative sleep patterns, but it is clear is that different sleep patterns have existed in various societies throughout history and may reflect local climate, seasons, day–night timing, and societal norms, among other factors. As modern sleep schedules change to accommodate different work schedules and sleep patterns, such differing sleep practices may offer alternatives to the unimodal sleep pattern that is currently most prevalent. However, the health benefits or detriments of these alternative sleep patterns have not been documented, and further study is needed.

Medical Perspectives of Sleep

The discipline of sleep medicine, while no longer new, is still a very recent one. It was 1952 when the first recordings of EEG and eye movements were made during sleep, prompting the realization that sleep was far from a time of brain inactivity and leading to greater scientific interest in sleep.[17] Thus, the birth of sleep science came with the discovery of the EEG. Since then, and especially in recent decades, there has been an explosion of scientific information in the field.

In its youth, sleep science was not segregated into body (medicine) and mind (behavioral/cognitive) components because both were regarded as integral to treatment. This unified approach to sleep disorders has gradually evolved, in part due to the discovery of sleep apnea and its treatments that have fueled the development of sleep medicine as its own discipline.

Obstructive sleep apnea (OSA) was discovered in 1965, but until the continuous positive airway pressure (CPAP) device was invented in 1981, the only known treatment was tracheostomy—a treatment that was not very palatable to patients. With the advent of CPAP and the uvulopalatopharyngoplasty (UPPP) surgical procedure, more acceptable treatment options became available. OSA was also found to be widely prevalent in an increasingly obese population, leading to broad public health implications. While interpreting polysomnograms as a whole remains a relatively complex diagnostic process, interpreting the severity of sleep apnea was straightforward, with well-defined parameters for the Apnea Hypopnea Index (AHI). A combination of these factors drove interest in OSA, but along with that came an interest in sleep disorders and sleep medicine as a whole.

As a result, sleep gradually became recognized as its own discipline. Established in 1975, the American Academy of Sleep Medicine (AASM) is a leading voice in the field of sleep medicine with the mission of advancing sleep care and enhancing sleep health to improve lives. *Principles and Practice of Sleep Medicine*, still considered the definitive textbook of sleep medicine and now in its sixth edition, was first published in 1989. The first *International Classification of Sleep Disorders* manual came out in 1990, and the American Board of Sleep Medicine was founded in 1991, which was the first organization to board certify physicians and doctorates in sleep medicine.

In 1998, Dr. William Dement, one of the fathers of sleep medicine, spoke on the history of sleep medicine and focused on the need to bring sleep into mainstream medicine, focusing particularly on OSA.[18] Now, more than 20 years since that address, it is safe to say that sleep medicine has indeed become a part of mainstream medicine. OSA is well recognized by primary care physicians and patients alike, and home sleep apnea testing is widely available throughout the United States, obviating the need for in-lab polysomnography for many patients.

Sleep medicine has joined the mainstream, but with that process has come an approach to sleep and sleep disorders that is reflective of conventional medicine. Conventional medicine relies heavily on diagnostic testing and pharmaceuticals to treat medical disorders. This method has strengths and benefits for some disorders but is less successful for others.

Sleep apnea, for which an objective quantifiable approach (the AHI) has been developed for diagnosis and determination of successful treatment, has been very successfully integrated into public consciousness and has made CPAP widely used and accepted. However, such an approach is not equally applicable to many other sleep disorders, such as insomnia and parasomnias, and how best to define and treat them remains elusive.

INSOMNIA: A LONG-NEGLECTED PROBLEM

Despite the increasing prevalence of sleep apnea, estimated at 12% of adults in the United States,[19] insomnia remains the most common sleep problem. The AASM estimates that short-term insomnia affects up to 50% of the population and chronic insomnia at least 5–15% of the population.[20] Insomnia is a subjective sleep complaint related to difficulty falling asleep or staying asleep despite adequate opportunities for sleep. Questionnaires such as the Insomnia Severity Index have been designed to objectively assess the severity of insomnia, but a comprehensive understanding of its pathogenesis and treatment have proved more challenging.

While insomnia has been declared a growing epidemic similar to sleep deprivation, it is difficult to know exactly how much insomnia has increased in the population. Diagnoses of insomnia have increased over the years, as have prescriptions for medications for sleep, but these may be influenced by heightened awareness through public health initiatives or promotions by pharmaceutical companies.

Medicalization is the process by which formerly normal biological processes or behaviors come to be described, accepted, or treated as medical problems. With the medicalization of sleep, insomnia has become increasingly viewed as a medical disorder for which medications are often used. Many insomnia patients seek relief through medications, often using over-the-counter remedies initially and subsequently obtaining prescription medications. It is interesting to note that prescriptions for sleep medications increased significantly after 1999[21] in concert with the acceptance of sleep medicine as a legitimate field.

The ideal medication for insomnia is a pill that puts a patient to sleep quickly, keeps the patient asleep through the night, and leaves the patient feeling alert and refreshed the following morning without any residual morning hangover effect. However, medications for insomnia fall far short of this ideal, and many patients experience side effects, some very serious. Moreover, the overall efficacy is poor. In one meta-analysis, hypnotic use in older patients was found to provide an average increase in sleep time of only 25 minutes.[22]

Benzodiazepines and the so called *Z drugs*—nonbenzodiazepine, benzodiazepine receptor agonists (BZRA)—work by affecting gamma-aminobutyric acid (GABA) receptors in the brain, which promote sleepiness. The hypnotic effects of many other medications used for insomnia, including antihistamines (such as diphenhydramine) and the sedating antidepressants (trazodone, mirtazapine, tricyclic antidepressants), are due at least in part to their blocking effect on histamine, a wakefulness-promoting neurotransmitter. But is the absence of wake the same as sleep?

Sleep is a complex process during which many neurotransmitters are active and inactive in different parts of the brain, and the full explanation for what happens during sleep has not yet been fully elucidated. Polysomnographic data show that medications can alter sleep architecture or cause EEG changes, such as increased spindle formation with benzodiazepine use. How these alterations impact the quality and function of sleep is not entirely clear, but they demonstrate that there are changes to what occurs normally during sleep.

Increasingly, the data suggest that sleep induced with medications is not the same as sleep that occurs naturally. Healthy sleep has been shown to improve memory, alertness, and health outcomes, whereas long-term use of antihistamines and benzodiazepines has been associated with an increased risk of dementia and death, with greater risk for the elderly. It is not clear if the newer hypnotics, such as the orexin antagonists (suvorexant, lemborexant) or melatonin receptor agonists, are safer longer term, but suvorexant has been associated with falls and driving impairment.[23] Sleep medications also foster a reliance that can be very difficult to terminate, thus undermining patients' self-efficacy for sleep.

The risks associated with benzodiazepines and BZRA's are wide-ranging, though not all are clearly demonstrated as cause and effect. Some of the stronger associations are related to the intended purpose of the medications themselves: sleepiness and the risks associated with excessive daytime sleepiness. Falls and fractures as well as motor vehicle accidents are increased in patients taking these medications.[23] BZRA's are well known to be associated with complex sleep behaviors, which are actions performed while a patient is still asleep and that have potentially serious repercussions. Other data suggest that though their efficacy may diminish over time, long term use may increase the likelihood of cancer, infections, and cognitive decline.[24] Due to concerns about the Z drugs in particular, a clinical practice guideline has been issued for de-prescribing these medications.[25]

Side effects from other medications, many of which can interfere with or alter sleep, can also affect insomnia patients. Beta blockers, for example, decrease the production of melatonin, and most antidepressants suppress rapid eye movement (REM) sleep. The long-term impact of many of these medication effects remains undetermined.

Nonpharmaceutical measures are often utilized by insomnia patients as well. *Sleep hygiene* is a series of sleep-supportive recommendations, such as avoiding alcohol and caffeine, sleeping in a quiet bedroom with appropriate lighting, etc. However, good sleep hygiene, though helpful for supporting healthy sleep, has not been shown to be a successful stand-alone treatment option for insomnia.

The greatest breakthrough for insomnia has been *cognitive-behavioral therapy for insomnia* (CBT-I). CBT-I focuses on behavioral modifications to alter patterns of sleep and has been shown to be more effective and longer lasting when compared to medications. In 2016, the American College of Physicians issued a clinical practice guideline recommending CBT-I as first-line therapy for insomnia,[26] which is supported by the latest AASM guidelines for the behavioral treatment for insomnia.[20] Though frequently confused with sleep hygiene, CBT-I has become more widely available over recent years, both online and in person.

While promoting a behavioral practice over prescription medications represents noteworthy progress, CBT-I is not a complete solution for insomnia. Many find it difficult to follow the behavioral practices required for successful treatment, and, though effective for most, CBT-I is not effective for a significant percentage of patients.[27] Mindfulness Based Therapy for Insomnia (MBTI), a newer modality that integrates mindfulness into the CBT-I framework, represents a step towards incorporating other aspects of healthy sleep into existing treatment regimens,[28] and more such developments are needed.

LIMITS OF CONVENTIONAL MEDICINE

As previously discussed, conventional medicine tends to rely heavily on testing and pharmaceuticals with quantifiable results. This approach often neglects the realm of healthy behaviors as well as cognitive and mind–body approaches to the treatment of sleep disorders, with the recent exception of CBT-I. Furthermore, sleep is often viewed in isolation of wake and vice versa. While conventional medicine tends to focus on either wake or sleep, it often fails to acknowledge the complex interplay between the two. Increasingly, data show that mood as well as health and wellness impact sleep quality at night, and this relationship is bidirectional. Stress reduction, physical fitness, appropriate light exposure—these are all important components of healthy sleep but are often given short shrift in the approach to sleep disorders. Even CBT-I, as successful as it has been for insomnia, focuses primarily on behavioral modifications but may fail to address all components of healthy sleep.

Treatment options for many other sleep disorders are even more limited than for insomnia. The literature for treatment of *parasomnias*, such as sleep walking or night terrors, is relatively sparse, and common suggestions include no treatment or the use of a few medications with largely unproved benefits.

Conventional medicine also has limited regard for the experience and individuality of sleep and sleep disorders. Attention is rarely paid to dreams other than to note them as "REM sleep," yet dreams may provide insight into the patient's frame of mind. At the very least, having patients relate their personal experience of sleep and dreaming provides the clinician with a greater understanding of the patient and allows the patient to better connect to the provider.

Integrative Sleep Medicine

Sleep medicine can be differentiated from most medical disciplines in that its focus is not on an organ or physical entity. Sleep is a process that impacts the entire body, with bidirectional relationships to every organ. It is perhaps most similar to mental health, which may help to explain its tight relationship with sleep. Sleep is also experiential. It is not just a biological process; it is subjective and personal, and it is not independent of wake.

Integrative medicine is healing-oriented medicine that takes account of the whole person, including all aspects of lifestyle. It is evidence-based and seeks the best of all appropriate therapeutic modalities, which includes conventional medicine but also complementary therapies from other cultures or times. The term "integrative sleep medicine" was first used by Rubin Naiman, who recognized a growing need to address sleep disorders from a holistic perspective. As such, the integrative approach to sleep medicine needs to utilize a whole-person perspective, acknowledging the roles of the mind and spirit, the physical, and the connection to the outside world through the circadian rhythm in the experience of sleep.

PRINCIPLES OF INTEGRATIVE SLEEP MEDICINE

Integrative sleep medicine recognizes all factors involved in healthy sleep. The following paragraphs describe the 10 principles underlying the integrative approach to sleep medicine.

1. *Utilizes the best of conventional and complementary medicine.* Integrative sleep medicine is based on efficacy of treatment regardless of discipline or origin. This includes all therapeutic modalities that have demonstrated benefit and/or low risk of harm. While conventional medicine excels at treating some sleep disorders, it has been less successful with others. Having additional treatment options provides greater therapeutic potential, and many have few if any adverse side effects. Depending on the sleep disorder, some of these options might include mind–body techniques, herbal remedies, clinical hypnosis, Traditional Chinese Medicine (TCM) or Ayurvedic medicine, tai chi, and dreamwork.

2. *Addresses sleep from the whole-patient perspective, including sleep phenomenology.* Effective treatment of patients requires a greater understanding of the patient's framework. The whole patient perspective restores regard for the sleeper by recognizing the importance of the subjective experience and its impact on a patient's life. Sleep is viewed from the context of the patient, including mood and well-being, lifestyle, family, and health. For any given individual, one or more of these aspects may take priority over the others, but all should be accounted for, and the focus should not be solely on what occurs at night. Sleep has an important mind–body component and is influenced by stress, anxiety, and mood, among other things. While this may seem readily apparent, it is frequently inadequately addressed.

3. *Partners with patients in the treatment of their sleep problems through education and engagement.* Patient centered care is a core tenet of integrative medicine and the foundation for successful treatment of sleep patients. Many therapies for sleep disorders require the patient to make a significant commitment, often altering long-standing habits and behaviors. It is therefore essential that the patient be a willing participant through education and partnering with their health care providers. Patients have many misconceptions about sleep, in large part due to the overabundance of readily available information. Most patients are unaware of what constitutes normal sleep and what treatment options are appropriate for their particular issues. CBT-I, for example, is often confused with sleep hygiene, and periodic and middle-of-the-night awakenings can be normal but provoke anxiety in many patients, which may exacerbate already existing insomnia. Successful

treatment requires engaging the patient in the process, ultimately empowering the patient to take control of their sleep issues.

4. *Evaluates for and addresses sleep disruptors.* Optimizing treatment regimens for sleep requires that all sleep disruptors be identified and treated as needed. Sleep disruptors include anything that may interfere with sleep. Many medical problems disrupt sleep, such as restless legs syndrome, gastroesophageal reflux disease, and pain from any cause. Mental health issues such as anxiety/depression are intricately tied to poor sleep as well, and both medical and mental health issues have bidirectional relationships with sleep. Medications and substances are also frequent sleep disruptors; steroids, for example, can cause insomnia. Common substances that disrupt sleep include caffeine and alcohol. These issues should be addressed as much as possible.

5. *Avoids sedatives and hypnotics when possible.* While sleep medications may be necessary in certain patients, this approach attacks the symptoms instead of seeking underlying or root causes. Sedatives and hypnotics should be avoided if possible, especially in the elderly and for long-term use. They are commonly associated with habituation and dependence and have been associated with serious long-term negative health consequences. The informed use of botanicals or nutraceuticals is preferred if needed, though ideally as part of an overall treatment regimen.

6. *Recognizes sleep and wake as complementary and interdependent processes.* Sleep and wake are a true *yin-yang* phenomenon; each affects the other, and together they form a harmonious whole. Reductively focusing on sleep in isolation from wake severs the involved and complex connection between the two. Yet, to fully discover effective therapies, it is essential to look at them as a whole. Benefits to avoiding a competing posture between them include decreased anxiety for the patient and the ability to construct patterns and behaviors that support one another. Analyzing sleep issues independent of wake neglects the interdependent relationship, promotes the use of medications as treatment, and limits the use of other therapies that may promote sleep.

7. *Recognizes the key role of rhythms, especially circadian and ultradian rhythms, in sleep and general health.* Human behavioral patterns developed in response to their surrounding environments, and the circadian rhythm reflects this evolution. Sleep is driven by both the circadian rhythm and homeostatic mechanisms. Just as food connects us to the ground and earth, the circadian rhythm connects us to the day–night cycle and thus the planet and solar system. Healthy sleep requires proper timing based on an individual's circadian rhythm, and sleep disorders may result from misalignment to natural biological rhythms. As people are increasingly separated from the physical world by decreased time outdoors and artificial lighting, methods to align sleep to the circadian rhythm need to be undertaken utilizing light, melatonin and other timing related activities.

8. *Affirms the critical importance of REM sleep/dreaming.* Dr. Naiman has long advocated for the importance of dreams in healthy sleep and views dreaming and dreaminess as the forgotten bridge to sleep. However, current approaches typically reduce dreaming to REM sleep, which is identified through EEG tracings, eye movements, and muscle tone. This simplistic view of dreaming disregards both the actual experience of dreaming and potential benefits beyond it simply being a part of sleep. Ancient societies may yield insight into how dreams can benefit patients or provide greater spirituality.

9. *Draws from practices in other cultures and times.* Scant regard has been paid to other views and practices of sleep in other cultures, yet these practices represent real-world information about how different peoples have found natural ways of optimizing sleep in various settings. Properly and scientifically studied, this data can provide stepping stones to sleep solutions for our current environment. Some avenues of potential study include TCM and Ayurvedic medicine but also extend to other sleep patterns and habits such as the siesta or first and second sleep. Different patterns of sleep have existed throughout history, but the current focus in sleep medicine has been on promoting a single consolidated period of sleep at night. Sleep patterns are affected by climate, environment, work schedules, physical activity, meals, etc., and, as a result, individuals may benefit from different sleep patterns depending on their personal circumstances. Further study of other cultural sleep practices, both current and historic, may yield greater insight and alternative therapies.

10. *Promotes sleep health and prevention of sleep disorders as a cornerstone of both individual and public health.* Sleep is pivotal to individual and societal health, but little has been done in the realm of prevention, nor has the important role that society plays in an individual's sleep health been widely acknowledged. Properly prioritized, healthy sleep may lead to the prevention of other health issues. However, sleep health cannot be fully addressed without looking beyond individuals, as collectively, sleep affects society, and society affects sleep. Sleep-deprived individuals have more motor vehicle and on-the-job accidents, impaired judgment, and absenteeism, but individuals' sleep schedules and sleep quality are influenced by work and school schedules, on-call requirements, and shift work, among others. When society recognizes the importance of healthy sleep, changes can be made that will positively impact many individuals' sleep health. An example of this is the recent trend to delay school start times for adolescents in high school who have a natural propensity to both fall asleep and wake up later.

The principles of integrative sleep medicine can serve as a guide for the field as well as for treating individuals. Now, more than ever, the need for improving sleep has become more pressing. While the scientific understanding of sleep has increased dramatically, successfully applying this science to the individual's and society's experience of sleep still requires further development. Improving sleep has the potential to benefit all involved: individuals, families, and society.

REFERENCES

1. Liu Y, Wheaton AG, Chapman DP, Cunningham TJ, Lu H, Croft JB. Prevalence of healthy sleep duration among adults: United States, 2014. *MMWR Morb Mortal Wkly Rep.* 2016 Feb 19;65(6):137–141.

2. Keyes KM, Maslowsky J, Hamilton A, Schulenberg J. The great sleep recession: Changes in sleep duration among US adolescents, 1991–2012. *Pediatrics.* 2015;135(3):460–468.

3. Jones JM. In U.S., 40% get less than recommended amount of sleep. December 9, 2013. https://news.gallup.com/poll/166553/less-recommended-amount-sleep.aspx

4. National Center for Statistics and Analysis. *Drowsy Driving 2015.* (Crash•Stats Brief Statistical Summary. Report No. DOT HS 812 446.) Washington, DC: National Highway Traffic Safety Administration; 2017.

5. Hafner M, Stepanek M, Taylor J, Troxel WM, van Stolk C. Why sleep matters: The economic costs of insufficient sleep: A cross-country comparative analysis. *Rand Health Q.* 2017;6(4):11.

6. Falchi F, Cinzano P, Duriscoe D, et al. The new world atlas of artificial night sky brightness. *Sci Adv.* 2016;2(6):e1600377.

7. Morgenthaler TI, Croft JB, Dort LC, Loeding LD, Mullington JM, Thomas SM. Development of the National Healthy Sleep Awareness Project sleep health surveillance questions. *J Clin Sleep Med.* 2015;11(9):1057–1062.

8. Hart GD. Asclepius, god of medicine. *Can Med Assoc J.* 1965;92(5):232–236.

9. Tedlock B. The poetics and spirituality of dreaming: A Native American enactive theory. *Dreaming.* 2004;14(2–3):183–189.

10. Hughes JD. Dream interpretation in ancient civilizations. *Dreaming.* 2000;10:7–18.

11. Naska A, Oikonomou E, Trichopoulou A, Psaltopoulou T, Trichopoulos D. Siesta in healthy adults and coronary mortality in the general population. *Arch Intern Med.* 2007;167(3):296–301.

12. Govan, F. Spanish scientists prove the siesta is good for you—and issue guidelines for a perfect nap. *The Telegraph.* August 2012. https://www.telegraph.co.uk/news/worldnews/europe/spain/9458799/Spanish-scientists-prove-the-siesta-is-good-for-you-and-issue-guidelines-for-a-perfect-nap.html

13. Foreman KJ, Marquez N, Dolgert A, et al. Forecasting life expectancy, years of life lost, and all-cause and cause-specific mortality for 250 causes of death: Reference and alternative scenarios for 2016–40 for 195 countries and territories. *Lancet.* 2018;392(10159):2052–2090.

14. Ekirch AR. *At day's close.* New York: W. W. Norton; October 2006.

15. Yetish G, Kaplan H, Gurven M, et al. Natural sleep and its seasonal variations in three pre-industrial societies. *Curr Biol.* 2015;25(21):2862–2868.

16. Samson DR, Manus MB, Krystal AD, Fakir E, Yu JJ, Nunn CL. Segmented sleep in a nonelectric, small-scale agricultural society in Madagascar. *Am J Hum Biol.* 2017;29(4):10–1002/ajhb.22979.

17. Shepard JW Jr, Buysse DJ, Chesson AL Jr, et al. History of the development of sleep medicine in the United States. *J Clin Sleep Med.* 2005;1(1):61–82.

18. Dement WC. The study of human sleep: A historical perspective. *Thorax.* 1998;53 (Suppl 3):S2–S7.

19. Hidden health crisis costing America billions: Underdiagnosing and undertreating obstructive sleep apnea draining healthcare system, a report commissioned by the American Academy of Sleep Medicine, 2016:5.

20. Edinger JD, Arnedt JT, Bertisch SM, Carney CE, Harrington JJ, Lichstein KL, Sateia MJ, Troxel WM, Zhou ES, Kazmi U, Heald JL, Martin JL. Behavioral and psychological treatments for chronic insomnia disorder in adults: an American Academy of Sleep Medicine clinical practice guideline. *J Clin Sleep Med.* 2021 Feb 1;17(2):255–262.

21. Bertisch SM, Herzig SJ, Winkelman JW, Buettner C. National use of prescription medications for insomnia: NHANES 1999–2010. *Sleep.* 2014;37(2):343–349. Published 2014 Feb 1. doi:10.5665/sleep.3410

22. Glass J, Lanctôt KL, Herrmann N, Sproule BA, Busto UE. Sedative hypnotics in older people with insomnia: Meta-analysis of risks and benefits. *BMJ.* 2005;331(7526):1169.

23. Schroeck JL, Ford J, Conway EL, Kurtzhalts KE, Gee ME, Vollmer KA, Mergenhagen KA. Review of safety and efficacy of sleep medicines in older adults. *Clin Ther.* 2016 Nov;38(11):2340–2372.

24. Kripke DF. Hypnotic drug risks of mortality, infection, depression, and cancer: but lack of benefit [version 3; referees: 2 approved] F1000Research 2018, 5:918.

25. Pottie K, Thompson W, Davies S, et al. Deprescribing benzodiazepine receptor agonists: Evidence-based clinical practice guideline. *Can Fam Physician.* 2018;64(5):339–351.

26. Qaseem A, Kansagara D, Forciea MA, Cooke M, Denberg TD; Clinical Guidelines Committee of the American College of Physicians. Management of chronic insomnia disorder in adults: A clinical practice guideline from the American College of Physicians. *Ann Intern Med.* 2016;165(2):125–133.

27. Matthews EE, Arnedt JT, McCarthy MS, Cuddihy LJ, Aloia MS. Adherence to cognitive behavioral therapy for insomnia: A systematic review. *Sleep Med Rev.* 2013;17(6):453–464.

28. Ong J, Sholtes D. A mindfulness-based approach to the treatment of insomnia. *J Clin Psychol.* 2010;66(11):1175–1184.

2

Sleep and Health

ANDREW S. TUBBS AND MICHAEL A. GRANDNER

Introduction

Sleep is an essential part of human existence and accounts for nearly a third of life. Despite being a critical element for human health, society continues to find new and innovative ways of avoiding or curtailing sleep, from stimulants to micro-naps and everything in between. Staying awake is associated with productivity and personal strength, while sleeping is attributed to weakness. The truth, however, is that time spent sleeping is not time wasted. Human physiology depends on this 7- to 8-hour period of inactivity to repair tissues, generate new cells, adjust metabolism, and synthesize necessary hormones. Sleep consolidates memories to secure facts and sensations that accrued throughout the day and process emotional wounds and psychological stressors that are otherwise suppressed.

The influence of sleep duration on human health includes both insufficient/ short sleep as well as excessive/long sleep. While the effects of excessive sleep on health have been studied in various contexts, the outcomes are often conflicting or difficult to interpret.[1] Most people do not choose to oversleep, but rather do so out of physiological or psychological necessity or as a result of pharmacological intervention. Therefore, excessive sleep will not be discussed as a behavioral risk factor.

The Epidemiology of Short Sleep

The optimal amount of sleep for an adult is at least 7 hours per night.[2] Unfortunately, many adults fall short of this goal. A 2005 survey of adults in 10 countries found that 25% of adults sleep 6–7 hours per night, while only 31% slept for an optimal

7–8 hours.[3] In the United States, the 2014 Behavioral Risk Factor Surveillance System (BRFSS), using average self-report sleep within 24 hours, reported that nearly 35% of adults sleep less than 7 hours.[4] Similarly, the 2007–2008 National Health and Nutrition Examination Survey (NHANES), which collected data on weeknight/worknight sleep, estimated that nearly 40% of adults sleep less than 7 hours.[5] The widespread prevalence of short sleep should be recognized as a major public health concern, especially given the impacts on human health discussed in the following sections.

Cardiometabolic Disease

Cardiometabolic disease refers to derangements in metabolic processes that affect cardiovascular function. While diet and exercise are commonly cited health behaviors, new research reveals sleep as critical to achieving cardiometabolic health. This section will examine how sleep is associated with major cardiometabolic diseases.

CLINICAL DISEASE

Obesity

Meta-analytic data clearly suggest a relationship between obesity and short sleep. Adults who chronically slept 5 hours or less were more strongly associated with obesity (odds ratio [OR] 1.55; [1.43, 1.68])[6] than those who slept 7–8 hours. Furthermore, for every additional hour of sleep, adults decreased their body mass index (BMI) by 0.35.[6] This relationship also applies to children, where the ORs of obesity among short sleepers range from 1.27 to 2.15.[6] Insufficient sleep also increases the risk of developing obesity by 30% (relative risk [RR] 1.30 [1.20, 1.42]),[7] while each additional hour of sleep decreases the association with obesity by 21% (OR 0.79 [0.70, 0.89]).[8]

On a behavioral level, sleep interferes with the normal homeostasis between energy intake and energy consumption. Energy homeostasis refers to the balance between energy intake (i.e., food consumption) and energy expenditure (i.e., exercise and basal metabolic rate). Sleep deprivation increases energy intake by as much as 500 kilocalories.[9,10] Sleep deprivation also affects food choices. Subjects who were sleep-deprived tended to eat fewer fruits and vegetables,[10–12] more fats,[10,11] less protein,[11,13] and more carbohydrate rich snack foods.[10–13] These dietary choices may be mediated by enhancing the hedonic perception of certain foods, which would drive food-seeking and consumption.[13] The result is a high-energy diet that, if maintained chronically, may lead to weight gain. While increased wakefulness may increase energy expenditure, subjects tended to consume far more calories than were needed to maintain energy homeostasis, resulting in a net positive intake.[14] Additionally, sleep and circadian timing significantly influence energy balance and weight gain. Individuals who are sleep-deprived tend to eat more after 8 PM, as well as more often throughout the day.[10–12,14] Since late eating reduces the effect of caloric restriction for weight loss,[11,12,14] sleep deprivation may influence weight gain through abnormally timed food intake.

So whose weight is most affected by insufficient sleep? The data suggest that blacks who sleep less than 5 hours a night have an increased risk of obesity over whites,[9] although there was no difference between whites and blacks for 5–6 hours per night. Additionally, young people, particularly children, appear most vulnerable to the effects of short sleep on obesity,[15] while the relationship between sleep and obesity is fairly attenuated, if not abolished, by age 65.[15,16] Interestingly, a meta-analysis of obesity and short sleep found that there was no significant difference between males and females.[16]

Diabetes

Diabetes mellitus is an endocrine disorder of the hormone insulin and glucose homeostasis. In Type I diabetes, autoimmune destruction of the beta cells of the pancreas results in loss of insulin. This blocks the extraction of glucose from the blood, resulting in hyperglycemia. In Type II diabetes (T2DM), insulin is present, but peripheral tissues are resistant to its action, resulting in hyperglycemia.

There is a wide body of evidence to support a relationship between short sleep and T2DM in adults. The prevalence of diabetes among short sleepers is twice that of normal sleepers.[17,18] Additionally, longitudinal data suggest that sleep shorter than 5–6 hours a night carries a 28% risk of incident diabetes (RR 1.28 [1.03, 1.60]) with the risk increasing 9% per hour lost (RR 1.09 [1.04, 1.15]) and 2% per year of short sleep (RR 1.02 [0.93, 1.12]).[19,20] Interestingly, current evidence does not support a differential effect of short sleep on diabetes risk among racial/ethnic groups after adjusting for socioeconomic status and obesity/BMI.[21,22] For short sleepers already diagnosed with T2DM, the risk of disease progression is elevated. Short sleep is associated with a 0.23% increase in hemoglobin A1c, a long-term measure of glucose control,[23] and a 34% increased risk of cardiovascular death (RR 1.34 [1.24, 1.46]).[24]

Coronary Heart Disease

The 2010 Behavioral Risk Factor Surveillance System reported the prevalence of coronary heart disease (CHD) among adults sleeping 6 hours or less was 11.1%, compared with 7.9% in the 7- to 9-hour group.[25] This suggests that short sleep may be a risk factor for CHD, although few studies have addressed this relationship.

However, insufficient sleep does exacerbate the health risks of CHD. A 2015 meta-analysis of patients with coronary artery disease found that morbidity was 10% higher in short sleepers (RR 1.10 [1.04, 1.17]) and mortality was 25% higher (RR 1.25 [1.06, 1.47]).[26] More specifically, short sleepers have a 19% increased risk of a heart attack (RR 1.19 [1.13, 1.26]),[24] with each hour of sleep lost increasing the risk of heart attack by 4% (RR 1.04 [1.01, 1.08]).[27] Future studies should determine if modifying short sleep in CHD decreases the risk of heart attack and death.

MECHANISMS OF CARDIOVASCULAR DISEASE

Inflammation

Insufficient sleep is associated with increased inflammatory markers such as C-reactive protein (CRP),[28-30] interleukin-6 (IL-6),[30-32] and tumor necrosis factor-alpha (TNFa).[32,33] Adjusting for comorbidities like obesity and apnea reduced the strength of the sleep–inflammation association.[31,33] So how could inflammation play a role in the development of cardiometabolic disease? Inflammatory cytokines increase insulin resistance,[34] resulting in difficulty controlling blood sugar and weight. Inflammation is also linked with T2DM and obesity and may influence sleep through neuroendocrine changes,[17]

Hypertension

Insufficient sleep increases the risk of developing hypertension by 20–30%.[35-37] Women who chronically sleep less than 5 hours a night are 68% more likely to also have hypertension (OR 1.68 [1.39, 2.03]); in contrast, there does not appear to be an association between sleep duration and hypertension in men.[36-38] Age is also a factor, as adults younger than 65 with insufficient sleep have a 61% increased association with hypertension (OR 1.61 [1.27, 2.04]).[37,38] By far the highest risk appears to be short sleeping premenopausal women, who are more associated with hypertension (OR 3.25 [1.37, 7.76]) than their normal sleeping peers.[34,39,40]

Hyperglycemia and Insulin Resistance

Observational studies of chronic short sleepers suggest that sleep deprivation disrupts glucose homeostasis. Individuals who slept less than 6.5 hours a night for at least 6 months required 50% more insulin to achieve the same glucose tolerance as normal sleepers.[41] Short sleep is associated with hyperglycemia, insulin resistance, and poor glycemic control[17, 18] and may produce a metabolic state akin to pre-diabetes.[42] Conversely, preliminary data suggest that increasing sleep returns glucose metabolism and insulin sensitivity to normal healthy levels.[14] Thus, sleep extension in pre-diabetes or T2DM patients may improve glucose control.

Cancer

One of the first epidemiological studies of sleep was the 1964 American Cancer Society study, which studied more than a million adults to find risk factors for cancer and mortality.[43] Hammond, however, made no comment on sleep duration as a risk factor for cancer, and subsequent meta-analyses support this.[44,45] Additionally, cancer mortality does not appear to differ between short and typical sleepers.[46]

In contrast to sleep duration, there is a small body of literature supporting an association between shift work and cancer. A large cross-sectional study found that prolonged shift work (20 or more years) was associated with an increased risk of any cancer (hazard ratio [HR] 1.27 [1.01, 1.59]) in men, but not women.[47] For men, there is an increased risk of prostate cancer in those who work rotating night shifts, although the effect size was small.[48] For women, an association between shift work and breast cancer was found when comparing never shift workers to ever shift workers, but not for other categories of shift work.[49] A different meta-analysis found that, while the overall association was marginal, the association in pre-menopausal women was more significant (OR 1.26 [1.05, 1.51]).[50] While no associations between shift work and other gynecological cancers currently exist, there are too few studies in this area to be sure.[51]

So how might shift work influence cancer risk? Several potential mechanisms exist, although there is insufficient evidence about which are actually involved.[52] Repeated disruption of the circadian system, which influences metabolic activity as well as cell division, may bring reactive oxygen species into contact with DNA during replication. Melatonin is a potent antioxidant, and so suppression of melatonin by light at night may impair the ability of the body to detoxify radicals. Additionally, sleep loss is known to suppress the immune system, and thus shift work may impair the immune response to cancer cells. Finally, disturbed sleep promotes obesity and inflammation, both of which contribute to increased cancer risk.

Cognitive Functioning

SLEEP AND COGNITIVE FUNCTION

Cognitive functioning is the conscious capacity of the individual to acquire, understand, and apply information through thoughts and actions. Cognitive functioning encompasses memory, language, attention, reasoning, and decision-making. This section explores the role of sleep in maintaining these processes and how deficits in sleep can produce profound and prolonged impairments.

Vigilant Attention

Vigilant attention is the ability to respond to a stimulus in the environment. In the laboratory, vigilant attention is tested by means of the psychomotor vigilance test (PVT), wherein subjects respond to a stimulus and their response times are recorded. Numerous studies have shown that when healthy subjects are sleep-deprived, their performance on the PVT worsens[53,54] and that objective deficits occur before subjects report feeling impaired.[55] Sleep deprivation affects the whole age spectrum, but young men appear particularly vulnerable.[56] Additionally, studies in minors suggest that insufficient sleep can contribute to poor attention, on both objective measures and subjective ratings by teachers and parents.[57]

Memory

Memory is a set of processes that store, recall, and compare stimuli to draw meaningful information and perform actions. Acute sleep deprivation compromises working memory.[53,54] Moreover, chronic sleep loss degrades working memory in both children[57,58] and adults.[59] Prospective memory, or the ability to recall information in the near future (e.g., providing a medication to a patient in half an hour), is also impaired in sleep-deprived states.[53,60,61] There is even evidence that sleep deprivation leads to the recall of erroneous information.[62]

IMPACT OF COGNITIVE FUNCTIONS ON HEALTH

Cognitive functions are not isolated laboratory phenomena or theoretical constructs, but actual tools used on a day-to-day basis. Humans solve problems, arrange priorities, interact with others, drive cars, ride bikes, and perform numerous other tasks, all of which depend on attention, memory, and executive function. Since sleep maintains these processes, chronic sleep loss not only deteriorates daytime functioning, but also increases the risk of accidents and injuries.

Occupational Accidents

Accidents happen when sleep is disturbed. Data gathered in the National Health Interview Survey between 2004 and 2013 suggest that 7–8 hours of sleep minimizes the risk of accidental injury and that every hour of sleep lost increases the association by 16% (OR 1.16 [1.12, 1.19]).[63] In general, insufficient sleep is associated with rates of injury ranging from 1.11 to 2.42 times that of normal sleepers,[64,65] although more dangerous occupations clearly carry higher risks[64] than desk jobs.[65]

Minors are also at risk. Surveys of high school students found that as sleep duration decreased, the rates of high-risk behaviors (e.g., driving without a seat belt or riding a bicycle without a helmet) increased.[66] Insufficient sleep increased the risk of bicycle accidents,[67] falls,[67,68] and occupational injuries.[69] Although untested, sleep interventions in this population may improve safety outcomes.

Drowsy Driving

By far the most dangerous interaction between sleep and injury occurs in drowsy driving. According to the American Academy of Sleep Medicine, drowsy driving is the operation of a motor vehicle while impaired by inadequate sleep and represents a "serious public health concern."[70] Impairment can be severe; studies of sleep deprivation and driving suggest that being awake for 17–19 hours results in performance equivalent to a blood alcohol content of 0.05.[71] Drowsy driving is common[72] and cannot be mitigated by professional training.[73] Of greater concern, impaired driving often occurs before drivers feel sleepy.[74] The result? One study estimated nearly 7% of all motor vehicle accidents and 16.5% of fatal accidents were due to drowsy driving.[75]

Mental Health

ANXIETY

Connecting anxiety with sleep loss is not a difficult task. Anyone who has taken an exam has probably experienced sleep disturbance the night before. Clinically speaking, sleep disturbance is one of the diagnostic features of generalized anxiety disorder, which affects roughly 3% of the US population.[76] For the purposes of this text, the general term "anxiety" will be used in place of a specific anxiety disorder since some studies do not differentiate between anxiety symptomatology and clinical diagnosis.

Anxiety is closely related to subjective sleep disturbance,[77] and longitudinal data suggest this relationship is bidirectional; insomnia can precede incident anxiety,[78–80] and anxiety can precede insomnia.[81] Insufficient sleep is also correlated with anxiety.[78,80,82] Fortunately, cognitive behavioral interventions for anxiety can improve sleep,[83,84] although the effects are modest and do not affect all domains of sleep. There is also evidence that cognitive-behavioral therapy for insomnia (C-BTI) reduces anxiety symptomatology.[85,86]

DEPRESSION

Depression affects millions of people globally. While the *Diagnostic and Statistical Manual of Mental Disorders* (DSM) describes a variety of depressive disorders, nearly all of them present with sleep disturbance as a core feature.[76] Sleeping less than 6 hours is associated with development of depressive symptoms.[82,87] Subjective symptoms of insomnia (difficulty falling asleep, awakening after sleep onset, early awakening, and nonrestorative sleep) also tended to predict depression onset.[78,79,87] Fortunately, current evidence shows that treating poor sleep improves non-sleep symptoms of depression.[88]

POSTTRAUMATIC STRESS DISORDER

Posttraumatic stress disorder (PTSD) is a psychopathologic response to an overwhelming threat which results in changes in health and behavior ranging from social interactions to cognitive functions.[76] Sleep disturbance is characteristic of PTSD and includes nightmares, mid-night awakenings, and insomnia.[81,89,90] In fact, there is evidence that subjective sleep disturbance immediately following the traumatic event is associated with development of PTSD[89] and that these disturbances in PTSD patients increase suicidality[91] and somatic/physical health problems.[90] Treating sleep disturbance in PTSD is crucial for restoring quality of life. Nightmares and subjective sleep quality are amenable to treatment,[92] and while insomnia symptoms tend to persist,[92] specific therapies targeting insomnia, such as CBT-I, improve both sleep and PTSD symptoms.[93]

SLEEP DISTURBANCE AND SUICIDE

Sleep serves as a modifiable risk factor for suicidality, a broad term referring to suicidal ideation, attempts, and completions. In case-control studies, individuals who attempted or completed suicide were more likely to have sleep disturbances than were controls,[94,95] even when controlling for comorbid psychiatric disease. In particular, subjects with suicidality were more likely to have interrupted sleep,[95] and increased severity of sleep disturbance conferred a higher OR of attempting or completing suicide.[94]

So what are the possible mechanisms relating sleep to suicidality? In a structured interview study, patients with depression and suicidal ideation identified several reasons.[96] First, sleep represents an alternative to suicide, and thus difficulty sleeping eliminates a potential coping mechanism for suicidal patients. Second, sleep disturbance results in patients being awake at night, when there is a reduced level of social support and an increased opportunity to commit suicide without interference. Finally, lack of good sleep was perceived as making life more difficult and contributing to depressed thinking.

A few studies suggest treating sleep disturbances may reduce suicidality. CBT-I in a community sample of depressed patients[88] correlated with decreased suicidality after treatment completion. Thus targeting patients' sleep behaviors may represent a useful intervention to reduce suicidality, particularly in vulnerable populations.

The Impact of Short Sleep

THE COST OF SHORT SLEEP

Sleeping less than 7 hours has negative outcomes on cardiometabolic, cognitive, and psychiatric well-being. What is less obvious is the impact on society. Insufficient sleep leads to reduced productivity, poor work performance, and adverse safety outcomes, which are estimated to cost $4.3 million annually.[97] Insufficient sleep also increases healthcare utilization and costs. Employees who reported frequent sleep difficulties consumed roughly $3,000 in healthcare more than those who never reported sleep difficulties.[98] Identifying and treating short sleep, therefore, is an issue of both individual and societal importance.

SHORT SLEEP AND MORTALITY

Short sleep carries a small but significant risk of increased all-cause mortality (ACM). Meta-analytic data estimate between 4% and 12% increased risk.[99] This represents a parabolic relationship between ACM and sleep duration, with chronic departures from roughly 7–8 hours of sleep per night possibly carrying an increased risk of mortality.[99]

Clinical Implications for Integrative Medicine

Sleep plays a critical role in relating social, environmental, and behavioral determinants to a wide range of metabolic, inflammatory, functional, and psychological outcomes and should be an important consideration in any integrative health practice. Patients often express concerns about sleep, and while many clinicians agree that sleep is important, most do not feel properly equipped to assess and treat sleep problems.[100] For these reasons, the following recommendations apply to clinical integrative medicine:

1. *Assess sleep in patients.* This can be as simple as a question, "How are you sleeping?" or as complex as using validated screening tools such as the Insomnia Severity Index to screen for insomnia, the STOP-BANG questionnaire to screen for sleep apnea, the Sleep Disorders Symptom Checklist to screen for sleep disorders in general, or another standard screening tool. Also, document sleep assessments and recommendations in clinical notes.
2. *Learn about sleep physiology and behavior,* as well as empirically supported (and empirically unsupported) treatments for sleep problems.
3. *Consider how social, environmental, physical, and behavioral factors influence sleep,* and how sleep can subsequently influence health.
4. *Consider sleep a vital sign,*[101] given the important role of healthy sleep in cardiovascular, metabolic, functional, and mental health.
5. *Include healthy sleep as an indicator of overall wellness,* and include healthy sleep as a goal of treatment.

REFERENCES

1. Grandner MA, Drummond SP. Who are the long sleepers? Towards an understanding of the mortality relationship. *Sleep Med Rev.* 2007;11(5):341–360.
2. Watson NF, et al. Recommended amount of sleep for a healthy adult: A joint consensus statement of the American Academy of Sleep Medicine and Sleep Research Society. *Sleep.* 2015;38(6):843–844.
3. Soldatos CR, et al. How do individuals sleep around the world? Results from a single-day survey in ten countries. *Sleep Med.* 2005;6(1):5–13.
4. Liu Y, et al. Prevalence of healthy sleep duration among adults: United States, 2014. *MMWR Morb Mortal Wkly Rep.* 2016;65(6):137–141.
5. Grandner MA, et al. Habitual sleep duration associated with self-reported and objectively determined cardiometabolic risk factors. *Sleep Med.* 2014;15(1):42–50.
6. Cappuccio FP, et al. Meta-analysis of short sleep duration and obesity in children and adults. *Sleep.* 2008;31(5):619–626.
7. Li L, et al. Sleep duration and obesity in children: A systematic review and meta-analysis of prospective cohort studies. *J Paediatr Child Health.* 2017;53(4):378–385.
8. Ruan H, et al. Habitual sleep duration and risk of childhood obesity: Systematic review and dose-response meta-analysis of prospective cohort studies. *Sci Rep.* 2015;5:16160.
9. Grandner MA. Sleep and obesity risk in adults: Possible mechanisms; contextual factors; and implications for research, intervention, and policy. *Sleep Health.* 2017;3(5):393–400.
10. St-Onge MP. The role of sleep duration in the regulation of energy balance: Effects on energy intakes and expenditure. *J Clin Sleep Med.* 2013;9(1):73–80.

11. Dashti HS, et al. Short sleep duration and dietary intake: Epidemiologic evidence, mechanisms, and health implications. *Adv Nutr.* 2015;6(6):648–659.

12. Baron KG, et al. Role of sleep timing in caloric intake and BMI. *Obesity (Silver Spring).* 2011;19(7):1374–1381.

13. Shechter A, Grandner MA, St-Onge MP. The role of sleep in the control of food intake. *Am J Lifestyle Med.* 2014;8(6):371–374.

14. McHill AW, Wright KP, Jr. Role of sleep and circadian disruption on energy expenditure and in metabolic predisposition to human obesity and metabolic disease. *Obes Rev.* 2017;18 Suppl 1:15–24.

15. Grandner MA, et al. Relationship between sleep duration and body mass index depends on age. *Obesity (Silver Spring).* 2015;23(12):2491–2498.

16. Itani O, et al. Short sleep duration and health outcomes: A systematic review, meta-analysis, and meta-regression. *Sleep Med.* 2017;32:246–256.

17. Barone MT, Menna-Barreto L. Diabetes and sleep: A complex cause-and-effect relationship. *Diabetes Res Clin Pract.* 2011;91(2):129–137.

18. Briancon-Marjollet, A, et al. The impact of sleep disorders on glucose metabolism: Endocrine and molecular mechanisms. *Diabetol Metab Syndr.* 2015;7:25.

19. Cappuccio FP, et al. Quantity and quality of sleep and incidence of type 2 diabetes: A systematic review and meta-analysis. *Diabetes Care.* 2010;33(2):414–20.

20. Shan Z, et al. Sleep duration and risk of type 2 diabetes: A meta-analysis of prospective studies. *Diabetes Care.* 2015;38(3):529–537.

21. Jackson CL, et al. Association between sleep duration and diabetes in black and white adults. *Diabetes Care.* 2013;36(11):3557–3565.

22. Zizi F, et al. Race/ethnicity, sleep duration, and diabetes mellitus: Analysis of the National Health Interview Survey. *Am J Med.* 2012;125(2):162–167.

23. Lee SW, Ng KY, Chin WK. The impact of sleep amount and sleep quality on glycemic control in type 2 diabetes: A systematic review and meta-analysis. *Sleep Med Rev.* 2017;31:91–101.

24. Krittanawong C, et al. Association between short and long sleep durations and cardiovascular outcomes: A systematic review and meta-analysis. *Eur Heart J Acute Cardiovasc Care.* 2017:2048872617741733.

25. Covassin N, Singh P. Sleep duration and cardiovascular disease risk: Epidemiologic and experimental evidence. *Sleep Med Clin.* 2016;11(1):81–89.

26. Yang X, et al. Association of sleep duration with the morbidity and mortality of coronary artery disease: A meta-analysis of prospective studies. *Heart Lung Circ.* 2015;24(12):1180–1190.

27. Yin J, et al. Relationship of sleep duration with all-cause mortality and cardiovascular events: A systematic review and dose-response meta-analysis of prospective cohort studies. *J Am Heart Assoc.* 2017;6(9).

28. Fernandez-Mendoza J, et al. Insomnia symptoms with objective short sleep duration are associated with systemic inflammation in adolescents. *Brain Behav Immun.* 2017;61:110–116.

29. Bakour C, Schwartz S, O'Rourke K, Wang W, Sappenfield W, Couluris M, Chen H. Sleep Duration Trajectories and Systemic Inflammation in Young Adults: Results From the National Longitudinal Study of Adolescent to Adult Health (Add Health). *Sleep.* 2017 Nov 1;40(11):zsx156. doi:10.1093/sleep/zsx156. PMID: 29155987; PMCID: PMC5806583.

30. Miller MA, et al. Gender differences in the cross-sectional relationships between sleep duration and markers of inflammation: Whitehall II study. *Sleep.* 2009;32(7):857–864.

31. Ferrie JE, et al. Associations between change in sleep duration and inflammation: Findings on C-reactive protein and interleukin 6 in the Whitehall II Study. *Am J Epidemiol.* 2013;178(6):956–961.

32. Hall MH, et al. Association between sleep duration and mortality is mediated by markers of inflammation and health in older adults: The Health, Aging and Body Composition Study. *Sleep.* 2015;38(2):189–195.

33. Patel SR, et al. Sleep duration and biomarkers of inflammation. *Sleep.* 2009;32(2):200–204.

34. Koren D, Dumin M, Gozal D. Role of sleep quality in the metabolic syndrome. *Diabetes Metab Syndr Obes.* 2016;9:281–310.

35. Meng L, Zheng Y, Hui R. The relationship of sleep duration and insomnia to risk of hypertension incidence: A meta-analysis of prospective cohort studies. *Hypertens Res.* 2013;36(11):985–995.

36. Guo X, et al. Epidemiological evidence for the link between sleep duration and high blood pressure: A systematic review and meta-analysis. *Sleep Med.* 2013;14(4):324–332.

37. Wang Q, et al. Short sleep duration is associated with hypertension risk among adults: A systematic review and meta-analysis. *Hypertens Res.* 2012;35(10):1012–1018.

38. Wang Y, et al. Relationship between duration of sleep and hypertension in adults: A meta-analysis. *J Clin Sleep Med.* 2015;11(9):1047–1056.

39. Stranges S, et al. A population-based study of reduced sleep duration and hypertension: The strongest association may be in premenopausal women. *J Hypertens.* 2010;28(5):896–902.

40. Gangwisch JE. A review of evidence for the link between sleep duration and hypertension. *Am J Hypertens.* 2014;27(10):1235–1242.

41. Knutson KL. Impact of sleep and sleep loss on glucose homeostasis and appetite regulation. *Sleep Med Clin.* 2007;2(2):187–197.

42. Gangwisch JE. Epidemiological evidence for the links between sleep, circadian rhythms and metabolism. *Obes Rev.* 2009;10 Suppl 2:37–45.

43. Hammond EC. Some preliminary findings on physical complaints from a prospective study of 1,064,004 men and women. *Am J Public Health Nations Health.* 1964;54:11–23.

44. Zhao H, et al. Sleep duration and cancer risk: A systematic review and meta-analysis of prospective studies. *Asian Pac J Cancer Prev.* 2013;14(12):7509–7515.

45. Lu Y, et al. Association between sleep duration and cancer risk: A meta-analysis of prospective cohort studies. *PLoS One.* 2013;8(9):e74723.
46. Ma QQ, et al. Sleep duration and total cancer mortality: A meta-analysis of prospective studies. *Sleep Med.* 2016;27–28:39–44.
47. Bai Y, et al. Association of shift-work, daytime napping, and nighttime sleep with cancer incidence and cancer-caused mortality in Dongfeng-tongji cohort study. *Ann Med.* 2016;48(8):641–651.
48. Mancio J, Leal C, Ferreira M, Norton P, Lunet N. Does the association of prostate cancer with night-shift work differ according to rotating vs. fixed schedule? A systematic review and meta-analysis. *Prostate Cancer Prostatic Dis.* 2018;21(3):337–344. doi:10.1038/s41391-018-0040-2. Epub 2018 Apr 27. PMID: 29700389.
49. Pahwa M, Labreche F, Demers PA. Night shift work and breast cancer risk: What do the meta-analyses tell us? *Scand J Work Environ Health.* 2018;44(4):432–435. doi:10.5271/sjweh.3738. Epub 2018 May 22. PMID: 29790566.
50. Cordina-Duverger E, et al. Night shift work and breast cancer: A pooled analysis of population-based case-control studies with complete work history. *Eur J Epidemiol.* 2018;33(4):369–379.
51. Schwarz C, et al. Gynaecological cancer and night shift work: A systematic review. *Maturitas.* 2018;110:21–28.
52. Haus EL, Smolensky MH. Shift work and cancer risk: Potential mechanistic roles of circadian disruption, light at night, and sleep deprivation. *Sleep Med Rev.* 2013;17(4):273–284.
53. Goel N, et al. Neurocognitive consequences of sleep deprivation. *Semin Neurol.* 2009;29(4):320–339.
54. Lim J, Dinges DF. A meta-analysis of the impact of short-term sleep deprivation on cognitive variables. *Psychol Bull.* 2010;136(3):375–389.
55. Franzen PL, Siegle GJ, Buysse DJ. Relationships between affect, vigilance, and sleepiness following sleep deprivation. *J Sleep Res.* 2008;17(1):34–41.
56. Urrila AS, et al. Psychomotor vigilance task performance during total sleep deprivation in young and postmenopausal women. *Behav Brain Res.* 2007;180(1):42–47.
57. Vriend JL, et al. Manipulating sleep duration alters emotional functioning and cognitive performance in children. *J Pediatr Psychol.* 2013;38(10):1058–1069.
58. Cho M, et al. Poor sleep and lower working memory in grade 1 children: Cross-sectional, population-based study. *Acad Pediatr.* 2015;15(1):111–116.
59. Lo JC, et al. Self-reported sleep duration and cognitive performance in older adults: A systematic review and meta-analysis. *Sleep Med.* 2016;17:87–98.
60. Grundgeiger T, Bayen UJ, Horn SS. Effects of sleep deprivation on prospective memory. *Memory.* 2014;22(6):679–686.
61. Esposito MJ, Occhionero M, Cicogna P. Sleep deprivation and time-based prospective memory. *Sleep.* 2015;38(11):1823–1826.
62. Lo JC, et al. Sleep deprivation increases formation of false memory. *J Sleep Res.* 2016;25(6):673–682.

63. Bhattacharyya N. Abnormal sleep duration is associated with a higher risk of accidental injury. *Otolaryngol Head Neck Surg.* 2015;153(6):962–965.

64. Lilley R, et al. The relationship between fatigue-related factors and work-related injuries in the Saskatchewan Farm Injury Cohort Study. *Am J Ind Med.* 2012;55(4):367–375.

65. Kucharczyk ER, Morgan K, Hall AP. The occupational impact of sleep quality and insomnia symptoms. *Sleep Med Rev.* 2012;16(6):547–559.

66. Wheaton AG, et al. Sleep duration and injury-related risk behaviors among high school students: United States, 2007–2013. *MMWR Morb Mortal Wkly Rep.* 2016;65(13):337–341.

67. Kim SY, et al. Sleep deprivation is associated with bicycle accidents and slip and fall injuries in Korean adolescents. *PLoS One.* 2015;10(8):e0135753.

68. Boto LR, et al. Sleep deprivation and accidental fall risk in children. *Sleep Med.* 2012;13(1):88–95.

69. Graves JM, Miller ME. Reduced sleep duration and history of work-related injuries among Washington State adolescents with a history of working. *Am J Ind Med.* 2015;58(4):464–471.

70. American Academy of Sleep Medicine, et al. Confronting drowsy driving: The American Academy of Sleep Medicine perspective. *J Clin Sleep Med.* 2015;11(11):1335–1336.

71. Williamson AM, Feyer AM. Moderate sleep deprivation produces impairments in cognitive and motor performance equivalent to legally prescribed levels of alcohol intoxication. *Occup Environ Med.* 2000;57(10):649–655.

72. Maia Q, et al. Short and long sleep duration and risk of drowsy driving and the role of subjective sleep insufficiency. *Accid Anal Prev.* 2013;59:618–622.

73. Howard ME, et al. Deterioration in driving performance during sleep deprivation is similar in professional and nonprofessional drivers. *Traffic Inj Prev.* 2014;15(2):132–137.

74. Abe T, Komada Y, Inoue Y. Short sleep duration, snoring and subjective sleep insufficiency are independent factors associated with both falling asleep and feeling sleepiness while driving. *Int Med.* 2012;51(23):3253–3260.

75. Tefft BC. Prevalence of motor vehicle crashes involving drowsy drivers, United States, 1999–2008. *Accid Anal Prev.* 2012;45:180–186.

76. Force D-VT. *Diagnostic and statistical manual of mental disorders* (DSM-5, 5th ed.). 2013. Washington, DC: American Psychiatric Association, xliv.

77. Ferre Navarrete F, et al. Prevalence of insomnia and associated factors in outpatients with generalized anxiety disorder treated in psychiatric clinics. *Behav Sleep Med.* 2016:1–11.

78. Gehrman P, et al. Predeployment sleep duration and insomnia symptoms as risk factors for new-onset mental health disorders following military deployment. *Sleep.* 2013;36(7):1009–1018.

79. Ford DE, Kamerow DB. Epidemiologic study of sleep disturbances and psychiatric disorders. An opportunity for prevention? *JAMA.* 1989;262(11):1479–1484.

80. Yu Y, Li M, Pu L, Wang S, Wu J, Ruan L, Jiang S, Wang Z, Jiang W. Sleep was associated with depression and anxiety status during pregnancy: A prospective longitudinal study. *Arch Womens Ment Health.* 2017;20(5):695–701. doi:10.1007/s00737-017-0754-5. Epub 2017 Jul 6. PMID: 28685391.

81. Marcks BA, et al. The relationship between sleep disturbance and the course of anxiety disorders in primary care patients. *Psychiatry Res.* 2010;178(173):487–492.

82. Chapman DP, et al. Frequent insufficient sleep and anxiety and depressive disorders among US community dwellers in 20 states, 2010. *Psychiatr Serv.* 2013;64(4):385–387.

83. Belleville G, et al. The impact of cognitive-behavior therapy for anxiety disorders on concomitant sleep disturbances: A meta-analysis. *J Anxiety Disord.* 2010;24(4):379–386.

84. Mason EC, Harvey AG. Insomnia before and after treatment for anxiety and depression. *J Affect Disord.* 2014;168:415–421.

85. Luik AI, et al. Treating depression and anxiety with digital cognitive behavioural therapy for insomnia: A real world NHS evaluation using standardized outcome measures. *Behav Cogn Psychother.* 2017;45(1):91–96.

86. Ye YY, et al. Internet-Based Cognitive Behavioral Therapy for Insomnia (ICBT-i) improves comorbid anxiety and depression: A meta-analysis of randomized controlled trials. *PLoS One.* 2015;10(11):e0142258.

87. Fernandez-Mendoza J, et al. Insomnia and incident depression: Role of objective sleep duration and natural history. *J Sleep Res.* 2015;24(4):390–398.

88. Manber R, et al. CBT for insomnia in patients with high and low depressive symptom severity: Adherence and clinical outcomes. *J Clin Sleep Med.* 2011;7(6):645–652.

89. McLay RN, Klam WP, Volkert SL. Insomnia is the most commonly reported symptom and predicts other symptoms of post-traumatic stress disorder in US service members returning from military deployments. *Mil Med.* 2010;175(10):759–762.

90. Mohr D, et al. The mediating effects of sleep in the relationship between traumatic stress and health symptoms in urban police officers. *Psychosom Med.* 2003;65(3):485–489.

91. Betts KS, et al. The role of sleep disturbance in the relationship between post-traumatic stress disorder and suicidal ideation. *J Anxiety Disord.* 2013;27(7):735–741.

92. Pruiksma KE, et al. Residual sleep disturbances following PTSD treatment in active duty military personnel. *Psychol Trauma.* 2016;8(6):697–701.

93. Ulmer CS, Edinger JD, Calhoun PS. A multi-component cognitive-behavioral intervention for sleep disturbance in veterans with PTSD: A pilot study. *J Clin Sleep Med.* 2011;7(1):57–68.

94. Jia CX, et al. Sleep disturbance and attempted suicide in rural China: A case-control study. *J Nerv Ment Dis.* 2015;203(6):463–468.

95. Koyawala N, et al. Sleep problems and suicide attempts among adolescents: A case-control study. *Behav Sleep Med.* 2015;13(4):285–295.

96. Littlewood DL, et al. Understanding the role of sleep in suicide risk: Qualitative interview study. *BMJ Open.* 2016;6(8):e012113.

97. Rosekind MR, et al. The cost of poor sleep: Workplace productivity loss and associated costs. *J Occup Environ Med.* 2010;52(1):91–98.
98. Hui SK, Grandner MA. Trouble sleeping associated with lower work performance and greater health care costs: Longitudinal data from Kansas State Employee Wellness Program. *J Occup Environ Med.* 2015;57(10):1031–1038.
99. Liu TZ, et al. Sleep duration and risk of all-cause mortality: A flexible, non-linear, meta-regression of 40 prospective cohort studies. *Sleep Med Rev.* 2017;32:28–36.
100. Papp KK, Penrod CE, Strohl KP. Knowledge and attitudes of primary care physicians toward sleep and sleep disorders. *Sleep Breath.* 2002;6(3):103–109.
101. Grandner MA, Malhotra A. Sleep as a vital sign: Why medical practitioners need to routinely ask their patients about sleep. *Sleep Health.* 2015;1(1):11–12.

3

Normal Sleep in Childhood

HOVIG K. ARTINIAN, MARY ANNE TABLIZO, AND MANISHA WITMANS

The role of restorative sleep is increasingly recognized as a critical factor for general health and well-being in children. Adequate restorative sleep is important to reduce risk of infection, optimize healing after infection, and support metabolism for normal childhood development, appropriate behavior, and good academic performance. Children who lack adequate and refreshing sleep show impaired learning and school performance, metabolic disorders, increased risk of future heart disease, behavioral and mood disturbances, and increased risk of sports injuries.[1-7] Sleep and rest are often prescribed as a way to heal many ailments, although the exact mechanisms by which the body heals during sleep remain elusive. The very purpose of sleep remains an unanswered question, with many theories proposed. Hypotheses include sleep for restoration, energy conservation, learning versus unlearning, evolutionary and adaptive theories, and more. The ultimate explanation is likely multifactorial and will require the integration of many proposed and as yet undetermined mechanisms. What is known, however, is that certain norms and patterns have emerged in children's sleep that are reproducible, essential, and beneficial for health. In this chapter, we discuss the pre-sleep behaviors and routines that optimally help children fall asleep, the neurophysiological changes associated with sleep, and how children's sleep architecture and duration change across the life span from infancy to adulthood. Additionally, the chapter highlights what are considered normal developmental sleep behaviors, their variants, and how the role of circadian rhythms also influence sleep, particularly in adolescence.

Neurophysiology of Sleep

Wakefulness and sleep are complex states of being controlled by a self-regulating network of interactions between the circadian system (process C; about 24 hours per cycle) and sleep–wake homeostasis (process S; equilibrium between drive to sleep and drive to wake), which are influenced by multiple exogenous and endogenous factors.[8-10] Humans have endogenous and physiologic circadian rhythms that are internally controlled and synchronized by the suprachiasmatic nuclei (SCN).[11-13] This intrinsic oscillation may apply to other physiological processes linked to sleep and wakefulness, such as diurnal blood pressure regulation. Sleepiness is managed by the anterior hypothalamus and preoptic area; wakefulness is managed by the posterior hypothalamus and rostral midbrain.[14]

The "master circadian pacemaker" is the SCN, which is regulated in its sleep–wake function by the hormone *melatonin*, produced in the pineal gland. Endogenous factors such as body temperature and hormonal influences, along with exogenous factors, such as darkness and subjective night, regulate the production of melatonin, which binds to MT_1 and MT_2 melatonin receptors at the SCN and regulates sleep and circadian rhythm.[15,16] Melatonin has been shown to promote sleep at any point in the 24-hour cycle but is only functional for phase shifting the circadian phase at certain periods of sensitivity (such as dawn and dusk).[17] The idea of a "master clock" that regulates a regular nocturnal sleep pattern is further supported by the fact that newborns do not have an established nocturnal pattern to their circadian rhythm. Rather, they have an ultradian rhythm characterized by periods of sleep interjected by periods of wakefulness over a 24-hour period. This is due in large part to the fact that the newborn infant does not produce melatonin and only a small amount of melatonin is maternally transferred at birth, which dissipates within about 1 week of life.[10] As the infant grows older and starts producing melatonin endogenously, they develop a more nocturnal pattern to their circadian rhythm, usually by around 10–12 weeks of age.[18] Establishing routines soon after birth helps expedite the development of these nocturnal sleep patterns in the infant.

Equally important in the development of normal sleep is the balance between the drive to wake and the drive to sleep in the central nervous system. Wakefulness is promoted by the reticular formation, whereby numerous neurotransmitters and inputs from sensory systems travel to the thalamus, hypothalamus, and basal forebrain to promote wakefulness and arousal.[19] Orexin/hypocretin neuropeptides are also released during wakefulness by neurons in the lateral and posterior hypothalamus, which innervate all ascending arousal systems to regulate wake and sleep.[20,21] This is believed to play a role in sustaining wakefulness as well as in stabilizing sleep during sleep periods. Significant sleep fragmentation is observed in patients with narcolepsy who have lower than normal levels of circulating orexin/hypocretin.[19,22]

As the hours of wakefulness accumulate, adenosine and prostaglandin increase, ultimately activating the ventrolateral preoptic area (VLPO) and median preoptic area (MNPO). When active, both VLPO and MNPO release inhibitory neurotransmitters gamma-aminobutyric acid (GABA) and galanin and act to essentially inhibit all the wake-promoting regions of the brain, thus resulting in the child entering non–rapid eye movement (NREM) sleep. MNPO neurons are noted to fire just before NREM sleep, suggesting they help initiate sleep. VLPO neurons are noted to fire during deep NREM sleep, suggesting they help maintain sleep.[19] Of note, there is a negative feedback loop during wakefulness whereby the high presence of monoaminergic and cholinergic activity inhibits the VLPO thus facilitating wakefulness. The back and forth inhibition between these two systems ensures stable wake or sleep while also ensuring efficient transitions between wake and sleep. However, in the newborn infant, the transition from wake to sleep occurs via rapid eye movement (REM) rather than NREM, as it does in older infants and beyond.

The pons and rostral projections from the midbrain play a significant role in promoting the cortical activation associated with REM sleep and muscle atonia through the release of acetylcholine from the lateral dorsal tegmentum and the pedunculopontine tegmentum.[23] Although these are the same cholinergic neurons that are involved in wakefulness, it is hypothesized that there are subpopulations that are active in both wakefulness and REM sleep or are only selectively active in REM sleep.[24] Additional contributions to sleep are provided by neurons in the lateral hypothalamus that are mixed in with the orexin neurons and produce melanin-concentrating hormone and GABA. Similar to the orexin/hypocretin neurons, they innervate all the similar wake-promoting regions of the central nervous system but act in an inhibitory way to promote sleep. Finally, somnogens, which are diffusible or circulating factors that act on diverse geographic areas of the brain to promote sleep, include adenosine, cytokines, and prostaglandins. These neurotransmitters and their respective locations are a well-orchestrated symphony that enables humans to have sleep and wake homeostasis. The failure of these systems to work effectively results in various sleep disorders, such as insomnia, narcolepsy, and both NREM and REM parasomnias, which can be seen in both pediatric and adult populations.

Circadian Rhythms

Circadian rhythms are endogenous biological rhythms that exist in all living organisms. As mentioned, sleep is governed by two processes, process C, which involves an approximately 24-hour circadian homeostasis, and process S, which is the drive for sleep. The internal circadian clock is synchronized to the 24-hour light–dark cycle in humans. The period of the clock and its length is genetically determined. In ideal circumstances, for optimal sleep, the internal circadian clock matches to the 24-hour clock time so that the periods of sleepiness and alertness coincide together perfectly. In circumstances where there is misalignment between the internal circadian clock and the 24-hour clock, there is a possibility of developing sleep and wake disturbances. If the internal circadian clock is not reset daily with routine and consistency, the misalignment can continue and the disharmony can lead to chronic sleep–wake disturbances. These changes result in individuals, particularly adolescents, being sleepy in the morning and unable to get up for school. It is also associated with alertness at inappropriate times when the individual should be sleeping. The lack of synchronization can lead to work or academic difficulties and may further exacerbate any other underlying psychological, neurodevelopmental, or psychiatric disorders. In teens, this has become such an epidemic, with its resultant school failure, that the American Academy of Sleep Medicine (AASM) has issued a position statement that recommends delaying school start times to 8:30 AM or later for middle school and high school students in an effort to promote alertness and optimal learning.[25] When evaluating an older child or adolescent, it is incumbent on the provider to differentiate what is true insomnia versus an abnormal circadian rhythm that results in inability to fall asleep at a desired time.

Normal Electroencephalographic Findings

One of the critical areas of knowledge related to monitoring physiological parameters during sleep is evaluating brain waves via electroencephalogram (EEG) signals. The overnight polysomnogram, which is the reference standard for monitoring sleep in children, involves monitoring the EEG. The transition from wake to sleep is associated with several activities, such as eyes closing, postural changes, breathing changes, decrease in responsiveness to the environment, and, ultimately, transition from consciousness to unconsciousness, which may not always be perceived by the individual.[26] The pediatric sleep study employs tools to observe these collateral behavioral changes in order to best identify wake versus sleep. The AASM recommends pediatric sleep staging rules be used to score sleep and wakefulness in children 2 months post-term or older; for infants less than 2 months post-term, infant sleep staging rules are recommended.[27]

EEG activity changes are age-dependent, and, in neonates, sleep–wake cycles can only be differentiated by EEG starting after 31 weeks conceptual age.[28] Knowing the infant's postmenstrual age (PMA) is crucial for interpreting the EEG patterns as neonates will have EEG activity that differs from that in an older infant. Differentiating between NREM and REM sleep in infants younger than 6 months post-term is enhanced through use of collateral behavioral observations, including regularity of respirations, chin muscle tone (EMG), and whether there are eye movements (EOG).

The scoring for sleep stages in infants younger than 2 months is limited to wake, NREM, REM, or transitional because they lack distinct EEG waveforms of the different NREM sleep stages. A summary of the sleep state characteristics in neonates is shown in Table 3.1. An infant is scored as awake when they have eyes open with blinking and scanning eye movements or rapid eye movements or are crying or feeding with irregular respirations, with mixed or low-voltage irregular background EEG pattern and high chin EMG. They are scored as NREM sleep when their activity starts to decline, they develop only periodic sucking and occasional startles, the eyes close and there are no eye movements, their respirations become regular, their chin EMG decreases or becomes absent, and their background EEG pattern shows trace alternant or high-voltage slow activity and possibly sleep spindles (these generally develop starting at 6 weeks of age). Finally, REM sleep is scored when the infant's eyes are closed with rapid eye movements or no eye movements and they have generally no muscle movements, an irregular respiratory pattern, and a low-voltage irregular or mixed-frequency background EEG. The EEG pattern in REM sleep has a dominant frequency that is slower and of higher voltage in younger infants and children, but which steadily increases in

Table 3.1 Summary of sleep characteristics in neonates

Stage	Behavioral	Respiration	EEG	EOG	Chin EMG
Wake	Eyes open, crying., feeding	Irregular	LVI or M	REMs, blinks, scanning eye movements	Present
N	Reduced movement relative to wake (Eyes closed, periodic sucking, occasional startle)	Regular	TA, HVS, sleep spindles, or M	Eyes closed with no EMs	Present or low
R	Eyes closed Small movements	Irregular	LVI or M (rarely HVS)	REMs or eyes closed with no EMs[N16]	Low, TMA may occur

HVS, high-voltage slow; LVI, low-voltage irregular; M, mixed; TA, trace alternant; REMs, rapid eye movements.

AASM Scoring Manual, Version 2.6.

frequency until 5 years, when the low-voltage mixed-frequency pattern is similar to that of adults, although with somewhat higher amplitude.[29]

Starting around 2 months of age, when an infant closes their eyes to enter sleep, a dominant posterior rhythm (DPR) is observed in the occipital leads in about 90% of the population. The DPR occurs when one is awake with eyes closed, and its EEG frequency changes with age and development (expected values as one ages are shown in Table 3.2). Identifying the DPR is beneficial to observing the transition from wake to sleep as the background EEG rhythm slows from DPR frequency to low-amplitude activity, predominantly theta frequency (about 4–7 Hz), as one enters stage N1. Another distinctive EEG pattern that emerges around 3–8 months of age and is rarely seen after 12 years of age is *hypnagogic hypersynchrony*; these are bursts of high-voltage delta EEG activity that begin and end abruptly and are best observed over the central, frontal, or frontocentral regions during drowsiness that signals transition to sleep. Vertex sharp waves can also be noted, which are less than 0.5 seconds in duration, typically over the central region, and distinguishable from background activity of N1. The background EEG of hypnagogic hypersynchrony and vertex sharp waves should not be confused with epileptiform activity. Additionally, activity in the frontocentral leads becomes more prominent on EEG, all signifying entrance into sleep stage N1. Typically, children spend about 2–5% of total sleep time in stage N1.[30] However, there are conditions which may result in an increase in sleep stage N1, including new sleep environment, such as the sleep lab; sleep disorders that cause sleep fragmentation; and medical conditions involving difficulty initiating or maintaining sleep.

Table 3.2 Initial age of waveform appearance

Waveform	Age of initial appearance
Sleep spindles	6 weeks–3 months post-term
K complexes	3–6 months post-term
Slow-wave activity	2–5 months post-term
Posterior dominant rhythm	
Frequency of 3.5–4.5 Hz	3–4 months post-term
Frequency of 5–6 Hz	5–6 months post-term
Frequency of 7.5–9.5 Hz	3 years
Mean frequency of 9 Hz	9 years
Mean frequency of 10 Hz	15 years
Vertex sharp waves	4–6 months post-term
Hypnagogic hypermachrony (HH)	3–6 months post-term

AASM Scoring Manual, Version 2.6.

The child transitions from stage N1 to stage N2 when spindles and K-complexes start to appear, as in the adult population. Typically children spend about 45–55% of total sleep time in stage N2. Spindles are 12–14 Hz bursts of EEG activity that first develop by 6 weeks to 3 months of age and remain asynchronous until 6–12 months of age. K-complexes on EEG develop between 3 and 6 months post-term.

In children, stage N3 occurs reasonably quickly after falling asleep and predominates in the first third to first half of the sleep period because the drive to sleep is maximal after wake periods. Children spend about 25% of total sleep time in stage N3. The large amount of stage N3 in early childhood makes children vulnerable to parasomnias, particularly if there is a family history or other factors that fragment sleep. There is a reduction in the amount of slow wave sleep in the second decade of life, associated with puberty, which is postulated to be associated with synaptic pruning.

REM sleep accounts for almost 50% of sleep in the newborn period but significantly decreases over time from newborn, through infancy, through the toddler stage, and into school age and adolescence. By school age, it accounts for about 20–25% of total sleep time, and this remains consistent throughout the remaining life span.

Physiological Changes During Sleep

A number of changes occur physiologically during sleep. As a general rule, the changes that occur in NREM sleep are typically the opposite of what occur during REM sleep.[31] Generally speaking, in NREM sleep, all the following physiological processes decrease as compared to when one is awake: brain activity, heart rate, blood pressure, sympathetic nerve activity, blood flow to the brain, and respiratory rate. Airway resistance increases from wakefulness, and body temperature is regulated at a lower set point than during wakefulness. However, there are examples of brief increases in blood pressure and heart rate that can occur with K-complexes in stage N2 and with arousals and large body movements. These are believed to be secondary to bursts of sympathetic nerve activity in NREM sleep after K-complexes.

In REM sleep, all the following physiological processes increase as compared to when one is awake: heart rate, blood pressure, sympathetic nerve activity, blood flow to the brain, respiratory rate, and airway resistance. Muscle tone is absent during REM sleep in all muscles except the extraocular muscles and diaphragm. Coughing is also suppressed. However, overall blood flow to the brain in REM sleep is comparable to wakefulness and, in fact, is increased to the limbic system and visual association areas.[32] Body temperature is not regulated during REM sleep, and the body becomes poikilothermic. Because of the physiological changes occurring in the REM sleep stage, the body is most vulnerable to respiratory instability; thus, any individual with respiratory difficulties is likely to struggle with sleep fragmentation and/or gas exchange limitations.

Overall it is felt that the adaptive responses to oxygenation and ventilation are less effective during sleep as compared to wakefulness due to the physiological changes in ventilatory parameters. As the child falls asleep, minute ventilation decreases as environmental and behavioral inputs to the brain that promote awake respiratory patterns terminate, metabolism decreases, and chemosensitivity to oxygen and carbon dioxide decrease.[33] Additionally, decrease in muscle tone occurs as one enters NREM and especially REM sleep (upper airway muscle tone is affected much more than intercostal or diaphragmatic muscle tone), and alterations in respiratory mechanics occur given positional changes associated with sleep. The combination of these changes in sleep results in inadequate ventilation, causing depression in oxygenation (typically observed as a fall in oxygen saturation of 1–2%) and elevation of pCO_2 (typically of 1–2 torr above baseline in NREM sleep and another 3–4 torr above baseline in REM sleep).

Hormonal changes also occur during sleep, including increased aldosterone release and decreased excretion of sodium, potassium, chloride, and calcium to allow for more concentrated and reduced urine flow. Additionally, growth hormone is typically released in the first few hours after sleep onset, coinciding with slow wave (N3) sleep. Thyroid hormone is secreted in the late evening. Cortisol typically peaks just before waking, in order to help one feel alert after awakening. Therefore, the physiological processes that occur during sleep are synchronized and linked to sleep and wakefulness. Their disruption can not only result in sleep disorders, but may also exacerbate any underlying organic or neuropsychiatric problems.

Normal Sleep Patterns

Systematic review of observational studies in infants and children (0–12 years) provided data for general sleep norms.[34] The need for sleep decreases from a high of 12–16 hours in a 24-hour period in newborns to 8–10 hours in adolescence. Figure 3.1 shows the consensus guidelines for amount of recommended sleep in each age group from infancy to adolescence. Neonates spend as much as 70–90% of their day sleeping up to 48 weeks conceptual age. Neonates usually transition into REM sleep following wakefulness until 2–3 months of age, and they spend the majority of their time in REM sleep (70–80% REM sleep in pre-term infants and 50% REM sleep in term infants, falling to 30% by 6 months of age).[35] Healthy infants cycle through sleep in 50–60 minutes, average (range: 30–70 minutes). In older children, sleep onset is normally into NREM sleep and typically occurs within about 20 minutes. The first REM period of the night typically occurs

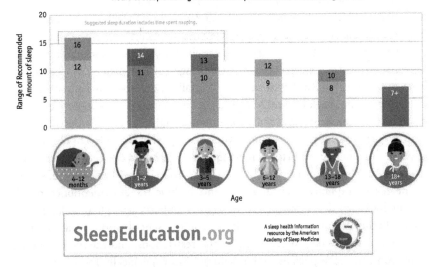

FIGURE 3.1 Consensus guidelines for amount of recommended sleep in each age group from infancy to adolescence.
Source: https://aasm.org/new-infographics-help-you-share-aasm-sleep-duration-recommendations/

70–110 minutes after sleep onset, and the remaining four to six cycles of alternating NREM and REM occur at intervals of 60–120 minutes.

Normative values have been determined for number of night wakings, sleep latency, longest sleep period overnight, and number of daytime naps.

1. *Night wakings*: Infants 0–2 months showed the highest number (mean 14.6), with a general decline in mean number of awakenings with increasing age to a low of 8.9 mean night wakings in 12-year-olds.
2. *Sleep latency*: Data show average value of 19 minutes for infants and a slight decline with increasing age to a low of 16 minutes in 5–6 year olds.
3. *Longest sleep period*: Data showed a trend for increasing sleep consolidation with age, with a low of 5.8 hours in the 0–5 months age range and a high of 8.4 hours in the 6–24 months age range.
4. *Number of daytime naps*: There was a mean of 1.7 naps per day in 0- to 2-year-olds, with a general decreasing trend in number of naps with increasing age. The majority of children give up napping by age 6 years.

Adolescent sleep patterns are more strongly affected by behavioral and environmental inputs. A hallmark behavioral change in sleep patterns of adolescents in preindustrial and industrial countries is a delay in sleep onset, with older teenagers reporting later bedtimes than younger peers.[36,37] While they require less sleep than young children, many adolescents self-report insufficient sleep not meeting recommendations for their age, with subsequent weekend "make-up sleep." There is an overall redistribution of sleep-stage variables noted in adolescence, including a decline in slow wave sleep and an increase stage 2 NREM sleep, as well as a tendency to skip the first REM episode.[38] Additionally, there is a decrease in process S, the sleep pressure that adolescents experience, and a delayed process C that results in adolescents not feeling sleepy until later in the night.

In the 2015 Youth Risk Behavior Surveillance report of US high school students, only 27.3% of students reported achieving 8 or more hours of sleep on an average school night, a significant linear decrease from 2007–2015.[39] Proposed causes for this decrease in quality sleep in adolescents include the aforementioned developmentally based decrease in sleep drive after puberty and phase delay in circadian rhythm, extracurricular activities, required school work, dietary choices (such as caffeine intake), decreased parental restrictions, and the increasing use of electronic media, especially in the evenings. Most specifically, those who spend more hours using their computer have been shown to have shorter sleep hours and lower sleep efficiency.[40] This decrease in quality sleep time has been documented to result in consequences including injuries, mental health issues, and poorer academic functioning.[41] Various policies, with varying efficacy and evidence, have been proposed to help adolescents achieve an appropriate length of sleep, including teaching adequate sleep hygiene and delaying school start times in the morning. The American Academy of Sleep Medicine has issued a position statement recommending delaying school start times to 8:30 am or later for middle school and high school students to promote alertness and optimal learning.[36]

Sleep Health

The American Academy of Pediatrics recommends that parents create a home environment that is conducive to good sleep for children through good sleep hygiene and consistent bedtime routines in infancy and throughout childhood. The concepts of healthy and good sleep refer to sleep habits and practices that are conducive to providing "ideal" and restorative sleep for children. The federal Office of Disease Prevention and Health Promotion has identified sleep health as a priority goal in its Healthy People 2020 guidelines and identified four main objectives for improvement. Among the objectives, one specifically targets the pediatric population, with the goal being to improve the proportion of adolescents in grades 9–12 who generally get insufficient sleep.[42] Like good nutrition and an active lifestyle, sleep that is of high quality and adequate duration is viewed as vital for development and learning in children. Figure 3.1 is the consensus statement by the AASM regarding generally accepted recommendations for sleep duration from infancy to adulthood based on a review of the literature.[43] Children and adolescents who regularly obtain these recommended hours of sleep display improved attention, behavior, learning, memory, emotional regulation, quality of life, and mental and physical health.[9]

Sleep problems in children are common and are among the most common behavioral issues brought up by parents to their pediatricians.[44] When predictable bedtime routines are implemented, they result in improved daytime behavior and less stress for both parent and child at bedtime.[45] Implementation of predictable and effective bedtime routines has also demonstrated a dose-dependent relationship, with improved outcomes in the younger age group when a consistent bedtime routine is carried out.[44] A growing body of research supports the importance of appropriate parental modeling in achieving desired behaviors in children. Just as the importance of proper parent modeling has been demonstrated for physical exercise, smoking, healthy eating, and bicycle helmet use, newer studies are also demonstrating the role parents play in healthy sleep behavior, such as avoiding technology use in bed.[46] The American Academy of Pediatrics website for parents, healthychildren.org, highlights best practices for parents when putting their children to bed. The recommendations appropriately highlight differences between infant, toddler, and older children in terms of how best to help a child fall asleep. Ultimately, the goal should be a short, consistent routine that is age-appropriate, implemented easily, and features minimal transitions or delays at bedtime. One such method highlighted is the "4 B's of Bedtime": Bathing, Brushing, Books, Bedtime.[47] Establishing routines in the newborn period can help newborns transition from an ultradian rhythm of sleep to a gradual nocturnal pattern of sleep much like older children and adults.[18]

Effective bedtime routines have been shown to improve sleep patterns in children, however the evidence for adequate sleep hygiene in adolescents is more complicated. A review of the various sleep hygiene recommendations, including exercise, stress, noise, sleep timing, and napping, revealed a lack of evidence showing efficacy in the general population.[48] This is not to say that individual components of sleep hygiene, when improved, won't lead to improved nocturnal sleep in individual patients when identified as a problem. Rather, the concept of sleep hygiene education as a whole has not been tested outside of highly controlled laboratory environments. Sleep hygiene must be considered in the context of the complex interplay between behavioral, environmental, and genetic factors. Ultimately, treatment plans must employ a personalized approach that shows understanding of individual differences between patients and how modifications to their sleep may result in changes to other behaviors, both intended and unintended.

Common Parasomnias

Most nocturnal physical events and experiences that occur in children do not signify a serious underlying medical, neurological, or neurodevelopmental problem. Parasomnias "encompass abnormal sleep related complex movements, behaviors, emotions, perceptions, dreams, and autonomic nervous system activity."[49] It is postulated that these behaviors occur as the sleep–wake cycle oscillates, placing the child in a temporary, unstable state of dissociation that manifests as behaviors that occur in the transition between wake and NREM sleep. The most common of the parasomnias in children are disorders of arousal, which include confusional arousals, sleepwalking, and sleep terrors.[50] They are all related to the asynchrony between wakefulness and sleep during N3 sleep. During a confusional arousal, which is a brief event at night within hours of sleep onset, the child may look confused and disoriented, and they will have no memory of the event the next morning. Sleepwalking, also known as *somnambulism*, occurs when a child can walk but is not awake and also has no recall of the event. Sleep terrors, also called *pavor nocturnus*, tend to be longer than confusional arousals and may involve an incoherent child sitting up in bed, screaming, apparently terrified and inconsolable, but again with no recall of the event. These are all NREM parasomnias, which typically occur in the first half of the night when NREM sleep is more predominant. They are characterized by the AASM's *International Classification of Sleep Disorders* (ICSD-3) as all sharing "similar genetics and familial patterns, similar pathophysiology of partial arousals from deep sleep, and similar priming by sleep deprivation and biopsychosocial stressors." These events generally resolve by adolescence and, apart from the risk of injury from lack of awareness or alertness during the event, no intervention other than parental reassurance is typically required. However, some individuals may develop parasomnias during adolescence, often related to underlying factors such as sleep deprivation in the context of genetic factors that make them susceptible. The family should be counseled about safety in order to prevent injuries. Optimizing sleep duration and schedule while addressing any associated sleep disorder, such as obstructive sleep apnea, can decrease the frequency and intensity of the parasomnias. Medications are very rarely used.

REM-related parasomnias can also occur in children, although true REM-behavior disorder (RBD; where sleepers act out their dreams) is quite uncommon in children. RBD can be seen in children taking psychotropic medications, such as a selective serotonin reuptake inhibitor (SSRI). More typically, children will experience nightmares. Because these are REM-related phenomena, they are more likely to occur in the second half of the night, when REM sleep is more predominant.

Conclusion

Sleep is an important and vital function in a child's life and changes from the newborn period to adulthood. There are factors that influence both circadian timing and the development of normal healthy sleep. Children require sleep, and their sleep needs change over time. Although there are features that are common in all children, certain differences are age specific. It is important to recognize normal sleep and variants in children as well as screen for any sleep disorders. Sleep disorders in children can lead to physical, psychological, and neurodevelopmental sequelae and therefore should be screened for at routine child visits.

REFERENCES

1. Redline S, Storfer-Isser A, Rosen CL, et al. Association between metabolic syndrome and sleep-disordered breathing in adolescents. *Am J Respir Crit Care Med.* 2007 Aug 15;176(4):401–408.
2. Milewski MD, Skaggs DL, Bishop GA, et al. Chronic lack of sleep is associated with increased sports injuries in adolescent athletes. *J Pediatr Orthop.* 2014;34:129–133.
3. Sarchiapone M, Mandelli L, Carli V, et al. Hours of sleep in adolescents and its association with anxiety, emotional concerns, and suicidal ideation. *Sleep Med.* 2014;15:248–254.
4. Baum KT, Desai A, Field J, Miller LE, Rausch J, Beebe DW. Sleep restriction worsens mood and emotion regulation in adolescents. *J Child Psychol Psychiatry.* 2014;55:180–190.
5. Cappuccio FP, Taggart FM, Kandala NB, et al. Meta-analysis of short sleep duration and obesity in children and adults. *Sleep.* 2008;31:619–626.
6. Van Cauter E, Knutson KL. Sleep and the epidemic of obesity in children and adults. *Eur J Endocrinol.* 2008;159: S59–S66.
7. Magee L, Hale L. Longitudinal associations between sleep duration and subsequent weight gain: A systematic review. *Sleep Med Rev.* 2012;16:231–241.
8. Borbely AA, Achermann P. Sleep homeostasis and models of sleep regulation. *J Biol Rhythms.* 1999;14(6):559–570.
9. Blunden S, Galland B. The complexities of defining optimal sleep: Empirical and theoretical considerations with a special emphasis on children. *Sleep Med Rev.* 2014;18(5):371–378.
10. Bathory E, Tomopoulos S. Sleep regulation, physiology and development, sleep duration and patterns, and sleep hygiene in infants, toddlers, and preschool-age children. *Curr Probl Pediatr Adolesc Health Care.* 2017;47:29–42.
11. Kleitman N. *Sleep and wakefulness.* Chicago: University of Chicago Press; 1963.
12. Ralph MR, Foster RG, Davis FC, Menaker M. Transplanted suprachiasmatic nucleus determines circadian period. *Science.* 1990;247:975.

13. Czeisler CA, Gooley JJ. Sleep and circadian rhythms in humans. *Cold Spring Harb Symp Quant Biol.* 2007;72:579–597.

14. Von Economo C. Sleep as a problem of localization. *J Nerv Ment Dis.* 1930;71:249–259.

15. Dubocovich M. Melatonin receptors: Role on sleep and circadian rhythm regulation. *Sleep Medicine.* 2007;8(3):34–42.

16. Zhdanova IV. Melatonin as a hypnotic: Pro. *Sleep Med Rev.* 2005;9:51–65.

17. Paul M, et al. Melatonin treatment for eastward and westward travel preparation. *Psychopharmacology.* 2010;208(3):377–386.

18. Davis KF, Parker KP, Montgomery GL. Sleep in infants and young children: Part one: Normal sleep. *J Pediatr Health Care.* 2004;18:65e71.

19. Espana R, Scammell T. Sleep neurobiology from a clinical perspective. *Sleep.* 2011;34(7):845–858.

20. Sakurai T, Amemiya A, Ishii M, et al. Orexins and orexin receptors: A family of hypothalamic neuropeptides and G protein-coupled receptors that regulate feeding behavior. *Cell.* 1998;92:1.

21. de Lecea L, Kilduff TS, Peyron C, et al. The hypocretins: Hypothalamus-specific peptides with neuroexcitatory activity. *Proc Natl Acad Sci USA.* 1998;95:322–327.

22. Mochizuki T, Crocker A, McCormack S, Yanagisawa M, Sakurai T, Scammell TE. Behavioral state instability in orexin knock-out mice. *J Neurosci.* 2004;24:6291–6300.

23. Weber F, Chung S, Beier KT, Xu M, Luo L, Dan Y. Control of REM sleep by ventral medulla GABAergic neurons. *Nature.* 2015;526:435–438.

24. El Mansari M, Sakai K, Jouvet M. Unitary characteristics of presumptive cholinergic tegmental neurons during the sleep-waking cycle in freely moving cats. *Exp Brain Res.* 1989;76:519–529.

25. Watson NF, et al. Delaying middle school and high school start times promotes student health and performance: An American Academy of Sleep Medicine position statement. *J Clin Sleep Med.* 2017;13(4):623–625.

26. Agnew HW, Wegg WB. Measurement of sleep onset by EEG criteria. *Am J EEG Technol.* 1972;12(3):127–134.

27. Berry RB, Albertario CL, Harding SM, et al.; for the American Academy of Sleep Medicine. *The AASM manual for the scoring of sleep and associated events: Rules, terminology and technical specifications.* Version 2.5. Darien, IL: American Academy of Sleep Medicine; 2018.

28. Britton JW, Frey LC, Hopp JL, et al. In St. Louis EK, Frey LC, eds. *Electroencephalography (EEG): An introductory text and atlas of normal and abnormal findings in adults, children, and infants* [Internet]. Chicago: American Epilepsy Society; 2016. https://www.ncbi.nlm.nih.gov/books/NBK390356/.

29. Sheldon, S, et al. *Principles and practice of pediatric sleep medicine,* 2nd ed. Elsevier. 2014.

30. Ohayon MM, et al. Meta-analysis of quantitative sleep parameters from childhood to old age in healthy individuals: Developing normative sleep values across the human lifespan. *Sleep.* 2004;27(7):1255–1273.

31. Colten HR, Altevogt BM. Sleep disorders and sleep deprivation: An unmet public health problem. Institute of Medicine (US) Committee on Sleep Medicine and Research. *National Academies Press (US).* 2006:33–54.

32. Madsen PL, Holm S, Vorstrup S, Friberg L, Lassen NA, Wildschiodtz G. Human regional cerebral blood flow during rapid-eye-movement sleep. *J Cerebr Blood Flow Metabol.* 1991;11(3):502–507.

33. Malik V, et al. Respiratory physiology during sleep. *Sleep Med Clin.* 2012;7:497–505.

34. Galland BC, et al. Normal sleep patterns in infants and children: A systematic review of observational studies. *Sleep Med Rev.* 2012;16:213–222.

35. Grigg-Damberger MM. The visual scoring of sleep in infants 0 to 2 months of Age. *J Clin Sleep Med.* 2016;12(3):429–445.

36. Carskadon MD. Maturation of processes regulating sleep in adolescents. In C. L. Marcus, J. L. Carroll, D. F. Donnelly, & G. M. Loughlin (Eds.), *Sleep in children: Developmental changes in sleep patterns*, 2nd ed. New York; Informa Healthcare. 2008: 95–114.

37. Crowley SJ, et al. Sleep, circadian rhythms, and delayed phase in adolescence. *Sleep Med.* 2007;8(6):602–612.

38. Tarokh L, Carskadon MA. Developmental changes in the human sleep EEG during early adolescence. *Sleep.* 2010;33(6):801–809.

39. Kann L, et al. Youth Risk Behavior Surveillance—United States, 2015. *Morb Mort Wkly Rep Surv Summ, CDC.* 2016;65(6):1–174. https://www.cdc.gov/mmwr/volumes/65/ss/ss6506a1.htm.

40. Tavernier R, et al. Adolescents' technology and face-to-face time use predict objective sleep outcomes. *Sleep Health.* 2017;3(4):276–283.

41. McKnight-Eily L, et al. Relationships between hours of sleep and health-risk behaviors in US adolescent students. *Prev Med.* 2011;53:271–273.

42. https://www.healthypeople.gov/2020/topics-objectives/topic/sleep-health/objectives.

43. Paruthi S, Brooks LJ, D'Ambrosio C, et al. Consensus statement of the American Academy of Sleep Medicine on the recommended amount of sleep for healthy children: Methodology and discussion. *J Clin Sleep Med.* 2016;12(11):1549–1561.

44. Mindell JA, Li AM, Sadeh A, Kwon R, Goh DY. Bedtime routines for young children: A dose-dependent association with sleep outcomes. *Sleep.* 2015;38(5):717–722.

45. Spagnola M, Fiese B. Family routines and rituals: A context for development in the lives of young children. *Infants Young Child.* 2007;20(4):284–299.

46. Buxton OM, et al. Sleep in the modern family: Protective family routines for child and adolescent sleep. *Sleep Health.* 2015(1):15–27.

47. Jana L, Shu J. *Food fights*, 2nd ed. AAP EBooks; 2012. Online.

48. Irish L, et al. The role of sleep hygiene in promoting public health: A review of empirical evidence. *Sleep Med Rev.* 2015;22:23–36.

49. ICSD-3, Parasomnia. Michael Sateia (Editor). AASM. Page 225–226.

50. Petit D, et al. Dyssomnias and parasomnias in early childhood. *Pediatrics.* 2007;119(5):e1016–1025.

4

Sleep Through the Ages: Adults and Older Adults

JOSEPH M. DZIERZEWSKI, TARAH RALDIRIS, AND SCOTT RAVYTS

Introduction

Thomas Dekker once described sleep as "that golden chain that ties health and our bodies together." The validity of his claim has been substantiated time and time again through both empirical investigation and clinical lore. Sleep serves many vital functions in humans, including facilitating the daily removal of metabolic waste (Xie et al., 2013), promoting brain health (Dzierzewski, Dautovich, & Ravyts, 2018), and nurturing mental and physical well-being (McCrae et al., 2008; Newman, Enright, Manolio, Haponik, & Wahl, 1997), among numerous other outcomes. Truth be told, it is tough to identify an area of functioning that does not rely on sleep for optimal performance. While sleep is of critical importance to individuals of any age, there are normative changes in the type, amount, and timing of sleep obtained from middle adulthood to late life. This chapter summarizes the typical changes in sleep architecture, sleep timing, sleep duration, and disordered sleep that occur in middle-aged to older adults. See Table 4.1 for a broad overview of sleep changes throughout the adult life span.

Disclosure: Dr. Dzierzewski was supported by a grant from the National Institute on Aging (K23AG049955). No other authors report commercial or financial conflicts of interest.

Table 4.1 Summary of sleep changes through the ages

Sleep parameter	Changes from middle age to late life
Sleep architecture	• Increase in N1 and N2 sleep • Decrease in N3 and REM sleep
Sleep timing	• Earlier bed times • Earlier rise times
Sleep duration	• Approximately 1 hour less of sleep per night
Sleep disorders	• Increased prevalence of circadian rhythm sleep disorder • Increased prevalence of sleep disordered breathing • Increased prevalence of insomnia

Sleep Architecture Throughout Adulthood and Aging

Sleep architecture is defined as the distribution of electrophysiologically distinct sleep states that occur throughout the night. Sleep can be broadly classified as either non–rapid eye movement (NREM) sleep or rapid eye movement (REM) sleep. NREM sleep can be further subdivided into three stages: N1, N2, and N3, with each stage corresponding to an increasing depth of sleep. NREM and REM sleep alternate intermittently throughout the night in approximately 90-minute cycles. In adulthood, individuals spend approximately 2–5% of sleep in N1, 45–55% in N2, 13–18% in N3, and 20–25% in REM sleep (Carskadon & Dement, 2011). NREM sleep therefore constitutes 75–80% of sleep, with the remaining 20–25% of REM sleep occurring in four to six discrete episodes.

Both polysomnography and actigraphy measures provide converging evidence for age-related changes in sleep architecture. For example, a meta-analysis of 65 studies with 3,577 participants across the life span found an increase in the proportion of N1 sleep and N2 sleep starting at midlife, as well as a decrease in the proportion of N3 sleep and REM sleep (Ohayon, Carskadon, Guilleminault, & Vitiello, 2004). Specifically, N3 sleep (deep sleep/slow wave sleep) was found to decline at a rate of approximately 2% per decade in young and middle-aged adults until plateauing around the age of 60 (Ohayon et al., 2004). See Figure 4.1 for a graphical depiction of sleep architecture changes across the life span. In addition to changes in the distribution of sleep stages, a shift in the occurrence of REM sleep toward the earlier part of the night occurs among older adults (Wauquier, van Sweden, Lagaay, Kemp, & Kamphuisen, 1992). Finally, in contrast to younger adults who are more susceptible to awake from REM sleep, older adults are more prone to arise from NREM sleep (Murphy, Rogers, & Campbell, 2000).

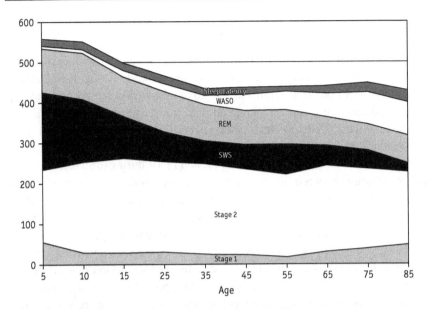

FIGURE 4.1 Time (in minutes) for sleep latency; wake after sleep onset (WASO); rapid eye movement (REM) sleep; sleep stages 1, 2, and 3 (SWS; slow wave sleep).
From Ohayon, M. M., Carskadon, M. A., Guilleminault, C., & Vitiello, M. V. (2004). Meta analysis of quantitative sleep parameters from childhood to old age in healthy individuals: developing normative sleep values across the human lifespan. *Sleep.* 2004, 27(7), 1255–1273.

Though age-related changes in sleep architecture are well-documented, their causes are not yet fully understood. Nevertheless, evidence suggests that changes in sleep architecture might occur as a result of age-related neural degeneration as well as a decrease in growth hormone secretion (Landolt & Borbély, 2001). Age-related changes in the human circadian pacemaker and sleep homeostatic mechanisms have also been identified as potential contributing factors to sleep architecture changes in late life (Dijk, Duffy, & Czeisler, 2000). Finally, preliminary evidence suggests that the presence of a health condition later in life, such as depression, may accelerate age-related changes in sleep architecture (Smagula et al., 2015). Changes in sleep architecture can have adverse consequences. For example, age-related changes in sleep architecture are associated with excessive daytime sleepiness which can subsequently lead to an increase in unintentional napping (Carskadon, Van den Hoed, & Dement, 1980). Preliminary evidence also suggests that increased N1 sleep and decreased REM sleep may predict poorer cognitive performance over time (Song et al., 2015). Specifically, age-related changes in sleep architecture may be a particularly salient factor related to memory consolidation during sleep (Harand et al., 2012).

Sleep Timing Throughout Adulthood and Aging

Sleep timing refers to one's desired bedtime based on circadian preferences (Tonetti, Fabbri, Filardi, Martoni, & Natale, 2015). In comparison to younger and middle-aged adults, older adults are more likely to go to sleep earlier at night and wake up earlier in the morning, with an average advance in sleep timing of 1 hour (Thomas, Lichstein, Taylor, Riedel, & Bush, 2014). According to the 2003 National Sleep Foundation's annual Sleep in America poll, 74% of adults between the ages of 54 and 84 years have a bedtime between 10 PM and 12 AM during the week compared to 69% of adults between the ages of 18 and 54 years with similar bedtimes. This difference in bedtimes greatly increases on weekends, however, with 75% of older adults going to bed between 10 PM and 12 AM, and only 63% of adults between the ages of 18 and 54 going to bed during these hours. Moreover, more than half (53%) of young/middle-aged adults wake up after 8 AM on weekends, whereas approximately 60% of older adults are already awake before 8 AM on weekends (National Sleep Foundation, 2003). Additional research supports these findings, indicating that retirees between the ages of 65 and 97 years have an average bedtime of 11:15 PM and an average wake time of 7:32 AM (Monk, Buysse, Schlarb, & Beach, 2012), whereas younger adults have an average bedtime of 12:17 AM and an average wake time of 8:11 AM (Yoon, Kripke, Youngstedt, & Elliott, 2003).

Changes in napping behavior across the life span are also evident. Research finds that napping episodes are more common among older than younger adults (Milner & Cote, 2009; Yoon et al., 2003), but there is no evidence that nap duration significantly varies with age (Campbell & Murphy, 2007). However, the timing of napping episodes does appear to vary between younger and older adults, with research indicating that older adults are more likely to nap during early evening hours, whereas younger adults take more afternoon naps (Yoon et al., 2003). Interestingly, the early evening nap times found for older adults occurred, on average, only 2 hours before their average bedtime and were associated with earlier wake times (Yoon et al., 2003).

Taken together, differences in sleep timing and napping behaviors suggest that older adults may experience circadian phase advances due to deterioration of the suprachiasmatic nucleus (SCN; Farajnia, Deboer, Rohling, Meijer, & Michel, 2014). Research on animal models supports a decline in functioning and neural firing of SCN cells with age (Farajnia et al., 2014). This finding is in line with research on older humans as well. For example, Czeisler and colleagues (1992) assessed circadian pacemakers in healthy younger and older adults by measuring core body temperature rhythms. Results indicated that the circadian pacemaker was found to be set earlier for older adults than younger adults (Czeisler et al., 1992). Moreover, research has found seriously damaged SCNs among older adults with Alzheimer's disease, a population that often displays circadian rhythm disturbances (Stopa et al., 1999).

More benign theories, including psychological and lifestyle changes, may further explain differences in sleep timing. In accordance with socioemotional selectivity theory (Carstensen, Isaacowitz, & Charles, 1999), older adults may deliberately shift their priorities to focus on more selective goals. As such, older adults may construct daily schedules that allow for earlier sleep times rather than planning events that may keep them awake later (Dillon et al., 2015). Likewise, older adults are more likely to be free from certain scheduling demands, including work, which may result in more opportunities to nap. Indeed, while 10% of adults between the ages of 55 and 64 years reported four to seven naps per week, this percentage increased to 15% among those between the ages of 65 and 74 years and to 24% among those between the ages of 75 and 84 years (National Sleep Foundation, 2003).

Sleep Duration Throughout Adulthood and Aging

Sleep duration refers to the total amount of time an individual sleeps per day. Based on a recent review of objectively recorded sleep duration, younger adults sleep approximately 7.5 hours per night compared to older adults who sleep roughly an hour less per night (Youngstedt et al., 2016). While it is a commonly held belief that sleep duration has been decreasing over time in the United States (and other industrialized societies), empirical evidence does not support this claim (Youngstedt et al., 2016). In fact, there is some evidence to suggest an increase in sleep duration over the previous decade of approximately 1 minute per year (Basner & Dinges, 2018). Importantly, although the observed trend toward increased sleep duration was observed for students, individuals currently employed, and those retired, older adults still reported sleeping less than their younger counterparts (Basner & Dinges, 2018).

Theories attempting to explain the observed age differences in sleep duration are wide ranging. Changes in health and the accompanying medications, life changes such as retirement and death of loved ones, and physiological changes resulting in decreased sleep needs have all been proposed as potential mechanisms responsible for the changes in sleep duration with age. It is most likely that a combination of these factors is responsible for the age-related changes in sleep duration.

Whatever its causes, it is clear that middle-aged and older adults are bordering on insufficient sleep. Short sleep duration is associated with a myriad of adverse health outcomes. In fact, a recent joint consensus statement from the American Academy of Sleep Medicine and the Sleep Research Society (Consensus Conference Panel et al., 2015) suggested between 7 and 9 hours of sleep per night for optimal health (along with avoiding numerous negative health consequences). Similarly, the National Sleep Foundation has recommended middle-aged adults obtain 7–9 hours of sleep per night, while older adults should obtain 7–8 hours of sleep per night (Hirshkowitz et al., 2015). As society continues to recognize the importance of sleep, perhaps actual sleep durations will begin to match those recommended by experts.

Sleep Disorders Throughout Adulthood and Aging

Approximately 67% of adults between the ages of 55 and 84 report having a sleep problem or disorder of some kind (National Sleep Foundation, 2003). One age-stratified, longitudinal study found that the prevalence of sleep disorders increases with age, with 19% of adults reporting a sleep disorder at 37 years of age compared to 30% at 52 years of age (Ribet & Derriennic, 1999). Research suggests that many sleep disorders and problems increase with age, including specific circadian rhythm disorders, sleep disordered breathing, and insomnia.

CIRCADIAN RHYTHM DISORDER

Although, as previously reviewed, older adults display circadian rhythm advances, this is not necessarily problematic unless desired bedtime conflicts with one's ability to fall asleep and causes significant daytime impairment. Circadian rhythm sleep–wake disorders (CRSWDs) can be conceptualized as a misalignment between sleep timing and sleep ability. Based on the *International Classification of Sleep Disorders*, 3rd Edition (ICSD-3; American Academy of Sleep Medicine, 2014), clinical diagnosis of a CRSD rests on three main criteria: (1) a chronic sleep–wake complaint due to the alteration of the circadian rhythm; (2) the sleep complaint leads to sleepiness, insomnia, or both; and (3) the sleep–wake complaint causes significant problems in at least one area of daily life, including social, occupational, and other important areas (American Academy of Sleep Medicine, 2014). There are seven subtypes of CRSWDs, yet all arise from problems in the circadian pacemaker or misalignments between the circadian pacemaker and the environment. The four primary subtypes, which include delayed sleep–wake phase disorder, advanced sleep–wake disorder, irregular sleep–wake disorder, and non–24-hour sleep–wake disorder, are all characterized by dysfunction within the circadian pacemaker (Toh, 2008). The two secondary CRSWDs, jet lag disorder and shift-work disorder, are not due to inherent issues with the circadian clock but rather arise from the misalignment of the clock with the external environment (Toh, 2008). There is also a circadian sleep–wake disorder not otherwise specified for symptoms not completely aligned with any of the previous diagnoses.

Between 3% (Schrader, Bovim, & Sand, 1993) and 10% (Barion & Zee, 2007) of adults suffer from a circadian rhythm disorder, but some subtypes are more common in older adults. For example, *advanced sleep–wake phase disorder,* which is characterized by sleep timing earlier than desired, and *irregular sleep–wake rhythm disorder* appear to be more common among older adults (Sack et al., 2007). Similarly, some research suggests that older adults are more likely to experience *non-24-hour sleep–wake rhythm disorder*, which involves sleep timing that moves later each night (Sack et al., 2007). However, it should be noted that the onset of non–24-hour sleep–wake disorder in late-life is likely comorbid with the onset of blindness, and irregular sleep–wake phase disorder occurs more often in nursing home residents, particularly among individuals with dementia. Thus, age alone does not appear to be a significant predictor of non–24-hour sleep–wake disorder or irregular sleep–wake rhythm disorder. In fact, diagnosis of primary CRSDs is relatively rare among healthy adults, with advanced sleep–wake phase disorder only occurring in about 1% of all middle-aged and older adults (Toh, 2008).

As discussed, the circadian timing system is coordinated by an area of the hypothalamus called the *suprachiasmatic nucleus* (Menaker, Takahashi, & Eskin, 1978). Although this internal rhythm is approximately 24 hours in humans, it is not exact and thus requires the system to regularly synchronize with conditions in the external environment, a process called *entrainment*. One way in which entrainment is achieved is through light–dark cycles in the environment (Duffy & Wright, 2005). Photoreceptors located within the eye communicate light information to the SCN, allowing the body to resynchronize daily (Duffy & Wright, 2005). The inability for blind individuals to entrain based on light cues explains why blindness is a risk factor for non–24-hour sleep–wake disorder. Furthermore, age-related deterioration of the SCN may cause an inability to successfully entrain, leading to primary CRSDs in older adults, including advanced sleep–wake phase disorder.

Treatment for CRSDs centers around resynchronizing the circadian rhythm. Given the importance of light–dark cycles for proper entrainment, artificial light exposure is one way to treat primary CRSDs (Richardson & Malin, 1996). In the case of advanced sleep–wake phase disorder, exposure to bright light in evening hours can help resynchronize the circadian timing system to a later phase. Conversely, exposure to bright light in early morning hours for those with delayed sleep–wake phase disorder appears effective. However, mixed results for the success of light exposure have been found for older adults with dementia suffering from irregular sleep–wake rhythm disorder (Mishima, Hishikawa, & Okawa, 1998; Satlin, Volicer, Ross, Herz, & Campbell, 1992). Therefore, the presence of comorbidities, such as blindness or dementia, may necessitate more complex plans for treatment.

The relationship between circadian rhythm disorders and neurodegeneration is not yet well understood, but recent evidence suggests that changes in the circadian rhythm may be an early indicator of neurodegenerative disease or cognitive decline (Tranah et al., 2011; Diem et al., 2016). Circadian phase delays in older adults are also related to increased memory problems (Haimov, 2006). Preliminary research suggests that in mouse models of Alzheimer's disease, disruption of neuronal activity in the SCN leads to circadian rhythm changes, thus serving as an indicator of early-stage dementia (Paul, Munir, van Groen, & Gamble, 2018). This suggests that, among older adults, changes in circadian rhythms may call for monitoring of their cognitive status.

SLEEP DISORDERED BREATHING

Sleep disordered breathing (SDB) is an umbrella term used to describe several chronic conditions in which partial or complete cessation of breathing occurs repeatedly during sleep. The term is most commonly associated with obstructive sleep apnea, but also refers to other conditions such as central sleep apnea and Cheyne–Stokes respiration. SDB is characterized by the presence of daytime sleepiness and abnormal respiratory events occurring during sleep, including apneas (complete cessation of breathing for >10 seconds), hypopneas (partial cessation of breathing resulting in a ≥30% reduction in airflow), and respiratory effort-related arousals (disruptions in sleep continuity associated with a breathing event not meeting criteria for either apneas or hypopneas). The severity of SDB is most commonly determined by the Apnea-Hypopnea Index (AHI), a measure of the average number of apnea and hypopnea events per hour. SBD is categorized as either none (AHI = 0–4), mild (AHI = 5–14), moderate (AHI = 15–30), or severe (AHI >30). Candidates for SDB treatment must have either an AHI index in the moderate to severe range or have an AHI in the mild range with concurrent daytime symptoms or other specific cormorbid conditions.

Among middle-aged adults, the prevalence of moderate to severe SDB (AHI ≥15) is estimated to be approximately 9.5% for men (confidence interval [CI]: 7.0–12.1) and 2.7% for women (CI: 1.7–4.0; Peppard et al., 2013). Similarly, approximately 11.7% of men (CI: 9.0–14.7) and 2.9% of women (CI: 1.7–4.3) have an AHI ≥5 and co-occurring symptoms of daytime sleepiness. SDB is well-known to increase with age (Durán, Esnaola, Rubio, & Iztueta, 2001); however, the prevalence of SDB among adults over the age of 60 varies widely based on setting and diagnostic criteria used. For example, the prevalence of SDB was found to be 27% among community-dwelling older adults and 42% among nursing home residents (Ancoli-Israel et al., 1991). In a recent community-based study, the prevalence of moderate to severe SDB (AHI ≥15) among older adults between the ages of 50 and 70 was estimated to be 17.4% for men (CI: 14.5–20.6) and 9.1% for women (CI: 6.8–11.4; Peppard et al., 2013). Approximately 17.6% of older adult males (CI: 14.7–20.3) and 7.5% of older adult females (CI: 5.9–9.7) are estimated to have both an AHI of 5 or greater and co-occurring symptoms of daytime sleepiness. While the rate of

SDB is known to increase with age, the prevalence of SDB is believed to plateau around the age of 65 (Young et al., 2002).

Several age-related physiological changes predispose older adults to SDB. For example, impairments in protective pharyngeal reflexes that occur as a part of normal aging increase the likelihood of upper airway collapse (Malhotra et al., 2006). Second, an increase in the deposition of adipose tissue around the pharynx that occurs independently of age-related changes in body fat compromises airway mechanics and increases the likelihood of SDB in late life (Schwartz et al., 2008).

SDB is associated with important adverse health consequences for adults throughout the life span. Studies examining SDB among younger adults show an increase in cardiovascular risk (Yaggi et al., 2005), although evidence regarding the consequences of SDB on cardiovascular events among older adults remains mixed (Javaheri et al., 2016). SDB also affects cognitive functioning of adults across the life span; however, the effects of SBD on cognitive functioning appear to be more pronounced among older adults (Dzierzewski et al., 2018). For example, SDB in older adults is more likely to be associated with an increased risk of cognitive impairment (Yaffe et al., 2011).

Positive airway pressure (PAP) is the first-line therapy for SDB and is associated with improvements in sleepiness, cognitive functioning, and quality of life for adults in mid- to late life (Giles et al., 2006). However, detection of SDB among older adults may go unnoticed given that symptoms such as sleepiness, daytime fatigue, and cognitive dysfunction may be incorrectly attributed to normal aging. Nevertheless, when adequately diagnosed and treated, older adults may require lower PAP levels compared to younger adults due to age-related physiological changes which enable greater reductions in airway resistance via treatment (Kostikas et al., 2006).

INSOMNIA

Broadly, *insomnia* is defined as difficulties in falling asleep, staying asleep, or nonrestorative sleep. The ICSD-3 criteria for a diagnosis of insomnia include reports of sleep initiation or maintenance difficulties, sufficient opportunity and environment for sleep, and some associated daytime consequences. A frequency of sleep difficulty at a rate of three times per week for at least 3 months in duration is required (American Academy of Sleep Medicine, 2014).

Rates of insomnia appear to increase across the life span. For example, among a sample between the ages of 25 and 45, approximately 12% reported symptoms of insomnia (Léger et al., 2011). For a sample of adults over the age of 65, though, roughly 55% reported at least one symptom of insomnia over the past month, and insomnia symptoms were found to be positively associated with age (Spira et al., 2014). Older adults appear to have particularly more issues with sleep maintenance and find themselves waking up more often during the night than desired (Leblanc, Desjardins, & Desgagné, 2015).

The higher prevalence of insomnia in older adults may be due to a multitude of reasons. One possibility for the increase of insomnia symptoms in later life is the presence of comorbid disorders. A study of nearly 9,000 American adults found nocturnal awakenings to be more frequent among those with organic diseases and psychiatric disorders (Ohayon, 2008), including heart failure, hypertension, and depression (Katz & McHorney, 1998; Kay & Dzierzewski, 2015). Likewise, prevalence rates of insomnia have been found to be higher in women, potentially due to estrogen deficiencies during menopause (Soares, 2005). Therefore, the presence of physical or psychological disorders may result in impaired sleep onset and maintenance outcomes.

Ancoli-Israel and Martin (2006) proposed that issues in circadian phases and napping behaviors may be to blame for increased insomnia in later life. As reviewed, napping episodes are more common in older adults than in younger or middle-aged adults (Milner & Cote, 2009). More frequent napping may lead to a cycle of poorer nocturnal sleep quality and greater impaired daytime functioning (Ancoli-Israel & Martin, 2006). Although causation has yet to be determined, this may be one piece of the puzzle toward understanding increased rates of insomnia in older adults.

Regardless of etiology, insomnia has detrimental impacts on older adults. One study of insomnia and well-being found that insomnia symptoms in older adults were associated with reduced overall well-being (Abell, Shipley, Ferrie, Kivimäki, & Kumari, 2016), increased psychiatric disturbances (Kay & Dzierzewski, 2015), reduced quality of life, and increased irritability (Léger et al., 2011). Moreover, for older adults, insomnia is especially concerning for cognitive functioning (Dzierzewski et al., 2018). Results from a sample of older adult men indicated that chronic insomnia was significantly predictive of cognitive decline (Cricco, Simonsick, & Foley, 2002).

Treatments for insomnia vary based on the underlying cause of the symptoms and include cognitive-behavioral therapy for insomnia (CBT-I), light therapy, mindfulness-based stress reduction, and pharmacologic options (Dzierzewski, Rodriguez Tapia, & Alessi, 2017). However, pharmacologic treatment options may be riskier for older adults than younger or middle-aged adults suffering from insomnia. Research suggests that although the use of sedatives in older adults marginally improved sleep, increases in cognitive difficulties, daytime drowsiness, and psychomotor problems were also evident (Glass, Lanctôt, Herrmann, Sproule, & Busto, 2005). Thus, any benefits of sedatives on sleep may be drastically outweighed by the negative impacts on daytime functioning and increased risk for falls and fractures (Rubenstein, 2006). In general, CBT-I is considered the gold standard and patient-preferred treatment for insomnia and includes stimulus control, sleep restriction, and sleep education (Dzierzewski et al., 2017).

Conclusion

Good sleep provides a solid foundation on which physical and mental health are built. However, like many areas of functioning, sleep changes throughout the life span. Sleep architecture changes with advanced age, resulting in less N3 sleep in late life. Older adults may experience a phase shift in their circadian rhythms, resulting in earlier bed and wake times. Similarly, older adults may also experience a gradual reduction in the overall duration of nocturnal sleep. Last, in late-life comes an increased prevalence of sleep disorders. Importantly, while these age-related changes in sleep may be associated with reductions in functioning, disturbed sleep is not the norm for older adults. The changes in sleep from middle adulthood to old age described throughout this chapter could be best characterized as gradual and subtle. Older adults are very capable of maintaining good sleep throughout the last decade of life, and, in the event that dysfunction in sleep develop, evidence-based treatments for late-life sleep disturbances abound. As such, there is no reason why sleep cannot continue to serve as the foundation for physical and mental health in older adults, or as Thomas Dekker put it—"that golden chain that ties health and our bodies together."

REFERENCES

Abell, J. G., Shipley, M. J., Ferrie, J. E., Kivimäki, M., & Kumari, M. (2016). Association of chronic insomnia symptoms and recurrent extreme sleep duration over 10 years with well-being in older adults: A cohort study. *BMJ Open, 6*(2), e009501. https://doi.org/10.1136/bmjopen-2015-009501

American Academy of Sleep Medicine. (2014). *International Classification of Sleep Disorders.* American Academy of Sleep Medicine. https://books.google.com/books?id=aXb7oAEACAAJ

Ancoli-Israel, S., Kripke, D. F., Klauber, M. R., Mason, W. J., Fell, R., & Kaplan, O. (1991). Sleep-disordered breathing in community-dwelling elderly. *Sleep, 14*(6), 486–495:

Ancoli-Israel, S., & Martin, J. L. (2006). Insomnia and daytime napping in older adults. *Journal of Clinical Sleep Medicine, 2*(3), 333–342.

Barion, A., & Zee, P. C. (2007). A clinical approach to circadian rhythm sleep disorders. *Sleep Medicine, 8*(6), 566–577. https://doi.org/10.1016/j.sleep.2006.11.017

Basner, M., & Dinges, D. F. (2018). Sleep duration in the United States 2003–2016: First signs of success in the fight against sleep deficiency? *Sleep.* https://doi.org/10.1093/sleep/zsy012

Campbell Scott S., & Murphy Patricia J. (2007). The nature of spontaneous sleep across adulthood. *Journal of Sleep Research, 16*(1), 24–32. https://doi.org/10.1111/j.1365-2869.2007.00567.x

Carskadon, M., & Dement, W. C. (2011). Normal human sleep: An overview. In Meir H. Kryger, Thomas Roth, William C. Dement (Eds.), *Principles and Practice of Sleep Medicine* (Fifth Edition, pp. 16–26), W.B. Saunders. ISBN 9781416066453, https://doi.org/10.1016/B978-1-4160-6645-3.00002-5

Carskadon, M. A., Van den Hoed, J., & Dement, W. C. (1980). Sleep and daytime sleepiness in the elderly. *Journal of Geriatric Psychiatry, 13*(2), 135–151.

Carstensen, L. L., Isaacowitz, D. M., & Charles, S. T. (1999). Taking time seriously. A theory of socioemotional selectivity. *American Psychologist, 54*(3), 165–181.

Consensus Conference Panel, Watson, N. F., Badr, M. S., Belenky, G., Bliwise, D. L., Buxton, O. M., . . . Tasali, E. (2015). Joint Consensus Statement of the American Academy of Sleep Medicine and Sleep Research Society on the recommended amount of sleep for a healthy adult: Methodology and discussion. *Journal of Clinical Sleep Medicine, 11*(8), 931–952. https://doi.org/10.5664/jcsm.4950

Cricco M., Simonsick E. M., & Foley D. J. (2002). The impact of insomnia on cognitive functioning in older adults. *Journal of the American Geriatrics Society, 49*(9), 1185–1189. https://doi.org/10.1046/j.1532-5415.2001.49235.x

Czeisler, C. A., Dumont, M., Duffy, J. F., Steinberg, J. D., Richardson, G. S., Brown, E. N., . . . Ronda, J. M. (1992). Association of sleep-wake habits in older people with changes in output of circadian pacemaker. *Lancet, 340*(8825), 933–936.

Diem, S. J., Blackwell, T. L., Stone, K. L., Yaffe, K., Tranah, G., Cauley, J. A., . . . Ensrud, K. E. (2016). Measures of sleep–wake patterns and risk of mild cognitive impairment or dementia in older women. *American Journal of Geriatric Psychiatry, 24*(3), 248–258. https://doi.org/10.1016/j.jagp.2015.12.002

Dijk, D.-J., Duffy, J. F., & Czeisler, C. A. (2000). Contribution of circadian physiology and sleep homeostasis to age-related changes in human sleep. *Chronobiology International, 17*(3), 285–311.

Dillon, H. R., Lichstein, K. L., Dautovich, N. D., Taylor, D. J., Riedel, B. W., & Bush, A. J. (2015). Variability in self-reported normal sleep across the adult age span. *The Journals of Gerontology: Series B, 70*(1), 46–56. https://doi.org/10.1093/geronb/gbu035

Duffy, J. F., & Wright, K. P. J. (2005). Entrainment of the human circadian system by light. *Journal of Biological Rhythms, 20*(4), 326–338. https://doi.org/10.1177/0748730405277983

Durán, J., Esnaola, S., Rubio, R., & Iztueta, Á. (2001). Obstructive sleep apnea-hypopnea and related clinical features in a population-based sample of subjects aged 30 to 70 yr. *American Journal of Respiratory and Critical Care Medicine, 163*(3), 685–689.

Dzierzewski, J. M., Dautovich, N., & Ravyts, S. (2018). Sleep and cognition in older adults. *Sleep Medicine Clinics, 13*(1), 93–106. https://doi.org/10.1016/j.jsmc.2017.09.009

Dzierzewski, J. M., Rodriguez Tapia, J. C., & Alessi, C. A. (2017). Synopsis of geriatric sleep disorders. In A. Y. Avidan (Ed.), *Review of Sleep Medicine* (4th ed., pp. 373–385). Philadelphia, PA: Elsevier.

Farajnia, S., Deboer, T., Rohling, J. H. T., Meijer, J. H., & Michel, S. (2014). Aging of the suprachiasmatic clock. *Neuroscientist, 20*(1), 44–55. https://doi.org/10.1177/1073858413498936

Giles, T. L., Lasserson, T. J., Smith, B., White, J., Wright, J. J., & Cates, C. J. (2006). Continuous positive airways pressure for obstructive sleep apnoea in adults. *Cochrane Library.* http://onlinelibrary.wiley.com/doi/10.1002/14651858.CD001106.pub3/full

Glass, J., Lanctôt, K. L., Herrmann, N., Sproule, B. A., & Busto, U. E. (2005). Sedative hypnotics in older people with insomnia: Meta-analysis of risks and benefits. *BMJ, 331*(7526), 1169. https://doi.org/10.1136/bmj.38623.768588.47

Haimov, I. (2006). Association between memory impairment and insomnia among older adults. *European Journal of Ageing, 3*(2), 107. https://doi.org/10.1007/s10433-006-0026-0

Harand, C., Bertran, F., Doidy, F., Guénolé, F., Desgranges, B., Eustache, F., & Rauchs, G. (2012). How aging affects sleep-dependent memory consolidation? *Frontiers in Neurology, 3.* https://doi.org/10.3389/fneur.2012.00008

Hirshkowitz, M., Whiton, K., Albert, S. M., Alessi, C., Bruni, O., DonCarlos, L., . . . Adams Hillard, P. J. (2015). National Sleep Foundation's sleep time duration recommendations: Methodology and results summary. *Sleep Health, 1*(1), 40–43. https://doi.org/10.1016/j.sleh.2014.12.010

Javaheri, S., Sharma, R. K., Wang, R., Weng, J., Rosen, B. D., Bluemke, D. A., . . . Redline, S. (2016). Association between obstructive sleep apnea and left ventricular structure by age and gender: The multi-ethnic study of atherosclerosis. *Sleep, 39*(3), 523–529. https://doi.org/10.5665/sleep.5518

Katz, D. A., & McHorney, C. A. (1998). Clinical correlates of insomnia in patients with chronic illness. *Archives of Internal Medicine, 158*(10), 1099–1107. https://doi.org/10.1001/archinte.158.10.1099

Kay, D. B., & Dzierzewski, J. M. (2015). Sleep in the context of healthy aging and psychiatric syndromes. *Sleep Medicine Clinics, 10*(1), 11–15.

Kostikas, K., Browne, H. A. K., Ghiassi, R., Adams, L., Simonds, A. K., & Morrell, M. J. (2006). The determinants of therapeutic levels of continuous positive airway pressure in elderly sleep apnea patients. *Respiratory Medicine, 100*(7), 1216–1225. https://doi.org/10.1016/j.rmed.2005.10.019

Landolt, H.-P., & Borbély, A. A. (2001). Age-dependent changes in sleep EEG topography. *Clinical Neurophysiology, 112*(2), 369–377. https://doi.org/10.1016/S1388-2457(00)00542-3

Leblanc, M.-F., Desjardins, S., & Desgagné, A. (2015). Sleep problems in anxious and depressive older adults. *Psychology Research and Behavior Management, 8*, 161–169. https://doi.org/10.2147/PRBM.S80642

Léger, D., Roscoat, E. du, Bayon, V., Guignard, R., Pâquereau, J., & Beck, F. (2011). Short sleep in young adults: Insomnia or sleep debt? Prevalence and clinical description of short sleep in a representative sample of 1004 young adults from France. *Sleep Medicine, 12*(5), 454–462. https://doi.org/10.1016/j.sleep.2010.12.012

Malhotra, A., Huang, Y., Fogel, R., Lazic, S., Pillar, G., Jakab, M., . . . White, D. P. (2006). Aging influences on pharyngeal anatomy and physiology: The predisposition to pharyngeal collapse. *American Journal of Medicine, 119*(1), 72.e9–72.14. https://doi.org/10.1016/j.amjmed.2005.01.077

McCrae, C. S., McNamara, J. P., Rowe, M. A., Dzierzewski, J. M., Dirk, J., Marsiske, M., & Craggs, J. G. (2008). Sleep and affect in older adults: Using multilevel modeling to examine daily associations. *Journal of Sleep Research, 17*(1), 42–53.

Menaker, M., Takahashi, J. S., & Eskin, A. (1978). The physiology of circadian pacemakers. *Annual Review of Physiology, 40*(1), 501–526. https://doi.org/10.1146/annurev.ph.40.030178.002441

Milner C. E., & Cote K. A. (2009). Benefits of napping in healthy adults: Impact of nap length, time of day, age, and experience with napping. *Journal of Sleep Research, 18*(2), 272–281. https://doi.org/10.1111/j.1365-2869.2008.00718.x

Mishima, K., Hishikawa, Y., & Okawa, M. (1998). Randomized, DIM light controlled, crossover test of morning bright light therapy for rest-activity rhythm disorders in patients with vascular dementia and dementia of Alzheimer's type. *Chronobiology International, 15*(6), 647–654. https://doi.org/10.3109/07420529808993200

Monk, T. H., Buysse, D. J., Schlarb, J. E., & Beach, S. R. (2012). Timing, duration and quality of sleep, and level of daytime sleepiness in 1166 retired seniors. *Healthy Aging & Clinical Care in the Elderly, 4*, 33–40. https://doi.org/10.4137/HACCE.S10596

Murphy, P. J., Rogers, N. L., & Campbell, S. S. (2000). Age differences in the spontaneous termination of sleep. *Journal of Sleep Research, 9*(1), 27–34.

National Sleep Foundation. 2003 Sleep in America Poll: Sleep and Aging. https://www.sleepfoundation.org/professionals/sleep-americar-polls/2003-sleep-and-aging. Published 2003. Accessed June 10, 2018.

Newman, A. B., Enright, P. L., Manolio, T. A., Haponik, E. F., & Wahl, P. W. (1997). Sleep disturbance, psychosocial correlates, and cardiovascular disease in 5201 older adults: The Cardiovascular Health Study. *Journal of the American Geriatrics Society, 45*(1), 1–7.

Ohayon, M. M. (2008). Nocturnal awakenings and comorbid disorders in the American general population. *Journal of Psychiatric Research, 43*(1), 48–54. https://doi.org/10.1016/j.jpsychires.2008.02.001

Ohayon, M. M., Carskadon, M. A., Guilleminault, C., & Vitiello, M. V. (2004). Meta-analysis of quantitative sleep parameters from childhood to old age in healthy individuals: Developing normative sleep values across the human lifespan. *Sleep, 27*(7), 1255–1273.

Paul, J. R., Munir, H. A., van Groen, T., & Gamble, K. L. (2018). Behavioral and SCN neurophysiological disruption in the Tg-SwDI mouse model of Alzheimer's disease. *Neurobiology of Disease, 114*, 194–200. https://doi.org/10.1016/j.nbd.2018.03.007

Peppard, P. E., Young, T., Barnet, J. H., Palta, M., Hagen, E. W., & Hla, K. M. (2013). Increased prevalence of sleep-disordered breathing in adults. *American Journal of Epidemiology, 177*(9), 1006–1014.

Ribet, C., & Derriennic, F. (1999). Age, working conditions, and sleep disorders: A longitudinal analysis in the French cohort E.S.T.E.V. *Sleep*, 22(4), 491–504. https://doi.org/10.1093/sleep/22.4.491

Richardson, G. S., & Malin, H. V. (1996). Circadian rhythm sleep disorders: Pathophysiology and treatment. *Journal of Clinical Neurophysiology*, 13(1), 17–31.

Rubenstein, L. Z. (2006). Falls in older people: Epidemiology, risk factors and strategies for prevention. *Age and Ageing*, 35(suppl_2), ii37–ii41. https://doi.org/10.1093/ageing/afl084

Sack, R. L., Auckley, D., Auger, R. R., Carskadon, M. A., Wright, K. P., Vitiello, M. V., & Zhdanova, I. V. (2007). Circadian rhythm sleep disorders: Part II, advanced sleep phase disorder, delayed sleep phase disorder, free-running disorder, and irregular sleep-wake rhythm. *Sleep*, 30(11), 1484–1501. https://doi.org/10.1093/sleep/30.11.1484

Satlin, A., Volicer, L., Ross, V., Herz, L., & Campbell, S. (1992). Bright light treatment of behavioral and sleep disturbances in patients with Alzheimer's disease. *The American Journal of Psychiatry*, 149(8), 1028–1032. https://doi.org/10.1176/ajp.149.8.1028

Schrader, H., Bovim, G., & Sand, T. (1993). The prevalence of delayed and advanced sleep phase syndromes. *Journal of Sleep Research*, 2(1), 51–55.

Schwartz, A. R., Patil, S. P., Laffan, A. M., Polotsky, V., Schneider, H., & Smith, P. L. (2008). Obesity and obstructive sleep apnea. *Proceedings of the American Thoracic Society*, 5(2), 185–192. https://doi.org/10.1513/pats.200708-137MG

Smagula, S. F., Reynolds, C. F., Ancoli-Israel, S., Barrett-Connor, E., Dam, T.-T., Hughes-Austin, J. M., . . . Osteoporotic Fractures in Men (MrOS) Research Group. (2015). Sleep architecture and mental health among community-dwelling older men. *Journals of Gerontology. Series B, Psychological Sciences and Social Sciences*, 70(5), 673–681. https://doi.org/10.1093/geronb/gbt125

Soares, C. N. (2005). Insomnia in women: An overlooked epidemic? *Archives of Women's Mental Health*, 8(4), 205–213. https://doi.org/10.1007/s00737-005-0100-1

Song, Y., Blackwell, T., Yaffe, K., Ancoli-Israel, S., Redline, S., & Stone, K. L. (2015). Relationships between sleep stages and changes in cognitive function in older men: The MrOS Sleep Study. *Sleep*, 38(3), 411–421.

Spira, A. P., Kaufmann, C. N., Kasper, J. D., Ohayon, M. M., Rebok, G. W., Skidmore, E., . . . Reynolds, C. F. (2014). Association between insomnia symptoms and functional status in US older adults. *Journals of Gerontology: Series B*, 69(Suppl_1), S35–S41. https://doi.org/10.1093/geronb/gbu116

Stopa, E. G., Volicer, L., Kuo-Leblanc, V., Harper, D., Lathi, D., Tate, B., & Satlin, A. (1999). Pathologic evaluation of the human suprachiasmatic nucleus in severe dementia. *Journal of Neuropathology & Experimental Neurology*, 58(1), 29–39. https://doi.org/10.1097/00005072-199901000-00004

Thomas, S. J., Lichstein, K. L., Taylor, D. J., Riedel, B. W., & Bush, A. J. (2014). Epidemiology of bedtime, arising time, and time in bed: Analysis of age, gender, and ethnicity. *Behavioral Sleep Medicine*, 12(3), 169–182. https://doi.org/10.1080/15402002.2013.778202

Toh, K. L. (2008). Basic science review on circadian rhythm biology and circadian sleep disorders. *Annals of the Academy of Medicine, Singapore, 37*(8), 662–668.

Tonetti, L., Fabbri, M., Filardi, M., Martoni, M., & Natale, V. (2015). Effects of sleep timing, sleep quality and sleep duration on school achievement in adolescents. *Sleep Medicine, 16*(8), 936–940. https://doi.org/10.1016/j.sleep.2015.03.026

Tranah G. J., Blackwell T., Stone K. L., Ancoli-Israel S., Paudel M. L., Ensrud K. E., . . . (2011). Circadian activity rhythms and risk of incident dementia and mild cognitive impairment in older women. *Annals of Neurology, 70*(5), 722–732. https://doi.org/10.1002/ana.22468

Wauquier, A., van Sweden, B., Lagaay, A. M., Kemp, B., & Kamphuisen, H. A. (1992). Ambulatory monitoring of sleep-wakefulness patterns in healthy elderly males and females (greater than 88 years): The "Senieur" protocol. *Journal of the American Geriatrics Society, 40*(2), 109–114.

Xie, L., Kang, H., Xu, Q., Chen, M. J., Liao, Y., Thiyagarajan, M., . . . Nedergaard, M. (2013). Sleep drives metabolite clearance from the adult brain. *Science, 342*(6156), 373–377. https://doi.org/10.1126/science.1241224

Yaffe, K., Laffan, A. M., Harrison, S. L., Redline, S., Spira, A. P., Ensrud, K. E., . . . Stone, K. L. (2011). Sleep-disordered breathing, hypoxia, and risk of mild cognitive impairment and dementia in older women. *JAMA, 306*(6), 613–619.

Yaggi, H. K., Concato, J., Kernan, W. N., Lichtman, J. H., Brass, L. M., & Mohsenin, V. (2005). Obstructive sleep apnea as a risk factor for stroke and death. *New England Journal of Medicine, 353*(19), 2034–2041.

Yoon, I. Y., Kripke, D. F., Youngstedt, S. D., & Elliott, J. A. (2003). Actigraphy suggests age-related differences in napping and nocturnal sleep. *Journal of Sleep Research, 12*(2), 87–93. https://doi.org/10.1046/j.1365-2869.2003.00345.x

Young, T., Shahar, E., Nieto, F. J., Redline, S., Newman, A. B., Gottlieb, D. J., . . . Samet, J. M. (2002). Predictors of sleep-disordered breathing in community-dwelling adults: The Sleep Heart Health Study. *Archives of Internal Medicine, 162*(8), 893–900. https://doi.org/10.1001/archinte.162.8.893

Youngstedt, S. D., Goff, E. E., Reynolds, A. M., Kripke, D. F., Irwin, M. R., Bootzin, R. R., . . . Jean-Louis, G. (2016). Has adult sleep duration declined over the last 50+ years? *Sleep Medicine Reviews, 28*, 69–85. https://doi.org/10.1016/j.smrv.2015.08.004

5

Circadian Rhythms and Homeostatic Mechanisms for Sleep Regulation

CASSIE J. HILDITCH AND ERIN E. FLYNN-EVANS

Introduction

Most people understand that sleep is important for health and well-being but less understood is the critical role that the mechanisms underlying sleep play in our lives. Sleep is regulated by the build-up of homeostatic sleep pressure and an internal drive to sleep controlled by the circadian rhythm. These two distinct sleep drives work together to consolidate sleep at night and allow people to maintain wakefulness during the day. Sleep pressure is intuitive; it is the build-up of sleep need over time. Most people recognize that staying up too late or not getting enough sleep is associated with a feeling of sleepiness. When people do not get enough sleep to alleviate sleep pressure, a sleep debt occurs and persists until sleep pressure is relieved through an extended sleep bout.

Unlike sleep pressure, the role of the circadian rhythm in sleep is not intuitive. Our circadian rhythms may be thought of as a central body clock that coordinates many aspects of biological function extending far beyond simply the drive to sleep. The circadian clock is intimately connected with the rotation of the Earth so that, under natural circumstances, the drive to sleep coincides with the solar night, and waking is promoted during the day. Circadian rhythms are ubiquitous to life and are the central timekeepers for animals and plants alike. Even ocean-dwelling bioluminescent single-celled organisms have an internal circadian clock that synchronizes the timing of their glow.[1] Importantly, the circadian clock is different between individuals, with some people having a longer than 24-hour circadian rhythm and other people having a shorter than 24-hour circadian rhythm. In order to stay synchronized with the 24-hour rotation of the Earth, our clocks must be reset each day to allow us to maintain sleep at night and wakefulness during the day. This resetting occurs through daily light exposure. Under normal circumstances, individuals do not need to do anything to stay synchronized with the 24-hour day other than experience the natural pattern of light exposure during the day and darkness at night.

Although the maintenance of sleep and waking occurs naturally, many aspects of modern society can lead to disruption of sleep pressure and the circadian rhythm, which can in turn lead to sleep complaints, sleep disorders, or even other seemingly unrelated chronic conditions. For example, when people look at light-emitting screens at night, such as from smartphones, that light exposure is interpreted by the circadian clock as a cue to promote wakefulness. This causes modest circadian misalignment, which can lead to a shortened sleep episode and the accumulation of a chronic sleep debt. A more extreme example of circadian misalignment is night shift work. When individuals stay awake at night and try to sleep during the day, their circadian rhythms become offset from their behavioral cycle. In these cases, peripheral clocks, such as in the stomach, pancreas, and reproductive organs, become desynchronized from the circadian clock. This can lead to short-term consequences, such as daytime sleepiness or overeating, and long-term consequences, such as an increased risk of obesity, diabetes, and breast and prostate cancers.

To understand and treat disorders arising from sleep loss and circadian misalignment, it is important to understand the underlying mechanisms driving sleep. This chapter describes how sleep pressure and the circadian rhythm interact to promote sleep. It covers the underlying mechanisms associated with sleep pressure and the circadian system and then describes the consequences of perturbing either of these sleep drives.

The Two-Process Model of Sleep Regulation

Understanding the mechanisms underlying the circadian rhythm and homeostatic drive for sleep is an important foundation for identifying and treating many sleep complaints and disorders. The interaction of these sleep drives has been described as the *two-process model of sleep regulation*,[2] with process S and process C used to describe the homeostatic sleep pressure and circadian components, respectively (see Figure 5.1). When an individual maintains regular sleep and wake timing, with approximately 8 hours in bed at night, process S and process C interact to promote a consolidated sleep episode. This process of synchronization to a light–dark cycle is called *entrainment*. When a person is entrained, the build-up of sleep pressure is very high at bedtime, while the circadian rhythm promotes sleep immediately prior to the habitual bedtime. The beginning of a normal sleep episode under entrained conditions is dominated by slow wave sleep (SWS), representing

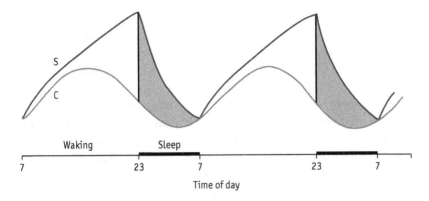

FIGURE 5.1 Two-process model of sleep: Process C, the circadian clock, and Process S, the homeostatic sleep drive.
From Kryger MH, Roth T, Dement WC, eds. *Principles and practice of sleep medicine*, 6th ed. Philadelphia, PA: Elsevier; 2017.

the payment of sleep debt accumulated through the waking day;[3] this is described in more detail later in the chapter. As SWS subsides and sleep pressure is relieved, the circadian drive for sleep peaks, coinciding with the peak of melatonin production, a nadir of body temperature, and an increase in rapid eye movement (REM) sleep.[4] At the end of a typical entrained sleep episode, sleep pressure is low, and the circadian rhythm begins to promote wakefulness coinciding with the habitual waketime and circadian peak in cortisol production.[5] Entrainment and consolidated sleep are maintained through regular wake-timing and regular light exposure following each sleep episode. The following sections describe how sleep homeostasis and the circadian rhythm are controlled and what happens when these processes are altered.

SLEEP HOMEOSTASIS

Insufficient sleep is pervasive in modern society. Social, domestic, and work pressures are increasingly cutting into the time we have available to sleep. Even seemingly inconsequential decisions to stay up an extra hour to finish watching a movie or get up an hour early to go to the gym before work can cut into valuable time that should otherwise be protected for sleep. Despite the focus on diet and exercise as pillars of health, a few hours' lost sleep can lead to both short- and long-term negative consequences for overall health. For example, chronic sleep restriction (i.e., getting less sleep than you need over the course of a week or more) can increase the risk of developing cardiometabolic diseases such as diabetes, obesity, and heart disease. In the short-term, a night of poor sleep can increase the risk of motor vehicle and occupational accidents and, if nothing else, can put you in a really bad mood. When we lose sleep, the only thing to replace it is recovery sleep. Until this need is met, we exist in a state of sleep debt. The following section describes the underlying processes of sleep need, or the homeostatic drive for sleep.

The homeostatic drive for sleep accumulates across hours of wakefulness and dissipates with time spent asleep. The biochemical process underlying the build-up and relief of sleep pressure is associated with the build-up of the neuromodulator adenosine in the brain. During wakefulness, energy use is high, resulting in the depletion of energy stores and the accumulation of associated metabolites.[6] For example, adenosine levels accumulate during wakefulness due to the use of adenosine triphosphate (ATP) by active neurons. This build-up of adenosine is associated with a feeling of sleepiness. Extracellular levels of adenosine are subsequently dissipated during sleep, particularly during slow wave sleep.[7-9] Although this build-up of sleepiness is best alleviated by sleep, millions of people worldwide do not get enough sleep and instead attempt to manage their sleepiness through the use of caffeine, which is an adenosine receptor antagonist. Caffeine doses of as little as 50 mg (the equivalent of a cup of tea or weak cup of coffee) can improve alertness and performance very quickly[10] and remain in the body for more than 6 hours. Despite the widespread cultural use and availability of caffeine, it should not be used as a replacement for sleep because adenosine continues to build even during caffeine use; after the effects of caffeine have worn off, many people experience a "crash" in alertness. In addition, habitual caffeine use diminishes mood, decreases sleep duration, and changes sleep architecture, making the sleep obtained while caffeine is circulating in the body less restorative than natural sleep.[11,12]

Biomarkers of Sleep Homeostasis

Early observations of the physiological markers of sleep homeostasis were derived from electroencephalographic (EEG) recordings of habitual sleep episodes. Slow wave sleep (SWS) was identified as a marker of process S based on the observation that, like sleep pressure, SWS is predominant during the first few sleep cycles and then diminishes across the sleep episode.[13] Furthermore, sleep pressure (e.g., under conditions of prior sleep loss and extended wakefulness) advances the onset of slow wave activity (SWA; EEG power density in the 0.75–4.5 Hz range) during non–rapid eye movement (NREM) sleep and increases the amount of SWA in the sleep episode.[13] For example, when people are allowed to take short naps during the day, the amount of prior wakefulness will determine the amount of SWA in the nap. That is, if you have been awake longer, you will have more SWA, or deeper sleep, in your nap.[14] Conversely, if you take a late afternoon nap, this can reduce the amount of sleep pressure preceding your nighttime sleep period and therefore reduce the amount of overnight SWA.[15,16] The homeostatic component of sleep is also evident under conditions of chronic sleep restriction. Under these conditions there is a conservation of SWS across restricted sleep episodes and a conservation or increase in SWA.[17] That is, if you only have 5 hours of sleep per night, your body will make sure to maintain the amount of SWA that would occur in an 8-hour sleep opportunity, sacrificing lighter sleep stages to preserve deep sleep.

While SWA is a primary biomarker of sleep homeostasis, it may not be practical to evaluate in a clinical setting. Other biomarkers of sleep pressure include self-reported sleepiness and sleep latency (the time it takes to fall asleep). Generally speaking, we know when we are tired, and self-reported sleepiness scales can be used to get a quick and easy subjective view of a person's sleep pressure at a given point in time (e.g., Karolinksa Sleepiness Scale, KSS), or over a longer term period (e.g., Epworth Sleepiness Scale, ESS). The KSS has been shown to correlate well with objective measures of sleepiness such as EEG and with performance measures such as standardized reaction time tests (e.g., psychomotor vigilance task, PVT).[18] It should be noted, however, that under some sleep loss conditions, self-reported sleepiness can be distorted, leading to a misleading view of underlying sleep pressure.[19] Therefore, where possible, an objective measure of sleepiness is preferable.

A relatively easy to administer test of objective sleepiness is called the Multiple Sleep Latency Task (MSLT). This task measures how long it takes someone to fall asleep on a comfortable bed in a dark, quiet room. The task is terminated after sleep onset or after 20 minutes, whichever is sooner, and is typically repeated every 2 hours across a day. Research suggests that falling asleep under these conditions within 8 minutes is indicative of clinically relevant sleepiness.[20]

CIRCADIAN SLEEP DRIVE

The circadian pacemaker is an endogenous oscillator located in the suprachiasmatic nucleus (SCN) of the hypothalamus that coordinates the action of many aspects of biological function. The term "circadian" was coined by Dr. Franz Halberg and comes from the Latin *circa* and *diem*, meaning "about a day."[21] The average circadian rhythm has a period of approximately 24.2 hours,[22] with about one-third of the population having a circadian period of less than 24 hours and two-thirds having a period of more than 24 hours.[23] The circadian rhythm is capable of resetting and entraining to periods that are close to the endogenous period through *zeitgebers* (time cues, from German, meaning "time giver"), with the strongest zeitgeber being light. The resetting capability of the circadian rhythm is important because it allows for the body clock to be flexible. Having a circadian rhythm that adapts to different light–dark cues allows us to be able to adapt to changes in time zones and to shift our sleep schedules when needed. Importantly, however, many people do not understand how the circadian rhythm works and, as a result, make choices that can cause sleep disruption. Understanding how the circadian rhythm works is an important component in treating modest sleep complaints.

Morningness-Eveningness Preference

Although daily light exposure is sufficient to synchronize the sleep–wake rhythms of most individuals to the 24-hour day, there is variation in how different individuals adapt to the day. Individuals with a longer circadian period tend to rate themselves as "night owls," while those who have a shorter circadian period tend to rate themselves as "morning larks."[24] Morningness-eveningness preference (also referred to as a person's *chronotype*) has also been shown to change throughout the life span. Post-adolescent children and young adults tend to prefer later bed- and waketimes, while older adults tend to prefer earlier bed- and wake times.

The underlying impact of morningness-eveningness preference on sleep relates to the differing phase angle of entrainment between larks and owls. Phase angle is the duration between bed- or waketime and a marker of circadian phase, such as the melatonin peak (i.e., at the circadian nadir, the strongest circadian drive to sleep). If an owl and a lark went to bed at the same clock time (say, 11:00 PM), the lark, with an earlier circadian phase (e.g., circadian nadir at 2:00 AM), would have a bedtime closer to their circadian nadir and, therefore, a smaller phase angle (3 hours), than the owl, which has a later circadian phase (e.g., circadian nadir at 4:00 AM) and, therefore, a larger phase angle (5 hour).[25] Although the modest differences in phase angle as observed in owls and larks allows for a stable sleep episode, larger differences can lead to sleep disruption. Morningness-eveningness preference can be evaluated clinically using questionnaires, such as the Horne-Ostberg Questionnaire or Munich Chronotype Questionnaire. A common example of how morningness-eveningness preference can interfere with lifestyle occurs in night owls. About two-thirds of the population have a longer than 24-hour circadian rhythm, which makes it relatively easy to stay up too late. This may not be a problem for a person who has a mid- to late-morning work start time, but if an early work time is required, night owls may have a very difficult time waking up and performing at work. This can be a major problem for high school and college students who are at an age where circadian preference is later and social pressures may lead to a desire to stay up late, yet early school start times prevent adequate sleep. These types of sleep complaints can be treated using light therapy (as described in the next section).

Light as a Zeitgeber

Light is the most potent synchronizer of the circadian rhythm. The light signal is transmitted to the SCN via a collection of intrinsically photosensitive retinal ganglion cells (ipRGCs) that contain the photopigment melanopsin.[26] These photoreceptors are separate from the visual photoreceptor system and project via the retino-hypothalamic tract to the SCN. The light signal is transmitted exclusively through the eyes,[27] and totally blind individuals lacking the ipRGCs in the outer retina cannot synchronize with a 24-hour light–dark cycle (entrain) via light cues (zeitgebers).[28] The action of light on the human circadian pacemaker depends on the timing, intensity, wavelength, pattern, and duration of the light stimulus. These properties of light can be manipulated for therapeutic intervention, but inappropriate light exposure can lead to sleep and circadian disruption. The importance of each of these aspects of light is described here.

Timing of light exposure. The action of light on circadian timing follows a phase response curve (PRC), where light administered in the biological morning causes a phase advance of the system (shifting circadian rhythms, including the drive to sleep and wake, earlier), while light in the biological evening causes a phase delay of the system (shifting circadian rhythms later)[29] (see Figure 5.2). In simple terms, this means that when traveling a few time zones eastward (or shifting bedtime earlier), morning light exposure and evening light avoidance will accelerate adaptation, while evening light exposure and morning darkness is required when traveling a few time zones westward (or for shifting bedtime later).

Light intensity. The magnitude of the effect of light depends on the intensity of the stimulus. Light levels as low as 1.5 lux (i.e., the equivalent of 1.5 candles burning 1 foot away) have been shown to facilitate entrainment in some individuals in laboratory environments,[23] while brighter light levels elicit faster circadian phase shifts and are better for maintaining stable entrainment. When individuals are exposed to dim light during waking, it can be difficult to entrain to day lengths that are far from an individual's endogenous circadian period. Conversely, bright light of 10,000 lux has been shown to elicit phase shifts of as much as 3 hours following a single, 6.7-hour light pulse.[29] In practice, this means that individuals who do not receive a sufficient daily light stimulus (e.g., miners, individuals in care homes or hospitals) or those who expose themselves to light during the biological night (e.g., while viewing computer screens) may experience circadian misalignment and subsequent sleep disruption.

Wavelength. The human circadian pacemaker is most sensitive to short-wavelength light in the 460–480 nm range.[30,31] Low-intensity blue light is capable of eliciting large phase shifts and melatonin suppression similar to those achieved with full-spectrum white light at much higher intensities.[32,33] In practice, these findings support the use of blue light for therapeutic interventions to improve the efficacy of treatment for disorders that involve shifting the circadian rhythm (e.g., advanced sleep phase syndrome, delayed sleep phase syndrome) but also highlight

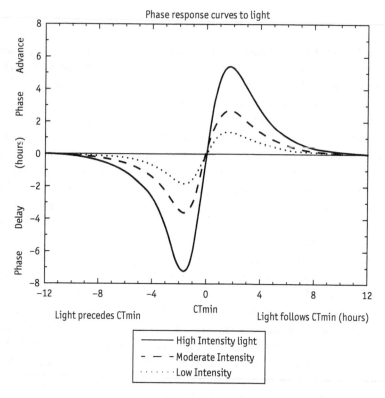

FIGURE 5.2 Phase response curves to light (CT_{min}: core body temperature minimum). From Lack, L. C. and Bootzin, R. R. (2003) Circadian rhythm factors in insomnia and their treatment. In *Treating sleep disorders: Principles and practice of behavioural sleep medicine*, pp. 305–343, Perlis M and Lichstein K (eds.), John Wiley, Hoboken NJ.

the importance of avoiding lights with blue peaks before and during the sleep episode.

Pattern and duration. The pattern and duration of light exposure can also influence the magnitude of the phase shift incurred. Long light exposures of 3–7 hours are capable of eliciting large phase shifts when timed near the circadian nadir,[29,34–36] while shorter light exposure sessions are capable of causing large phase shifts if the light is of sufficient intensity or spectral content.[37] Recent evidence suggests that even millisecond flashes of light, pulsed between 2.5 and 30 seconds over an hour during wake or sleep, are capable of causing phase shifts of up to 2 hours.[38,39] Together, these data support the importance of educating patients on how very short light exposures are capable of causing phase shifts and suggest that even very brief light exposure during sleep can influence the circadian system (e.g., checking a brightly lit phone screen or turning on a bright bathroom light). These studies also highlight the importance of considering the timing and duration of light exposure regimes when administering light therapy to patients.

Many people expose themselves to light in ways that can cause sleep disruption. The prevalence of handheld tablets and phones in modern society can be blamed for many modest sleep complaints. Historically, one way people used to wind down for bed was by reading a book in bed by candle light or a bedside table lamp but now, what was formerly an appropriate bedtime routine, has been replaced by people effectively staring at bright blue lights just before bed. The light generated from a tablet screen has been shown to cause a circadian phase shift by as much as 1.5 hours, leading to elevated sleepiness upon waking, relative to reading a book with a table lamp.[40] Furthermore, looking at screens before bed doesn't simply cause a problem at the time of the exposure. The circadian pacemaker interprets the light signal from one night and uses that information to change the timing of the sleep drive for the next night. This means that if a person looks at a screen for 1 hour before bed tonight, it will be very difficult to go to bed at that time tomorrow. From a treatment perspective, simply teaching people to change their evening routines and turn off screens within 2 hours of their desired bedtime has the potential to greatly improve sleep outcomes for those with complaints of sleep onset difficulties and early morning sleepiness.

Influence of Non-Photic Cues

As described previously, light is recognized as the strongest resetting agent, but there are several other "non-photic" zeitgebers capable of shifting circadian phase in animal models, many of which have yet to be demonstrated in humans. It should also be noted that among the human studies that have been conducted to evaluate the impact of non-photic cues, no non-photic stimulus has been shown to be as strong as even dim light exposure. The primary non-photic cues that have been explored are described here.

Meal timing. Despite popular media articles suggesting scheduled meal timing as a panacea to jet lag, there is currently scarce evidence in humans that meal timing can enhance acute phase shifting beyond photic effects.[41] To date, little is known about the efficacy of scheduled meal timing to shift circadian rhythms in humans, although meals misaligned with the circadian rhythm are associated with adverse health outcomes, as discussed in later in this chapter. It is difficult to assess the impact of meal timing in humans due to the influence of other exposures such as light and activity. Therefore, it is hard to say whether there is an independent effect of meal timing on human circadian phase, peripheral or otherwise. A study of morning versus evening carbohydrate-rich meals demonstrated that the core body temperature rhythm but not the melatonin rhythm shifted earlier in the morning meal condition compared to the evening meal.[42] This study suggests that there is the potential for meal timing to aid in shifting peripheral clocks (discussed later in this chapter), but it appears to have less of an effect on central oscillations.

Exercise. Several studies have assessed the ability to entrain the circadian system through scheduled bouts of exercise. Early studies suggested that exercise might be capable of shifting the circadian rhythm; however, in those early studies light exposure was not strictly controlled and measures of circadian phase were not reliable, potentially confounding results. Recent studies have shown modest effects of exercise on circadian phase shifting, but only when individuals were kept in dim light. In addition, the influence of exercise on the circadian pacemaker is a short-term effect, with repeated cycles of exercise being required to maintain entrainment. Although there is evidence for exercise to produce a non-photic phase shift in humans, the duration and intensity of exercise required to make a significant contribution may not be viable in real-world settings such as the workplace.

Independent of phase shifting, of note, it has been shown that regular exercise can improve sleep in humans,[43] and short bursts of moderate to high intensity exercise can improve subjective alertness and objective cognitive performance in the short term,[44] which may be a more useful way of improving sleep and alertness than direct phase resetting.

Social and behavioral cues. Before light was accepted as a critical zeitgeber in humans, evidence of co-habitating individuals synchronizing circadian rhythms under conditions of self-selected bedtimes was interpreted as being driven by behavioral and social cues.[45] It has since been shown that the self-selected light schedules in that study were probably the main driving force behind these observations. Co-habitation in dim light (<8 lux), by contrast, did not show any synchrony in circadian phases between subjects.[46,47] Social cues, therefore, are not a consistent entraining factor.[48] Choosing to engage in social activities (or mandatory events, such as early work starts) is more likely to change circadian timing through other exposures such as light, food intake, and physical activity or by changing sleep–wake timing itself.

There is some evidence, however, that social cues and sleep–wake cycles alone can entrain circadian rhythms. Although rare, some blind individuals with no response to photic cues still exhibit a 24-hour rhythm.[49] In these case studies, it is unknown which non-photic cues are responsible for entrainment. It is likely that only individuals with an endogenous period close to 24-hours are able to entrain to non-photic zeitgebers.

Melatonin and pharmacological agents. Studies of treatment of non–24-hour circadian rhythm disorders, particularly in the blind, have shown exogenous melatonin administration to be successful in entraining circadian rhythms.[50] Similarly, a clinical trial of tasimelteon, a melatonin receptor agonist, was successfully used to advance circadian rhythms more rapidly than placebo[51] and to entrain blind individuals.[52] Melatonin has also proved useful in shift workers to help adapt to daytime sleep patterns.[53] The effects of melatonin, like light, follow a phase response curve, with greater efficacy when delivered during naturally low levels of endogenous melatonin (i.e., during the day/light period for humans).[54]

Until recently the phase shifting effects of caffeine had only been investigated in animal studies and with mixed results.[55,56] Recently, however, caffeine has been shown to shift circadian rhythms in humans.[57,58] The phase shifting properties of stimulants (i.e., methamphetamines) and hypnotics (i.e., benzodiazepines) may be due to their effects on behavior (increase activity or sleep, respectively). While changes in sleep–wake patterns are only weak zeitgebers, this may be enhanced through pharmacological agents, which may also act through additional pathways to enhance re-entrainment.

OUTPUTS OF THE CIRCADIAN RHYTHM

Many people understand that the circadian pacemaker controls the drive to sleep at specific times of day; less known are the other aspects of biological function that are under circadian control. One important feature of the circadian rhythm is that it also controls the drive to be awake. The strongest drive to be awake occurs in the hours just before one's habitual bedtime and has been dubbed the "wake maintenance zone." The purpose of the wake maintenance zone is to dampen the high homeostatic sleep pressure that occurs near the end of the day in order for people to make it to a bedtime that will allow for a consolidated nightly sleep episode. Under normal circumstances, the wake maintenance zone is important in helping to maintain entrainment. However, the wake maintenance zone can lead to sleep complaints when individuals try to sleep during it. For example, when an individual needs to wake up at 4:00 AM to work or catch a flight, she would need to go to bed at 8:00 PM in order to have 8 hours available for sleep. If that person normally goes to bed at 10:00 PM, then 8:00 PM will fall during the wake maintenance zone and it will be very difficult to sleep at that time. Similarly, a 3-hour advance in bedtime, such as the phase shift that occurs during jet lag when crossing three time zones eastward, can lead to sleep fragmentation at the beginning of the sleep episode due to the intersection of the imposed bedtime with the wake maintenance zone.[59]

Although the circadian pacemaker controls many aspects of biological function, melatonin is the hormone most often measured as a biomarker of circadian phase. When a person is entrained, melatonin is produced just prior to one's habitual bedtime. Optimal sleep initiation follows the onset of melatonin production. On average, melatonin peaks approximately 6 hours after sleep onset and is not produced during the waking day (see Figure 5.3). The timing of the melatonin onset or peak can be used to determine whether an individual's circadian rhythm is optimally timed relative to their sleep opportunity. Many researchers and clinicians use the dim light melatonin onset (DLMO) to assess circadian phase in individuals who are suspected of having circadian rhythm sleep issues. DLMO is collected by asking an individual to remain in dim light for up to 6 hours before

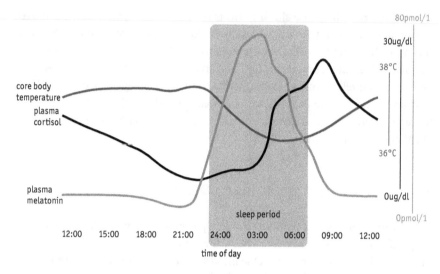

FIGURE 5.3 Circadian rhythms in physiology.
From Hickie, I. B., Naismith, S. L., Robillard, R., Scott, E. M., & Hermens, D. F. (2013). Manipulating the sleep-wake cycle and circadian rhythms to improve clinical management of major depression. *BMC Medicine, 11*(1), 79.

and up to 3 hours after their habitual bedtime. Melatonin is typically measured by taking hourly saliva or blood samples (although urine samples can be used to evaluate the melatonin peak over a 24-hour duration). Clinicians may find it beneficial to measure DLMO for confirmation of diagnosis in individuals suspected of having advanced or delayed sleep phase disorder. It may also be beneficial to measure DLMO in individuals who have sleep onset or early waking insomnia. Modest circadian misalignment is apparent in as many as 20% of individuals diagnosed with insomnia.[60] In these cases, if the timing of DLMO occurs very late (e.g., after midnight in someone who desires to sleep at 10:00 PM), then the person has a phase delayed circadian rhythm and will require either exogenous melatonin treatment before bed, or bright light therapy in the morning, or both to align the circadian rhythm with the individual's desired sleep time. In cases where the timing of DLMO occurs very early (e.g., before 7:00 PM in a person who desires to sleep at 10:00 PM), then the person has a phase-advanced circadian rhythm. In this case, bright light treatment in the evening would be required to align the circadian rhythm with the sleep opportunity.

Although melatonin is the output rhythm most commonly associated with the circadian pacemaker, the production of many other hormones and body temperature are also under circadian control. For example, there is a daily rhythm in the production of cortisol, which peaks in association with waking in entrained individuals. This morning cortisol peak is referred to as the *cortisol awakening response* (CAR). The hormone leptin, which is associated with appetite suppression, is also under circadian control, with a peak during the night. Similarly, body temperature follows a predictable circadian rhythm. Core body temperature drops in conjunction with an individual's habitual bedtime and reaches a nadir during the night, approximately 6 hours after sleep onset, coinciding with the strongest circadian drive to sleep. Skin temperature follows an opposite pattern and reaches a peak during the night. These daily patterns can only shift in conjunction with careful control of light and darkness, so if a person who is normally entrained stays up all night, she will still experience these fluctuations in biological rhythms.

PERIPHERAL CLOCKS

The central circadian pacemaker in the SCN is the master clock of the body, but many organs and tissues also contain circadian clock genes that organize their activities in conjunction with the master clock. When the SCN is removed, these clocks continue to oscillate but become desynchronized from one another.[61] Peripheral clocks control a myriad of processes including the circadian secretion of myokines (e.g., interleukin-6) by skeletal muscle, through to daily fluctuations in gene expression in reproductive organs. The importance of these peripheral clocks is increasingly being recognized. For example, disruption of peripheral clock genes in reproductive organ tissue leads to a decrease in fertility in animal models. Many metabolic functions are also under circadian control through peripheral clocks in the pancreas, gut, and liver. There is a peripheral clock in the pancreas that coordinates the timing of insulin secretion, thus promoting insulin production approximately 4 hours after the peak in melatonin (early morning).[62] Similarly, the conversion of glucose to glycogen in the liver is controlled by a peripheral clock that synchronizes glucose regulation and storage. This coordination and synchrony across organs and tissues within the body allows for an appropriate metabolic response to food consumed during the day, with better glucose tolerance occurring in the morning compared to the evening.[63]

Under conditions of shift work, meal timing often occurs out of phase with these coordinated circadian clocks. Peripheral clocks are more sensitive to phase changes induced by non-photic cues such as food intake and can shift at rates different from the SCN and other tissues. This can lead to desynchrony across tissues and between the peripheral and central clocks, essentially disrupting the otherwise synchronized physiological functions coordinated for processing of food. This can lead to reduced insulin sensitivity and impaired glucose tolerance when eating at night. Recent studies suggest that avoiding large meals on night shift can help to reduce the impact of circadian misalignment on these metabolic outcomes.[64]

CIRCADIAN MISALIGNMENT

Circadian misalignment occurs when a sleep–wake or light–dark cycle is desynchronized from the body's internal circadian clock. This desynchrony can lead to a host of short- and long-term neurobehavioral and physiological changes. Shift work is a common example of circadian misalignment as workers are often required to be active during the night, leading to desynchrony between the work–rest cycle and their endogenous circadian rhythms. Other common examples of circadian misalignment include jet lag due to transmeridian travel, social jet lag resulting from changing sleep behaviors on weekends compared to weekdays, or extreme chronotypes (i.e., night owls) forced to keep regular office hours.[65] The impact of circadian misalignment on short- and long-term health and well-being is far reaching, as described here.

Performance and Alertness (Neurobehavioral Effects)

The neurobehavioral outcomes of atypical working hours have been well-documented. Shift work is associated with sleep loss, sleepiness, and increased error rates. Circadian misalignment affects neurobehavioral outcomes in two ways: (1) attempting to maintain wakefulness at times when the circadian pressure for sleep is high (e.g., 02:00–06:00 AM) and (2) attempting to sleep during the day when the circadian rhythm is promoting wakefulness.[66] Workers on both permanent night shifts and rotating night shifts only partially adapt to the nocturnal work pattern and maintain a degree of misalignment between their endogenous rhythms and the work–rest cycle.[67,68] Those who do partially adapt to night work may have better alertness on shift [69] but may also find it harder to revert to being awake during the day on days off, therefore experiencing misalignment during both work days and days off.[70,71] It is worth noting that, although the sleep loss caused by circadian disruption plays a role in the consequences observed in shift work, the desynchrony of circadian and environmental cycles has independent effects on physiological factors and has been shown to further exacerbate the effects of sleep loss itself.[72,73] Therefore, even though a nightshift worker might report being able to sleep relatively well during the day, they may still suffer from the effects of circadian misalignment on other physiological outcomes such as gastrointestinal complaints from eating at night.

Cardiometabolic Disorders

A higher incidence of metabolic and cardiovascular disorders such as obesity, type 2 diabetes, and coronary heart disease have been observed in shift work populations compared to daytime workers.[74-76] There is some evidence to suggest that shift workers eat more poorly, consuming foods with higher fat content and higher calories per day compared to day workers, which may explain this epidemiological observation.[77] However, a meta-analysis comparing the 24-hour energy intake of shift workers versus day workers found no difference between these two populations, suggesting that other factors may be contributing to this epidemic.[78] The timing, rather than content, of meals has since been the focus of research to probe the physiological mechanisms underlying the pathologies seen in the shift-working population. Indeed, laboratory studies of simulated shift work have shown that eating at night can impair glucose tolerance and metabolism,[79,80] which is a risk factor for obesity and type 2 diabetes. Furthermore, young adults who eat closer to their biological night have a higher percent body fat and body mass index (BMI).[81] These studies suggest that the misalignment of meal timing with internal circadian rhythms can lead to metabolic dysfunction, with effects observed after both acute and chronic misalignment.

Cancer

Epidemiological studies have shown modest yet inconsistent associations between shift work and cancer risk.[82-85] While breast cancer has received the most attention, studies of colorectal, endometrial, and prostate cancer have also emerged. In 2007, based on a review of both animal and human studies, the International Agency for Research on Cancer (IARC) classified shift work associated with circadian disruption or chronodisruption (CD) as a "probable human carcinogen."[86]

The primary mechanistic link between circadian misalignment and cancer appears to involve the increased exposure to light during the biological night, which leads to the suppression of melatonin.[87] Melatonin has been shown to exhibit tumor-suppressing actions and acts as a mediator in estrogen signaling pathways.[88] In rodents, studies have shown that light at night (LAN) reduces melatonin and increases markers of tumor progression, whereas exogenous replacement of melatonin in LAN conditions rescued these effects.[89,90] In humans, the association between LAN and cancer is less consistent. A recent prospective study of 105,866 participants in the UK Generations Study found no significant association between LAN exposure and cancer risk.[91] However, an earlier meta-analysis showed an increased relative risk of breast cancer with high artificial light exposure but not ambient light exposure.[87] Therefore, the intensity of the light exposure and relative reduction in melatonin may account for discrepancies in reported associations. Furthermore, increased methylation of tumor-suppression factors[92] and shortened telomere length,[93] both risk factors for cancer, were only observed in workers with long and/or intense shift work exposure, suggesting greater exposure to LAN. Epigenetic studies suggest that interactions between circadian genotypes and shift work exposure may put some shift workers at a greater risk of developing cancer, further obscuring the effects of circadian misalignment due to shift work in the general population.[92,94] Together these studies suggest that the effects of light-suppressed melatonin due to shift work on cancer risk may be mediated by genotype (e.g., light sensitivity, chronotype).[94]

Mental Health

Surveys of shift workers report greater negative impacts on stress,[95,96] mental health,[97] mood,[8] and family and life satisfaction.[99] Controlled laboratory studies of rats suffering from circadian misalignment show expression of depressive behaviors during the active period, suggesting a direct link between circadian desynchrony and mental health.[100] In humans, the independent contribution of circadian misalignment on depression and other mood disorders has yet to be disentangled from the myriad factors contributing to overall mental health.

Conclusion

A daily, consolidated sleep episode is achieved through stable entrainment of the circadian rhythm to a robust light–dark cycle. Such entrainment, with regular sleep–wake timing, allows for the predictable build-up of homeostatic sleep pressure during the waking day and maintenance of sleep during the night, as described by the two-process model of sleep regulation. Light is the most potent synchronizer of the circadian rhythm, while timed feeding, exercise, and social interaction have a weak to no influence on circadian entrainment in humans. Desynchronization of the homeostatic and circadian drives for sleep, such as that which occurs with jet lag, shift work, or insufficient light exposure, leads to sleep loss and sleep fragmentation. Persistent circadian misalignment, such as occurs during many years of shift work, can lead to an increased risk of an array of negative health outcomes including metabolic syndrome, cancer, and negative mental health effects. Together, these findings support the importance of encouraging patients to maintain stable sleep timing in addition to sleep of adequate duration in order to realize short- and long-term health benefits.

REFERENCES

1. Hastings JW. The Gonyaulax clock at 50: Translational control of circadian expression. *Cold Spring Harbor Symp Quantit Biol.* 2007;72:141–144.
2. Borbely AA. A two process model of sleep regulation. *Hum Neurobiol.* 1982;1(3):195–204.
3. Dijk DJ, Brunner DP, Beersma DG, Borbely AA. Electroencephalogram power density and slow wave sleep as a function of prior waking and circadian phase. *Sleep.* 1990;13(5):430–440.

4. Dijk DJ, Shanahan TL, Duffy JF, Ronda JM, Czeisler CA. Variation of electroencephalographic activity during non-rapid eye movement and rapid eye movement sleep with phase of circadian melatonin rhythm in humans. *J Physiol.* 1997;505 (Pt 3):851–858.

5. Orth DN, Island DP, Liddle GW. Experimental alteration of the circadian rhythm in plasma cortisol (17-OHCS) concentration in man. *J Clin Endocrinol Metabol.* 1967;27(4):549–555.

6. Scharf MT, Naidoo N, Zimmerman JE, Pack AI. The energy hypothesis of sleep revisited. *Prog Neurobiol.* 2008;86(3):264–280.

7. Benington JH, Heller HC. Restoration of brain energy metabolism as the function of sleep. *Prog Neurobiol.* 1995;45:347–360.

8. Porkka-Heiskanen T, Strecker RE, Thakkar M, Bjorkum AA, Greene RW, McCarley RW. Adenosine: A mediator of the sleep-inducing effects of prolonged wakefulness. *Science.* 1997;276:1265–1268.

9. Landolt HP. Sleep homeostasis: A role for adenosine in humans? *Biochem Pharmacol.* 2008;75(11):2070–2079.

10. Wyatt JK, Cajochen C, Ritz-De Cecco A, Czeisler CA, Dijk DJ. Low-dose repeated caffeine administration for circadian-phase-dependent performance degradation during extended wakefulness. *Sleep.* 2004;27(3):374–381.

11. Yanik G, Glaum S, Radulovacki M. The dose-response effects of caffeine on sleep in rats. *Brain Res.* 1987;403(1):177–180.

12. Biggs SN, Smith A, Dorrian J, Reid K, Dawson D, van den Heuvel C, et al. Perception of simulated driving performance after sleep restriction and caffeine. *J Psychosom Res.* 2007;63(6):573–577.

13. Webb WB, Agnew HW. Stage 4 sleep: Influence of time course variables. *Science.* 1971;174:1354–1356.

14. Dijk DJ, Beersma DGM, Daan S. EEG power density during nap sleep: Reflection of an hourglass measuring the duration of prior wakefulness. *J Biol Rhythms.* 1987;2:207–219.

15. Werth E, Dijk DJ, Achermann P, Borbély AA. Dynamics of the sleep EEG after an early evening nap: Experimental data and simulations. *Am J Physiol.* 1996;271:R501–R10.

16. Centofanti SA, Dorrian J, Hilditch CJ, Banks S. Do night naps impact driving performance and daytime recovery sleep? *Accident Analysis Prevention.* 2017;99(Pt B):416–421.

17. Brunner DP, Dijk DJ, Borbely AA. Repeated partial sleep deprivation progressively changes in EEG during sleep and wakefulness. *Sleep.* 1993;16(2):100–113.

18. Kaida K, Takahashi M, Akerstedt T, Nakata A, Otsuka Y, Haratani T, et al. Validation of the Karolinska sleepiness scale against performance and EEG variables. *Clin Neurophysiol.* 2006;117(7):1574–1581.

19. Van Dongen HP, Maislin G, Mullington JM, Dinges DF. The cumulative cost of additional wakefulness: Dose-response effects on neurobehavioral functions and sleep physiology from chronic sleep restriction and total sleep deprivation. *Sleep.* 2003;26(2):117–126.

20. American Academy of Sleep Medicine. *International classification of sleep disorders.* 3rd ed. Darien, IL: American Academy of Sleep Medicine; 2014.

21. Halberg F, Cornelissen G, Katinas G, Syutkina EV, Sothern RB, Zaslavskaya R, et al. Transdisciplinary unifying implications of circadian findings in the 1950s. *J Circadian Rhythms.* 2003;1(1):2.

22. Czeisler CA, Duffy JF, Shanahan TL, Brown EN, Mitchell JF, Rimmer DW, et al. Stability, precision, and near-24-hour period of the human circadian pacemaker. *Science.* 1999;284(5423):2177–2181.

23. Wright KP, Jr., Hughes RJ, Kronauer RE, Dijk DJ, Czeisler CA. Intrinsic near-24-h pacemaker period determines limits of circadian entrainment to a weak synchronizer in humans. *Proc Natl Acad Sci U S A.* 2001;98(24):14027–14032.

24. Lack L, Bailey M, Lovato N, Wright H. Chronotype differences in circadian rhythms of temperature, melatonin, and sleepiness as measured in a modified constant routine protocol. *Nat Sci Sleep.* 2009;1:1–8.

25. Dijk DJ, Lockley SW. Integration of human sleep–wake regulation and circadian rhythmicity. *J Appl Physiol.* 2002;92(2):852–862.

26. Morin LP. Neuroanatomy of the extended circadian rhythm system. *Exp Neurol.* 2013;243:4–20.

27. Wright KP, Jr., Czeisler CA. Absence of circadian phase resetting in response to bright light behind the knees. *Science.* 2002;297(5581):571.

28. Flynn-Evans EE, Tabandeh H, Skene DJ, Lockley SW. Circadian rhythm disorders and melatonin production in 127 blind women with and without light perception. *J Biolog Rhythms.* 2014;29(3):215–224.

29. Khalsa SB, Jewett ME, Cajochen C, Czeisler CA. A phase response curve to single bright light pulses in human subjects. *J Physiol.* 2003;549(Pt 3):945–952.

30. Brainard GC, Sliney D, Hanifin JP, Glickman G, Byrne B, Greeson JM, et al. Sensitivity of the human circadian system to short-wavelength (420-nm) light. *J Biol Rhythms.* 2008;23(5):379–386.

31. Lockley SW, Evans EE, Scheer FA, Brainard GC, Czeisler CA, Aeschbach D. Short-wavelength sensitivity for the direct effects of light on alertness, vigilance, and the waking electroencephalogram in humans. *Sleep.* 2006;29(2):161–168.

32. West KE, Jablonski MR, Warfield B, Cecil KS, James M, Ayers MA, et al. Blue light from light-emitting diodes elicits a dose-dependent suppression of melatonin in humans. *J Appl Physiol.* 2011;110(3):619–626.

33. Ruger M, St Hilaire MA, Brainard GC, Khalsa SB, Kronauer RE, Czeisler CA, et al. Human phase response curve to a single 6.5 h pulse of short-wavelength light. *J Physiol.* 2013;591(1):353–363.

34. Minors DS, Waterhouse JM, Wirz-Justice A. A human phase-response curve to light. *Neurosci Lett.* 1991;133(1):36–40.

35. Czeisler CA, Kronauer RE, Allan JS, Duffy JF, Jewett ME, Brown EN, et al. Bright light induction of strong (type o) resetting of the human circadian pacemaker. *Science.* 1989;244(4910):1328–1333.

36. Van Cauter E, Sturis J, Byrne MM, Blackman JD, Leproult R, Ofek G, et al. Demonstration of rapid light-induced advances and delays of the human circadian clock using hormonal phase markers. *Am J Physiol.* 1994;266(6 Pt 1):E953–E963.

37. St Hilaire MA, Gooley JJ, Khalsa SB, Kronauer RE, Czeisler CA, Lockley SW. Human phase response curve to a 1 h pulse of bright white light. *J Physiol.* 2012;590(Pt 13):3035–3045.

38. Zeitzer JM, Fisicaro RA, Ruby NF, Heller HC. Millisecond flashes of light phase delay the human circadian clock during sleep. *J Biol Rhythms.* 2014;29(5):370–376.

39. Najjar RP, Zeitzer JM. Temporal integration of light flashes by the human circadian system. *J Clin Invest.* 2016;126(3):938–947.

40. Chang AM, Aeschbach D, Duffy JF, Czeisler CA. Evening use of light-emitting eReaders negatively affects sleep, circadian timing, and next-morning alertness. *Proc Natl Acad Sci USA.* 2015;112(4):1232–1237.

41. Mistlberger RE, Skene DJ. Nonphotic entrainment in humans? *J Biol Rhythms.* 2005;20(4):339–352.

42. Kräuchi K, Cajochen C, Werth E, Wirz-Justice A. Alteration of internal circadian phase relationships after morning versus evening carbohydrate-rich meals in humans. *J Biol Rhythms.* 2002;17(4):364–376.

43. Youngstedt SD. Effects of exercise on sleep. *Clin Sports Med.* 2005;24(2):355–365, xi.

44. Horne JA, Staff LHE. Exercise and sleep: Body-heating effects. *Sleep.* 1983;6:36–46.

45. Wever R. Autonomous circadian rhythms in man. Singly versus collectively isolated subjects. *Die Naturwissenschaften.* 1975;62(9):443–444.

46. Middleton B, Arendt J, Stone BM. Human circadian rhythms in constant dim light (8 lux) with knowledge of clock time. *J Sleep Res.* 1996;5:69–76.

47. Middleton B, Stone BM, Arendt J. Human circadian phase in 12:12 h, 200: < 8 lux and 1000: < 8 lux light–dark cycles, without scheduled sleep or activity. *Neurosci Lett.* 2002;329:41–44.

48. Mistlberger RE, Skene DJ. Social influences on mammalian circadian rhythms: Animal and human studies. *Biol Rev Camb Philos Soc.* 2004;79(3):533–556.

49. Klerman EB, Rimmer DW, Dijk DJ, Kronauer RE, Rizzo JF, III, Czeisler CA. Nonphotic entrainment of the human circadian pacemaker. *Am J Physiol.* 1998;274:R991–R996.

50. Arendt J, Skene DJ. Melatonin as a chronobiotic. *Sleep Med Rev.* 2005;9(1):25–39.

51. Rajaratnam SM, Polymeropoulos MH, Fisher DM, Roth T, Scott C, Birznieks G, et al. Melatonin agonist tasimelteon (VEC-162) for transient insomnia after sleep-time shift: Two randomised controlled multicentre trials. *Lancet.* 2008;373(9662):482–491.

52. Lockley SW, Dressman M, Licamele L, Xiao C, Fisher DM, Flynn-Evans E, et al. Tasimelteon for non-24-hour sleep–wake disorder in totally blind people (SET and RESET): Two multicentre, randomised, double-masked, placebo-controlled phase 3 trials. *Lancet.* 2015;386(10005):1754–1764. doi:10.1016/S0140-6736(15)60031-9. Epub 2015 Aug 4. PMID: 26466871.

53. Sharkey KM, Fogg LF, Eastman CI. Effects of melatonin administration on daytime sleep after simulated night shift work. *J Sleep Res.* 2001;10:181–192.

54. Wyatt JK, Dijk DJ, Ritz-De Cecco A, Ronda JM, Czeisler CA. Effects of physiologic and pharmacologic doses of exogenous melatonin on sleep propensity and consolidation in healthy young men and women are circadian phase-dependent. *Sleep Res Online.* 1999;2(Suppl 1):636.

55. Ding JM, Buchanan GF, Tischkau SA, Chen D, Kuriashkina L, Faiman LE, et al. A neuronal ryanodine receptor mediates light-induced phase delays of the circadian clock. *Nature.* 1998;394:381–384.

56. Diaz-Munoz M, Dent MA, Granados-Fuentes D, Hall AC, Hernandez-Cruz A, Harrington ME, et al. Circadian modulation of the ryanodine receptor type 2 in the SCN of rodents. *Neuroreport.* 1999;10(3):481–486.

57. McHill AW, Smith BJ, Wright KP, Jr. Effects of caffeine on skin and core temperatures, alertness, and recovery sleep during circadian misalignment. *J Biol Rhythms.* 2014;29(2):131–143.

58. Burke TM, Markwald RR, McHill AW, Chinoy ED, Snider JA, Bessman SC, et al. Effects of caffeine on the human circadian clock in vivo and in vitro. *Science Translatl Med.* 2015;7(305):305ra146.

59. Strogatz SH, Kronauer RE, Czeisler CA. Circadian pacemaker interferes with sleep onset at specific times each day: Role in insomnia. *Am J Physiol.* 1987;253(1 Pt 2):R172–178.

60. Flynn-Evans EE, Shekleton JA, Miller B, Epstein LJ, Kirsch D, Brogna LA, et al. Circadian phase and phase angle disorders in primary insomnia. *Sleep.* 2017;40(12).

61. Mohawk JA, Green CB, Takahashi JS. Central and peripheral circadian clocks in mammals. *Annu Rev Neurosci.* 2012;35:445–462.

62. McHill AW, Hull JT, McMullan CJ, Klerman EB. Chronic insufficient sleep has a limited impact on circadian rhythmicity of subjective hunger and awakening fasted metabolic hormones. *Front Endocrinol (Lausanne).* 2018;9:319.

63. Morris CJ, Yang JN, Garcia JI, Myers S, Bozzi I, Wang W, et al. Endogenous circadian system and circadian misalignment impact glucose tolerance via separate mechanisms in humans. *Proc Natl Acad Sci USA.* 2015;112(17):E2225–2234.

64. Centofanti S, Banks S, Colella A, Dingle C, Devine L, Galindo H, et al. Coping with shift work-related circadian disruption: A mixed-methods case study on napping and caffeine use in Australian nurses and midwives. *Chronobiol Int.* 2018;35(6):853–864.

65. Wittmann M, Dinich J, Merrow M, Roenneberg T. Social jetlag: Misalignment of biological and social time. *Chronobiol Int.* 2006;23(1–2):497–509.

66. Borbély AA. A two process model of sleep regulation. *Hum Neurobiol.* 1982;1:195–204.

67. Rajaratnam SM, Arendt J. Health in a 24-h society. *Lancet.* 2001;358(9286):999–1005.

68. McHill AW, Melanson EL, Higgins J, Connick E, Moehlman TM, Stothard ER, et al. Impact of circadian misalignment on energy metabolism during simulated nightshift work. *Proc Natl Acad Sci USA.* 2014;111(48):17302–17307.

69. Ftouni S, Sletten TL, Nicholas CL, Kennaway DJ, Lockley SW, Rajaratnam SM. Ocular measures of sleepiness are increased in night shift workers undergoing a simulated night shift near the peak time of the 6-sulfatoxymelatonin rhythm. *J Clin Sleep Med.* 2015;11(10):1131–1141.

70. Bjorvatn B, Kecklund G, Åkerstedt T. Rapid adaptation to night work at an oil platform, but slow readaptation after returning home. *JOEM.* 1998;40(7):601–608.

71. Van Dongen HP, Belenky G, Vila BJ. The efficacy of a restart break for recycling with optimal performance depends critically on circadian timing. *Sleep.* 2011;34(7):917–929.

72. Leproult R, Holmback U, Van Cauter E. Circadian misalignment augments markers of insulin resistance and inflammation, independently of sleep loss. *Diabetes.* 2014;63(6):1860–9.

73. Morris CJ, Yang JN, Garcia JI, Myers S, Bozzi I, Wang W, et al. Endogenous circadian system and circadian misalignment impact glucose tolerance via separate mechanisms in humans. *Proc Natl Acad Sci USA.* 2015;112(17):E2225–34.

74. Biggi N, Consonni D, Galluzzo V, Sogliani M, Costa G. Metabolic syndrome in permanent night workers. *Chronobiol Int.* 2008;25(2):443–454.

75. Chen JD, Lin YC, Hsiao ST. Obesity and high blood pressure of 12-hour night shift female clean-room workers. *Chronobiol Int.* 2010;27(2):334–344.

76. Li Y, Sato Y, Yamaguchi N. Shift work and the risk of metabolic syndrome: A nested case-control study. *Int J Occup Environ Health.* 2011;17(2):154–160.

77. Atkinson G, Fullick S, Grindey C, Maclaren D. Exercise, energy balance and the shift worker. *Sports Med.* 2008;38(8):671–685.

78. Bonham MP, Bonnell EK, Huggins CE. Energy intake of shift workers compared to fixed day workers: A systematic review and meta-analysis. *Chronobiol Int.* 2016;33(8):1086–1100.

79. Grant CL, Dorrian J, Coates AM, Pajcin M, Kennaway DJ, Wittert GA, et al. The impact of meal timing on performance, sleepiness, gastric upset, and hunger during simulated night shift. *Industrial Health.* 2017;55(5):423–436.

80. Centofanti SA, Dorrian J, Hilditch C, Grant CL, Coates AM, Banks S. Eating on nightshift: A big vs small snack impairs glucose response to breakfast. *Neurobiol Sleep Circadian Rhythms.* 2017;4(January 2018):44–48.

81. McHill AW, Phillips AJ, Czeisler CA, Keating L, Yee K, Barger LK, et al. Later circadian timing of food intake is associated with increased body fat. *Am J Clin Nutrition.* 2017;106(5):1213–1219. doi: 10.3945/ajcn.117.161588. Epub 2017 Sep 6. PMID: 28877894; PMCID: PMC5657289

82. Schernhammer ES, Laden F, Speizer FE, Willett WC, Hunter DJ, Kawachi I, et al. Night-shift work and risk of colorectal cancer in the nurses' health study. *J Natl Cancer Inst.* 2003;95(11):825–828.

83. Flynn-Evans EE, Mucci L, Stevens RG, Lockley SW. Shiftwork and prostate-specific antigen in the National Health and Nutrition Examination Survey. *J Natl Cancer Inst.* 2013;105(17):1292–1297.

84. Travis RC, Balkwill A, Fensom GK, Appleby PN, Reeves GK, Wang XS, et al. Night shift work and breast cancer incidence: Three prospective studies and meta-analysis of published studies. *J Natl Cancer Inst.* 2016;108(12).

85. Wang F, Yeung KL, Chan WC, Kwok CC, Leung SL, Wu C, et al. A meta-analysis on dose-response relationship between night shift work and the risk of breast cancer. *Ann Oncol.* 2013;24(11):2724–2732.

86. Straif K, Baan R, Grosse Y, Secretan B, El Ghissassi F, Bouvard V, et al. Carcinogenicity of shift-work, painting, and fire-fighting. *Lancet Oncol.* 2007;8(12):1065–1066.

87. Yang WS, Deng Q, Fan WY, Wang WY, Wang X. Light exposure at night, sleep duration, melatonin, and breast cancer: A dose-response analysis of observational studies. *Eur J Cancer Prev.* 2014;23(4):269–276.

88. Viswanathan AN, Schernhammer ES. Circulating melatonin and the risk of breast and endometrial cancer in women. *Cancer Lett.* 2009;281(1):1–7.

89. Dauchy RT, Xiang S, Mao L, Brimer S, Wren MA, Yuan L, et al. Circadian and melatonin disruption by exposure to light at night drives intrinsic resistance to tamoxifen therapy in breast cancer. *Cancer Res.* 2014;74(15):4099–4110.

90. Xiang S, Dauchy RT, Hauch A, Mao L, Yuan L, Wren MA, et al. Doxorubicin resistance in breast cancer is driven by light at night-induced disruption of the circadian melatonin signal. *J Pineal Res.* 2015;59(1):60–69.

91. Johns LE, Jones ME, Schoemaker MJ, McFadden E, Ashworth A, Swerdlow AJ. Domestic light at night and breast cancer risk: A prospective analysis of 105 000 UK women in the Generations Study. *Br J Cancer.* 2018;118(4):600–606.

92. Liu R, Jacobs DI, Hansen J, Fu A, Stevens RG, Zhu Y. Aberrant methylation of miR-34b is associated with long-term shiftwork: A potential mechanism for increased breast cancer susceptibility. *Cancer Causes Control.* 2015;26(2):171–178.

93. Samulin Erdem J, Noto HO, Skare O, Lie JS, Petersen-Overleir M, Reszka E, et al. Mechanisms of breast cancer risk in shift workers: Association of telomere shortening with the duration and intensity of night work. *Cancer Med.* 2017;6(8):1988–1997.

94. Rabstein S, Harth V, Justenhoven C, Pesch B, Plottner S, Heinze E, et al. Polymorphisms in circadian genes, night work and breast cancer: Results from the GENICA study. *Chronobiol Int.* 2014;31(10):1115–1122.

95. Dorrian J, Tolley C, Lamond N, van den HC, Pincombe J, rogers AE, et al. Sleep and errors in a group of Australian hospital nurses at work and during the commute. *Appl Ergon.* 2008;39(5):605–613.

96. Parent-Thirion A, Vermeylen G, Van Houten G, Biletta I, Cabrita J. *Eurofound* (2012), *Fifth European Working Conditions Survey*. Luxemborg: Publications Office of the European Union, Luxembourg; 2012.

97. Thun E, Bjorvatn B, Torsheim T, Moen BE, Mageroy N, Pallesen S. Night work and symptoms of anxiety and depression among nurses: A longitudinal study. *Work Stress.* 2014;28(4):376–386.

98. Smith-Coggins R, Rosekind MR, Hurd S, Buccino KR. Relationship of day versus night sleep to physician performance and mood. *Ann Emerg Med.* 1994;24(5):928–934.

99. Grosswald B. The effects of shift work on family satisfaction. *Families in Society: J Contemp Soc Serv.* 2004;85(3):413–423.

100. Ben-Hamo M, Larson TA, Duge LS, Sikkema C, Wilkinson CW, de la Iglesia HO, et al. Circadian forced desynchrony of the master clock leads to phenotypic manifestation of depression in rats. *eNeuro.* 2016;3(6):ENEURO.0237-16.2016. doi: 10.1523/ENEURO.0237-16.2016. PMID: 28090585; PMCID: PMC5216685.

6

Sleep Duration, Timing, and Napping as Components of Healthy Sleep

NATALIE D. DAUTOVICH, JANNA L. IMEL, AND JOSEPH M. DZIERZEWSKI

Introduction

Sleep is recognized as an important determinant of overall health, just as important to our health as good diet and adequate physical activity.[1] Unfortunately, an estimated 50–70 million Americans experience chronic sleep and wakefulness disorders.[2] Beyond addressing sleep disorders, however, there is a need to quantify and optimize healthy sleep.[3] Accordingly, in the spirit of defining healthy sleep, in this chapter we provide an overview of optimum sleep duration, optimum sleep timing, and optimum napping behaviors. Napping fits nicely into the larger conversation about sleep duration and timing because daytime naps can influence both nighttime sleep duration and timing. Each of these sleep characteristics has implications for sleep health and, consequently, overall health and well-being. Throughout this review, it is our hope that the information provided will help individuals to more effectively plan for optimal sleep health.

Optimum Sleep Duration

Obtaining a sufficient amount of sleep each night is important for overall health and well-being. Inadequate sleep duration is associated with a number of adverse health outcomes including an increased risk of cardiovascular disease,[4] obesity,[5] diabetes,[6] cancer,[7] and liver disease.[8] In addition, chronic levels of inadequate sleep are associated with significantly higher mortality risks.[9] Inadequate sleep duration is also closely associated with adverse mental health outcomes. For example, short sleep duration is associated with a significantly greater risk of depression[10] and suicidal ideation.[11] Moreover, inadequate sleep duration is linked with impaired emotion regulation, diminished emotional expressivity, and decreased emotion recognition.[12] Relatedly, inadequate sleep duration is also predictive of poorer levels of social functioning.[13]

Despite overwhelming evidence for the importance of obtaining sufficient sleep there has been a lack of consensus as to what qualifies as "sufficient." To answer this question, the National Sleep Foundation convened an expert panel in 2015 to review the state of the science regarding sleep duration and to make sleep duration recommendations.[14] This expert panel put forth recommendations for sleep duration grouped by chronological age, with babies and young children needing more sleep than adults, who need more sleep than older adults (see Figure 6.1). In addition to the recommended sleep durations, the National Sleep Foundation also presented duration recommendations that may be appropriate for a small number of individuals who have an unusually small or large sleep need (data available in referenced publication). At the same time, the American Academy of Sleep Medicine and Sleep Research Society also convened an expert panel to generate a consensus statement regarding recommended sleep durations necessary for optimal health across numerous health conditions.[15] Generally speaking, this expert panel recommended approximately 7–9 hours of sleep per night to promote optimal health across numerous health disorders (e.g., cardiovascular

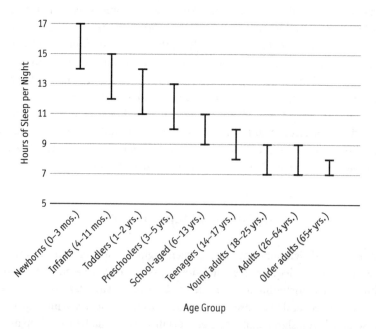

FIGURE 6.1 Sleep duration recommendations by age group.

health, metabolic health, mental health, immune health, and pain). Obtaining less than 7 hours of sleep per night was viewed as potentially detrimental to optimal health, while no consensus was reached regarding the effects of obtaining more than 9 hours of sleep per night (except in the case of mortality, where more than 9 hours of sleep per night was viewed negatively).[15]

Despite the importance of sufficient sleep for our health and well-being, inadequate sleep duration appears to be quite common. Short sleep duration is typical of the general population, with 28.3% of adults sleeping 6 hours or fewer.[16] When compared to other health conditions, poor sleep is among the most prevalent health issues in the United States, impacting individuals from every socioeconomic strata, race/ethnicity, age group, and sexual orientation. Furthermore, racial and ethnic minority populations may have disproportionally higher rates of inadequate sleep duration.[16] For example, blacks are significantly more likely to report very short (<5 hours) and short (5–6 hours) sleep durations compared to white individuals.[17] There also appear to be geographic variations in typical sleep experience, with the Southeastern region of United States being associated with disproportionately higher amounts of insufficient sleep duration compared to other parts of the country.[18] Optimistically, recent reports have questioned whether sleep duration is continuing to decline within the United States or whether the historical decline has plateaued or even reversed.[19,20] Future longitudinal investigations employing well-validated measures of sleep duration are needed to better address this question. Given the established relationships among sleep duration and numerous health outcomes, routine achievement of 7–9 hours of sleep per night is recommended for healthy adults.

Optimum Timing of Sleep

In addition to obtaining sleep that is of sufficient duration, the timing of the sleep period in the 24-hour day has important implications for health and well-being. The timing of the sleep cycle is governed by circadian rhythms, one of two processes governing the sleep–wake cycle. According to the two-process model of sleep regulation,[21] the circadian process (process C) interacts continuously with the sleep-homeostasis process (process S) to help regulate when we sleep and when we wake. The circadian process functions on a roughly 24-hour rhythm that is synced to the natural light–dark cycle governed by the Earth's daily rotation. This synchronization with the environment is referred to as *entrainment* and is driven by cues known as *zeitgebers* that signal our biological clocks.[22] Light is the most dominant zeitgeber driving the circadian process.[22] With the dawn of a new day, the circadian alerting process begins. With the ending of daylight, the alerting process recedes. Synchronization to the light–dark environment allows us to anticipate and prepare for sleep and wake. Light enters the retina and is conveyed to the brain through specialized retinal ganglion cells known as *intrinsically photo-sensitive retinal ganglion cells* (ipRGCs).[22] These ipRGCs project to the suprachiasmatic nucleus, the circadian pacemaker that governs the body's internal clock. The suprachiasmatic nucleus, in turn, projects to several brain regions implicated in sleep regulation, such as the lateral hypothalamus and the ventrolateral preoptic nucleus[23,24] and cues the release and suppression of melatonin in response to light input.[25]

As a result of the circadian process, the optimum timing of the sleep period is during natural darkness. In fact, engaging in sleep during the period from 2–4 AM has been identified as an indicator of sleep health.[3] Of course, the optimum timing of sleep during the nocturnal period depends on a number of different factors including age, sleep duration needs, and chronotype. With aging, the timing of the sleep–wake period advances such that, as individuals age they become sleepier earlier in the evening and wake earlier in the morning.[26] This phase advance is the opposite of what is seen in young adulthood, with a delay in the sleep period occurring across late adolescence until the peak delay is reached around age 20.[27] In addition to changes in sleep timing due to age, sleep duration needs will affect the timing of the sleep period (e.g., waking earlier due to a shorter sleep need; see discussion in section on "Optimum Sleep Duration"). Last, differences in sleep timing emerge based on an individual's chronotype, with "lark" or morning types preferring an earlier bedtime and wake time and "owls" or evening types preferring a later bedtime and wake time.[28] Regardless of individual differences in the precise timing of the sleep–wake cycle, for the majority of individuals, sleep is designed to occur during natural darkness.

When a sleep cycle is misaligned with the natural light–dark cycle, the consequences are many. Whether due to shift work obligations, individual preferences (e.g., chronotype), or a sleep disorder (e.g., delayed sleep phase disorder), individuals who sleep during the solar day are at higher risk for health conditions such as metabolic syndrome,[29] coronary heart disease,[30] diabetes,[31] and even mortality.[32] Furthermore, sleep obtained during the light part of the day is not as healthy as sleep occurring during darkness and increases the risk of accidents.[33]

If sufficient sleep cannot be obtained during a typical night, individuals may engage in compensatory sleep behaviors such as napping (discussed later) or sleeping longer on "free days" (e.g., sleeping longer on weekends vs. weekdays). As a result of these compensatory behaviors, sleep may become biphasic or polyphasic, with multiple sleep periods occurring during a 24-hour period as opposed to a single monophasic sleep period at night. A small body of research has evaluated "catching up on sleep" by sleeping longer during free days. The number of studies examining this approach are limited as sleep is typically averaged across weekdays and weekends or participants respond to single-item questions asking about their typical sleep by referencing their weekday sleep rather than their weekend sleep.[34] Regardless, the effects of sleeping longer on free days to compensate for insufficient sleep are mixed. Insufficient sleep, even for short periods of time, can have lasting negative neurobehavioral effects that are not reversed by recovery sleep.[1] Conversely, weekend compensatory sleep has shown potential to counter the effects of insufficient weekday sleep on hypertension levels[35] and cardiometabolic risk.[36] The architecture of compensatory sleep may not exactly match the architecture of an optimum night's sleep for an individual, which could explain some of the negative effects of relying on compensatory sleep (e.g., less time spent in restorative sleep[37]). Engaging in compensatory sleep on free days contradicts common sleep hygiene recommendations to maintain a regular sleep schedule (even on weekends[38]) and is associated with social jet lag (e.g., a discrepancy between work and free day sleep that has negative mental and physical health consequences).[39] However, if sufficient sleep cannot be regularly obtained during workdays, compensatory sleep strategies may alleviate some associated consequences.

Napping

Napping is a unique sleep behavior that does not fit the recommendations for optimum duration and timing of nocturnal sleep. However, napping remains a common practice throughout the United States and abroad, and, consequently, there is a need to identify the characteristics of healthy nap behaviors. A 2013 National Sleep Foundation poll found that 51% of Americans take at least one nap within a 2-week period, with the majority napping three to four times during this timeframe.[40] The amount of Americans engaging in daytime napping is parallel to reported napping in Japan at just over half of respondents.[40] The prevalence of napping in the United States is higher compared to Canada, Mexico, the United Kingdom, and Germany.[40] Napping in the United States is not limited to weekdays as recent data show that 44% of adults report weekend napping, with Baby Boomers and members of Generation Y reporting the highest amount of weekend napping.[41] In recent decades, "power naps"—naps of less than 20 minutes—have become increasingly prevalent to fight drowsiness at work and in daily life.[42] Fighting fatigue through napping may happen more among younger adults. A 2011 National Sleep Foundation poll found that younger adults in Generation Z (i.e., "Millennials") nap more during the week versus the weekend, likely to make up for sleep debt incurred on weekdays.[41] However, it is important to note that naps are not limited to individuals with drowsiness. Even adults without sleep debt endorse napping during the daytime.[42] Overall, napping is a common behavior that is associated with both benefits and costs.[43]

Daytime napping during both weekdays and weekends has been linked to many positive outcomes including enhanced performance, better emotional states, a decrease in sleepiness, and an ability to sustain arousal levels throughout the day.[43–45] Napping not only helps in the short term, but napping also has long-term implications including decreased mortality risk depending on time spent napping and frequency of napping. Specifically, individuals who nap multiple times a week for less than 30 minutes in duration show the most favorable health outcomes, including lower risk for myocardial infarction, cardiovascular disease, and Alzheimer's disease.[46,47] Conversely, individuals engaging in frequent, but longer naps (i.e., 45 minutes or greater) appear to be at a higher risk for adverse health outcomes.[43]

Napping is also beneficial to shift workers, who frequently use napping as a coping behavior to address regular sleep debt, sleep restriction, and circadian misalignment.[48] Shift workers often sleep at a time when their circadian rhythm is peaking in wakefulness (e.g., early and late morning). Sleeping in the early to late morning is associated with insufficient and poorer sleep as well as increased sleepiness, fatigue, and deficits in performance.[48,49] To make up for deficient sleep, workers often compensate by napping both at home and on the job.[50] To decrease fatigue, some shift workers engage in planned naps at work or naps before driving home. Such scheduled napping is associated with an increase in performance at work as well as lower levels of fatigue.[50] Some workplaces have even recommended that their workers engage in scheduled napping to decrease sleepiness (e.g., health-care workers and flight crews).[51,52] Overall, napping has the potential benefits of supplementing sleep, increasing performance, reducing fatigue, increasing safety at the workplace, and buffering the adverse health effects (e.g., cardiovascular disease) associated with sleep deprivation among shift workers.[53–55]

Although daytime napping has been connected to multiple benefits, drawbacks to napping also exist. Other than the apparent loss of productivity while napping, other downsides to daytime napping include sleep inertia and a potential negative impact on sleep at night. *Sleep inertia* is defined by feeling "groggy" and having impaired alertness immediately following a nap, which can last for up to 30 minutes after awakening.[56] Sleep inertia is linked to a temporary dip in mood, impaired performance, and slower cognitive speed.[43] Sleep inertia is most likely to occur following longer versus shorter naps, as discussed in more detail later.[43]

Napping during the day is also frequently attributed to poorer sleep at night by disrupting the body's homeostatic sleep drive. The homeostatic sleep drive is process S of the two-process model of sleep regulation.[21] This process refers to an accumulated drive to sleep the longer one is awake.[21] Once an individual sleeps, the drive to sleep is relieved until they are awake long enough for the pressure to sleep to build again.[21] This process is cyclic because the drive to sleep increases during wakefulness and declines while the individual is asleep.[21] Napping has the potential to disrupt this cycle, as taking a nap during the day would reduce an individual's drive to sleep, potentially upsetting their nighttime sleeping pattern. Accordingly, daytime napping has been linked to increased sleep onset latency and decreased depth of nighttime sleep in normal conditions.[57,58]

Despite the theoretical support for daytime napping disrupting nocturnal sleep, the empirical support for the association between daytime napping and nighttime sleep is mixed. Specifically, younger adults napping later in the day report worse subjective ratings of sleep, including an increased number of nighttime awakenings.[59] Contrastingly, older adults (age 65 and older) report fewer awakenings at nighttime and higher subjective sleep ratings after having engaged in napping later in the day.[59,60] It is plausible that late-day napping may be an extension of sleep cycles in older individuals given that older individuals tend to sleep 1 hour less each night when compared to younger adults, and the wake and bedtimes of older individuals shift forward with age.[59,61] In one study examining the effects of daytime napping on nightly sleep in older individuals via polysomnography, daytime nappers slept an average of 7.4 hours throughout a 24-hour period, compared to non-nappers who slept only 6.2 hours.[62] The older adults gained the extra hour via napping. Although daytime napping was associated with increased sleep onset latency for the older adults, the study found no differences in sleep efficiency or time spent in each sleep stage.[62]

Overall, daytime napping appears to be less disruptive for the sleep of older individuals given the changes seen with sleep as age increases. The association between daytime napping and nighttime sleep for younger and middle-aged adults is less clear. However, it should be noted that with short daytime naps (i.e., <20 minutes), subjective reports of nocturnal sleep quantity and sleep quality did not differ in daytime nappers versus non-nappers across the life span.[42] More research is needed to fully understand the relationship between napping and nighttime sleep in younger populations.

In addition to the body's homeostatic sleep drive, the circadian process (described in the section "Optimal Sleep Timing") affects the timing of sleep during the day and night. Unsurprisingly, many factors can affect the timing of one's circadian rhythm, including light and temperature.[21,63] As such, it is essential to consider the timing of the body's internal clock as well as the environment when choosing the most optimal time to nap. Overall, the ideal time to take a daytime nap is in the mid-afternoon. During this time individuals experience "post-lunch sleepiness," a drop in alertness that occurs even without the consumption of lunch.[64] Given decreasing daytime arousal levels by mid-afternoon, napping at this time is also most beneficial for increasing alertness.[65] Napping during the mid-afternoon is linked to improved cognitive performance and restored energy.[66,67] As daytime napping may meet sleep needs, reduce the drive to sleep, and make it more difficult to fall and stay asleep at night, napping should not occur in the late afternoon or evening.[59] In fact, subjective sleep reports indicate that later napping is predictive of poorer subjectively rated sleep quality, although these associations may be dependent on age.[68]

Regarding duration of napping, individuals should either nap for less than 20 minutes or more than 90 minutes to avoid the highest risk of sleep inertia.[43] The shorter nap enables the individual to awaken before entering deep non–rapid eye movement (NREM) sleep, while the longer nap allows enough time to complete one sleep cycle before awakening.[43] However, prior night sleep losses in the form of staying awake for extended periods of time can affect the likelihood of experiencing sleep inertia.[45] For example, individuals who were kept awake for 20 continuous hours, 64 continuous hours, or 64 hours with 20-minute naps every 6 hours, were shown to experience significant sleep inertia despite taking a nap shorter than 30 minutes following the sleep loss.[69,70] As such, the more sleep loss an individual has accumulated before the nap, the higher the risk of sleep inertia.[45] Given the potential impact of prior sleep loss, sleep–wake history must be taken into consideration when estimating the likelihood of sleep inertia. Overall, the recommended duration of napping to avoid the greatest chance of sleep inertia is 10–20 minutes in individuals who are well rested and have not had sleep restrictions in previous nights.[45]

Given the benefits associated with napping and the parameters surrounding what constitutes a "beneficial nap," we have summarized the following tips to help individuals nap better and experience the full effects of napping (also see Table 6.1). Daytime napping should occur no later than 4:00 PM to prevent the possibility of the nap interrupting nightly sleep.[59,68] Napping during the mid-afternoon is ideal as this is the natural time the body's alertness begins to dip. The nap should be no more than 20 minutes in length to help avoid sleep inertia. If a nap longer than 20 minutes is needed, the nap should last 90 minutes to complete a full sleep cycle and decrease the chances of sleep inertia upon awakening. As with sleep, brief napping can be improved if napping is undertaken at a regular time each day.

Table 6.1 Tips for better napping

Timing and duration	• Nap during the mid-afternoon
	• Avoid late-afternoon/evening naps
	• Nap less than 20 minutes *or* nap for a full 90 minutes
	• Set a scheduled nap time
	• Create a napping routine (e.g., engage in relaxing activities prior to napping)
Environment	• Remove entertainment
	• Reduce bright light
	• Consider a white-noise machine or fan to block noise
	• Set the thermostat between 60°F and 67°F
	• Create a comfortable place to sleep (i.e., comfortable sheets, blankets, and pillows)

Tips referenced from National Sleep Foundation's website page "Healthy Sleep Tips." https://www.thensf.org/sleep-tips/

Creating a napping routine will help the body have time to unwind before the nap. For example, individuals may engage in deep breathing, progressive muscle relaxation, or other relaxing activities before beginning a daytime nap.

Effective napping is also dependent on a good sleeping environment. According to the National Sleep Foundation, the sleeping environment should be cool, comfortable, and free of distractions.[71] To create this space, individuals should remove entertainment (e.g., light and sound from computers, televisions, and cell phones) and other distractions (e.g., loud noises and bright light). A white noise machine or fan creates a consistent background noise throughout the nap, which can be soothing and block other noise. Individuals tend to sleep best when the thermostat is set between 60°F and 67°F as the air temperature helps to cool the body and prepare the individual for sleep. Finally, a comfortable place to sleep is important for both napping and sleep. As such, an individual should invest in sheets, pillows, and a mattress that fit their needs. If napping in the workplace, making the sleep surface as comfortable as possible by adding a blanket and pillow.

Last, to further enhance a daytime nap, consider consuming caffeine before the nap. Drinking a cup of coffee immediately before a 20-minute nap has been shown to increase alertness following a nap, as the caffeine begins to take its effect on awakening.[72] In fact, the combination of a nap and caffeine is superior to a nap or caffeine alone, as the nap and caffeine combination further enhances the alleviation of sleepiness and increases performance.[72] However, it is worth noting that caffeine consumption, even in the afternoon, can be disruptive for sleep at night for some individuals and should be avoided.[73]

Conclusion

Although optimal sleep is essential for overall health and well-being, questions often abound regarding the sufficient duration of sleep, appropriate timing of sleep, and whether or not naps are helpful or harmful. This chapter reviewed information pertaining to optimal sleep duration, optimal sleep timing, and napping. Generally speaking, for optimal sleep health, adults should aim for obtaining between 7 and 9 hours of sleep per day. The optimal timing of this daily sleep is during the nocturnal hours. In regards to napping, evidence is mixed regarding whether napping represents a detriment to optimal sleep behavior. For those who engage in napping, the duration, timing, regularity, and environment of napping are important factors to consider. In sum, there are many ways we can optimize our sleep behaviors to promote better sleep health. By prioritizing our sleep health, hopefully we, too, can end the day like the English poet Thomas Hood and exclaim, "Oh bed! oh bed! delicious bed."

REFERENCES

1. Luyster FS, Strollo PJ, Zee PC, Walsh JK. Sleep: A health imperative. *Sleep.* 2012;35(6):727–734. doi:10.5665/sleep.1846

2. Institute of Medicine. *Sleep disorders and sleep deprivation: An unmet public health problem.* Washington, DC: Institute of Medicine; 2006.

3. Buysse DJ. Sleep health: Can we define it? Does it matter? *Sleep.* 2014;37(1):9–17. doi:10.5665/sleep.3298

4. Meisinger C, Heier M, Löwel H, Schneider A, Döring A. Sleep duration and sleep complaints and risk of myocardial infarction in middle-aged men and women from the general population: The MONICA/KORA Augsburg Cohort study. *Sleep.* 2007;30(9):1121–1127.

5. Cappuccio FP, Taggart FM, Kandala N-B, et al. Meta-analysis of short sleep duration and obesity in children and adults. *Sleep.* 2008;31(5):619–626.

6. Gangwisch JE, Heymsfield SB, Boden-Albala B, et al. Sleep duration as a risk factor for diabetes incidence in a large US sample. *Sleep.* 2007;30(12):1667–1673.

7. Sigurdardottir LG, Valdimarsdottir UA, Fall K, et al. Circadian disruption, sleep loss, and prostate cancer risk: A systematic review of epidemiologic studies. *Cancer Epidemiol Prev Biomark.* May 2012. doi:10.1158/1055-9965.EPI-12-0116

8. Kim C-W, Yun KE, Jung H-S, et al. Sleep duration and quality in relation to non-alcoholic fatty liver disease in middle-aged workers and their spouses. *J Hepatol.* 2013;59(2):351–357. doi:10.1016/j.jhep.2013.03.035

9. Grandner MA, Hale L, Moore M, Patel NP. Mortality associated with short sleep duration: The evidence, the possible mechanisms, and the future. *Sleep Med Rev.* 2010;14(3):191–203. doi:10.1016/j.smrv.2009.07.006

10. Zhai L, Zhang H, Zhang D. Sleep duration and depression among adults: A meta-analysis of prospective studies. *Depress Anxiety.* 2015;32(9):664–670. doi:10.1002/da.22386

11. Pigeon WR, Pinquart M, Conner K. Meta-analysis of sleep disturbance and suicidal thoughts and behaviors. *J Clin Psychiatry.* 2012 Sep;73(9):e1160–e1167. doi:10.4088/JCP.11r07586. PMID: 23059158.

12. Gruber R, Cassoff J. The interplay between sleep and emotion regulation: Conceptual framework empirical evidence and future directions. *Curr Psychiatry Rep.* 2014;16(11):500. doi:10.1007/s11920-014-0500-x

13. Beattie L, Kyle SD, Espie CA, Biello SM. Social interactions, emotion and sleep: A systematic review and research agenda. *Sleep Med Rev.* 2015;24:83–100. doi:10.1016/j.smrv.2014.12.005

14. Hirshkowitz M, Whiton K, Albert SM, et al. National Sleep Foundation's sleep time duration recommendations: Methodology and results summary. *Sleep Health.* 2015;1(1):40–43. doi:10.1016/j.sleh.2014.12.010

15. Consensus Conference Panel, Watson NF, Badr MS, et al. Joint consensus statement of the American Academy of Sleep Medicine and Sleep Research Society on the recommended amount of sleep for a healthy adult: Methodology and discussion. *J Clin Sleep Med.* 2015;11(8):931–952. doi:10.5664/jcsm.4950

16. Krueger PM, Friedman EM. Sleep duration in the United States: A cross-sectional population-based study. *Am J Epidemiol.* 2009;169(9):1052–1063. doi:10.1093/aje/kwp023

17. Whinnery J, Jackson N, Rattanaumpawan P, Grandner MA. Short and long sleep duration associated with race/ethnicity, sociodemographics, and socioeconomic position. *Sleep.* 2014;37(3):601–611. doi:10.5665/sleep.3508

18. Grandner MA, Smith TE, Jackson N, Jackson T, Burgard S, Branas C. Geographic distribution of insufficient sleep across the United States: A county-level hotspot analysis. *Sleep Health J Natl Sleep Found.* 2015;1(3):158–165.

19. Basner M, Dinges DF. Sleep Duration in the United States 2003–2016: First signs of success in the fight against sleep deficiency? *Sleep.* January 2018. doi:10.1093/sleep/zsy012

20. Ogilvie RP, Patel SR. Changing national trends in sleep duration: Did we make America sleep again? *Sleep.* 2018;41(4). doi:10.1093/sleep/zsy055

21. Borbély AA, Daan S, Wirz-Justice A, Deboer T. The two-process model of sleep regulation: A reappraisal. *J Sleep Res.* 2016;25(2):131–143. doi:10.1111/jsr.12371

22. LeGates TA, Fernandez DC, Hattar S. Light as a central modulator of circadian rhythms, sleep and affect. *Nat Rev Neurosci.* 2014;15(7):443–454. doi:10.1038/nrn3743

23. Saper CB, Chou TC, Scammell TE. The sleep switch: Hypothalamic control of sleep and wakefulness. *Trends Neurosci.* 2001;24(12):726–731.

24. Gaus SE, Strecker RE, Tate BA, Parker RA, Saper CB. Ventrolateral preoptic nucleus contains sleep-active, galaninergic neurons in multiple mammalian species. *Neuroscience.* 2002;115(1):285–294.

25. Kalsbeek A, Cutrera RA, Van Heerikhuize JJ, Van Der Vliet J, Buijs RM. GABA release from suprachiasmatic nucleus terminals is necessary for the light-induced inhibition of nocturnal melatonin release in the rat. *Neuroscience.* 1999;91(2):453–461.

26. Duffy JF, Zitting K-M, Chinoy ED. Aging and circadian rhythms. *Sleep Med Clin.* 2015;10(4):423–434. doi:10.1016/j.jsmc.2015.08.002

27. Roenneberg T, Kuehnle T, Pramstaller PP, et al. A marker for the end of adolescence. *Curr Biol.* 2004;14(24):R1038–R1039. doi:10.1016/j.cub.2004.11.039

28. Roenneberg T, Kuehnle T, Juda M, et al. Epidemiology of the human circadian clock. *Sleep Med Rev.* 2007;11(6):429–438. doi:10.1016/j.smrv.2007.07.005

29. Karlsson B, Knutsson A, Lindahl B. Is there an association between shift work and having a metabolic syndrome? Results from a population based study of 27 485 people. *Occup Environ Med.* 2001;58(11):747–752. doi:10.1136/oem.58.11.747

30. Kawachi I, Colditz GA, Stampfer MJ, et al. Prospective study of shift work and risk of coronary heart disease in women. *Circulation.* 1995;92(11):3178–3182.

31. Pan A, Schernhammer ES, Sun Q, Hu FB. Rotating night shift work and risk of type 2 diabetes: Two prospective cohort studies in women. *PLoS Med.* 2011;8(12):e1001141. doi:10.1371/journal.pmed.1001141

32. Akerstedt T, Kecklund G, Johansson S-E. Shift work and mortality. *Chronobiol Int.* 2004;21(6):1055–1061.

33. Folkard S, Åkerstedt T. Trends in the risk of accidents and injuries and their implications for models of fatigue and performance. *Aviat Space Environ Med.* 2004;75(3 Suppl):A161–167.

34. Åkerstedt T, Ghilotti F, Grotta A, et al. Sleep duration and mortality: Does weekend sleep matter? *J Sleep Res.* May 2018:e12712. doi:10.1111/jsr.12712

35. Hwangbo Y, Kim W-J, Chu MK, Yun C-H, Yang KI. Association between weekend catch-up sleep duration and hypertension in Korean adults. *Sleep Med.* 2013;14(6):549–554. doi:10.1016/j.sleep.2013.02.009

36. Pizinger TM, Aggarwal B, St-Onge M-P. Sleep extension in short sleepers: An evaluation of feasibility and effectiveness for weight management and cardiometabolic disease prevention. *Front Endocrinol.* 2018;9:392. doi:10.3389/fendo.2018.00392

37. Kitamura S, Katayose Y, Nakazaki K, et al. Estimating individual optimal sleep duration and potential sleep debt. *Sci Rep.* 2016;6:35812. doi:10.1038/srep35812

38. Perlis ML, Jungquist C, Smith MT, Posner D. *Cognitive behavioral treatment of insomnia: A session-by-session guide.* 2nd ed. New York: Springer; 2008.

39. Wittmann M, Dinich J, Merrow M, Roenneberg T. Social jetlag: Misalignment of biological and social time. *Chronobiol Int.* 2006;23(1–2):497–509. doi:10.1080/07420520500545979

40. National Sleep Foundation. 2013 International Bedroom Poll first to explore sleep differences among six countries. https://sleepfoundation.org/media-center/press-release/national-sleep-foundation-2013-international-bedroom-poll

41. National Sleep Foundation. Sleep in America Poll: Communications technology in the bedroom. 2011. https://sleepfoundation.org/sites/default/files/sleepinamericapoll/SIAP_2011_Summar y_of_Findings.pdf Published 2011

42. Pilcher JJ, Michalowski KR, Carrigan RD. The prevalence of daytime napping and its relationship to nighttime sleep. *Behav Med.* 2001;27(2):71–76. doi:10.1080/08964280109595773

43. Dhand R, Sohal H. Good sleep, bad sleep! The role of daytime naps in healthy adults. *Curr Opin Pulm Med.* 2006;12(6):379. doi:10.1097/01.mcp.0000245703.92311.do

44. Luo Z, Inoué S. A short daytime nap modulates levels of emotions objectively evaluated by the emotion spectrum analysis method. *Psychiatry Clin Neurosci.* 54(2):207–212. doi:10.1046/j.1440-1819.2000.00660.x

45. Hilditch CJ, Dorrian J, Banks S. A review of short naps and sleep inertia: Do naps of 30 min or less really avoid sleep inertia and slow-wave sleep? *Sleep Med.* 2017;32:176–190. doi:10.1016/j.sleep.2016.12.016

46. Asada T, Motonaga T, Yamagata Z, Uno M, Takahashi K. Associations between retrospectively recalled napping behavior and later development of Alzheimer's disease: Association with APOE genotypes. *Sleep.* 2000;23(5):629–634.

47. Campos H, Siles X. Siesta and the risk of coronary heart disease: Results from a population-based, case-control study in Costa Rica. *Int J Epidemiol.* 2000;29(3):429–437.

48. Ruggiero JS, Redeker NS. Effects of napping on sleepiness and sleep-related performance deficits in night-shift workers: A systematic review. *Biol Res Nurs.* 2014;16(2):134–142. doi:10.1177/1099800413476571

49. Belenky G, Åkerstedt T. Occupational sleep medicine: Introduction. In Kryger MH, Roth T, Dement WC, eds. *Principles and practice of sleep medicine.* 5th ed. St. Louis, MO: Elsevier; 2011: 734–737.

50. Martin-Gill C, Barger LK, Moore CG, et al. Effects of napping during shift work on sleepiness and performance in emergency medical services personnel and similar shift workers: A systematic review and meta-analysis. *Prehosp Emerg Care.* 2018;22(sup1):47–57. doi:10.1080/10903127.2017.1376136

51. Caldwell JA, Mallis MM, Caldwell JL, Paul MA, Miller JC, Neri DF. Fatigue countermeasures in aviation. *Aviat Space Environ Med.* 2009;80(1):29–59.

52. The Joint Commission. Health care worker fatigue and patient safety. *Sentin Event Alert.* 2011;(48):1–4.

53. Drake CL, Wright KPJ. Shift work, shift work disorder, and jet lag. In Kryger MH, Roth T, Dement WC, eds. *Principles and practice of sleep medicine.* 5th ed. St. Louis, MO: Elsevier Saunders; 2011: 784–798. https://www.researchgate.net/profile/Christopher_Drake2/publication/279721280_Shift_Work_Shift-Work_Disorder_and_Jet_Lag/links/5a0dcddfaca27244d2858000/Shift-Work-Shift-Work-Disorder-and-Jet-Lag.pdf

54. Geiger-Brown J, McPhaul KM. Sleep promotion in occupational health settings. In Redeker NS, McEnany GP, eds. *Sleep disorders and sleep promotion in nursing practice.* New York: Springer; 2011: 355–369.

55. Petrie KJ, Powell D, Broadbent E. Fatigue self-management strategies and reported fatigue in international pilots. *Ergonomics.* 2004;47(5):461–468. doi:10.1080/0014013031000085653

56. Tassi P, Muzet A. Sleep inertia. *Sleep Med Rev.* 2000;4(4):341–353. doi:10.1053/smrv.2000.0098

57. Stepanski EJ, Wyatt JK. Use of sleep hygiene in the treatment of insomnia. *Sleep Med Rev.* 2003;7(3):215–225.

58. Werth E, Dijk DJ, Achermann P, Borbely AA. Dynamics of the sleep EEG after an early evening nap: Experimental data and simulations. *Am J Physiol-Regul Integr Comp Physiol.* 1996;271(3):R501–R510. doi:10.1152/ajpregu.1996.271.3.R501

59. Shoji KD, Tighe CA, Imel JL, Dautovich ND, McCrae CM. Napping in older and college-aged adults. *J Am Geriatr Soc.* 64(4):896–898. doi:10.1111/jgs.14056

60. Dautovich ND, McCrae CS, Rowe M. Subjective and objective napping and sleep in older adults: Are evening naps "bad" for nighttime sleep? *J Am Geriatr Soc.* 56(9):1681–1686. doi:10.1111/j.1532-5415.2008.01822.x

61. Foley DJ, Monjan AA, Brown SL, Simonsick EM, Wallace RB, Blazer DG. Sleep complaints among elderly persons: An epidemiologic study of three communities. *Sleep.* 1995;18(6):425–432. doi:10.1093/sleep/18.6.425

62. Campbell SS, Murphy PJ, Stauble TN. Effects of a nap on nighttime sleep and waking function in older subjects. *J Am Geriatr Soc.* 2005;53(1):48–53. doi:10.1111/j.1532-5415.2005.53009.x

63. Czeisler CA, Duffy JF, Shanahan TL, et al. Stability, precision, and near-24-hour period of the human circadian pacemaker. *Science.* 1999;284(5423):2177–2181. doi:10.1126/science.284.5423.2177

64. Stahl ML, Orr WC, Bollinger C. Postprandial sleepiness: Objective documentation via polysomnography. *Sleep*. 1983;6(1):29–35. doi:10.1093/sleep/6.1.29

65. Corskadon MA. Ontogeny of human sleepiness as measured by sleep latency. In Dinges DF, Broughton RJ, eds. *Sleep and alertness: Chrono-biological, behavioral, and medical aspects of napping*. New York: Raven Press; 1989: 53–69.

66. Tietzel AJ, Lack LC. The short-term benefits of brief and long naps following nocturnal sleep restriction. *Sleep*. 2001;24(3):293–300. doi:10.1093/sleep/24.3.293

67. Hayashi M, Watanabe M, Hori T. The effects of a 20 min nap in the mid-afternoon on mood, performance and EEG activity. *Clin Neurophysiol*. 1999;110(2):272–279. doi:10.1016/S1388-2457(98)00003-0

68. Ye L, Johnson SH, Keane K, Manasia M, Gregas M. Napping in college students and its relationship with nighttime sleep. *J Am Coll Health*. 2015;63(2):88–97. doi:10.1080/07448481.2014.983926

69. Naitoh P, Kelly T, Babkoff H. Sleep inertia: Best time not to wake up? *Chronobiol Int*. 1993;10(2):109–118. doi:10.1080/07420529309059699

70. Signal TL, Berg MJ van den, Mulrine HM, Gander PH. Duration of sleep inertia after napping during simulated night work and in extended operations. *Chronobiol Int*. 2012;29(6):769–779. doi:10.3109/07420528.2012.686547

71. National Sleep Foundation. Healthy Sleep Tips. https://sleepfoundation.org/sleep-tools-tips/healthy-sleep-tips

72. Hayashi M, Masuda A, Hori T. The alerting effects of caffeine, bright light and face washing after a short daytime nap. *Clin Neurophysiol*. 2003;114(12):2268–2278. doi:10.1016/S1388-2457(03)00255-4

73. Clark I, Landolt HP. Coffee, caffeine, and sleep: A systematic review of epidemiological studies and randomized controlled trials. *Sleep Med Rev*. 2017;31:70–78. doi:10.1016/j.smrv.2016.01.006

7

Light and Sleep

MORGAN P. REID, NATALIE D. DAUTOVICH, AND
JOSEPH M. DZIERZEWSKI

Introduction

Sleep has been consistently demonstrated as a key component of overall health,[1] and poor sleep is associated with various negative physical,[2] cognitive,[3] and mental health outcomes.[4] In a poll conducted by the National Sleep Foundation,[5] 45% of Americans reported that poor or insufficient sleep affected their daily activities at least once in the previous week. Although some individuals may experience poor sleep due to sleep disorders such as insomnia and obstructive sleep apnea, still others may be experiencing less than optimal sleep due to factors in the environment. Light plays a key role in the sleep–wake cycle,[6] and exposure to particular light sources may be preventing individuals from achieving the healthy sleep that they need. This chapter explores the biological association between light and sleep, how light may impact sleep in the home environment, and how light may be used to best optimize healthy sleep. We also explore how light has been effectively used in the treatment of sleep disorders.

Importance of Light in Regulating Sleep

In order to maintain a 24-hour sleep–wake cycle, the body relies on several *zeitgebers*, or environmental cues, to synchronize its rhythm.[7] Without these cues,

Disclosure: Dr. Dzierzewski was supported by a grant from the National Institute on Aging (K23AG049955). No other authors report commercial or financial conflicts of interest.

the sleep–wake cycle would be greater than 24 hours, leading to drifting wake and sleep times.[7] Non-entrainment of the sleep–wake cycle to the 24-hour day has also been associated with endocrine, neurobehavioral, and sleep dysfunctions.[8] Social interaction, meals, exercise, and other activities all have the ability to *entrain*, or synchronize, a circadian rhythm and are thus considered zeitgebers.[9] Light serves as one of the most dominant zeitgebers in regulating the sleep–wake cycle,[6] and exposure to light within and outside of the bedroom may influence sleep timing, quality, and other important sleep outcomes.

Underlying Biological Mechanisms

To understand the impact of light on sleep, it is first necessary to examine the biological mechanisms that enable light to affect the circadian rhythm. Light enters the retina and is absorbed by melanopsin, a photopigment that is located in specialized retinal ganglion cells called *intrinsically photosensitive retinal ganglion cells* (ipRGCs).[10] These cells are distinct from other retinal cells in that they do not play a role in forming visual images.[11] The ipGRCs project to the suprachiasmatic nucleus, a region of the hypothalamus that is positioned above the optic chiasm.[12] The suprachiasmatic nucleus then projects to several brain regions implicated in sleep regulation, including the ventrolateral preoptic nucleus and the lateral hypothalamus.[12,13] In response to the presence or absence of light, the suprachiasmatic nucleus sends cues for the release or suppression of melatonin, a hormone made by the pineal gland.[14] With increasing levels of darkness, the suprachiasmatic nucleus cues greater release of melatonin, which in turn produces less alertness.[15] This decreased alertness enables sleep onset.

Natural daylight helps to synchronize the circadian rhythm to a 24-hour period in most locations. However, advances in technology lead to greater exposure to artificial light, including lighting sources in homes and office buildings, street lamps, exterior house lighting, and light emanating from devices within the home. Increased exposure to artificial light heightens the risk of desynchronization of the circadian rhythm from the natural light–dark cycle. This desynchronization, as occurs in individuals engaged in shift work, has been associated with negative sleep and physical health outcomes. In order to understand how varying light sources may impact the sleep–wake circadian rhythm,[16–18] it is important to assess which characteristics of light directly affect the sleep–wake cycle.

Characteristics of Light

Several characteristics of light have been found to influence sleep outcomes. The rate of change of light exposure affects the strength of the light's impact as abrupt changes in light amounts have a greater impact on alertness and vigilance than more gradual changes.[19] Similarly, the impact of light can depend on the individual's prior light exposure history immediately preceding the stimulus.[19] The duration and spectrum of light also differentially impacts sleep, with light enriched in blue wavelengths having the most significant impact on sleep due to the sensitivity of both melanopsin and the ipRGCs to these shorter wavelengths.[20,21]

Perhaps the most researched characteristics of light that influence sleep are the amount and timing of light exposure. The amount of light exposure, or illuminance level, is measured in *lux units* and refers to the amount of light measured in a specific area.[22] Less than 100 lux is generally considered to be dim light. An example of dim light would be twilight, which is approximately 10 lux.[23] The living area of a home, approximately 300 lux, would be considered moderate light (approximate range: 100–1,000 lux). Bright light, such as sunlight (100,000 lux) is light that is greater than 1,000 lux.[24] In general, higher levels of light exposure throughout the day are positively associated with sleep outcomes.[25] Exposure to bright light throughout the day is associated with shorter sleep onset latency,[26] fewer overall awakenings,[27] decreased awakenings during the first third of sleep, increased awakenings during the last third of sleep,[28] and reduced motor activity during sleep.[28] However, studies also have found that bright light exposure was associated with more fragmented sleep, lower sleep efficiency,[26] and shorter sleep duration[27] in comparison with dim light. The reason for these discrepant findings is somewhat unclear; however, individual differences such as age and mood may cause light to differentially impact sleep.[24]

The timing of light exposure also seems particularly important. Timing of light exposure is linearly associated with the timing of the sleep period, such that later timing of light is associated with a later sleep midpoint.[29] Light exposure in the beginning of the night can cause a delay in the sleep period, whereas light exposure at the end of the night can cause an advance in the sleep period.[30,31]

Many studies support the idea that there is an interaction between the amount and timing of light resulting in differential impacts on sleep. Brighter morning light was associated with sleep changes indicative of an advance of the sleep period, including longer total sleep time and shorter sleep onset latency as measured by polysomnography.[32] In addition, brighter morning light exposure was associated with better self-reported sleep outcomes in comparison to dimmer morning light.[33] Brighter evening light was associated with sleep outcomes consistent with a delay of the sleep period. Individuals who were exposed to 3,800–6,000 lux emitted from light racks during the evening had longer sleep onset latency than individuals who were exposed to 300 lux emitted from a desk lamp during the evening.[34] Bright light exposure in the evening was also associated with a greater delay to stages 1 and 2 sleep and REM sleep than was evening dim light exposure.[35] Evening bright light exposure was also associated with more superficial sleep, with greater time spent in stages 1 and 2 and more frequent arousals than was dim evening light exposure.[36] Bright evening light was associated with negative subjective sleep outcomes as well, with participants exposed to bright evening light reporting longer sleep initiation and poorer sleep quality than participants exposed to moderate evening light.[37]

This research suggests that there is an interaction effect between the amount and timing of light exposure, such that bright morning light is advantageous for sleep outcomes, while bright evening light can have detrimental effects. Several individual variables may serve as confounding factors in this interaction effect, accounting for some of the mixed research in this area. In a study of older adults, bright evening light was associated with shorter sleep onset latency, contrary to the expected negative effects.[38] Age may influence the associations between amount and timing of light exposure and sleep as the older adults in this study were most likely experiencing a natural age-related phase advance of the sleep period. Mood may also impact the effects of amount and timing of light exposure. Negative associations between average lux exposure and sleep time have been found in post-menopausal[32,39] and postpartum women,[40] such that exposure to bright morning light is associated with short sleep. Those with short sleep duration were less likely to be depressed and also experienced better overall sleep.[39] Future research should continue to explore how mood impacts the association between light characteristics and sleep outcomes.

Although the majority of research on the association between light and sleep has been conducted in laboratory settings, researchers have also been interested in applying these findings to the home environment. The following section explores how light characteristics and sleep may interact within the home.

The Home Environment

As stated in the previous section, exposure to bright light in the evening is more likely to delay the sleep period than is exposure to dim light.[24] Research investigating naturalistic light sources demonstrates a similar pattern. In one experiment, participants were exposed to either room lighting (approximately 200 lux) or dim light (less than 3 lux) in the late evening, and their ability to synthesize melatonin was measured.[41] Brighter room lighting shortened melatonin duration by approximately 90 minutes compared to exposure to dim lighting. Moreover, exposure to electrical light between dusk and bedtime was associated with a 12.5% reduction of total daily melatonin levels and a 71.4% reduction of presleep melatonin levels. When participants were exposed to room lighting throughout the night, daily melatonin levels were reduced by more than 50% in most participants.[41] These results suggest that exposure to regular room lighting of moderate intensity in the evening is associated with a significant reduction of melatonin. However, advancing technology makes it likely that there are other sources of light, including televisions, cell phones, and computers, in the bedroom that could influence sleep as well.

Use of Electronics and Sleep

According to a poll conducted by the National Sleep Foundation, the majority of participants reported having an alarm clock (89%), table lamp (73%), phone or cell phone (72%), and television (71%) in their bedroom.[5] Moreover, 11% of participants reported that they leave their television on overnight, 46% reported leaving a nightlight on, and 39% reported leaving their phone/cell phone on while sleeping. Device use prior to bedtime was also common, with 47% of participants reporting that they watch television within an hour of bedtime at least a few nights a week and more than half of participants using their cell phones within an hour of bedtime. Although less common, participants also reported computer/laptop (39%) and video game (19%) use within an hour of bedtime as well.[5]

All of these devices share a common feature: a *light emitting diode* (LED) screen that emits short wavelengths of light, often called "blue light." As stated previously, the photosensitive retinal ganglion cells that project to the suprachiasmatic nucleus and regulate the sleep–wake cycle are particularly sensitive to these shorter wavelengths of light. Indeed, exposure to as little as less than 1 lux of monochromatic blue light has been found to suppress nighttime melatonin synthesis.[42] In one experiment, participants were seated in front of a 22-inch computer screen between 9 PM and 11 PM.[43] Participants were exposed to a combination of high and low light amounts as well as short and long wavelengths. Regardless of the amount of light present, exposure to shorter wavelengths of light was associated with negative sleep outcomes, including decreased sleep efficiency, shorter total sleep time, and longer wake time after falling asleep as measured by polysomnography Although shorter wavelengths of light were a strong predictor of poor sleep outcomes, the amount of light also negatively impacted sleep outcomes, as exposure to shorter wavelengths and higher amounts were both independently associated with increased time spent in the earlier stages of sleep (stages 1 and 2) and decreased time spent in slow wave sleep.[43]

These findings suggest that both room lighting and the light that emanates from electronic devices impact melatonin synthesis and other sleep processes. These factors are all within the individual's immediate environment. In addition, there are other sources of light outside the home that may have a detrimental impact on sleep. These sources will be discussed in the following section.

Environmental Light Pollution

Light pollution refers to the alteration of natural lighting levels by human-made lighting sources.[44] Approximately 80% of the world lives under a light-polluted sky. In America, approximately 99% of the population is exposed to daytime light pollution, with at least half continuing to be exposed to light pollution throughout the night.[45] Sources of this pollution may include streetlamps and exterior house lighting, as well as light emanating from advertisements, commercial properties, office buildings, and factories.[46] These light sources tend to be in constant use and overly bright. Moreover, they are often not adequately shielded, causing light to spread over an unnecessarily wide area.[46]

Due to their energy efficiency, many environmental policy groups have been advocating for the replacement of halogen and incandescent light bulbs with LED bulbs.[47] The consumer marketplace has mirrored this trend, with LED bulbs accounting for 65% of the consumer lamp market and halogen incandescent lamps accounting for only 28% of the market in 2018.[47]

The shorter wavelength emitted by LED bulbs, however, may be detrimental for sleep outcomes. The American Medical Association (AMA) reported that LED streetlights may suppress melatonin release and desynchronize the sleep–wake cycle. Although conventional streetlights may impact the regulation of melatonin as well, the impact of LED streetlights is up to five times greater than the impact of more traditional bulbs.[48] Due to these findings, the AMA declared that overexposure to light sources at night can be considered a form of environmental pollution due to its negative impact on biological processes.[48]

How to Optimize Light in the Sleeping Environment

The previous sections discussed how light in the sleeping environment, including room lighting, electronic devices, streetlights, and exterior house lighting can negatively impact sleep. However, there are several steps that individuals can take to optimize light in their sleeping environment.

To avoid the harmful effects of blue light, it is important to have warmer wavelengths of light in the bedroom.[49] In the living area and other spaces that may be used for multiple purposes, it may be helpful to purchase dimmer switches that allow the consumer to change the intensity of the light from daytime to nighttime. It is also important to evaluate sources of light from outside the bedroom and home. Unnecessary hallway lights and nightlights may be turned off, and room-darkening curtains may be purchased to block out exterior lighting.[50]

With regard to electronic usage, the National Sleep Foundation recommends setting a "digital curfew," when all family members turn off electronic devices for the night. Although it is best that this curfew is several hours before bed, even 30 minutes may provide sleep benefits. Many devices also have a "night mode" feature that softens the light emanated from the device at a certain time.[49]

Use of Light in Treatment for Sleep Disorders

Although certain intensities and timing of light exposure may have detrimental effects on the sleep–wake cycle, researchers have also used the benefits of light to create evidence-based treatments for several sleep disorders. Circadian rhythm sleep disorders occur when there is a dysfunction of the circadian pacemaker or when there is a misalignment between the circadian rhythm and the socially desired sleep–wake cycle.[51] There are several types of circadian rhythm sleep disorders, including delayed sleep phase disorder, advanced phase sleep disorder, and shift work sleep disorder.

Individuals with delayed sleep phase disorder have delayed sleep onset and wake times. They may experience academic or occupational impairment due to excessive morning sleepiness or the inability to wake up at the desired time.[52] Evidence has suggested that exposure to bright light for 2 hours in the morning can phase advance the circadian rhythm of core body temperature, thereby improving circadian rhythm synchronization.[53] In contrast, individuals with advance phase sleep disorder experience fatigue in the early evening hours and wake earlier than the desired time.[54] This disorder is most common in older adults,[55] although the exact mechanisms underlying the development of this disorder are unclear.[51] Exposure to bright light between 7:00 PM and 9:00 PM has been associated with improved sleep and daytime performance among older adults with this disorder.[56,57]

Shift work sleep disorder occurs in individuals whose work schedules are not consistent with the average sleep–wake cycle. Work schedules may also vary from week to week, causing consistent irregularities in an individual's sleep.[54] Shift work sleep disorder has been associated with excessive sleepiness and insomnia as well as numerous other physical and mental health concerns.[58] The timing of light exposure for patients with shift work sleep disorder depends on the timing of their work schedules. For those who work at night, exposure to bright light throughout the work shift successfully delayed the circadian rhythm.[59] In addition, it may be helpful for individuals working the night shift to avoid exposure to morning bright light as much as possible when commuting home in order to facilitate quicker sleep onset.[60]

Although there is evidence that light therapy has been effective in the treatment of these various sleep disorders, most studies resulted in only small to medium effect sizes.[61] Further research should be conducted that examines how to optimally apply light therapy for patients with circadian rhythm sleep disorders.

Conclusion

Light is the dominant environmental cue that enables the synchronization of the sleep–wake circadian rhythm to the 24-hour period. The amount and timing of light exposure can impact various sleep outcomes, including sleep onset latency, sleep duration, efficiency, and number of nighttime awakenings. By understanding the impact of light on sleep, we can take steps to enhance the sleeping environment by optimizing light usage and eliminating environmental light pollution. We can also harness the power of light to create empirically based treatments for various sleep disorders.

REFERENCES

1. Matricciani L, Bin YS, Lallukka T, Kronholm E, Wake M, Paquet C, et al. Rethinking the sleep-health link. *Sleep Health*, 2018;4:339–348. doi:10.1016/j.sleh.2018.05.004.
2. Grandner MA. Addressing sleep disturbances: An opportunity to prevent cardiometabolic disease? *Int Rev Psychiatry*. 2014;26:155–176. doi:10.3109/09540261.2014.911148.
3. Nebes RD, Buysse DJ, Halligan EM, Houck PR, Monk TH. Self-reported sleep quality predicts poor cognitive performance in healthy older adults. *J Gerol: Psychol Sci*. 2009;64B:180–187. doi:10.1093/geronb/gbn037.
4. Zhai L, Zhang H, Zhang D. Sleep duration and depression among adults: A meta-analysis of prospective studies. *Depress Anxiety*. 2015;32:664–670. doi:10.1002/da.22386.
5. Sleep in America Poll: Communications Technology in the Bedroom. Sleepfoundation.org. 2011. https://www.sleepfoundation.org/sites/default/files/inline-files/SIAP_2011_Summary_of_Findings.pdf
6. Mistlberger RE, Skene DJ. Nonphotic entrainment in humans? *J Biol Rhythms*. 2005;20(4):339–352. doi:10.1177/0748730405277982.
7. Baron KG, Reid KJ. Circadian misalignment and health. *Int Rev Psychiatry*. 2014;26:139–154. doi:3109/09540261.2014.911149.
8. Gronfier C, Wright KP, Kronauer RE, Czeisler CA. Entrainment of the human circadian pacemaker to longer-than-24-h days. *Proc Natl Acad Sci*. 2007;104:9081–9086. doi:10.1073/pnas.0702835104.
9. Grandin LD, Alloy LB, Abramson LY. The social zeitgeber theory, circadian rhythms, and mood disorders: Review and evaluation. *Clin Psychol Rev*. 2006;26:679–694. doi:10.1016/j.cpr.2006.07.001.
10. Provencio I, Rodriguez IR, Jiang G, Hayes WP, Moreira EF, Rollag MD. A novel human opsin in the inner retina. *J Neurosci*. 2000;20:600–605. doi:10.1523/jneurosci.20-02-00600.2000.

11. Dijk DJ, Archer SN. Light, sleep, and circadian rhythms: Together again. *PLoS Biol.* 2009;7(6). doi:10.1371/journal.pbio.1000145.

12. Gaus SE, Strecker RE, Tate BA, Parker RA, Saper CB. Ventrolateral preoptic nucleus contains sleep-active, galaninergic neurons in multiple mammalian species. *Neurosci.* 2002;115:285–294. doi:10.1016/s0306-4522(02)00308-1.

13. Saper CB, Chou TC, Scammell TE. The sleep switch: Hypothalamic control of sleep and wakefulness. *Trends Neurosci.* 2001;24:726–731. doi:10.1016/s0166-2236(00)02002-6.

14. Kalsbeek A, Cutera RA, van Heerikhuize JJ, van der Vliet J, Buijs RM. GABA release from suprachiasmatic nucleus terminals is necessary for the light-induced inhibition of nocturnal melatonin release in the rat. *Neurosci.* 1999;91:453–461. doi:10.1016/s0306-4522(98)00635-6.

15. Scheer FAJL, Czeisler CA. Melatonin, sleep, and circadian rhythms. *Sleep Med Rev.* 2005;9:5–9. doi:10.1016/j.smrv.2004.11.004.

16. Zee PC, Turek FW. Respect the clock. *Sleep Med Rev.* 2013;17:395–397. doi:10.1016/j.smrv.2013.08.001.

17. Haus EL, Smolensky MH. Shift work and cancer risk: Potential mechanistic roles of circadian disruption, light at night, and sleep deprivation. *Sleep Med Rev.* 2013;17:273–284. doi:10.1016/j.smrv.2012.08.003.

18. Irwin MR. Why sleep is important for health: A psychoneuroimmunology perspective. *Annu Rev Psychol.* 2015;66:143–172. doi:10.1146/annurev-psych-010213-115205.

19. Chang A-M, Scheer FAJL, Czeisler CA, Aeschbach D. Direct effects of light on alertness, vigilance, and the waking electroencephalogram in humans depend on prior light history. *Sleep.* 2013;36:1239–1246. doi:10.5665/sleep.2894.

20. Altimus CM, Guler AD, Villa KL, McNeill DS, LeGates TA, Hattar S. Rods-cones and melanopsin detect light and dark to modulate sleep independent of image formation. *Proc Natl Sci Acad.* 2008;105:19998–20003. doi:10.1073/pnas.0808312105.

21. Tsai JW, Hannibal J, Hagiwara G et al. Melanopsin as a sleep modulator: Circadian gating of the direct effects of light on sleep and altered sleep homeostasis in Opn4 -/- mice. *PLoS Biol.* 2009;7(6):e1000125. doi:10.1371/journal.pbio.1000125.

22. Stevens RG, Rea MS. Light in the built environment: Potential role of circadian disruption in endocrine disruption and breast cancer. *Cancer Causes Control.* 2001;12(3):279–287. doi:10.1023/A:1011237000609.

23. Druzik JR, Michalski S. Guidelines for selecting solid-state lighting for museums. Canadian Conservation Institute; 2011.

24. Dautovich ND, Schreiber DR, Imel JL, Tighe CA, Shoji KD, Cyrus J, et al. A systematic account of the amount and timing of light in association with objective and subjective sleep outcomes in community-dwelling adults. *Sleep Health.* 2019;5:31–48. doi:10.1016/j.sleh.2018.09.006.

25. Ohayon MM, Milesi C. Artificial outdoor nighttime lights associate with altered behavior in the American general population. *Sleep.* 2016;39:1311–1320. doi:10.5665/sleep.5860.

26. Kobayashi R, Kohsaka M, Fukuda N, Sakakibara S, Honma H, Koyama T. Effects of morning bright light on sleep in healthy elderly women. *Psychiatry Clin Neurosci.* 1999;53:237–238. doi:10.1046/j.1440-1819.1999.00486.x.

27. Dijk DJ. Beersma DG, Daan S, Lewy AJ. Bright morning light advances the human circadian system without affecting NREM sleep homeostasis. *Am J Physiol.* 1989;256(1 Pt 2):R106-R111. doi:10.1152/ajpregu.1989.256.1.r106.

28. Kohsaka M, Fukuda N, Kobayashi R, Honma H, Sakakibara S, Koyama E, et al. Effect of short duration morning bright light in elderly men: Sleep structure. *Psychiatry Clin Neurosci.* 2000;54:367–368. doi:10.1046/j.1440-1819.2000.00718.x.

29. Thompson A, Jones H, Gregson W, Atkinson G. Effects of dawn stimulation on markers of sleep-inertia and post-waking performance in humans. *Eur J Appl Physiol.* 2014;114:1049–1056. doi:10.1007/s00421-014-2831-z.

30. Minors DS, Waterhouse JM, Wirz-Justice A. A human phase-response curve to light. *Neurosci Lett.* 1991;133:36–40. doi:10.1016/0304-3940(91)90051-t.

31. Khalsa SBS, Jewett ME, Cajochen C, Czeisler CA. A phase response curve to single bright light pulses in human subjects. *J Physiol.* 2003;549(Pt. 3):945–952. doi:10.1113/jphysiol.2003.040477.

32. Cho C-H, Lee H-J, Yoon H-K, Kang S-G, Bok K-N, Jung K-Y, et al. Exposure to dim artificial light at night increases REM sleep and awakenings in humans. *Chronobiol Int.* 2016;33:117–123. doi:10.3109/07420528.2015.1108980.

33. Youngstedt SD, Leung A, Kripke DF, Langer RD. Association of morning illumination and window covering with mood and sleep among post-menopausal women. *Sleep Biol Rhythms.* 2004;2(3):174–182. doi:10.1111/j.1479-8425.2004.00139.x.

34. Campbell SS, Dawson D. Aging young sleep: A test of the phase advance hypothesis of sleep disturbance in the elderly. *J Sleep Res.* 1992;1:205–210. doi:10.1111/j.1365-2869.1992.tb00040.x.

35. Burgess HJ, Sletten T, Savic N, Gilbert SS, Dawson D. Effects of bright light and melatonin on sleep propensity, temperature, and cardiac activity at night. *J Appl Physiol.* 2001;91:1214–1222.

36. Dijk DJ, Cajochen C, Borbely AA. Effect of a single 3-hour exposure to bright light on core body temperature and sleep in humans. *Neurosci Lett.* 1991;121(2):59–62. doi:10.1016/0304-3940(91)90649-e.

37. Kubota T, Uchiyama M, Hirokawa G, Ozaki S, Hayasi M, Okawa M. Effects of evening light on body temperature. *Psychiatry Clin Neurosci.* 1998;52:248–249. doi:10.1111/j.1440-1819.1998.tb01057.x.

38. Gordijn MCM, Beersma DGM, Korte HJ, Hoofdakker RH. Effects of light exposure and sleep displacement on dim light melatonin onset. *J Sleep Res.* 1999;8(3):163–174. doi:10.1046/j.1365-2869.1999.00156.x.

39. Kohsaka M, Fukuda N, Honma H, Koboyashi R, Sakakibara S, Koyama E, et al. Effects of moderately bright light on subjective evaluations in elderly healthy women. *Psychiatry Clin Neurosci.* 1999;53(2):239–241. doi:10.1046/j.1440-1819.1999.00539.x.

40. Park D-H, Kripke DF, Louis GJ et al. Self-reported sleep latency in postmenopausal women. *J Korean Med Sci.* 2007;22:1007–1014. doi:10.3346/jkms.2007.22.6.1007.

41. Gooley JJ, Chamberlain K, Smith KA, Khalsa SBS, Rajaratnam SMW, Van Reen E, et al. Exposure to room light before bedtime suppresses melatonin onset and shortens melatonin duration in humans. *Endocrinology.* 2011;152:742. doi:10.1210/endo.152.2.zee742.

42. Smolensky MH, Sackett-Lundeen LL, Portaluppi F. Nocturnal light pollution and underexposure to daytime sunlight: Complementary mechanisms of circadian disruption and related diseases. *Chronobiol Int.* 2015;32:1029–1048. doi:10.3109/07420528.2015.1072002.

43. Green A, Cohen-Zion M, Haim A, Dagan Y. Evening light exposure to computer screens disrupts human sleep, biological rhythms, and attention abilities. *Chronobiol Int.* 2017;34:855–865. doi:10.1080/07420528.2017.1324878.

44. Cinzano P, Falchi F, Elvidge CD, Baugh KE. The artificial night sky brightness mapped from DMSP satellite Operational Linescan System measurements. *Mon Not R Astron Soci.* 2000;318:641–657. doi:10.1046/j.1365-8711.2000.03562.x.

45. Falchi F, Cinzano P, Duriscoe D, Kyba CCM, Elvidge CD, Baugh K, et al. The new world atlas of artificial night sky brightness. *Sci Advances.* 2016;2(6):e1600377. doi:10.1126/sciadv.1600377.

46. Falchi F, Cinzano P, Elvidge CD, Keith DM, Haim A. Limiting the impact of light pollution on human health, environment and stellar visibility. *J Environ Manage.* 2011;92:2714–2722. doi:10.1016/j.jenvman.2011/06.029.

47. Bhambhani D. How many administrations does it take to screw in a light bulb rule? Forbes.com. 2019. https://www.forbes.com/sites/dipkabhambhani/2019/02/11/how-many-administrations-does-it-take-to-screw-in-a-light-bulb-rule/#166e93abc4bc

48. American Medical Association. AMA adopts guidance to reduce harm from high intensity street lights. Ama-assn.org. 2016. https://www.ama-assn.org/press-center/press-releases/ama-adopts-guidance-reduce-harm-high-intensity-street-lights

49. National Sleep Foundation. Why electronics may stimulate you before bed. Sleepfoundation.org. 2019. https://www.sleepfoundation.org/articles/why-electronics-may-stimulate-you-bed

50. National Sleep Foundation. Healthy sleep tips. Sleepfoundation.org. 2019. https://www.sleepfoundation.org/articles/healthy-sleep-tips

51. Dodson ER, Zee PC. Therapeutics for circadian rhythm sleep disorders. *Sleep Med Clinics.* 2010;5:701–715. doi:10.1016/j.jsmc.2010.08.001.

52. Weitzman ED, Czeisler CA, Coleman RM, Spielman AJ, Zimmerman JC, Dement W, et al. Delayed sleep phase syndrome: A chronobiological disorder with sleep onset insomnia. *Arch Gen Psychiatry.* 1981;38:737–746.

53. Rosenthal NE, Joseph-Vanderpool JR, Levendosky AA, Johnston SH, Allen R, Kelly KA, et al. Phase-shifting effects of bright morning light as treatment for delayed sleep phase syndrome. *Sleep.* 1990;13:354–361.

54. American Academy of Sleep Medicine. *The international classification of sleep disorders: Diagnostic and coding manual.* Westchester, IL: American Academy of Sleep Medicine; 2005.

55. Ebisawa T. Circadian rhythms in CNS and peripheral clock disorders: Human sleep disorders and clock genes. *J Pharmacol Sci.* 2007;103:150–154. doi:10.1254/jphs.fmj06003x3.

56. Lack L, Wright H. The effect of evening bright light in delaying the circadian rhythms and lengthening the sleep of early morning awakening insomniacs. *Sleep.* 1993;16:436–443. doi:10.1093/sleep/16.5.436.

57. Lack L, Wright H, Kemp K, Gibbon S. The treatment of early-morning awakening insomnia with 2 evenings of bright light. *Sleep.* 2005;28:616–623. doi:10.1093/sleep/28.5.616.

58. Drake CL, Roehrs T, Richardson G, Walsh JK, Roth T. Shift work sleep disorder: Prevalence and consequences beyond that of symptomatic day workers. *Sleep.* 2004;27:1453–1462. doi:10.1093/sleep/27.8.1453.

59. Burgess HJ, Sharkey KM, Eastman CI. Bright light, dark and melatonin can promote circadian adaptation in night shift workers. *Sleep Med Rev.* 2002;6:407–420. doi:10.1053/smrv.2001.0215.

60. Eastman CI, Stewart KT, Mahoney MP, Liu L, Fogg LF. Dark goggles and bright light improve circadian rhythm adaptation to night-shift work. *Sleep.* 1994;17:535–543. doi:10.1093/sleep/17.6.535.

61. van Maanen A, Meijer AM, van der Heijden KB, Oort FJ. The effects of light therapy on sleep problems: A systematic review and meta-analysis. *Sleep Med Rev.* 2016;29:59–62. doi:10.1016/j.smrv.2015.08.009.

8

Sleep Hygiene

SMITA PATEL

etter sleep habits can improve quality of sleep, and studies show that instruction on healthy sleep habits results in more peaceful sleep with fewer nighttime awakenings. Sleep hygiene, or the variety of different practices and habits that are supportive of good nighttime sleep quality and full daytime alertness, is recommended as an initial intervention for adults with insomnia so that personal habits and environmental factors that negatively impact sleep can be identified and corrected.[1,2]

Typically, recommendations about sleep requirements are based on surveys of Western populations.[3,4,5] Most adults require 7–9 hours of sleep a night.[3] Less than that, and sleep deprivation begins to starve the brain of glucose. After 24 hours of sleep deprivation, there is a 6% reduction in glucose that reaches the brain, specifically the prefrontal cortex, or the area most needed for complex cognitive thinking.[6] Additionally, the glymphatic system, a recently discovered system that rids the brain of accumulated waste metabolites, is most active during sleep and least active during wakefulness.[7] During deep sleep, accumulated proteins and other metabolites are transferred from the brain via glymphatic vessels to the body for management by the lymphatic system. Research suggests that lack of sleep or disrupted sleep leads to an increase in accumulated proteins in the brain, which affects cognition and thinking. These proteins include those that accumulate in Alzheimer's disease (beta amyloid and tau), Lewy body dementia, and Parkinson's disease (alpha synuclein). A recent systematic review suggests that 15% of Alzheimer's disease may be directly attributable to sleep problems.[9] Chronic lack of adequate sleep may help fuel the epidemic of Alzheimer's disease as well as the epidemics of obesity and diabetes.[8,9,10]

Parents tend to establish bedtime rituals for babies and young children to improve the likelihood of quality sleep. Many new mothers give their infant a relaxing massage and then a warm bath prior to bedtime. As adults, developing a personalized evening ritual, or preparing for bedtime, remains an important strategy to achieve better sleep. Treatment should start with attention to the sleep environment and personal habits.[11] According to the American Academy of Sleep Medicine's 2021 Practice Guideline for Chronic Insomnia Disorder in Adults, sleep hygiene alone is not considered a primary therapy for chronic insomnia, it can be an important adjunctive measure to improve sleep quality along with cognitive behavioral therapy and therapeutics.[12,13] What follows are common recommendations regarding good sleep hygiene and the evidence behind them.

Address Environmental Factors

A comfortable bed in a quiet, darkened room at a cool temperature has been found to promote sleep. Researchers have found that the optimal room temperature for sleep is actually quite cool; around 60°F to 67°F.[11,14] Sleep is typically initiated during the time when body temperature starts to decline secondary to decreased heat production and increased heat loss.[15] It is suggested that a rapid decline in core body temperature increases the likelihood of sleep initiation and may facilitate an entry into the deeper stages of sleep.[16] Sleeping in a hot environment has also been shown to increase wakefulness and decrease slow wave sleep, and the addition of high humidity can intensify the effect of heat.[16] In studies looking at quality of sleep in patients with sleep apnea, sleep quality improved as temperature moved from 75.2°F to 60.8°F. Cooler temperatures facilitated longer sleep times and greater alertness the following morning.[17] In addition, sleeping on a high heat capacity mattress has been shown in a randomized trial to increase body heat loss and improve slow wave sleep.[18]

The ideal bedroom to induce sleep is not only cool, but also dark and quiet. Simple environmental changes to achieve this include hanging heavy draperies or black-out curtains to prevent noise and light from entering the bedroom, wearing a comfortable eye mask, and placing rugs or carpets to soak up sound. White noise machines and smartphone apps can help mask sounds with soothing white noise or serene soundscapes. Research on listening to white noise at bedtime has shown that subjects fall asleep faster and report improved sleep quality when compared to normal environmental noise.[19]

Studies show that people may experience increased deep sleep by sleeping alone compared to sleeping next to a partner, even though many couples like the intimacy and comfortable feeling of having their partner close. Mattress selection is an important part of creating an optimal sleep environment. The right mattress should provide support in roughly the same position as when standing with good posture. If the mattress is too firm, it will push on pressure points and cause problems with alignment. If the mattress is too soft, those pressure points will not be properly supported either. Both of these scenarios can lead to back pain or nonrestorative sleep in the morning. Also mattresses do need to be replaced after 10–15 years. Mattresses collect dust mites, fungus, and other germs that can exacerbate allergies and negatively impact sleep patterns.[20]

Develop Evening Rituals

A hot bath may be beneficial for sleep as sleep onset typically occurs when core body temperature decreases. The gradual reduction in body temperature after a hot bath may help trigger sleep onset.[15] Warm milk or herbal noncaffeinated tea may work in a similar manner, but a trial-and-error approach is best for any given individual. Writing down immediate problems and worries and an action plan to tackle them is a beneficial tool to improve sleep, in addition to talking over mutual concerns with a partner. This "worry time" is designed to alleviate the stress of carrying problems to bed. A recent study aimed to determine whether making a list of future "to-do's" versus creating a list of recently accomplished tasks would affect sleep latency (the time it takes to fall asleep) differently. Five minutes ahead of bedtime at a polysomnography (PSG) center, subjects were randomized to journaling a to-do list or a completed tasks list. Results showed that subjects creating to-do lists had significantly shorter sleep latency compared to subjects creating lists of completed tasks. Additionally, the more specific the to-do lists, the shorter the sleep latency observed.[21] In addition, research shows that journaling is an effective stress-relieving exercise and that those who participate in journaling reap both physical and emotional benefits.[22]

Other evening rituals may be reading, yoga or gentle stretches, meditation, or quiet time. The following studies were done on patients with insomnia and demonstrate how a variety of different practices and habits (Table 8.1) are supportive of good nighttime sleep quality. There is good evidence for cognitive and physiological arousal in chronic insomnia. Accordingly, clinical trial studies of insomnia treatments aimed at reducing arousal, including relaxation and meditation, have reported positive results. Certain types of yoga may be effective in reducing arousal, although yoga has not been well evaluated as a treatment for insomnia. In a preliminary study, a simple daily yoga treatment was evaluated in a chronic insomnia population. Participants maintained sleep–wake diaries during a pretreatment 2-week baseline and a subsequent 8-week yoga intervention in which they practiced the treatment on their own following a single in-person training session with subsequent brief in-person and telephone follow-ups. Sleep efficiency (SE), or how much time is spent sleeping versus awake, total sleep time (TST), total wake time (TWT), sleep onset latency (SOL), wake time after sleep onset (WASO), number of awakenings, and sleep quality measures were derived from

Table 8.1 Ten techniques to get a better night's sleep

1	Address environmental factors	Optimal sleep environment is cool, dark, and quiet, with a properly supportive mattress
2	Develop sleep-promoting evening rituals	Hot bath, herbal tea, journal to-do lists, relaxing yoga, mindful meditation
3	Avoid screens prior to bedtime	Blue light from smartphones, tablets, and computers trigger biological processes that maintain wakefulness
4	Avoid using the bedroom for activities not related to sleep	Stimulus control—conditioning oneself to associate the bedroom with only activities that promote sleep
5	Maintain regular bedtime and wake times	Promote circadian rhythm and optimal hormone regulation
6	Maintain a healthy diet	Avoid diets high in sugar and refined carbohydrate, avoid unhealthy fats; choose whole foods and healthy fats
7	Limit caffeine	Caffeine significantly disrupts sleep and should be avoided during the 6 hours preceding bedtime
8	Limit alcohol	Alcohol significantly disrupts sleep even after it is fully metabolized from the body
9	Get regular exercise	Exercise improves many aspects of sleep
10	Avoid watching the clock during sleeplessness	Stimulus control—engage in a relaxing activity outside of the bedroom until sleepy to associate the bedroom with sleep onset as opposed to restlessness

diary entries. Statistically significant improvements were observed in SE, TST, TWT, SOL, and WASO at end-treatment as compared with pretreatment.[23]

A meditation routine may also positively impact sleep among those with insomnia. One clinical trial randomized older adults with insomnia to receive either a mindful awareness meditation intervention plus written information on good sleep hygiene or to receive only written information on good sleep hygiene. Those randomized to mindfulness meditation practice showed significant improvement in insomnia outcomes, depressive symptoms, and fatigue compared to the group not receiving the meditation intervention.[24] Another recent meta-analysis on mindfulness meditation for insomnia found that mindfulness meditation significantly improved sleep quality and can be considered an adjunctive treatment to medications.[25] Intense meditation practices have helped to achieve a harmony between body and mind. Meditation practices influence brain functions; induce various intrinsic neural plasticity events; and modulate autonomic, metabolic, endocrine, and immune functions and thus mediate global regulatory changes in various behavioral states including sleep.[26] The effect of meditation on sleep was first reported by Mason in practitioners of transcendental meditation.[27] The main objective was to evaluate the neurophysiological correlates of the higher states of consciousness during sleep. In this study, senior meditators spent more time in slow wave sleep with higher theta–alpha power with background delta activity, together with reduced electromyogram (EMG). Rapid eye movement (REM) sleep was also found to be enhanced. The distinct theta–alpha pattern observed during sleep was considered an electrophysiological correlate of a stabilized state of higher consciousness in sleep.

Avoid Screens Prior to Bedtime

Exposure to bright screens during the evening hours has been found to be particularly harmful to a good night's sleep. Light-emitting screens are detrimental to sleep patterns due to the blue light (of a wavelength of ~470 nm) that is emitted by these devices. Light-exposed retinal ganglion cells send signals to the suprachiasmatic nucleus (SCN) in the brain, which is also know as the "master clock." The SCN is responsible for daily sleep–wake cycles, body temperature regulation, and the production of hormones including melatonin. When artificial light hits the retina, the SCN undergoes processes designed to keep the body alert and awake, including lowering production of melatonin. Melatonin synchronizes the body's circadian rhythms with the real-life cycle of day and night experienced by the body, and this system can be easily fooled by exposure to artificial light. There is published experimental data demonstrating that just 2 hours of evening exposure to bright computer screens emitting blue light decreases sleep duration and, more importantly, dramatically reduces sleep quality. People exposed to computer screens were awakening during the night more often compared to those who did not use computers in the evening. The data also demonstrated that both the type of light emitted by the screens and its intensity is important for nighttime sleep quality. Screens with low brightness were less disturbing for sleep quality, and screens emitting red light did not affect nighttime sleep.[28–31] Additionally, a recent study found that unrestricted evening use of light-emitting devices delayed self-selected bedtime by 30 minutes, depressed melatonin levels, delayed timing of melatonin production, decreased self-ratings of sleepiness at night and increased self-ratings of low-alertness the following morning when compared to unrestricted use of printed reading materials before bed.[32]

Avoid Using the Bedroom for Activities Not Related to Sleep

Conditioning oneself to use the bedroom for only relaxation activities that promote sleep is known as *stimulus control*, a technique from cognitive behavioral therapy. It is recommended to avoid sustained television viewing, paperwork from the office or home, paying bills, or using your smartphone in the bedroom. It is best practice to associate the bedroom only with rest, sleep, and time with a partner. Avoiding mentally stimulating activities in bed has arguably become more difficult with the introduction of smartphones and other hand-held mobile devices and social media. A recent observational study examined the relationship between use of mobile device-based electronic social media (ESM) in bed and insomnia, mood, sleep duration, and daytime sleepiness in adults. The researchers found that roughly 70% of subjects engaged in ESM in bed before sleep, with 15% of subjects spending at least 1 hour engaged in this stimulating activity. Results showed that, compared to non-use, use was associated with short sleep duration, anxiety, and insomnia.[33]

Keep Regular Bedtimes and Wake Times

Sleep is optimized when the sleep period is aligned with an individual's circadian body clock and when sleep times are kept fairly regular.[34] Timing is key to good sleep and health. In the following study, the melatonin levels of shift workers working nights and sleeping days were significantly lower compared with those of daytime workers sleeping nights. Night shift workers had 57% lower urinary 6-sulfatoxymelatonin levels during daytime sleep compared with day shift-working men during nighttime sleep. Additionally, night shift workers had 16% higher urinary cortisol levels during daytime sleep.[35]

Evidence suggests that various hormones and metabolic processes are affected by sleep quality and circadian rhythms. Hormones such as growth hormone, melatonin, cortisol, leptin (which regulates fat storage in the body), and ghrelin (which triggers the appetite) are closely associated with sleep and circadian rhythms, and endogenous circadian-regulating mechanisms play an important role in glucose and lipid homeostasis, which are vital for health. Sleep disturbances and, particularly, sleep deprivation are associated with an increased risk of obesity, diabetes, and insulin insensitivity, and with dysregulation of leptin and ghrelin, which negatively impacts human health.[36] Additionally, in a study of 1,978 older adults, published in *Scientific Reports*, researchers at Duke Health and the Duke Clinical Research Institute found people with irregular sleep patterns weighed more and had higher blood sugar, higher blood pressure, and a higher projected risk of having a heart attack or stroke within 10 years than those who slept and woke at the same times every day.[37]

Research on sleep timing has uncovered associations between irregular sleep schedules and increased daytime sleepiness and poor subjective sleep quality, and reports show improvements in subjective sleep quality with the adoption of regular sleep schedules.[38,39] Clinical trial evidence also suggests decreased daytime sleepiness when participants are assigned to a regular sleep schedule versus controls.[40] While trying to find the ideal sleep schedule, researchers recommend aiming for 7.5 hours of sleep per night with regular bedtime and wake times.[34]

Maintain a Healthy Diet

An overall healthy diet is important for good sleep as well as all-around good health. Although no conclusive studies point to one particular diet that is best for sleep, various sources suggest that a variety of whole foods and a low-glycemic diet is helpful in improving sleep quality.[41,42] Research published in the *Journal of Clinical Sleep Medicine* found that people who eat diets high in sugar and refined carbs tend to take longer to fall asleep and wake more frequently during the night.[43] In the Women's Health Initiative study, the researchers observed the deleterious effects of sugar and the benefits of fiber. Sugar intake was linked with more excessive daytime sleepiness. Increased fiber resulted in less difficulty maintaining sleep, less difficulty with nonrestorative sleep, and less daytime sleepiness.[44] Another study associated sugar and high-glycemic load with fatigue. A high-glycemic load diet is linked with more depression symptoms, total mood disturbance, and fatigue compared to a low-glycemic load diet, especially in people who are overweight or obese.[45] Meanwhile, unhealthy fats could negatively affect the body's normal sleep–wake cycle, increasing sleep latency and reducing sleep efficiency.[43] In another study, researchers investigated the effects of fatty fish on sleep, daily functioning, and biomarkers such as vitamin D status (serum 25-hydroxyvitamin D [25OHD]), eicosapentaenoic acid (EPA, 20:5n-3), and docosahexaenoic acid (DHA, 22:6n-3) in red blood cells and heart rate variability (HRV). (Low HRV is associated with poor health outcomes.) Fatty fish seemed to have a positive impact on sleep in general and on daily functioning. Sufficient vitamin D status and high HRV seemed to be positively related to the beneficial effects.[46]

In addition to the diet's effect on sleep, the opposite is true as well: sleep also affects diet. It is now well established that short sleep duration is associated with obesity and risk of future weight gain.[47] In the journal *Sleep*, a study reported that sleep deprivation cranks up the pleasurable effects of salty, sugary, and fatty foods. In addition, when one doesn't get enough sleep, the body prompts one to eat more calories and burn fewer of them.[48]

Limiting Caffeine

Caffeine is a powerful nervous system stimulant. A study published in the *Journal of Clinical Sleep Medicine* shared some critical insights about the effect of caffeine on sleep. In this study, 12 healthy normal sleepers were asked to maintain their normal sleep routine. They gave each participant three pills to take each day for 4 days. One pill was to be taken 6 hours before bedtime, the second at 3 hours before, and the third at bedtime. One of the three pills contained 400 mg of caffeine (equivalent to 2 or 3 cups of coffee) and the other two looked identical to the caffeine pill but were only placebo. On one of the days, all three pills were placebos. Sleep disturbance was measured in two ways: objectively by means of a sleep monitor used at home and subjectively from diaries kept by the participants. The results showed that consuming caffeine 3 and even 6 hours before bedtime significantly disrupted sleep.[49] A recent systematic review of epidemiological studies and randomized controlled trials reported that caffeine reduces total sleep time, reduces sleep efficiency, delays sleep latency, worsens perceived sleep quality, increases wakefulness and number of arousals, and reduces slow wave sleep.[50]

Limit Alcohol

Alcohol consumed at bedtime, after an initial stimulating effect, may decrease the time required to fall asleep, and, because of its sedating effect, many people with insomnia consume alcohol to promote sleep; however, alcohol consumed within an hour of bedtime disrupts the second half of the sleep period.[51] Research shows that subjects sleep fitfully during the second half of sleep, awakening from dreams and returning to sleep with difficulty if they had consumed alcohol before bed. With continued consumption just before bedtime, alcohol's sleep-inducing effect may decrease, while its disruptive effects continue or increase.[52] This sleep disruption may lead to daytime fatigue and sleepiness.

Alcoholic beverages are often consumed in the late afternoon (e.g., at "happy hour" or with dinner) without further consumption before bedtime. Studies show that a moderate dose of alcohol consumed as much as 6 hours before bedtime can increase wakefulness during the second half of sleep.[53] By the time this effect occurs, the dose of alcohol consumed earlier has already been eliminated from the body, suggesting a relatively long-lasting change in the body's mechanisms of sleep regulation via alcohol consumption.[51,52]

Adverse effects of sleep deprivation combined with alcohol consumption have also been reported. Subjects administered very low doses of alcohol following a night of reduced sleep perform poorly in a driving simulator, even with no alcohol left in the body.[54] Reduced alertness may potentially increase alcohol's sedating effect in situations such as rotating sleep–wake schedules (e.g., shift work) and rapid travel across multiple time zones (i.e., jet lag).[55] A person may not recognize the extent of sleep disturbance and impairment that occur under these circumstances when sleepiness and alcohol consumption co-occur.

Get Regular Exercise

Aerobic exercise has been tested in multiple studies as a nonpharmacological intervention for improving sleep in older adults that has general health benefits and is readily accessible to most individuals.[56,57] The benefits of exercise on insomnia symptoms are most consistent for self-reported sleep quality and sleep diary–based measures. A systematic review of six randomized trials of exercise in older adults (with and without insomnia) demonstrated improvements in self-reported sleep quality, decreased self-reported sleep latency, and decreased need to use sleep medications.[58] King and colleagues demonstrated that 12 months of moderate-intensity aerobic activity led to improvements in self-rated and diary-based measures of sleep quality, as well as modest improvement in PSG measures, including fewer awakenings in the first third of the night, in a sample of older adults with poor sleep quality.[57] A recent study conducted in Brazil demonstrated improvements in both self-reported sleep quality and PSG measures in a sample of middle-aged adults with insomnia. In this study, 6 months of aerobic exercise (50 min, 3 times/week) led to objective and subjective improvements, including decreased SOL as measured by PSG and by sleep diary, decreased wakefulness after sleep onset, increased sleep efficiency (the amount of time spent sleeping as opposed to awake during the night), and increased ratings of sleep quality and of feeling rested.[59]

Patients with insomnia should be encouraged to exercise regularly and monitor improvement in sleep over longer periods of time rather than focusing on daily improvement. Understanding the relationship between exercise and sleep may help inform the development of behavioral interventions for insomnia.[60]

Avoid Watching the Clock During Phases of Sleeplessness

Staying in bed and watching the clock during periods of sleeplessness may associate the bed with anxiety and restlessness, and it is widely recommended, as another example of stimulus control behavioral modification, to get out of bed if one is unable to sleep within 30 minutes. Whether wakefulness occurs while trying to go to sleep or during the middle of the sleep period, one should leave the bedroom, go into another room, and do a relaxing activity like reading (avoiding blue-light emitting screens) or listening to the radio. Return to bed only when feeling tired again. This aims to associate the bed with sleep onset as opposed to restlessness.[61,62]

Conclusion

Sleep hygiene is recommended as an initial intervention for all adults with insomnia so that personal habits and environmental factors that negatively impact sleep can be identified and corrected. The effectiveness of sleep hygiene as a single therapy is unclear but is superior to placebo.[63,64] Sleep hygiene education seeks to optimize sleep quality by teaching patients about good sleep habits. Examples of concepts to discuss with patients include realistic expectations about sleep requirements, realistic consequences of insomnia, and healthy strategies to promote sleep. Regardless of the cause, most patients with insomnia benefit from approaches that focus on good sleep habits, especially when combined with other cognitive behavioral therapy approaches.

REFERENCES

1. Morin CM, Vallieres A, Guay B, et al. Cognitive behavioral therapy, singly and combined with medication, for persistent insomnia: a randomized controlled trial. *JAMA*. 2009;301(19):2005–2015.
2. www.sleepfoundation.org/sleep-topics/sleep-hygiene
3. Hirshkowitz M, Whiton K, Albert SM, et al. National Sleep Foundation sleep time duration recommendations: methodology and results summary. *Sleep Health*. 2015;1(1):40–43.
4. Paruthi S, Brooks LJ, D'Ambrosio C, et al. Recommended amount of sleep for pediatric populations: A consensus statement of the American Academy of Sleep Medicine. *J Clin Sleep Med*. 2016;12(6):785–786.
5. Iglowstein I, Jenni OG, Molinari L, Largo RH. Sleep duration from infancy to adolescence: reference values and generational trends. *Pediatrics*. 2003;111(2):302–307.
6. Pomplun M, Silva EJ, Ronda JM, Cain SW, Munch MY, Czeisler CA, Duffy JF. The effects of circadian phase, time awake, and imposed sleep restriction on performing complex visual tasks: Evidence from comparative visual search. *J Vis*. 2013;12(7):1–19
7. Jessen NA, Finmann Munk AS, Lundgaard I, Nedergaard M. The glymphatic system—a beginner's guide. *Neurochem Res*. 2015;40(12):2583–2599.
8. Morselli L, Leproult R, Balbo M, Spiegel K. Role of sleep duration in the regulation of glucose metabolism and appetite. *Best Pract Res Clin Endocrinol Metab*. 2010;24(5):687–702.
9. Bubu OM, Brannick M, Mortimer J, et al. Sleep, cognitive impairment, and Alzheimer's disease: A systematic review and meta-analysis. *Sleep*. 2017 Jan 1;40(1).
10. Musiek ES, Xiong DD, Holtzman DM. Sleep, circadian rhythms, and the pathogenesis of Alzheimer's disease. *Exp Mol Med*. 2015;47(3):e148.https://doi.org/10.1038/emm.2014.121

11. Onen SH, Onen F, Bailly D, Parquet P. Prevention and treatment of sleep disorders through regulation of sleeping habits. *Presse Med.* 1994;23(10):485–489.

12. Edinger JD, Arnedt JT, Bertisch SM, et al. Behavioral and psychological treatments for chronic insomnia disorder in adults: an American Academy of Sleep Medicine clinical practice guideline. *J Clin Sleep Med.* 2021;17(2):255–262.

13. Asok A, Sreekumar S, Tk R, et al. Effectiveness of zolpidem and sleep hygiene counseling in the treatment of insomnia in solid tumor patients. *J Oncol Pharm Pract.* 2019;25(7):1608–1612.

14. National Sleep Foundation. The sleep environment. http://www.sleepfoundation.org/article/how-sleep-works/the-sleep-environment

15. Murphy PJ, Campbell SS. Nighttime drop in body temperature: A physiological trigger for sleep onset? *Sleep.* 1997 Jul;20 (7):505–511.

16. Jordan J, Montgomery I, Trinder J. The effect of afternoon body heating on body temperature and slow wave sleep. *Psychophysiology.* 1990 Sep;27(5):560–566.

17. Valham F, Sahlin C, Stenlund H, Franklin KA. Ambient temperature and obstructive sleep apnea: Effects on sleep, sleep apnea, and morning alertness. *Sleep.* 2012 Apr 1;35(4):513–517.

18. Kräuchi K, Fattori E, Giordano A, et al. Sleep on a high heat capacity mattress increases conductive body heat loss and slow wave sleep. *Physiol Behav.* 2018 Mar 1;185:23–30.

19. Messineo L, et al. Broadband sound administration improves sleep onset latency in healthy subjects in a model of transient insomnia. *Front Neurol.* 2017;8:718.

20. Leger D, Annesi-Maesano I, Carat F, et al. Allergic rhinitis and its consequences on quality of sleep: An unexplored area. *Arch Intern Med.* 2006 Sep 18;166(16):1744–1748.

21. Scullin MK, Krueger ML, Pruett N, Bilwise DL. The effects of bedtime writing on difficulty falling asleep: A polysomnographic study comparing to-do lists and completed activity lists. *J Exp Psychol Gen.* 2018 Jan;147(1):139–146.

22. Pennebaker JW. Writing about emotional experiences as a therapeutic process. *Psychol Sci.* 1997;8(3):162–166.

23. Khalsa SB. Treatment of chronic insomnia with yoga: A preliminary study with sleep-wake diaries. *Appl Psychophysiol Biofeedback.* 2004 Dec;29(4):269–278.

24. Black DS, O'Reilly GA, Olmstead R, et al. Mindfulness meditation and improvement in sleep quality and daytime impairment among older adults with sleep disturbances: A randomized clinical trial. *JAMA Intern Med.* 2015 Apr;175(4):494–501

25. Gong H, Ni CX, Liu YZ et al. Mindfulness meditation for insomnia: A meta-analysis of randomized controlled trials. *J Psychosom Res.* 2016 Oct;89:1–6.

26. Nagendra RP, Maruthai N, Kutty BM. Meditation and its regulatory role on sleep. *Front Neurol.* 2012;3:54.

27. Mason LI, Alexander CN, Travis FT, et al. Electrophysiological correlates of higher states of consciousness during sleep in long-term practitioners of the transcendental meditation program. *Sleep.* 1997;20:102–110.

28. Figueiro MG, Wood B, Plitnick, Rea MS. The impact of light from computer monitors on melatonin levels in college students. *Neuro Endocrinol Lett.* 2011;32(2):158–163.

29. Skene DJ, Arendt J. Human circadian rhythms: physiological and therapeutic relevance of light and melatonin. *Ann Clin Biochem*. 2006;43(Pt 5):344–353.

30. Wright HR, Lack LC, Kennaway DJ. Differential effects of light wavelength in phase advancing the melatonin rhythm. *J Pineal Res*. 2004;36(2):140–144.

31. Wilhelmsen-Langeland A, Saxvig IW, Pallesen S, et al. A randomized controlled trial with bright light and melatonin for the treatment of delayed sleep phase disorder. *J Biol Rhythms*. 2013;28(5):306–321.

32. Chinoy ED, Duffy JF, Czeisler CA. Unrestricted evening use of light-emitting tablet computers delays self-selected bedtime and disrupts circadian timing and alertness. *Physiol Rep*. 2018;6(10):e13692. doi:10.14814/phy2.13692.

33. Bhat S, Pinto-Zipp G, Upadhyay H, et al. To sleep, perchance to tweet": In-bed electronic social media use and its association with insomnia, daytime sleepiness, mood, and sleep duration in adults. *Sleep Health*. 2018 Apr;4(2):166–173.

34. https://sleep.org/articles/circadian-rhythm-body-clock/

35. Mirick DK, Bhatti P, Chen C, Nordt F, Stanczyk FZ, Davis S. Night shift work and levels of 6-sulfatoxymelatonin and cortisol in men. *Cancer Epidemiol Biomarkers Prev*. 2013 Jun;22(6):1079–1087.

36. Kim TW, Jeong JH, Hong SC. The impact of sleep and circadian disturbance on hormones and metabolism. *Int J Endocrinol*. 2015:591729.

37. Lunsford-Avery JR, Engelhard MM, Navar AM, Kollins SH. Validation of the Sleep Regularity Index in older adults and associations with cardiometabolic risk. *Sci Rep*. 2018 Sep 21;8(1):14158.

38. Carney CE, Edinger JD, Meyer B, Lindman L, Istre T. Daily activities and sleep quality in college students. *Chronobiol Int*. 2006;23:623–637.

39. Monk TH, Buysse DJ, Billy BD, Fletcher ME, Kennedy KS, Schlarb JE, et al. Circadian type and bed-timing regularity in 654 retired seniors: Correlations with subjective sleep measures. *Sleep*. 2011;34:235–239.

40. Manber R, Bootzin RR, Acebo C, Carskadon MA. The effects of regularizing sleep-wake schedules on daytime sleepiness. *Sleep*. 1996;19:432–441.

41. Arora T. Sleep doesn't waste time, it's good for the waist line. *Sleep*. 2015 Aug 1;38(8):1159–1160.

42. Grandner MA, Kripke DF, Naidoo N, Langer RD. Relationships among dietary nutrients and subjective sleep, objective sleep, and napping in women. *Sleep Med*. 2010 Feb;11(2):180.

43. St-Onge MP, Roberts A, Shechter A, Choudhury AR. Fiber and saturated fat are associated with sleep arousals and slow wave sleep. *J Clin Sleep Med*. 2016;12 (1):19–24.

44. Grandner MA, Jackson N, Gerstner JR, Knutson KL. Sleep symptoms associated with intake of specific dietary nutrients. *J Sleep Res*. 2014 Feb;23(1):22–34.

45. Breymeyer KL, Lampe JW, McGregor BA, Neuhouser ML. Subjective mood and energy levels of healthy weight and overweight/obese healthy adults on high-and low-glycemic load experimental diets. *Appetite*. 2016 Dec 1;107:253–259.

46. Hansen AL, Dahl L, Olson G, et al. Fish consumption, sleep, daily functioning, and heart rate variability. *J Clin Sleep Med*. 2014;10(5):567–575.

47. Patel SR, Hu FB. Short sleep duration and weight gain: A systematic review. *Obesity (Silver Spring).* 2008;16:643–653.
48. Dennis LE, Spaeth AM, Goel N. Energy balance responses show phenotypic stability to sleep restriction and total sleep deprivation in healthy adults. *Sleep.* 2017;40(Suppl 1):A71–A72.
49. Drake C, Roehrs T, Shambroom J, Roth T. Caffeine effects on sleep taken 0,3, or 6 hours before going to bed. *J Clin Sleep Med.* 2013;9(11):1195–1200.
50. Clark I, Landolt HP. Coffee, caffeine, and sleep: A systematic review of epidemiological studies and randomized controlled trials. *Sleep Med Rev.* 2017 Feb;31:70–78.
51. Landolt HP, Roth C, Dijk DJ, Borbely AA. Late-afternoon ethanol intake affects nocturnal sleep and the sleep EEG in middle-aged men. *J Clin Psychopharmacol.* 1996;16(6):428–436.
52. Vitiello MV. Sleep, alcohol and alcohol abuse. *Addict Biol.* 1997;2 (2):151–158.
53. Roehrs T, Roth T. Alcohol-induced sleepiness and memory function. *Alcohol Health Res World.* 1995;19(2):130–135.
54. Roehrs T, Beare D, Zorick F, Roth T. Sleepiness and ethanol effects on simulated driving. *Alcohol Clin Exp Res.* 1994;18(1):154–158.
55. Krull KR, Smith LT, Sinha R, Parsons OA. Simple reaction time event-related potentials: Effects of alcohol and sleep deprivation. *Alcohol Clin Exp Res.* 1993;17(4):771–777.
56. Baron KG, Reid KJ, Zee PC. Exercise to improve sleep in insomnia: Exploration of the bidirectional effects. *J Clin Sleep Med.* 2013;9(8):819–824.
57. King CR, Knutson KL, Rathouz PJ, Sidney S, Liu K, Lauderdale DS. Short sleep duration and incident coronary artery calcification. *JAMA.* 2008;300(24):2859–2866.
58. Yang PY, Ho KH, Chen HC, Chien MY. Exercise training improves sleep quality in middle-aged and older adults with sleep problems: A systematic review. *J Physiother.* 2012;58:157–163.
59. Passos GS, Poyares DL, Santana MG, Tufik S, Mello MT. Is exercise an alternative treatment for chronic insomnia? *Clinics (Sao Paulo).* 2012;67:653–660.
60. Passos GS, Poyares D, Santana MG, et al. Effects of moderate aerobic exercise training on chronic primary insomnia. *Sleep Med.* 2011;12(10):1018–1027.
61. Morin CM, Cognitive-behavioral approaches to the treatment of insomnia. *J Clin Psychiatry.* 2004;65(Suppl 16):33–40.
62. Budur K, Rodriguez C, Foldvary-Schaefer N. Advances in treating insomnia. *Cleve Clinic J Med.* 2007;74(4):251–266.
63. Ringdahl EN, Pereira SL, Delzell JE Jr. Treatment of primary insomnia. *J Am Board Fam Pract.* 2004;17(3):212–219.
64. Schutte- Rodin S, Broch L, Buysse D, Dorsey C, Sateia M. Clinical guideline for the evaluation and management of chronic insomnia in adults. *J Clin Sleep Med.* 2008;4(5):487–504.

9

Physical Activity, Sleep, and Sleep Disorders

PATRICK J. O'CONNOR AND CARLY L. A. WENDER

Introduction

The benefits of both physical activity and sleep for health have been suggested since ancient times.[1] Over the past 50 years, hundreds of research studies have documented that physical activity improves cardiorespiratory fitness, flexibility, muscular strength, and physical function in children and adults. During this time, convincing scientific evidence has been generated showing that physical activity helps prevent the development of several chronic diseases including coronary heart disease, osteoporosis, and cancers of the breast and colon. Regular physical activity has been established as an effective treatment for numerous medical conditions including diabetes, back pain, and depression, and it is commonly considered one of the foundations of optimal health.[2]

Sleep also benefits physical and mental health. Sleep that habitually is either short (≤5 hours per night) or long (≥9 hours per night) has been linked to numerous health maladies including affective disorders, obesity, diabetes, coronary heart disease, strokes, and all-cause mortality.[3,4] Yet as fundamental as exercise and sleep are to overall health and well-being, the association between the two has not been well established. The hunch that exercise promotes longer sleep duration or better quality sleep has existed for decades, and recent scientific evidence generally supports this notion. A newer idea, that good sleep impacts daytime physical activity, has only recently been examined scientifically.

This chapter addresses bidirectional relationships between physical activity and sleep. While the body of evidence on this topic is somewhat limited, it is instructive to recognize that knowledge of physical activity and sleep is expanding. As shown in Figure 9.1, the amount of scientific evidence about sleep and physical activity has increased dramatically during the past decade. We estimate that about 50%

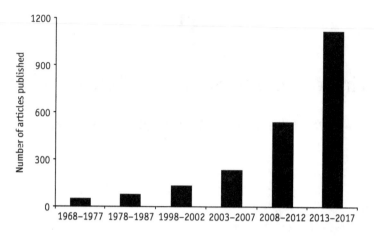

FIGURE 9.1 Number of scholarly papers focused on physical activity and sleep during six 5-year time periods. Data based on a Google Scholar search performed December 12, 2017. The search identified papers in which the title included the word "sleep" combined with at least one of the following words: "cardiorespiratory fitness," "exercise," "gardening," "muscular strength," "physical activity," "strengthening," "stretching," "weight lifting," and "yoga."

of all published science-based papers about physical activity and sleep have been published in the past 5 years. This growing body of evidence increasingly supports the supposition that sleep and physical activity have bidirectional relationships. Overall, health professionals should continue to promote regular physical activity as a potential contributor to healthy sleep and consider the possibility that healthy sleep may be a contributor to regular physical activity.

This chapter begins by reviewing what is known about relationships between acute and chronic physical activity and sleep in healthy people. When possible, characteristics of exercise that may moderate these effects are also discussed. This is followed by summaries of what is known about physical activity and several major sleep disorders: insomnia, apnea, restless legs syndrome (RLS), narcolepsy, circadian rhythm sleep–wake disorders, and parasomnias. There are more than 100 sleep disorders described in the most recent *International Classification of Sleep Disorders*,[5] but we refrained from commenting on most sleep disorders in this chapter because of a lack of science-based information about how they are impacted by physical activity.

Acute Physical Activity and Sleep in Healthy Adults

The effect of acute physical activity on sleep in healthy adults has been examined in dozens of experiments. In 2015, Kredlow and colleagues summarized 41 of these studies using meta-analytic techniques.[6] Four studies were randomized controlled trials while 37 employed "within-participant open trial designs," where sleep measures were compared on days with and without exercise. As illustrated in Figure 9.2, acute exercise had small, generally beneficial effects on sleep. Specifically, wakefulness after sleep onset, stage 1 sleep, rapid eye movement (REM), and sleep onset latency were reduced after acute exercise while total sleep time, sleep efficiency, and slow wave sleep were increased.

Several factors moderated the size of these effects of acute exercise on sleep in healthy adults. Exercise of greater duration was associated with larger effects for almost every sleep outcome measured, including total sleep time, slow wave sleep, and sleep onset latency. Meta-analytic results suggest that the effects of physical activity on sleep is greatest when the duration of a single exercise session exceeds 1 hour[7]; however, this possibility requires confirmation from experiments in which participants are randomized to different durations of exercise. Moreover, exercise durations longer than 1 hour are impractical for many people.

The results of the Kredlow et al. meta-analysis also showed that slow wave sleep increased after acute exercise to a greater extent among active compared to sedentary participants and for those who performed cycling compared to running exercise.[6] A single bout of weight lifting had unclear effects on sleep based on the results of three studies.[8] No studies have made direct comparisons between different modes of exercise while controlling for potentially confounding features

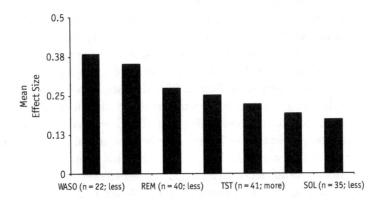

FIGURE 9.2 Mean standardized statistically significant effects of acute exercise on polysomnographic measures of sleep based on the results of 41 studies. The effects are in standard deviation units. Effect sizes of ~0.25 are commonly judged as clinically small effects. The number of studies that provided data for each outcome and the direction of the effect is given in parentheses.

REM, rapid eye movement; SOL, sleep onset latency; SWS, slow wave sleep; WASO, wakefulness after sleep onset.

Adapted from Kredlow et al., 2015.

of the exercise, such as the duration of active muscle contractions, the exercise intensity, or the time of day it was completed. Time of day relative to bedtime was a significant moderator in the Kredlow meta-analysis[6]; the greatest effects of acute exercise on sleep were observed when exercise occurred more than 8 hours or less than 3 hours before bedtime. It is important to note that despite the belief among many sleep clinicians that exercise should be avoided shortly before bed, the evidence indicates that late night exercise generally benefits sleep.[9]

Exercise intensity does not moderate the effects of acute exercise on sleep according to the meta-analysis conducted by Kredlow and colleagues.[6] Nevertheless, it is possible that expectations, preferences for, or perceptions about exercise intensity could influence the effects of exercise on sleep. A study conducted by Brand and colleagues[10] found that 52 young adults who regularly participated in sports in the evening slept better after nights in which the exercise intensity was perceived as being higher than on nights when the exercise intensity was perceived as being lower. Correlational analysis revealed a positive association between greater self-perceived exercise intensity and higher sleep efficiency, decreased sleep onset latency, fewer and shorter awakenings during sleep, less stage 1 and 2 sleep, and more stage 3 and 4 sleep. Additionally, greater perceived exertion during the previous night's exercise was associated with better self-perceived sleep quality the following morning.[10] Research with larger and more diverse samples is necessary to draw reliable conclusions about the extent to which, and how, exercise expectations, preferences, and perceptions influence sleep.

It seems plausible that the small benefits healthy individuals accrue from acute exercise could be augmented in adults with health problems that may directly or indirectly affect sleep. This was not found in a study of acute resistance exercise on sleep in institutionalized older adults. Specifically, there were no changes in sleep efficiency, time in non–REM (NREM) sleep, time in REM sleep, time awake, time until sleep onset, total sleep stage shifts, or REM sleep stage latency the night after daytime weight lifting compared to a control condition without exercise.[11] Kurka[12] examined the effects of two consecutive days of high-intensity and moderate-intensity exercise performed 4–6 hours before bedtime on subsequent nights of sleep in 11 middle-aged women with self-report subclinical symptoms of insomnia. Overall there were no differences in actigraphy-measured sleep outcomes between the exercise condition and non-exercise control. However, total sleep time was increased on the fourth night in the high-intensity condition, and sleep onset latency was increased on the third and fourth nights in the moderate-intensity condition. Contradictory to the findings of the Kredlow meta-analysis showing that exercise intensity does not moderate the influence of exercise on sleep,[6] only the high-intensity exercise condition showed increases in total sleep time, and only the moderate-exercise condition showed worse sleep onset latency.[12] It is unclear if these results are due to small sample size bias or if acute exercise has delayed effects on sleep in those with insomnia.

While acute exercise generally confers small sleep benefits, in some groups with medical illness it is plausible that exercise could produce sleep problems. A single bout of aerobic, but not resistance, exercise performed by patients with type 1 diabetes resulted in significant sleep loss compared to a day without exercise.[13] Exercise-induced reductions in glucose are plausible contributors to this effect and to the fact that the effects of single bouts of exercise on sleep are generally larger with longer duration exercise that is more likely to deplete brain glycogen stores. Even without exercise, brain glycogen is depleted during the day and resynthesized at night, and it appears to be a marker of the drive for homeostatic sleep.[14]

Chronic Physical Activity and Sleep in Healthy Adults

Community-based cross-sectional studies consistently show that regular physical activity is associated with better sleep and fewer sleep complaints among both apparently healthy and overweight adults,[15,16] but it is unclear whether alternative explanations, such as better health among those who exercise, account for these findings. A smaller number of prospective studies also show that regular physical activity can contribute to the prevention of new sleep complaints.[17]

Experiments involving random assignment to exercise training or non-exercise conditions provide information about whether regular physical activity causes changes in sleep in healthy adults. A meta-analysis of 25 experiments, all of which included non-exercise controls, provides quantitative information about the influence of exercise training on sleep.[6] About 91% of the samples analyzed consisted of participants who were free of sleep complaints. As illustrated in Figure 9.3, exercise training programs resulted in a large mean improvement in sleep quality and small mean improvements in sleep onset latency, sleep efficiency, and total sleep time. Moderator analysis showed that (1) sleep onset latency improvements were greater for younger than older adults and for longer exercise durations, (2) total sleep time was improved more after exercise training programs that were shorter in duration (programs ranged from 2 to 52 weeks), and (3) sleep quality was better when exercise adherence was better. Recent randomized trials show that exercise training benefits sleep quality when performed by breast cancer survivors,[18] resistance exercise can improve sleep quality,[8] and night-to-night variability in wakefulness after sleep onset is reduced after the adoption of either a low-dose or a higher dose of walking among older women.[19] Studies investigating the effects of chronic physical activity on sleep in individuals with sleep disorders are discussed in the next sections.

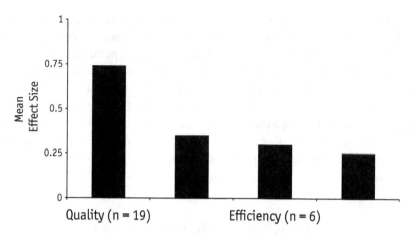

FIGURE 9.3 Mean standardized effects of exercise training on sleep quality, sleep onset latency, sleep efficiency, and total sleep time. The number of studies that provided data for each outcome is given in parentheses. The effects are in standard deviation units. Effect sizes of ~0.25 and ~0.50 are commonly judged as clinically small and moderate-sized effects, respectively. Positive values show beneficial effects.
Adapted from Kredlow et al., 2015.

Physical Activity, Insomnia, and Its Symptoms

Insomnia is characterized by the inability to fall asleep or stay asleep. Insomnia is a common problem, more prevalent in women than men, with about one-third of the population reporting symptoms and about 6% with a confirmed diagnosis.[20] Insomnia contributes to daytime sleepiness, reduced work productivity, and accidents, and it is associated with mental and physical health problems including cardiovascular disease and depression.[21,22] Insomnia is currently treated primarily with psychological, behavioral, or pharmacotherapy. Exercise not only has been left out of practice guidelines for the management of insomnia,[23] but clinicians providing sleep hygiene advice frequently recommend that physical activity be avoided 4–5 hours prior to usual sleep time because of the transient impact of exercise on physiological arousal. However, the weight of the currently available evidence shows that evening exercise is not associated with worse sleep for most people.[24]

More than a dozen epidemiologic studies have shown that participation in regular physical activity is associated with fewer symptoms of insomnia.[25] The effect is consistent across age and has been observed in multiple countries including China, Finland, Japan, Taiwan, and the United States. The beneficial effect of regular exercise for symptoms of insomnia has been documented in prospective studies even after adjusting for potential confounders such as age, smoking, snoring status, alcohol use, and body mass index.[26]

Exercise mode has rarely been considered in the epidemiological studies of physical activity and insomnia symptoms. However, in one study of 4,386 adults who completed the 2005–2006 National Health and Nutrition Examination Survey, those who engaged in regular muscle strengthening exercise, compared to those not engaging in resistance exercise, had a 19% greater odds of sleeping for 7–8 hours per night.[27]

A limitation of most epidemiological studies is that both physical activity and sleep are measured using brief survey questions with uncertain validity. Consequently, epidemiology studies with objective measures can be especially informative. One cross-sectional study of 3,081 healthy adults measured physical activity objectively for 7 days using accelerometers and found a 40% reduction in risk of daytime sleepiness among those participants who met or exceeded the US government physical activity recommendations designed to maintain or improve health (75 minutes of vigorous or 150 minutes of moderate-intensity exercise per week).[28] No epidemiological studies with an objective measure have obtained data from diagnosed insomnia patients. One cross-sectional study of 3,489 female and male Norwegian adults found a significant, modest negative association between insomnia symptoms and objectively measured cardiorespiratory fitness, which is typically achieved by being regularly physically active and/or not gaining fat mass, after adjusting for self-reported physical activity and cardiovascular risk factors.[29] One prospective study of more than 8,000 subjects tested initially at about age 50 and prospectively followed for about 25 years found that maintaining objectively measured cardiorespiratory fitness protected against the odds of developing sleep complaints made to a physician.[30]

Exercise training is associated with improvements in sleep quality in middle-aged and older adults with symptoms of insomnia. Much of this evidence involves integrative types of exercise, primarily yoga.[31] At least 11 clinical trials have examined the influence of yoga on sleep quality among cancer patients, individuals who are at increased risk for symptoms of insomnia. Yoga, a diverse practice that often adds regulated breathing and an emphasis on cognition (such as mindfulness techniques) to the completion of physical postures, appears to be well-tolerated and promising for improving sleep in cancer patients. Seven trials showed improvements in sleep among cancer patients, while in 4 studies the findings were null.[32] The largest study, a multicenter trial involving 410 cancer patients who completed a standardized yoga intervention twice per week for 4 weeks, found significant reductions in sleep medication use as well as improvements in self-reported wakefulness after sleep onset and sleep efficiency.[33]

At least four experiments have examined the influence of 4–26 weeks of stationary cycling or treadmill walking on small samples of patients diagnosed with insomnia. Each of these investigations show that the adoption of regular exercise by patients with an insomnia disorder (primary or psychophysiological) resulted in significant improvements in sleep onset latency, sleep efficiency, and sleep quality.[34-37] The weight of the available evidence supports that regular physical activity improves sleep quality in those with symptoms of insomnia.

Physical Activity and Obstructive Sleep Apnea

Complete or partial blockage of the airway during sleep results in obstructive sleep apnea (OSA). OSA is highly prevalent in the United States, although rates vary based on how it is defined. When OSA is defined by five or more apneas or hypopneas per hour (an apnea-hypopnea index [AHI] of ≥5), as is most common, the prevalence has been estimated to be between 9% and 38%. OSA is more prevalent among those who snore, are excessively sleepy during the daytime, have a family history of OSA, or are overweight/obese. Acute risk factors include nasal congestion and alcohol consumption. Most studies show dose-response effects with greater alcohol use producing more apneas and hypopneas. OSA is associated with several chronic diseases, including hypertension, diabetes, and mortality from all causes.[38] Common treatments for OSA include continuous positive airway pressure (CPAP), mandibular advancement devices, and weight loss.

Several cross-sectional studies show an association between physical inactivity and increased risk of OSA.[39,40] One study that measured sleep objectively in 1,104 middle-aged men and women, as illustrated in Figure 9.4, found a negative

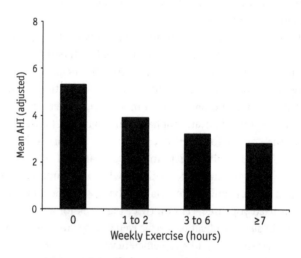

FIGURE 9.4 Cross-sectional relationship between hours of weekly exercise reported and the mean apnea-hypopnea index (AHI) in 1,104 middle-aged men and women after statistical adjustments were made for multiple potential confounding variables such as age and body mass.
Adapted from Peppard and Young, 2004.

dose-dependent association between the number of hours of weekly exercise and the AHI, even after adjusting for multiple potential confounding variables.[41] At least seven experiments have examined the influence of exercise training on OSA. All these 3- to 6-month experiments showed that exercise training reduced apneas or hypopneas compared to non-exercise control conditions. The average magnitude of the improvement was about six fewer apneas or hypopneas per hour, which signifies a moderate, clinical meaningful benefit.[42,43] The improvements were not dependent on the duration of each exercise session or weight loss determined from changes in body mass index. When exercise training was compared to other treatments for sleep apnea, mean AHI reductions were largest for CPAP followed by exercise and mandibular advancement device, and smallest for dieting, either alone or in combination with exercise. Improvements in daytime sleepiness were greatest for exercise training compared to the other treatments measured. In sum, the available evidence supports that exercise training can produce clinically meaningful improvements in sleep apnea and daytime sleepiness either alone or as an adjunct therapy.

Physical Activity and Restless Legs Syndrome

RLS refers to uncomfortable perceptions in the legs combined with an irresistible urge to move the legs that is attenuated with movement. When this occurs at night, it can disrupt sleep onset. More than 80% of people with RLS also experience periodic limb movements during sleep, which can negatively affect many aspects of their sleep. The prevalence of RLS ranges from about 5% to 12% in North America and Europe and is higher among older adults, in women, during pregnancy, and in some medical conditions, such as kidney disease.[44] Medications that influence central nervous system dopaminergic neurons, such as ropinirole and levodopa, are the most common recommendation for patients with moderate to severe RLS. Exercise increases dopamine release and upregulates striatal dopamine D_2 receptors in rats but the effects of acute and chronic exercise on dopaminergic neural function in humans is poorly understood.[45] When RLS is secondary to hemodialysis treatment, there is more evidence to support the use of vitamins C and E supplementation but ropinirole, levodopa, and exercise also are recommended.[46]

The relationship between RLS and physical activity has been inconsistent in cross-sectional studies. In a sample of adult residents of Kentucky, the odds of frequent restless legs symptoms was 3.3 times higher in those reporting less than 3 hours per month of exercise compared to those doing more.[47] However, in a study of 8,980 European adults, an increased probability of meeting diagnostic criteria for RLS was found for those who performed either regular daytime exercise (an 18% increase in odds) or regular exercise close to bed time (a 34% increase in odds) compared to those reporting no physical exercise.[48] The prevalence of RLS was relatively high (13%) in a sample of 54 Brazilian distance runners despite high levels of activity.[49] Other community-based studies have shown weak associations between physical activity and RLS.[50,51]

Unlike epidemiological results, small exercise training studies have resulted in consistent positive effects on symptoms of RLS. Progressive, moderate-intensity leg cycling performed 3 times per week for 6 months during hemodialysis in patients with kidney disease ($n = 12$) reduced the severity of RLS symptoms compared to patients ($n = 12$) who performed the same number of cycling bouts for the same duration but at a very low intensity (against no resistance).[52] Similar results were reported in other randomized trials in patients with kidney disease involving moderate-intensity and shorter duration (4 months) leg cycling exercise during hemodialysis.[53,54] Treadmill walking combined with lower body resistance exercises for 16 weeks improved restless legs symptoms in adults with RLS as their primary disorder,[55] and periodic limb movements were reduced among 11 patients who performed 72 exercise training sessions.[56] Acute exercise also may impact RLS. One small study found that leg movements during sleep were lower the night following a single graded maximal arm exercise test performed by athletes with a complete spinal cord injury compared to a day that did not involve exhaustive arm exercise.[57] This body of evidence suggests that physical activity is an effective treatment for restless leg syndrome in people with kidney disease. More research is required to make this same assertion for other affected populations.

Physical Activity and Narcolepsy

Narcolepsy is a sleep disorder characterized by the sudden onset of extreme sleepiness that is not caused by disturbed sleep at night. Narcolepsy can be accompanied by *cataplexy*, the sudden loss of muscle control and tone during wakefulness, which is often triggered by surprising events eliciting a strong emotional reaction. Environmental and genetic factors are thought to play a role in narcolepsy. Both autoimmune processes and the hypocretin system have been implicated in narcolepsy. Pharmacological therapies that promote wakefulness, such as modafinil and stimulants, are most commonly used in the treatment of narcolepsy.

Narcolepsy reduces many aspects of quality of life, including participation in sports. A survey of 305 adult members of the United Kingdom Association of Narcolepsy found that 40% of the sample reported that their symptoms made playing sports difficult.[58] In a study of 109 narcolepsy patients with cataplexy and hypocretin-1 deficiency, about half indicated that exercise could trigger cataplexy, and, when this occurred, 59% of the sample showed clear associations with a strong emotion (e.g., making or anticipating a winning shot in tennis).[59] Physical activity was lower and sedentary time was higher, according to wrist-worn accelerometers, during a 4-day unmedicated period in a study of nine middle-aged narcoleptics compared to age- and sex-matched controls.[60] These observations are generally consistent with data from a rodent model of narcolepsy. Mice lacking hypocretin engage in less spontaneous wheel running than do normal mice, and wheel running increased the amount of cataplexy in mice lacking hypocretin.[61] In sum, the evidence suggests that people with narcolepsy are physically inactive, but the size, number, and type of studies conducted to date are insufficient to determine whether physical activity reliably attenuates or exacerbates narcolepsy or cataplexy in the majority of these patients.

Physical Activity and Circadian Rhythm Sleep–Wake Disorders

Circadian rhythm sleep–wake disorders occur when the circadian timing system malfunctions or endogenous 24-hour rhythms become desynchronized from the external environment in response to shift work or air travel across time zones. Specific disorders of this type include advanced sleep–wake phase disorder, delayed sleep–wake phase disorder, non–24-hour sleep–wake disorder, irregular sleep–wake rhythm disorder, shift work disorder, and jet lag disorder. Appropriately timed bright light or melatonin have been recommended to treat these disorders. Despite the potential for physical activity to treat circadian rhythm sleep–wake disorders, no studies have yet documented the influence of physical activity on groups with advanced sleep–wake phase disorder, delayed sleep–wake phase disorder, non–24-hour sleep–wake disorder, or irregular sleep–wake rhythm disorder. This may be one reason that the American Academy of Sleep Medicine currently does not recommend that timed physical activity be used to treat these disorders.

Physical activity has the potential to aid in the treatment of circadian rhythm sleep–wake disorders. Multiple experiments in rodents and humans have shown that a single bout of exercise can cause circadian phase shifts.[62,63] Moderate intensity physical activity of 1–3 hours completed in the late night/early morning produces phase delays in the human circadian system, while evening exercise produces phase advances. The largest study conducted in this area showed that the average magnitude of both the phase advance and phase delay after 1 hour of stair walking was about 45 minutes.[64] It has been hypothesized that this effect is caused by exercise-induced changes in melatonin acting on melatonin receptors on the suprachiasmatic nuclei (SCN) or exercise-stimulated serotonergic input to the SCN from the median raphe.[65] Late night bright light 4 hours prior to early morning exercise has an additive phase-delaying effect.[66] The influence of exercise training on circadian rhythms is less well studied and understood. In one study, ten 70-year-old healthy men adopted a 3-month supervised aerobic exercise program and circadian rest–activity rhythms were assessed using wrist actigraphy. Compared to a control group of 8 healthy men who did not adopt the exercise program, the active men showed a significant reduction in the fragmentation of the rest–activity rhythm.[67]

Shift workers frequently have disturbed sleep–wake cycles, and they engage in less sustained moderate and vigorous leisure time physical activity.[68] At least one study found that exercise during work is likely to be beneficial for shift workers. Compared to sedentary controls, experimental participants who cycled for 15-minutes every hour during the first 3 of 8 consecutive simulated night shifts more frequently exhibited large, appropriate phase delays (63% of the exercisers vs. 38% of the controls).[69]

A limited amount of evidence suggests that physical activity may be able to treat jet lag. Physical activity hastened entrainment to a simulated phase advance of 8 hours in hamsters.[70] In humans, one study of urinary corticosteroid rhythms in 10 airline crewmembers found that outdoor exercise facilitated rhythm resynchronization 4 days after a return flight across eight time zones from Tokyo to Los Angeles.[71] The absence of large field studies and the modest effect sizes of the studies conducted to date have led some clinicians to question the usefulness of exercise in the management of jet lag[72]; more data are needed from well-designed studies to resolve the issue.

Physical Activity and Parasomnias

Parasomnias, characterized by abnormal activity of the nervous system during sleep, can emerge during REM or NREM sleep. NREM parasomnias, including sleep terrors, sleepwalking disorder, and confusional arousals, can occur when the cortex incompletely activates from slow wave sleep. REM sleep behavior disorder is a clinically important REM parasomnia because it may herald the onset of neurodegenerative diseases and is associated with the lack of usual atonia in REM, which can result in physically "acting out" dreams. Medications and cognitive-behavioral therapies can be used to treat parasomnias, but there is an absence of high-level evidence documenting the efficacy of any treatment for parasomnias.

The influence of acute or chronic physical activity on parasomnias has been infrequently researched. At least two studies suggest benefits of physical activity for parasomnias. The risk of a parasomniac event was reduced by 40% when sleep was preceded by "heavy" daytime physical activity in Nigerian university students who self-reported sleep and physical activity in a diary for 14 continuous days.[73] Fewer parasomniac events were reported in a sample of 207 regularly active middle-aged Japanese women compared to a group of 567 inactive women.[74] Conversely, at least two studies showed no strong association between physical activity and parasomniac events. Self-reported parasomnias were not significantly more or less common in physically active compared to inactive groups in a study of Brazilian elementary school children.[75] The prevalence of apparent REM behavior disorder did not differ between physically active and inactive groups in a community sample of 3,635 older adult residents of Shanghai who were free of dementia and Parkinson's disease.[76] In sum, the available evidence, which is correlational and shows mixed results, is insufficient to determine whether physical activity influences parasomnias.

Effects of Integrative Exercise on Sleep

Physical activity is a complex stimulus, the features of which can be difficult to measure and isolate in real-world settings. Most of the published research on physical activity and sleep has used modes of physical activity that permit relatively easy scientific quantification of some aspects of the stimulus, such as leg cycling (or treadmill walking) at a specified power output (or treadmill speed and grade) for a specific amount of time and over a certain number of weeks. Integrative exercise modes, such as yoga, Tai Chi, and Qigong, add additional layers of complexity. These modes of physical activity combine movement with controlled breathing, a dimension of focused attention (meditation, mindfulness, relaxation), and at times are performed with the addition of chanting or activity partners or in unique environments such as heated rooms.

Integrative exercise modes have become increasingly popular among Western practitioners and researchers in recent years. However, it is important to acknowledge that results from integrative exercise studies are more difficult to interpret because it is less certain which feature of the experience caused the outcome, even when a randomized controlled trial design is used. For example, if patients with attention deficit hyperactivity disorder perform a single bout of hot yoga in a group setting and sleep better compared to a non-exercise control condition in which sleep was unchanged, it would be unclear if the positive effects on sleep were attributable to the heat, the exercise, the mindfulness, the social interaction, or some combination of these factors. In this section, we will not reiterate the information about yoga presented in an earlier section of this chapter, but rather what follows is a succinct summary of what is known about sleep and the traditional Chinese exercises of Tai Chi and Qigong based on available quantitative reviews.

One meta-analysis examined the influence of adopting 1–4 months of Qigong on sleep quality. The analysis looked at 14 prospective studies involving 1,182 adult Chinese participants with insomnia symptoms. All the studies involved Baduanjin, a popular form of Qigong in China, which involves low-intensity movements, postures, and stretches combined with controlled breathing and meditation. Large post-intervention improvements were found in self-reported sleep quality as measured by the Pittsburgh Sleep Quality Index.[77]

A separate meta-analysis quantified the influence of Tai Chi on sleep quality in adults. Tai Chi is a traditional Chinese activity that has substantial overlap with Qigong; both practices involve a series of flowing low-impact, low-intensity movements combined with attention being paid to breathing, coordination, and relaxation.[78] The influence of 6–24 weeks of Tai Chi on self-reported sleep quality was quantified in a meta-analysis of nine randomized controlled trials with 660 adults. Most of the participants were older adults, and about one-third of the samples had chronic medical conditions such as fibromyalgia or a cerebrovascular disorder. Compared to non-exercise controls, a large mean post-intervention improvement (standardized mean effect of 0.89) was found in self-reported sleep quality.[79]

These meta-analyses support the idea that integrative exercises, including yoga, Qigong, and Tai Chi, improve sleep quality, and the results are generally consistent with previous literature reviews.[80] These results should be interpreted with caution, however, because of weaknesses in the study designs and the absence of compelling placebo conditions or objective measures of sleep.

Influence of Sleep on Physical Activity

Over the past decade, researchers have begun to examine whether sleep influences the next day's physical activity. The weight of the available evidence is mixed because studies have found that greater sleep duration or sleep quality is associated with more,[81,82] less,[83–86] and no change[87–90] in the next day's physical activity. Reasons for the differences among results are unclear but likely stem in part from variations in the samples tested (e.g., children vs. adults), the analytic procedures used, and the methods by which both sleep and physical activity were measured (e.g., subjective vs. objective). The effect of sleep on physical activity appears to be small in the larger studies that used objective measures. For example, longer sleep duration was associated with a next-day reduction in sedentary time and an increase in both light and moderate to vigorous physical activity in a study of 5,779 children aged 9–11 years who wore accelerometers. However, for every hour increase in sleep duration, sedentary behavior decreased by 3 minutes, while low and moderate/vigorous activity increased by only 2 minutes and less than 1 minute, respectively.[91]

There is increasing interest in whether changes in sleep can enhance the performance of athletes. A small body of research indicates that one night of sleep deprivation has little effect on maximal strength or performance in short-duration, high-power/high-output tasks, such as an all-out 15- or 30-second cycling sprint, while detrimental effects on performance were more likely with endurance tasks.[92,93] For example, one well-designed study showed that the distance covered during an all-out 30-minute treadmill run was 2.9% worse (the distance run was less for 9 of 11 participants) after a night of sleep deprivation compared to a full night of sleep.[94] A few studies of short-term partial sleep deprivation (e.g., 3 days of 5 hours sleep per night) showed little effect on athletic performance.[95-97] One study of 112 adolescent athletes found that those who slept an average of less than 8 hours per night were 1.7 times more likely to suffer from a sports-related injury compared with athletes who slept 8 or more hours per night.[98] Experiments that increased sleep duration (sleep extension) in athletes for 1–6 weeks showed associated improvements in basketball shooting and tennis serve accuracy.[99,100] The accuracy of these studies is uncertain, however, because of major flaws in the design of these studies, including the failure to use a control group. The tennis study failed to document if serve speed was maintained, which is important because it is well-established that greater accuracy can be obtained by reducing movement speed. More well-designed studies are needed to confirm whether sleep extension improves athletic performance.

Conclusion

The available evidence supports that acute and chronic physical activity is associated with small improvements in sleep in healthy adults. The evidence also implies that clinicians can safely recommend the adoption and maintenance of regular physical activity as an adjunctive therapy for insomnia and obstructive sleep apnea patients. Integrative exercise modes, such as yoga, Tai Chi, and Qigong, are associated with improvements in sleep quality. Worse sleep after exercise has occasionally been documented, for example in a small sample of type 1 diabetics, but none of the dozens of other studies reviewed reported a consistent pattern of adverse effects of physical activity on sleep. Clinicians, who should consider probable benefits and harms in deciding whether to prescribe exercise, are generally aware of the large body of literature showing health benefits of physical activity, including in the management of diabetes.

Based on the available research, the specific conclusions were that (1) healthy people who engage in a single bout of physical activity show small sleep benefits compared to a day in which no physical activity was performed; (2) healthy sedentary people who adopt a program of regular physical activity show improvements in sleep after the exercise training, especially in perceived sleep quality; (3) physical activity and cardiorespiratory fitness are associated with reduced sleep complaints, while a small number of randomized trials with insomnia patients supports that regular physical activity can improve their sleep; (4) regular physical activity reduces the severity of obstructive sleep apnea and improves daytime sleepiness in these patients; (5) the adoption of an exercise training program reduces symptoms of RLS in patients with kidney disease, but the evidence is uncertain whether physical activity improves RLS in other patient groups; (6) physical activity has the potential to treat circadian rhythm sleep–wake disorders because a single bout of appropriately timed exercise can cause circadian phase shifts, although experiments testing this possibility in sleep disorder patients remain to be conducted; and (7) it is uncertain if physical activity impacts the sleep of patients with narcolepsy or parasomnias.

REFERENCES

1. Berryman JW. Motion and rest: Galen on exercise and health. *Lancet.* 2012;380(9838):210–211. doi:10.1016/s0140-6736(12)61205-7. PMID: 22826836.
2. Physical Activity Guidelines Advisory Committee. *Physical activity guidelines advisory committee scientific report.* Washington, DC: US Department of Health and Human Services;2018.
3. Shan Z, Ma H, Xie M, et al. Sleep duration and risk of type 2 diabetes: A meta-analysis of prospective studies. *Diabetes Care.* 2015;38(3):529–537.
4. Sofi F, Cesari F, Casini A, Macchi C, Abbate R, Gensini GF. Insomnia and risk of cardiovascular disease: A meta-analysis. *Eur J Prevent Cardiol.* 2014;21(1):57–64.
5. Sateia MJ. International classification of sleep disorders-third edition. *Chest.* 2014;146(5):1387–1394.
6. Kredlow MA, Capozzoli MC, Hearon BA, Calkins AW, Otto MW. The effects of physical activity on sleep: A meta-analytic review. *J Behav Med.* 2015;38(3):427–449.
7. Youngstedt SD, O'Connor PJ, Dishman RK. The effects of acute exercise on sleep: A quantitative synthesis. *Sleep.* 1997;20(3):203–214.
8. Kovacevic A, Mavros Y, Heisz JJ, Fiatarone Singh MA. The effect of resistance exercise on sleep: A systematic review of randomized controlled trials. *Sleep Med Rev.* 2018;39:52–68. doi:10.1016/j.smrv.2017.07.002. Epub 2017 Jul 19. PMID: 28919335.
9. Youngstedt S, Kripke D, Elliott J. Is sleep disturbed by vigorous late-night exercise? *Med Sci Sports Exercise.* 1999;31(6):864–869.
10. Brand S, Kalak N, Gerber M, Kirov R, Pühse U, Holsboer-Trachsler E. High self-perceived exercise exertion before bedtime is associated with greater objectively assessed sleep efficiency. *Sleep Med.* 2014;15(9):1031–1036.
11. Herrick JE, Puri S, Richards KC. Resistance training does not alter same-day sleep architecture in institutionalized older adults. *J Sleep Research.* 2018;27(4):e12590. doi:10.1111/jsr.12590. Epub 2017 Aug 10. PMID: 28795452; PMCID: PMC5809228.
12. Kurka JM. *Effects of physical activity on sleep in sedentary adults with sleep problems.* Tucson: Arizona State University; 2016.
13. Reddy R, El Youssef J, Winters-Stone K, et al. The effect of exercise on sleep in adults with type 1 diabetes. *Diabetes Obesity Metabol.* 2017:1–5.
14. Petit J-M, Burlet-Godinot S, Magistretti PJ, Allaman I. Glycogen metabolism and the homeostatic regulation of sleep. *Metabol Brain Dis.* 2015;30(1):263–279.
15. Buman MP KA. Exercise as a treatment to enhance sleep. *Am J Lifestyle Med.* 2010;4(6):500–514.

16. Cassidy S, Chau JY, Catt M, Bauman A, Trenell MI. Low physical activity, high television viewing and poor sleep duration cluster in overweight and obese adults: A cross-sectional study of 398,984 participants from the UK Biobank. *Int J Behav Nutrit Phys Act*. 2017;14(1):57.

17. Gerber M, Lindwall M, Börjesson M, Hadzibajramovic E, Jonsdottir IH. Low leisure-time physical activity, but not shift-work, contributes to the development of sleep complaints in Swedish health care workers. *Mental Health Physical Act*. 2017;13(Suppl C):22–29.

18. Rogers L, Hopkins-Price P, Vicari S, et al. A randomized trial to increase physical activity in breast cancer survivors. *Med Sci Sports Exercise*. 2009;41:935–946.

19. Breneman CB, Kline CE, West DS, et al. The effect of moderate-intensity exercise on nightly variability in objectively measured sleep parameters among older women. *Behav Sleep Med*. 2017:1–11.

20. Ohayon MM. Epidemiology of insomnia: What we know and what we still need to learn. *Sleep Med Rev*. 2002;6(2):97–111.

21. Baglioni C, Battagliese G, Feige B, et al. Insomnia as a predictor of depression: A meta-analytic evaluation of longitudinal epidemiological studies. *J Affect Dis*. 2011;135(1):10–19.

22. Francesco S, Francesca C, Alessandro C, Claudio M, Rosanna A, Gian Franco G. Insomnia and risk of cardiovascular disease: A meta-analysis. *Eur J Prevent Cardiol*. 2012;21(1):57–64.

23. Qaseem A, Kansagara D, Forciea M, Cooke M, Denberg TD, for the Clinical Guidelines Committee of the American College of P. Management of chronic insomnia disorder in adults. *Ann Intern Med*. 2016;165(2):125–133.

24. Buman MP, Phillips BA, Youngstedt SD, Kline CE, Hirshkowitz M. Does nighttime exercise really disturb sleep? Results from the 2013 national sleep foundation sleep in America poll. *Sleep Med*. 2014;15(7):755–761.

25. Youngstedt SD, Kline CE. Epidemiology of exercise and sleep. *Sleep Biol Rhythms*. 2006;4(3):215–221.

26. Chen L-J, Steptoe A, Chen Y-H, Ku P-W, Lin C-H. Physical activity, smoking, and the incidence of clinically diagnosed insomnia. *Sleep Med*. 2017;30(Suppl C):189–194.

27. Loprinzi PD, Loenneke JP. Engagement in muscular strengthening activities is associated with better sleep. *Prevent Med Rep*. 2015;2(Suppl C):927–929.

28. Loprinzi PD, Cardinal BJ. Association between objectively-measured physical activity and sleep, NHANES 2005–2006. *Mental Health Physical Act*. 2011;4(2):65–69.

29. Strand LB, Laugsand LE, Wisløff U, Nes BM, Vatten L, Janszky I. Insomnia symptoms and cardiorespiratory fitness in healthy individuals: The Nord-Trøndelag Health Study (Hunt). *Sleep*. 2013;36(1):99–108C.

30. Dishman RK, Sui X, Church TS, Kline CE, Youngstedt SD, Blair SN. Decline in cardiorespiratory fitness and odds of incident sleep complaints. *Med Sci Sports Exercise*. 2015;47(5):960–966.

31. Rubio-Arias JÁ, Marín-Cascales E, Ramos-Campo DJ, Hernandez AV, Pérez-López FR. Effect of exercise on sleep quality and insomnia in middle-aged women: A systematic review and meta-analysis of randomized controlled trials. *Maturitas.*100:49–56.

32. Mustian KM, Janelsins M, Peppone LJ, Kamen C. Yoga for the treatment of insomnia among cancer patients: Evidence, mechanisms of action, and clinical recommendations. *Oncol Hematol Rev.* 2014;10(2):164–168.

33. Mustian KM, Sprod LK, Janelsins M, et al. Multicenter, randomized controlled trial of yoga for sleep quality among cancer survivors. *J Clin Oncol.* 2013;31(26):3233–3241.

34. Guilleminault C, Clerk A, Black J, Labanowski M, Pelayo R, Claman D. Nondrug treatment trials in psychophysiologic insomnia. *Arch Intern Med.* 1995;155(8):838–844.

35. Passos GS, Poyares D, Santana MG, et al. Effects of moderate aerobic exercise training on chronic primary insomnia. *Sleep Med.* 2011;12(10):1018–1027.

36. Reid KJ, Baron KG, Lu B, Naylor E, Wolfe L, Zee PC. Aerobic exercise improves self-reported sleep and quality of life in older adults with insomnia. *Sleep Med.* 2010;11(9):934–940.

37. Tan X, Alén M, Wiklund P, Partinen M, Cheng S. Effects of aerobic exercise on home-based sleep among overweight and obese men with chronic insomnia symptoms: A randomized controlled trial. *Sleep Med.* 2016;25(Suppl C):113–121.

38. Kendzerska T, Mollayeva T, Gershon AS, Leung RS, Hawker G, Tomlinson G. Untreated obstructive sleep apnea and the risk for serious long-term adverse outcomes: A systematic review. *Sleep Med Rev.* 2014;18(1):49–59.

39. Moreno CRC, Carvalho FA, Lorenzi C, et al. High risk for obstructive sleep apnea in truck drivers estimated by the Berlin questionnaire: Prevalence and associated factors. *Chronobiol Int.* 2004;21(6):871–879.

40. Hong S, Dimsdale J. Physical activity and perception of energy and fatigue in obstructive sleep apnea. *Med Sci Sports Exercise.* 2003;35(7):1088–1092.

41. Peppard PE, Young T. Exercise and sleep-disordered breathing: An association independent of body habitus. *Sleep.* 2004;27(3):480–484.

42. Aiello KD, Caughey WG, Nelluri B, Sharma A, Mookadam F, Mookadam M. Effect of exercise training on sleep apnea: A systematic review and meta-analysis. *Respir Med.* 2016;116(Suppl C):85–92.

43. Iftikhar IH, Kline CE, Youngstedt SD. Effects of exercise training on sleep apnea: A meta-analysis. *Lung.* 2014;192(1):175–184.

44. Koo BB. Restless leg syndrome across the globe: Epidemiology of the restless legs syndrome/Willis-Ekbom Disease. *Sleep Med Clin.* 2015;10(3):189–205.

45. Dishman RK, Berthoud H-R, Booth FW, et al. Neurobiology of exercise. *Obesity.* 2006;14(3):345–356.

46. Winkelman JW, Armstrong MJ, Allen RP, Chaudhuri KR, Ondo W, Trenkwalder C, Zee PC, Gronseth GS, Gloss D, Zesiewicz T. Practice guideline summary: Treatment of restless legs syndrome in adults. Report of the Guideline Development, Dissemination, and Implementation Subcommittee

of the American Academy of Neurology. *Neurology.* 2016;87(24):2585–2593. doi:10.1212/WNL.0000000000003388. Epub 2016 Nov 16. PMID: 27856776; PMCID: PMC5206998.

47. Phillips B, Young T, Finn L, Asher K, Hening WA, Purvis C. Epidemiology of restless legs symptoms in adults. *Arch Intern Med.* 2000;160(14):2137–2141.

48. Ohayon MM, Roth T. Prevalence of restless legs syndrome and periodic limb movement disorder in the general population. *J Psychosomatic Res.* 2002;53(1):547–554.

49. Fagundes SBR, Fagundes DJL, Luna AA, Bacci A, Waisberg M. Prevalence of restless legs syndrome in runners. *Sleep Med.* 2012;13(6):771.

50. Högl B, Kiechl S, Willeit J, et al. Restless legs syndrome: A community-based study of prevalence, severity, and risk factors. *Neurology.* 2005;64(11):1920–1924.

51. Kim J, Choi C, Shin K, et al. Prevalence of restless legs syndrome and associated factors in the Korean adult population: The Korean Health and Genome Study. *Psychiatry Clin Neurosci.* 2005;59–3):350–353.

52. Giannaki CD, Hadjigeorgiou GM, Karatzaferi C, et al. A single-blind randomized controlled trial to evaluate the effect of 6 months of progressive aerobic exercise training in patients with uraemic restless legs syndrome. *Nephrol Dialysis Transplant.* 2013;28(11):2834–2840.

53. Mortazavi M, Vahdatpour B, Ghasempour A, et al. Aerobic exercise improves signs of restless leg syndrome in end stage renal disease patients suffering chronic hemodialysis. *Sci World J.* 2013;2013:4.

54. Sakkas GK, Hadjigeorgiou GM, Karatzaferi C, et al. Intradialytic aerobic exercise training ameliorates symptoms of restless legs syndrome and improves functional capacity in patients on hemodialysis: A pilot study. *ASAIO J.* 2008;54(2):185–190.

55. Aukerman MM, Aukerman D, Bayard M, Tudiver F, Thorp L, Bailey B. Exercise and restless legs syndrome: A randomized controlled trial. *J Am Board Fam Med.* 2006;19(5):487–493.

56. Esteves AM, De Mello MT, Pradell-Hallinan M, Tufik S. Effect of acute and chronic physical exercise on patients with periodic leg movements. *Med Sci Sports Exercise.* 2009;41(1):237–242.

57. Mello MTD, Lauro FAA, Silva AC, Tufik S. Incidence of periodic leg movements and of the restless legs syndrome during sleep following acute physical activity in spinal cord injury subjects. *Spinal Cord.* 1996;34:294.

58. Daniels E, King MA, Smith IE, Shneerson JM. Health-related quality of life in narcolepsy. *J Sleep Res.* 2001;10(1):75–81.

59. Overeem S, van Nues SJ, van der Zande WL, Donjacour CE, van Mierlo P, Lammers GJ. The clinical features of cataplexy: A questionnaire study in narcolepsy patients with and without hypocretin-1 deficiency. *Sleep Med.* 2011;12(1):12–18.

60. Bruck D, Kennedy GA, Cooper A, Apel S. Diurnal actigraphy and stimulant efficacy in narcolepsy. *Hum Psychopharmacol Clin Exp.* 2005;20(2):105–113.

61. España RA, McCormack SL, Mochizuki T, Scammell TE. Running promotes wakefulness and increases cataplexy in orexin knockout mice. *Sleep.* 2007;30(11):1417–1425.

62. Edgar DM DW. Regularly scheduled voluntary exercise synchronizes the mouse circadian clock. *Am J Physiol Regulatory, Integrative Comparative Physiol.* 1991;261(4):R928–R933.

63. Van Reeth O SJ, Byrne MM. Nocturnal exercise phase delays circadian rhythms of melatonin and thyrotropin secretion in normal men. *Am J Physiol Endocrinology Metabol.* 1994;266(6):E964–E974.

64. Buxton OM LC, l'Hermite-Baleriaux M, Turek FW. Exercise elicits phase shifts and acute alterations of melatonin that vary with circadian phase. *Am J Physiol Regulatory, Integrative Comparative Physiol.* 2003;284(3):R714–R724.

65. Cuesta M, Boudreau P, Boivin DB. Basic circadian timing and sleep–wake regulation. In Chokroverty S, ed. *Sleep disorders medicine: Basic science, technical considerations and clinical aspects.* New York: Springer New York; 2017: 79–102.

66. Youngstedt SD, Kline CE, Elliott JA, Zielinski MR, Devlin TM, Moore TA. Circadian phase-shifting effects of bright light, exercise, and bright light + exercise. *J Circadian Rhythms.* 2016;14:2.

67. Someren EJWV, Lijzenga C, Mirmiran M, Swaab DF. Long-term fitness training improves the circadian rest-activity rhythm in healthy elderly males. *J Biol Rhythms.* 1997;12(2):146–156.

68. Loprinzi PD. The effects of shift work on free-living physical activity and sedentary behavior. *Prevent Med.* 2015;76(Suppl C):43–47.

69. Eastman CI, Hoese EK, Youngstedt SD, Liu L. Phase-shifting human circadian rhythms with exercise during the night shift. *Physiol Behav.* 1995;58(6):1287–1291.

70. Mrosovsky N, Salmon PA. A behavioural method for accelerating re-entrainment of rhythms to new light-dark cycles. *Nature.* 1987;330(6146):372–373.

71. Shiota M SM, Ohshima M. Using outdoor exercise to decrease jet lag in airline crewmembers. *Aviation Space Environ Med.* 1996;67(12):1155–1160.

72. Sack RL. Jet lag. *N Engl J Med.* 2010;362(5):440–447.

73. Oluwole OSA. Lifetime prevalence and incidence of parasomnias in a population of young adult Nigerians. *J Neurol.* 2010;257(7):1141–1147.

74. Mizuno KOH, Kunii M, Seita T, Ono S, Komada Y, Shirakawa S. Effects of habitual exercise on sleep habits and sleep health in middle-aged and older japanese women. *Jap J Phys Fitness Sports Med.* 2004;53(5):527–536.

75. Ruotolo F, Prado LBF, Ferreira VR, Prado GF, Carvalho LBC. Intake of stimulant foods is associated with development of parasomnias in children. *Arquivos de Neuro-Psiquiatria.* 2016;74:62–66.

76. Ma J-F, Qiao Y, Gao X, et al. A community-based study of risk factors for probable rapid eye movement sleep behavior disorder. *Sleep Med.* 2017;30(Suppl C):71–76.

77. Jiang Y-H, Tan C, Yuan S. Baduanjin exercise for insomnia: A systematic review and meta-analysis. *Behav Sleep Med.* 2017:1–13.

78. Abbott R, Lavretsky H. Tai chi and qigong for the treatment and prevention of mental disorders. *Psychiatric Clin N Am.* 2013;36(1):109–119.

79. Raman G, Zhang Y, Minichiello VJ, D'Ambrosio CM, Wang C. Tai chi improves sleep quality in healthy adults and patients with chronic conditions: A systematic review and meta-analysis. *J Sleep Dis Therapy*. 2013;2(6):141.

80. Sarris J, Byrne GJ. A systematic review of insomnia and complementary medicine. *Sleep Med Rev*. 2011;15(2):99–106.

81. Hart CN, Hawley N, Davey A, et al. Effect of experimental change in children's sleep duration on television viewing and physical activity. *Pediatr Obesity*. 2017;12(6):462–467.

82. Dzierzewski JM, Buman MP, Giacobbi PR, et al. Exercise and sleep in community-dwelling older adults: Evidence for a reciprocal relationship. *J Sleep Res*. 2014;23(1):61–68.

83. Sorić M, Starc G, Borer KT, et al. Associations of objectively assessed sleep and physical activity in 11-year old children. *Ann Hum Biol*. 2015;42(1):31–37.

84. Pesonen A-K, Sjöstén NM, Matthews KA, et al. Temporal associations between daytime physical activity and sleep in children. *PloS One*. 2011;6(8):e22958.

85. McNarry MA, Stevens D, Stone M, Roberts S, Hall S, Mackintosh KA. Physical activity, sedentary time and sleep in cystic fibrosis youth: A bidirectional relationship? *Pediatr Pulmonol*. 2021;56(2):450–456. doi:10.1002/ppul.25185. Epub 2020 Dec 8. PMID: 33236848.

86. Bouwmans MEJ, Oude Oosterik NAM, Bos EH, de Groot IW, Oldehinkel AJ, de Jonge P. The temporal order of changes in physical activity and subjective sleep in depressed versus nondepressed individuals: Findings from the Moovd Study. *Behav Sleep Med*. 2018;16(2):154–168.

87. Ekstedt M, Nyberg G, Ingre M, Ekblom Ö, Marcus C. Sleep, physical activity and BMI in six to ten-year-old children measured by accelerometry: A cross-sectional study. *Int J Behav Nutrit Phys Act*. 2013;10(1):82.

88. Vincent GE, Barnett LM, Lubans DR, Salmon J, Timperio A, Ridgers ND. Temporal and bidirectional associations between physical activity and sleep in primary school-aged children. *Appl Physiol Nutrit Metabol*. 2016;42(3):238–242.

89. Youngstedt SD, Perlis ML, O'Brien PM, et al. No association of sleep with total daily physical activity in normal sleepers. *Physiol Behav*. 2003;78(3):395–401.

90. Nixon GM, Thompson JMD, Han DY, et al. Short sleep duration in middle childhood: Risk factors and consequences. *Sleep*. 2008;31(1):71–78.

91. Lin Y, Tremblay MS, Katzmarzyk PT, Fogelholm M, Hu G, Lambert EV, Maher C, Maia J, Olds T, Sarmiento OL, Standage M, Tudor-Locke C, Chaput JP; ISCOLE Research Group. Temporal and bi-directional associations between sleep duration and physical activity/sedentary time in children: An international comparison. *Prevent Med*. 2018;111:436–441. doi:10.1016/j.ypmed.2017.12.006. Epub 2017 Dec 7. PMID: 29223790.

92. Reilly T, Piercy M. The effect of partial sleep deprivation on weight-lifting performance. *Ergonomics*. 1994;37(1):107–115.

93. Thun E, Bjorvatn B, Flo E, Harris A, Pallesen S. Sleep, circadian rhythms, and athletic performance. *Sleep Med Rev*. 2015;23:1–9.

94. Oliver SJ, Costa RJS, Laing SJ, Bilzon JLJ, Walsh NP. One night of sleep deprivation decreases treadmill endurance performance. *Eur J Appl Physiol.* 2009;107(2):155–161.

95. Vardar SA, Öztürk L, Kurt C, Bulut E, Sut N, Vardar E. Sleep deprivation induced anxiety and anaerobic performance. *J Sports Sci Med.* 2007;6(4):532–537.

96. Mougin F, Bourdin H, Simon-Rigaud ML, Didier JM, Toubin G, Kantelip JP. Effects of a selective sleep deprivation on subsequent anaerobic performance. *Int J Sports Med.* 1996;17(02):115–119.

97. Souissi N, Souissi M, Souissi H, et al. Effect of time of day and partial sleep deprivation on short-term, high-power output. *Chronobiol Int.* 2008;25(6):1062–1076.

98. Milewski MD, Skaggs DL, Bishop GA, et al. Chronic lack of sleep is associated with increased sports injuries in adolescent athletes. *J Pediatr Orthopaed.* 2014;34(2):129–133.

99. Schwartz J, Simon RD. Sleep extension improves serving accuracy: A study with college varsity tennis players. *Physiol Behav.* 2015;151:541–544.

100. Mah CD, Mah KE, Kezirian EJ, Dement WC. The effects of sleep extension on the athletic performance of collegiate basketball players. *Sleep.* 2011;34(7):943–950.

10

The Gastrointestinal System, Nutrition, and Sleep

JOSÉ COLÓN

Sleep and watchfulness, both of them, when immoderate, constitute disease.

—Hippocrates

Earth and life have rhythms. The sun rises in the morning and sets in the evening, forming the basis of the circadian rhythm. Innumerable other rhythms exist as well, including temperature, seasons, and atmospheric pressure. Over hundreds of millions of years, humans have evolved in concert with these rhythms, and our bodies are physiologically attuned to them. Estrogen and progesterone cycles mirror the lunar cycle; core body temperature and cortisol levels are influenced by our sleep cycles, and melatonin levels influence sleep.

Melatonin is thought of primarily as a sleep hormone secreted by the pineal gland and regulated by the suprachiasmatic nucleus, the body's circadian pacemaker. Interestingly, the gut contains 400 times the amount of melatonin than the pineal gland. Just as our bodies have a sleep–wake cycle, so does our gastrointestinal (GI) tract and the microbiota within it. It is perhaps no wonder, then, that circadian rhythm disruptions affect the gut. This relationship is bidirectional as well: GI disturbances are associated with sleep disturbances, and alimentation of nutrients affect our sleep. Ingesting substances that harm this delicate ecosystem may lead to increased intestinal permeability and dysbiosis.[1] Disease shows up not only in the form of specific GI disorders such as gastro-esophageal reflux disease (GERD), inflammatory bowel disease (IBD), and gastroenteritis but also as systemic problems.

Sleep and the GI Tract

Traditionally, the GI system has been viewed as a means for transport of food, absorption of nutrients, and excretion of waste. These functions are regulated largely by the enteric nervous system, but, during sleep, GI function is controlled by both the autonomic nervous system and the enteric nervous system. Advancements in science have revealed that the GI tract serves other functions beyond its traditional view. The GI tract's enteric nervous system houses more neurotransmitters than the brain and makes up 70% of the entire immune system. The GI tract also contains an entire ecosystem that constitutes its microbiome. This ecosystem contains more than 400 different species, leading to approximately 100 trillion bacteria, 10 times more than the amount of cells we have in our entire body. The microbiome assists in the breakdown of food to make nutrients more available, and it also serves to inhibit pathogenic bacteria, protect the intestinal lining through formation of a gut mucosal layer, and communicate with the enteric immune system.

The GI tract is one of the largest organs in our body, and its surface area has been argued to equal the size of tennis court. In a lifetime, literally tons of food are ingested, and this food must be broken down, processed, sorted, and then used or eliminated. In the esophagus, there is little absorption but rapid movement, whereas greater absorption occurs in the small bowel and colon and transit is slower. Changes in GI function occur during sleep, and patients with GI disease may complain of sleep disorders. The opposite is true as well: patients with disrupted sleep may exhibit GI symptoms.[2]

Gastric acid secretion occurs in a circadian pattern, with peak secretion between 10 PM and 2 AM, while the nadir occurs around the time of morning awakening. This is influenced by vagal tone. During sleep, swallowing, motility, and acid clearance are reduced, as is the production of saliva that acts as a buffer to acid. These factors may lead to an increase in symptoms of GERD, which in turn may lead to more frequent arousals.

Sleep also has effects on upper GI function. Tonic activity of the stomach and small bowel is reduced during sleep. This decrease appears to be secondary to circadian rhythm rather that to sleep cycles.[3]

Intestinal activity may affect sleep. An example of this would be postprandial somnolence, which is likely related to a combination of intestinal activity and macronutrient composition, as sleep onset latency after a solid meal is shorter than that of equal volume of water.[4]

Similar to upper GI function, colonic tone is diminished during sleep, with inhibition of colonic contractions and myoelectric activity. The decrease in colonic activity appears to be more pronounced in slow wave sleep, which occurs in the first half of the night. Upon awakening from sleep, colonic activity significantly increases, which may provide a potential explanation for the common urge to defecate in the morning. Although colonic activity and tone is decreased during sleep, rectal motor activity is actually increased during sleep, though in a retrograde rather than anterograde manner.[5] These factors help explain why, in the absence of GI ailment, the urge to defecate is uncommon during sleep.

Sleep disturbances have been linked to both upper and lower GI symptoms in the general population. In one study, waking up once nightly at least four times a month was significantly associated with pain, nausea, dysphagia, diarrhea, loose stools, urgency, and a feeling of anal blockage. Trouble falling asleep was significantly associated with rectal urgency.[6]

The digestive system has intrinsic rhythms that interact dynamically with circadian rhythms. It has been demonstrated that sleep and circadian factors influence appetite, nutrient absorption, and metabolism. Disruption of sleep and circadian rhythms influence the vulnerability of digestive disorders, including reflux, ulcers, inflammatory bowel issues, irritable bowel disease, and GI cancer.[7] These disturbances have also been noted in jet lag, a circadian desynchrony, as travelers usually experience symptoms after air travel across at least two time zones. Symptoms may include disturbed sleep, daytime fatigue, decreased ability to perform mental and physical tasks, reduced alertness, and GI disturbances.

Historically, many herbal treatments used to improve sleep have also been used for GI ailments. Chamomile use dates back to ancient Egypt, and, over the ages, chamomile has had broad use, including to relieve stress, anxiety, upset stomach, and insomnia. In the United States, chamomile is best known as an ingredient in herbal teas. Similarly, passion flower has been used for both sleep and digestion. The use of passion flower goes back to Native Americans, who used the leaves to make a tea for insomnia and hysteria; it was noted to have pain relief properties as well. Modern day use of passion flower includes treating anxiety and insomnia, and it may have antispasmodic effects that promotes digestion. Interestingly, recent research suggests that melatonin may be beneficial for certain GI ailments. Though not a herb but a hormone, melatonin for GI disorders nevertheless supports an association between the gut and sleep.

Sleep and GI Disease: GERD, IBS, IBD

GERD is perhaps the best studied GI disorder during sleep. Nocturnal GERD is associated with prolonged acid contact with the mucosa during sleep, leading to greater risk of mucosal damage. Complications of nighttime GERD can lead to the development of esophagitis and acid secretion into the bronchioles, which can contribute to asthma, chronic cough, and sleep disturbances. Gastric acid secretion also plays a role in ulcers, and nocturnal acid suppression has been found to be a significant factor in healing ulcers.

Nighttime heartburn commonly results in disturbed sleep due to more frequent awakenings from pain, coughing, and choking. Patients who report heartburn at least twice per week have increased symptoms of coughing, wheezing, and daytime sleepiness.[8] This disturbed sleep may affect mood and function the following day, and nighttime GERD is associated with an increased use of sleeping pills. The use of hypnotics may lead to maladaptive behavior as it fails to address the underlying cause of poor sleep, and it may also contribute to prolonged contact of gastric acid with esophageal mucosa.

GERD has been associated with insomnia, and this is a bidirectional finding. Population studies show that the risk of reflux symptoms in insomnia patients is three times greater than in those without insomnia.[9] Overall sleep quality is negatively correlated with longer recumbent reflux events,[10] and increased nocturnal acid contact time is associated with more severe sleep complaints. Treatment of GERD has been shown to improve sleep quality. Most studies on treatment of GERD to improve sleep have been conducted with antacids such as proton pump inhibitors (PPIs). However, the pathophysiology of GERD is not due to excess acid production, but due to the presence of acid in the esophagus rather than the stomach. PPIs reduce GERD symptoms by blocking the secretion of acid but do not address the underlying problem of regurgitation of gastric lumen contents into the esophagus. While PPIs can provide valuable short-term treatment of GERD, long-term use may lead to complications, including increased risk of pneumonia, *Clostridium difficile* colitis, and decreased absorption of micronutrients such as vitamin B_{12}, calcium, magnesium, and iron.[11] Furthermore, PPI use may be detrimental to a healthy gut microbiome.[12]

Obstructive sleep apnea (OSA) is associated with reflux, and patients with OSA are often obese, another risk factor for reflux. The negative intrathoracic pressure associated with upper airway obstruction is a risk factor for GERD, and treatment of sleep apnea with continuous positive airway pressure (CPAP) has been demonstrated to reduce heartburn complaints.[13]

Positional sleeping is an effective nonpharmaceutical approach to reduce recumbent esophageal acid exposure. Sleeping with an elevated head of the bed reduces GERD, as does lying on the left versus right side or supine. When measured on impedance-pH tests, the combination of these two using a sleep positioning device is associated with less reflux.[14]

Other common integrative medicine treatment approaches to GERD include practicing relaxation techniques, keeping a food log to determine which foods trigger symptoms, eating a diet rich in fiber, reducing alcohol, and avoiding caffeine and tobacco, as well as using herbs such as deglycyrrhizinated licorice (DGL). Licorice has been shown to have anti-*Helicobacter pylori* effects.[15] Licorice extract has also been used as an alternative to bismuth for peptic ulcer disease, and it has a protective role against acid and pepsin secretions by covering the site of lesion and promoting mucous secretion.[16] Other herbal and naturopathic methods exist to treat GERD as well, beyond the scope of this chapter.

Sleep disturbances are a common complaint of patients with irritable bowel syndrome (IBS). Up to 40% of patients with IBS can have sleep complaints, and in these patients poor sleep can predict next-day symptoms.[17] The sleep disturbance is more pronounced in constipation-predominant IBS.

IBD consist of two predominant diseases: *Crohn's disease* and *ulcerative colitis*. Symptoms of IBD may include bloody diarrhea, abdominal pain, urgency and fecal incontinence, fatigue, and fever, and sleep complaints are common as well. Disturbed sleep can even be a trigger for exacerbation of symptoms, and IBD patients have a higher incidence of sleep symptoms than do controls. Interestingly, melatonin has been found to have powerful antioxidant properties and to decrease levels of inflammation. It has been proposed as a potential treatment for IBD, though more research is needed.

As previously mentioned, melatonin levels in the GI tract are noted to be 400 times higher than in the pineal gland, and there is evidence that melatonin may help treat GI disorders. Melatonin receptors can be found in the gut, and their involvement in the regulation of GI motility, inflammation, and pain has been reported in numerous basic and clinical studies. These human studies include patients with lower GI diseases, especially patients with IBS, IBD, and colorectal cancer.[18]

Sleep and the Microbiome

Rhythmicity of the intestinal microbiota is regulated by the host circadian clock. In mammals, disruption of clock gene expression through changes in the light–dark cycle have been found to alter rhythmicity in the fecal microbiota as well as its composition.[19] Intestinal dysbiosis and circadian disruption are associated with chronic diseases including obesity, metabolic syndrome, type 2 diabetes, and IBD. Restless legs syndrome (RLS), which has a circadian component, has been associated with IBS and small intestinal bacterial overgrowth.

Just as the microbiome is sensitive to the light–dark cycle, so is it sensitive to melatonin. Melatonin can influence the growth and function of certain organisms in the microbiome, and probiotics may act by influencing melatonin production.[20] In patients with irritable bowel syndrome, treatment with probiotics has been noted to increase salivary morning melatonin, and GI symptom improvement correlated with this rise in morning melatonin.

The microbiome has interconnections with mood and sleep. Depression has long been associated with sleep disorders. Depression is a complex chronic mood disorder associated with many factors, including genetics and the environment. It has recently been linked to alterations of the gut microbiota. Indeed, mood disorders are found to be associated with sleep symptoms including insomnia, excessive sleep, or loss of energy. Some improvement in objective sleep parameters and mood were found in participants treated for microbiota imbalance.[21] Evidence supports the idea that intestinal dysbiosis can profoundly affect multiple aspects of sleep, mood, and cognitive function. The delicate balance between the human microbiome and the development of psychopathologies is particularly interesting given the ease with which the microbiome can be altered by external factors such as disrupted sleep.[22]

Sleep and Appetite

Sleep doesn't waste time, it's good for the waistline.

—*Teresa Arora, PhD*[23]

The period of hunger and satiety is controlled by the central pacemaker residing in the suprachiasmatic nucleus of the hypothalamus, and it communicates with tissues via bidirectional neuronal and humoral pathways.[24] Sleep loss has effects on appetite regulation. The Sleep Debt Study showed that leptin levels and amplitude were decreased after sleep restriction when compared to sleep extension. Furthermore, sleep restriction alters the ability of leptin to accurately signal caloric needs. Sleep loss also further leads to elevated ratios of ghrelin to leptin. These factors lead to a misperception of insufficient caloric intake, leading to increased appetite.[25] Sleep loss further alters hormones that affect weight, including increased cortisol, decreased insulin sensitivity, and reduced leptin and elevated ghrelin.

Food intake studies show that when comparing sleep-restricted individuals to those with sleep extension, there is a significant increase of caloric intake from snacks in the short sleep condition.[26] One study found that short sleep of less than 6 hours' duration in young adults was associated with a particularly strong increase in appetite for foods with high carbohydrate content. The sleep-deprived brain craved its primary fuel, glucose, which the body produces from carbohydrates.[27] In a society with readily available foods and beverages, longer wake times may lead to an increased likelihood of eating or drinking. Thus, sleeping more may reduce caloric intake, especially in a nighttime snacker. It has been suggested that eliminating just 125 calories a day by sleeping instead of snacking can result in weight loss of 10 pounds in 1 year with no other dietary modification of any kind.[28] These findings are not isolated to sleep loss. As previously mentioned, GI disturbances are associated with circadian disruption and jet lag. It should be duly noted that "social jet lag" is also associated with obesity.[29]

Nutrition and Sleep

Nutrition is often an overlooked contributor to sleep disorders, but micronutrients, macronutrients, and diet can impact sleep and fatigue. It is important to consider fatigue as well, as many patients who complain of nonrestorative sleep symptoms complain of insomnia when in fact they may have a medical-nutritional cause for their fatigue.

Let food be thy medicine, and medicine be thy food.

—*Hippocrates*

B VITAMINS

B vitamins are necessary for converting food into energy. Cofactors in the mito-chondrial respiratory chain include B_1, B_2, B_3, B_5, B_6, B_{12}, and folate.[30]

Vitamin B₁ (Thiamine)

In clinical trials, thiamine supplementation of healthy elderly individuals with marginal thiamine deficiency improved their sleep. Studies of elderly women who were given thiamine supplements demonstrated a trend toward improved sleep patterns. One study showed reduced daytime sleep and increased activity, while another found a trend toward increased activity and energy.[31,32] A study looking at adults in India showed that people with insomnia consumed significantly lower quantities of nutrients as compared to normal sleepers. Differences in intakes of thiamine, folic acid, and B_{12} were noted.[33]

Vitamin B₉ (Folate)

Vitamin B_6 and folate are both cofactors for several neurotransmitters in the brain, many of which regulate sleep patterns. Folate is a water-soluble B vitamin neces-sary for the proper biosynthesis of the monoamine neurotransmitters serotonin and dopamine. Folate is one of several nutrients that have been suggested to im-prove mood and sleep.[34] Folate is equally important for GI health, as folate defi-ciency increases the risk of colorectal cancer.[35]

Vitamin B₆

Research suggests that deficiencies in vitamin B_6 promote psychological distress and ensuing sleep disturbance. Pyridoxine is a cofactor for 5-hydroxytryptophan decarboxylase, an enzyme in the biosynthesis pathway of serotonin, and serotonin levels in the brain are implicated as a mediating factor. Vitamin B_6 may improve dream recall. One study on dream salience suggests that vitamin B_6 may act by increasing cortical arousal during periods of rapid eye movement (REM) sleep.[36] Vitamin B_6 is also important for GI health as deficiency is also linked with a higher risk of developing colon cancer.[37]

Vitamin B$_{12}$ (Methylcobalamin)

Vitamin B$_{12}$ influences circadian rhythms. Therapeutic benefits of B$_{12}$ supplementation, both oral and intravenous, have been documented. Case reports document that vitamin B$_{12}$ administration has improved circadian rhythm disorders. High-dose B$_{12}$ (3,000 mcg/day) has been used to treat a 15-year-old girl with delayed sleep phase syndrome and a 17-year-old boy with free running sleep–wake disorder. Neither had clinical or laboratory evidence of B$_{12}$ deficiency or hypothyroidism, but both responded to treatment.[38] Animal models have also demonstrated that B$_{12}$ may affect polysomnographic findings.[39] It is important to note that antacid treatment with PPIs depletes B$_{12}$.

Vitamin B$_{12}$ is also important for GI health as deficiency results in the development of gastric dysmotility and its clinical consequences. Subsequent replacement therapy can improve gastric emptying in some patients with dyspepsia.

METABOLITES

Carnitine

Carnitine has been found to have a role in fatigue. Carnitine transports fatty acids into mitochondria. Carnitine decreases both mental and physical fatigue in clinical trials.[40] Carnitine also plays an important function in GI health as it has been found to be beneficial in people with colitis due to its role in fatty acid metabolism, which is often impaired in GI disorders.[41]

MINERALS

Minerals are important to quality sleep. They have been found to have a role in sleep apnea, and the trace minerals zinc, copper, magnesium, manganese, and selenium are critical cofactors for the major antioxidant enzymes, which are important in repairing cellular damage caused by hypoxemia in sleep apnea.[42]

Magnesium

Magnesium mimics the action of melatonin, and magnesium status has been correlated with quality of sleep. The widespread use of PPIs may have increased the prevalence of low magnesium levels in the population as long-term use of PPIs can lead to hypomagnesemia.

Magnesium may alleviate insomnia related to RLS. One study found that magnesium treatment may be a useful alternative therapy in patients with mild or moderate RLS- or periodic leg movement syndrome (PLMS)-related insomnia.[43] Polysomnographic data in patients with RLS and magnesium deficiency show frequent periods of nocturnal awakenings, increase of the durations and percentages of light slow wave sleep (using older polysomnographic data), a decrease of duration and percentage of deep slow wave sleep, and a decrease of duration and percentage of REM sleep.

Balanced magnesium status is required for maximal efficiency of the suprachiasmatic nucleus and the pineal gland, whose actions regulate the circadian clock. In one study, the administration of nightly melatonin, magnesium, and zinc (5 mg melatonin, 225 mg magnesium, and 11.25 mg zinc) appeared to improve the quality of sleep and the quality of life in long-term care facility residents with primary insomnia.[44] Magnesium supplementation has also been associated with improving sleep quality in adults with poor sleep at baseline, though more studies are needed.

Magnesium plays a role in fatigue. Magnesium is required to store the energy molecule adenosine triphosphate (ATP), and repletion of magnesium in chronic fatigue patients showed clinical improvement in energy levels.[45] Magnesium is equally important for GI health as it has been found that magnesium deficiency affects the microbiome.[46] This phenomenon may affect inflammation and metabolic disorders.

Zinc and Copper

Zinc and copper have roles in regulating sleep. They interact with N-methyl-D-aspartate (NMDA) receptors in the brain that regulate sleep. A higher zinc-to-copper ratio is linked to longer sleep duration, and a supplement of magnesium, zinc, and melatonin has been demonstrated to improve quality of sleep in long-term care residents with insomnia.[44] Sufficient levels of zinc are associated with good sleep quality in school-aged children, and low blood zinc concentrations in preschool-aged children predict poor sleep efficiency and quality in adolescence.[47]

In the gut, zinc supplements have been found to ameliorate Crohn's disease symptoms and decrease intestinal permeability in colitis.[48] Furthermore, zinc deficiency may exacerbate alcohol-induced intestinal barrier dysfunction.[49] This is important because some people with difficulty sleeping may misuse alcohol for its sedating effects.

ANTIOXIDANTS

It is well documented that sleep apnea patients have both reduced antioxidant capacity and higher levels of oxidative stress than controls. In one study, antioxidants with vitamin C and E were found to improve Epworth scores and increase slow wave sleep in patients with sleep apnea.[50]

Several studies have also confirmed that the symptoms related to oxidative stress include fatigue, and chronic fatigue patients have been found to have unusually low levels of glutathione.[51] Mitochondrial dysfunction (inefficient energy metabolism) can be treated therapeutically with antioxidants such as selenium, cysteine, a-lipoic acid, and glutathione.

Cysteine

Oral supplementation with cysteine, the precursor to glutathione, has therapeutic potential for sleep apnea. The number and duration of snoring episodes were significantly reduced for patients treated with N-acetyl cysteine compared to untreated sleep apnea patients.[52]

In an animal model, intermittent hypoxia was associated with a decrease in sternohyoid muscle endurance. In separate experiments, daily treatment with the antioxidant N-acetyl cysteine blocked the deleterious effects of intermittent hypoxia on respiratory muscle function. It is suggested that oxidative stress contributes to impaired upper airway muscle endurance and that endogenous glutathione may be especially important in limiting free radical-induced muscle dysfunction.[53]

CoQ10

CoQ10 has a known role in fatigue. CoQ10 deficiency causes fatigue due to its role in mitochondrial energy metabolism; therapeutic benefits are particularly noticeable in chronic fatigue syndrome.[54]

Vitamin C

Vitamin C has a known role in fatigue. It assists iron uptake and transport, and it is a precursor to carnitine and several hormones that affect energy levels. Supplementation has been found to reduce fatigue in some trials.[55] Vitamin C also has a role in sleep apnea, and it may improve endothelial function (blood vessel health) in sleep apnea patients to levels seen in people without sleep apnea.[56]

IBD is associated with higher levels of oxidative stress, and vitamin C supplementation has been found to be beneficial. Vitamin C may promote tissue healing in the GI tract, and an animal model has demonstrated that vitamin C supplementation can improve intestinal anastomosis healing.[57]

Vitamin E

Vitamin E has a role in sleep apnea. Vitamin E mitigates the oxidative stress seen in sleep apnea patients, and it works synergistically with vitamin C.[58] An inverse correlation between fatigue and vitamin E levels has also been noted.[59]

Selenium

Selenium may play a role in sleep apnea. In one case report, selenium supplementation completely stopped snoring caused by non–obesity-related sleep apnea.[60] Selenium's role as a potent antioxidant may reduce the oxidative stress seen in sleep apnea patients.[61]

Selenium also plays a role in GI health. It functions as a cofactor to glutathione peroxidase (GPx), which protects the intestinal wall from inflammatory damage.[62] Lower GPx activity due to selenium deficiency is very common in people with gut inflammation.

FATTY ACIDS

Oleic acid, a monounsaturated omega-9 fatty acid, is a precursor of oleamide, which may mediate the drive for sleep.[63] Oleamide has been shown to accumulate in the spinal fluid of sleep-deprived animals, and it induces sleep when administered experimentally to animals. Oleic acid also facilitates the absorption of vitamin A.

Sleep disturbances are one of the most frequent symptoms of depression. Low concentrations of omega-3-fatty acids might represent one determinant within that process. Negative correlations have been demonstrated between the degree of sleep disturbances and fatty acid concentrations (myristic, palmitic, palmitoleic, oleic, linoleic, eicosadienoic, and docosahexaenoic acid). Palmitoleic and oleic acid seem to be especially important for sleep disorders, possibly due to their function as precursors of the sleep-inducing oleamide. Linoleic and eicosadienoic acid may also be helpful for maintaining sleep because they are precursors of the sleep mediator PGD2.[64]

OTHER VITAMINS

Vitamin A

Studies suggest that vitamin A deficiency alters brains waves in NREM sleep, causing sleep to be less restorative. Vitamin A is the parent compound of retinoids, which regulate gene transcription by binding to nuclear retinoid receptors. Retinoid signaling mechanisms may be involved in the homeostatic component of the sleep electroencephalogram (EEG)[65] as vitamin A deficiency induces a decrease in EEG delta power during sleep in mice. The action of retinoic acid may regulate several rhythms in the brain and body, from circadian to seasonal.[66]

Vitamin A has been found to have associations with sleep apnea, and sleep apnea patients have low retinol levels (vitamin A). Retinol suppresses the growth of vascular smooth muscle, a process that causes blood vessels to clog. This may be the mechanism by which low vitamin A levels are associated with cardiovascular complications seen in sleep apnea patients.[67]

Vitamin A deficiency has been implicated in fatigue because when cellular levels of vitamin A are low, mitochondrial respiration and ATP production decreases. Vitamin A is also important to GI health as it regulates growth of epithelial cells, including those that line the GI tract.

Vitamin D

Inadequate vitamin D levels are associated with the symptoms of wake impairment commonly associated with sleep disorders. Persistent deficiency of vitamin D may also increase the risk for OSA via promotion of adenotonsillar hypertrophy, airway muscle myopathy, and/or chronic rhinitis. Additionally, emerging evidence suggests that low vitamin D levels increase the risk for autoimmune disease, chronic rhinitis, cardiovascular disease, and diabetes. These conditions are mediated by altered immunomodulation, increased propensity to infection, and increased levels of inflammatory substances, including those that regulate sleep, such as tumor necrosis factor alpha (TNF-a), interleukin (IL)-1, and prostaglandin D2 (PD2).[68]

People with sleep apnea have a high prevalence of vitamin D deficiency, and the worse the apnea, the more severe the deficiency. Evidence suggests that low vitamin D levels increase the risk of sleep apnea in heart disease.[69]

Vitamin D is important to gut health, and a deficiency of vitamin D has been linked to IBD, a greater likelihood of needing steroids for treatment of IBD, and decreased quality of life in IBD patients.[70] Vitamin D deficiency can affect the microbiome as well by reducing B vitamin production in the gut. The resulting lack of pantothenic acid adversely affects the immune system, producing a pro-inflammatory state associated with atherosclerosis and autoimmunity.[71]

MACRONUTRIENTS AND WHOLE FOODS ON SLEEP

The previous micronutrient summary demonstrates some of the myriad effects that micronutrients have on sleep and fatigue. Equally important, macronutrient intake may impact sleep. An analysis of the literature, however, does not demonstrate conclusively that one particular diet is best for sleep. Nonetheless, various literature sources suggest that a low-glycemic diet may be helpful in improving sleep quality. Based on the information presented on micronutrients, a low-glycemic diet with a high variety of whole foods is advised.

In an ancillary study of the Women's Health Initiative, food frequency questionnaires were analyzed to examine dietary intake and sleep quality. An optimal sleep time of 7–8 hours was associated with the highest variety of foods. Both short sleep time and long sleep time were associated with decreased food variety. Short sleep time was defined as less than 5 hours, and long sleep time was defined as greater than 9 hours.[72] Interestingly, these results parallel a meta-analysis that showed that both short and long sleep times are associated with cancer.[73] Though long sleep time may superficially sound desirable, studies consistently demonstrate that excessive sleep time is associated with chronic or debilitating illnesses.

In the Women's Health Initiative study, lower protein intake was associated with both short and long sleep time. Increased protein intake was associated with less difficulty falling asleep, less difficulty maintaining sleep, and less nonrestorative sleep. Another study showed protein intake at 20% of calories produced the best Global Sleep Score (GSS) regardless of quality of protein from either animal or vegetable sources.[74]

Carbohydrate consumption was also associated with less difficulty maintaining sleep, but it is important to note that this benefit is associated with complex carbohydrates as sugar intake was associated with excessive daytime sleepiness. Another study found sugar and high glycemic load to be associated with fatigue as well. A high-glycemic load diet is associated with higher depression symptoms, total mood disturbance, and fatigue compared to a low-glycemic load diet, especially in overweight/obese but otherwise healthy adults.[75] It is important to note that mood disturbances are associated with poor sleep as well. Conversely, increased fiber intake resulted in less difficulty maintaining sleep, lower likelihood of nonrestorative sleep, and less daytime sleepiness.

Although simple carbohydrates may be sedating and even decrease sleep latency,[76] consuming a high glycemic load does not equate to better sleep. It is important to remember that after surges in blood sugar, there is a subsequent drop in blood sugar 4–5 hours later. The body's homeostatic response is an increase in appetite as well as a surge of norepinephrine, which is a stimulating neuro-transmitter associated with alertness.[77] This is the same phenomena that leads to overeating and obesity. Therefore, milk and cookies before bed, though possibly-sleep inducing, are less than ideal for sleep quality. Indeed, studies evaluating high- and low-glycemic index drinks on children's sleep patterns demonstrate more sleep disturbances in the children receiving high-glycemic drinks, with polysomnography data showing more NREM over REM sleep and higher arousal indexes.[78] These data parallels findings related to the use of alcohol, in which its sedating properties can shorten sleep onset but then disrupt the second half of the sleep period.

The role of fat in the diet is controversial, in part because many studies lump all fats into one category while other studies don't account for other macronutrient composition. In the previous discussion of micronutrients, it was noted that low levels of oleic acid are associated with insomnia. In the Women's Health Initiative study, increased fat consumption was not associated with any adverse sleep symptoms, but a low-fat diet was associated with nonrestorative sleep and excessive daytime sleepiness.

Ketogenic diets have been associated with improved sleep quality and decreased fatigue. It is unclear if this is due to high fat intake or a result of a low-glycemic diet. One study found that a ketogenic diet improved sleep quality in children with therapy-resistant epilepsy. In this study, the authors found that REM sleep was increased while slow wave sleep was preserved. Daytime sleepiness was reduced, and improvements in quality of life were noted.[79] In another study, the effects of a ketogenic diet on quality of life was studied in 16 patients with advanced cancer, and an improvement in emotional functioning and less insomnia was found.[80] Last, a study looking at a very low carbohydrate (VLC) diet had mixed findings as it showed short-term increases in the percentage of slow wave sleep with a reduction in the percentage of REM sleep.[81]

As previously mentioned, high-glycemic diets are associated with fatigue. Interestingly, dietary therapy utilizing a low-carbohydrate, ketogenic diet (LCKD) have been found to be effective in improving symptoms of narcolepsy. Narcolepsy patients treated with LCKD therapy experienced modest improvements on Narcolepsy Symptoms Status Questionnaire (NSSQ).[82] The use of diet therapy in the treatment of narcolepsy is not a new concept because medications alone may not completely resolve excessive daytime sleepiness, and fewer than 15% of patients with narcolepsy rely on medications alone.[83] Dietary manipulation has been found to be a common treatment approach used by narcolepsy patients, the majority of whom did not receive counseling by their treating physician.[84]

Narcolepsy type I is a disorder of sleepiness associated with a deficiency of orexin neurons. Interestingly, high glucose levels inhibit lateral hypothalamic neurons that contain orexin.[85] The lateral hypothalamic area (LHA) is known to contain neurons that are stimulated by falls in circulating glucose but inhibited by feeding-related signals from the viscera. In diagnosing disorders of central hypersomnia such as narcolepsy, sleep clinicians are trained to keep sleep logs documenting total sleep time, but nutrition logs might also be of utility.

Other studies have shown the effects of whole foods on sleep. Phytonutrient consumption has been associated with better sleep. In a cross-sectional study of Japanese adults, higher daily isoflavone intake was positively associated with optimal sleep duration and quality.[86] Consumption of fish has also been associated with improved sleep, with one study finding that fish consumption has a positive impact on sleep in general and also on daily functioning, which may be related to vitamin D status and heart rate variability.[87] While it is well-known that melatonin affects sleep, it is important to note that it can be found in plant foods including tomatoes, walnuts, barley, strawberries, olive oil, and wine. The synthesis of melatonin requires the precursor tryptophan as well as a smoothly functioning cascade of several enzyme-based reactions, first to compose serotonin and subsequently melatonin. Several vitamins and minerals act as co-factors and activators in these processes, and a clear deficiency of needed nutrients may restrict the synthesis of melatonin.[88]

Tart cherry juice concentrate provides an increase in exogenous melatonin and may be of benefit in managing disturbed sleep. In one study, tart cherry juice was found to be beneficial in improving sleep duration and quality in healthy men and women.[89] In another pilot study, CherryPharm, a tart cherry juice blend, was noted to have modest beneficial effects on sleep in older adults with insomnia.[90]

A review of the previously described data leads to the conclusion that nutrition impacts sleep quality and fatigue. It does not appear that one isolated vitamin or mineral or macronutrient plays a definitive role in optimizing sleep, but rather that they all work together in concert. Studying individual nutrients may therefore not account for this complexity of interactions while studying dietary patterns may be more revealing.

Adherence to a Mediterranean Diet pattern has been associated with a lower risk of shortened sleep duration and better sleep quality in older adults.[91] The Mediterranean Diet is not associated with an increase of any one particular micronutrient or macronutrient. Rather it is associated with a low-glycemic index, minimally processed whole fresh foods abundant in plant-based phytonutrients, moderate protein intake with an emphasis on fish over red meat, and healthy fats such as olive oil and nuts and seeds. This variety of food intake better supplies an appropriate distribution of macronutrients and micronutrients that, as a whole, may be beneficial for sleep.

Conclusion

Sleep and the GI system are linked in numerous ways in a bidirectional fashion. While our understanding of this relationship is still not well delineated, cumulatively, the data clearly demonstrate that nutrition and GI health are impacted by the circadian rhythm and sleep, and vice versa. Intriguing areas of research remain, including in the areas of the microbiome and sleep, melatonin and its role in the GI tract, and nutrition and sleep. Though insufficient data exist to make many recommendations, a well-rounded whole foods low-glycemic diet such as the Mediterranean Diet may be beneficial to sleep health. Further studies are needed to better understand the interdependent relationship of sleep and GI health.

REFERENCES

1. Mullin GE. *Integrative gastroenterology*. New York: Oxford University Press; 2011.
2. Orr WC, Chen CL. Sleep and the gastrointestinal tract. *Neurol Clin.* 2005;23: 1007–1024.
3. Kumar D, Idzikowski C, Wingate DL, et al. Relationship between enteric migrating motor complex and the sleep cycle. *Am J Physiol.* 1990;259(6 pt 1):G983–990.
4. Orr WC, Shadid G, Harnish MJ, et al. Meal composition and its effect on postprandial sleepiness. *Physiol Behav.* 1997;62:709–712.
5. Orkin BA, Hanson RB, Kelly KA, et al. Human anal motility while fasting, after feeding, and during sleep. *Gastroenterology.* 2000;95:1195–1200.
6. Cremonini F, Camilleri M, Zinsmeister AR, Herrick LM, Beebe T, Talley NJ. Sleep disturbances are linked to both upper and lower gastrointestinal symptoms in the general population. *Neurogastroenterol Motil.* 2009 Feb;21(2):128–135.
7. Vaughn B, Rotolo S, Roth H. Circadian rhythm and sleep influences on digestive physiology and disorders. *ChronoPhysiol Therapy.* 2014 Sep;4:67–77.
8. Gisalson T, Janson C, Vermeire P, et al. Respiratory symptoms and nocturnal gastroesophageal reflux. *Chest.* 2002;121:158–163.
9. Jansson et. al. A population-based study showing an association between gastroesophageal reflux disease and sleep problems. *Clin Gastroenterol Hep.* 2009:960–965.
10. Dickman et. al. Relationships between sleep quality and pH monitoring findings in persons with gastroesophageal reflux disease. *J Clin Sleep Med.* 2007:3;505–513.
11. Hess MW, et al. Systematic review: Hypomagnesaemia induced by proton pump inhibition. *Aliment Pharma Ther.* 2012;36:405.
12. Imhann F, Bonder MJ, Vich Vila A, et al. Proton pump inhibitors affect the gut microbiome. *Gut.* 2015. doi:10.1136/gutjnl-2015-310376.

13. Green BT, Broughton WA, O'Connor JB. Marked improvement in nocturnal gastro-esophageal reflux in a large cohort of patients with obstructive sleep apnea treated with continuous positive airway pressure. *Arch Intern Med.* 2003;163:341–345.

14. Person E, Rife C, Freeman J, Clark A, Castell DO. A novel sleep positioning device reduces gastroesophageal reflux: A randomized controlled trial. *J Clin Gastroenterol.* 2015 Sep;49(8):655–659.

15. Rahnama M, Mehrabani D, Japoni S, Edjtehadi M, Firoozi MS. The healing effect of licorice (*Glycyrrhiza glabra*) on *Helicobacter pylori* infected peptic ulcers. *J Res Med Sci.* 2013 Jun;18(6):532–533.

16. Asl MN, Hosseinzadeh H. Review of pharmacological effects of Glycyrrhiza sp. and its bioactive compounds. *Phytother Res.* 2008 Jun;22(6):709–724.

17. Bellini M. Evaluation of latent links between irritable bowel syndrome and sleep quality. *World J Gastrol.* 2011;17:5089–5096.

18. Chen CQ, Fichna J, Bashashati M, Li YY, Stor M. Distribution, function and physiological role of melatonin in the lower gut. *World J Gastroenterol.* 2011 Sep 14;17(34):3888–3898.

19. Voigt RM, Forsyth CB, Green SJ, et al. Circadian disorganization alters intestinal microbiota. PLoS ONE. 2014;9(5):e97500.

20. Wong RK, Yang C, Song GH, Wong J, Ho KY. Melatonin regulation as a possible mechanism for probiotic (VSL#3) in irritable bowel syndrome: A randomized double-blinded placebo study. *Dig Dis Sci.* 2015 Jan;60(1):186–194.

21. Jackson ML, Butt H, Ball M, Lewis DP, Bruck D. Sleep quality and the treatment of intestinal microbiota imbalance in Chronic Fatigue Syndrome: A pilot study. *Sleep Science.* 2015;8(3):124–133. doi:10.1016/j.slsci.2015.10.001.

22. Thaiss CA, Zeevi D, Levy M, et al. Transkingdom control of microbiota diurnal oscillations promotes metabolic homeostasis. *Cell.* 2014;159:514–529.

23. Arora T. Sleep doesn't waste time, it's good for the waist line. *Sleep.* 2015;38(8):1159–1160.

24. Konturek PC, Brzozowski T, Konturek SJ. Gut clock: Implication of circadian rhythms in the gastrointestinal tract. *J Physiol Pharmacol.* 2011 Apr;62(2):139–50.

25. Zee P. *Sleep and endocrinology. Basics of sleep guide*, 2nd ed. Darien, IL: Sleep Research Society; 2009.

26. Nedeltcheva AV, Kilkus JM, Imperial J, Kasza K, Schoeller DA, Penev PD. Sleep curtailment is accompanied by increased intake of calories from snacks. *Am J Clin Nutr.* 2009;89(1):126–133.

27. Van Cauter E. Sleep and the epidemic of obesity in children and adults. *Eur J Endocrinol.* 2008;159(S1):S59–S66.

28. Sivak M. Sleeping more as a way to lose weight. *Obesity Rev.* 2006;7(3):295–296.

29. Till Roenneberg KV, Allebrandt MM, Vetter C. Social jet lag and obesity. *Curr Biol.* 2012;22:939–943.

30. Huskisson E, Maggini S, Ruf M. The role of vitamins and minerals in energy metabolism and well-being. *J Int Med Res.* 2007;35:277–289.

31. Smidt L, Cremin F, Grivetti L, et al. Influence of thiamine supplementation on the health and general well-being of an elderly Irish population with marginal thiamine deficiency. *J Gerontol.* 1991;46:M16–M22.

32. Wilkinson T, Hanger H, Elmslie J, et al. The response to treatment of subclinical thiamine deficiency in the elderly. *Am J Clin Nutr.* 1997;66:925–928.

33. Zadeh S, Begum K. Comparison of nutrient intake by sleep status in selected adults in Mysore, India. *Nutr Res Pract.* 2011;5:230–235.

34. Larzelere M, Wiseman P. Anxiety, depression and insomnia. *Prim Care.* 2002;19:339–360.

35. Knock E, Deng L, Wu Q, et al. Low dietary folate initiates intestinal tumors in mice, with altered expression of G2-M checkpoint regulators polo-like kinase 1 and cell division cycle 25c. *Cancer Res.* 2006;66:10349–10356.

36. Ebben M, Lequerica A, Spielman A. Effects of pyridoxine on dreaming: A preliminary study. *Percept Mot Skills.* 2002;95:135–140.

37. Larsson S, Orsini N, Wolk A. Vitamin B6 and risk of colorectal cancer: A meta-analysis of prospective studies. *JAMA.* 2010;303:1077–1083.

38. Ohta T, Ando K, Iwata T, et al. Treatment of persistent sleep–wake schedule disorders in adolescents with methylcobalamin (vitamin B12). *Sleep.* 1991;14:414–418.

39. Ebihara S, Mano N, Kurono N, et al. Vitamin B12 affects non-photic entrainment of circadian locomotor activity rhythms in mice. *Brain Res.* 1996;727:31–39.

40. Malaguarnera M, Cammalleri L, et al. L-Carnitine treatment reduces severity of physical and mental fatigue and increases cognitive functions in centenarians: A randomized and controlled clinical trial. *Am J Clin Nutr.* 2007;86:1738–1744.

41. Mikhailova T, Sishkova E, Poniewierka E, et al. Randomised clinical trial: The efficacy and safety of propionyl-L carnitine therapy in patients with ulcerative colitis receiving stable oral treatment. *Aliment Pharmacol.* 2011;34:1088–1097.

42. Sadasivam K, Patial K, Vijayan V, et al. Anti-oxidant treatment in obstructive sleep apnoea syndrome. *Indian J Chest Dis Allied Sci.* 2011;53:153–162.

43. Hornyak M, Voderholzer U, Hohagen F, et al. Magnesium therapy for periodic leg movements-related insomnia and restless legs syndrome: An open pilot study. *Sleep.* 1998;21:501–505.

44. Rondanelli M, Opizzi A, Monteferrario F, et al. The effect of melatonin, magnesium, and zinc on primary insomnia in long-term care facility residents in Italy: A double-blind, placebo-controlled clinical trial. *J Am Geriatr Soc.* 2011;59:82–90.

45. Moorkens G, Manuel Y, et al. Magnesium deficit in a sample of the Belgium population presenting with chronic fatigue. *Magnes Res.* 1997;10:329–337.

46. Pachikian BD, Neyrinck AM, Deldicque L, et al. Changes in intestinal bifidobacteria levels are associated with the inflammatory response in magnesium-deficient mice. *J Nutr.* 2010;140:509–514.

47. Ji X, Liu J. Associations between blood zinc concentrations and sleep quality in childhood: A cohort study. *Nutrients.* 2015;7(7):5684–5696. doi:10.3390/nu7075247.

48. Tawil A. Zinc supplementation tightens leaky gut in Crohn's disease. *Inflamm Bowel Dis.* 2012;18:E399.

49. Zhong W, McClain C, Cave M, et al. The role of zinc deficiency in alcohol-induced intestinal barrier dysfunction. *Am J Physiol Gastrointest Liver Physiol.* 2010;298:G625–633.

50. Lee D, Badr M, Mateika J, et al. Progressive augmentation and ventilatory long-term facilitation are enhanced in sleep apnoea patients and are mitigated by anti-oxidant administration. *J Physiol.* 2009;587:5451–5467.

51. Bounous G, Molson J. Competition for glutathione precursors between the immune system and the skeletal muscle: Pathogenesis of chronic fatigue syndrome. *Med Hypotheses.* 1999;53:347–349.

52. Sadasivam K, Patial K, Vijayan V, et al. Anti-oxidant treatment in obstructive sleep apnoea syndrome. *Indian J Chest Dis Allied Sci.* 2011;53:153–162.

53. Dunleavy M, Bradford A, O'Halloran K. Oxidative stress impairs upper airway muscle endurance in an animal model of sleep-disordered breathing. *Adv Exp Med Biol.* 2008;605:458–462.

54. Maes M, Mihaylova I, et al. Coenzyme Q10 deficiency in myalgic encephalo-myelitis/chronic fatigue syndrome (ME/CFS) is related to fatigue, autonomic and neurocognitive symptoms and is another risk factor explaining the early mortality in ME/CFS due to cardiovascular disorder. *Neuro Endocrinol Lett.* 2009;30(4):470–476.

55. Suh S, Bae W, et al. Intravenous vitamin C administration reduces fatigue in office workers: A double-blind randomized controlled trial. *Nutr J.* 2012;11:7.

56. Grebe M, Eisele HJ, Weissmann N, et al. Antioxidant vitamin C improves endothelial function in obstructive sleep apnea. *Am J Respir Crit Care Med.* 2006;173:897–901.

57. Cevikel MH, Tuncyurek P, Ceylan F, et al. Supplementation with high-dose ascorbic acid improves intestinal anastomotic healing. *Eur Surg Res.* 2008;40:29–33.

58. Singh T, Patial K, Vijayan K, et al. Oxidative stress and obstructive sleep apnoea syndrome. *Indian J Chest Dis Allied Sci.* 2009;51:217–224.

59. Vecchiet J, Cipollone F, et al. Relationship between musculoskeletal symptoms and blood markers of oxidative stress in patients with chronic fatigue syndrome. *Neurosci Lett.* 2003;335:151–154.

60. Dekok H. Case report: The medical treatment of obstructive sleep apnoea syndrome (OSAS) with selenium. *Med Hypotheses.* 2005;65:817–818.

61. Albuquerque RG, Hirotsu C, Tufik S, Andersen ML. Why should we care about selenium in obstructive sleep apnea? *J Clin Sleep Med.* 2017;13(7):931–932.

62. Nagy D, Fülesdi B, Hallay J. Role of selenium in gastrointestinal inflammatory diseases. *Orv Hetil.* 2013;154:1636–1640.

63. Mueller G, Driscoll W. Biosynthesis of oleamide. *Vitam Horm.* 2009;81:55–78.

64. Irmisch G, Schläfke D, Gierow W, Herpertz S, Richter J. Fatty acids and sleep in depressed inpatients. *Prostaglandins Leukot Essent Fatty Acids.* 2007 Jan;76(1):1–7.

65. Sei H. Vitamin A and sleep regulation. *J Med Invest.* 2008;55:1–8.

66. Ransom J, Morgan PJ, McCaffery PJ, Stoney PN. The rhythm of retinoids in the brain. *J. Neurochem.* 2014;129:366–376.

67. Barcelo A, Barbe F, de la Pena M, et al. Antioxidant status in patients with sleep apnoea and impact of continuous positive airway pressure treatment. *Eur Respir J.* 2006;27:756–760.

68. McCarty DE, Chesson AL Jr, Jain SK, Marino AA. The link between vitamin D metabolism and sleep medicine. *Sleep Med Rev.* 2014 Aug;18(4):311–319.

69. Mete T, Yalcin Y, Berker D, et al. Obstructive sleep apnea syndrome and its association with vitamin D deficiency. *J Endocrinol Invest.* 2013;36(9):681–685.

70. Ulitsky A, Ananthakrishnan AN, Naik A, et al. Vitamin D deficiency in patients with inflammatory bowel disease: Association with disease activity and quality of life. *J Parenter Enteral Nutr.* 2011 May;35:308–316.

71. Gominack SC. Vitamin D deficiency changes the intestinal microbiome reducing B vitamin production in the gut. The resulting lack of pantothenic acid adversely affects the immune system, producing a "pro-inflammatory" state associated with atherosclerosis and autoimmunity. *Med Hypotheses.* 2016 Sep;94:103–107.

72. Grandner MA, Jackson N, Gerstner JR, Knutson KL. Sleep symptoms associated with intake of specific dietary nutrients. *J Sleep Res.* 2014 Feb;23(1):22–34.

73. Zhao H, Yin JY, Yang WS, et al. Sleep duration and cancer risk: A systematic review and meta-analysis of prospective studies. *Asian Pac J Cancer Prev.* 2013;14(12):7509–7515.

74. Zhou J, Kim JE, Armstrong CL, Chen N, Campbell WW. Higher-protein diets improve indexes of sleep in energy-restricted overweight and obese adults: Results from 2 randomized controlled trials. *Am J Clin Nutr.* 2016;103:766–774.

75. Breymeyer KL, Lampe JW, McGregor BA, Neuhouser ML. Subjective mood and energy levels of healthy weight and overweight/obese healthy adults on high-and low-glycemic load experimental diets. *Appetite.* 2016 Dec 1;107:253–259.

76. Afaghi A, O'Connor H, Chow CM. High-glycemic-index carbohydrate meals shorten sleep onset. *Am J Clin Nutr.* 2007 Feb;85(2):426–430.

77. Ludwig DS, Majzoub JA, Al-Zahrani A, Dallal GE, Blanco I, Roberts SB. High glycemic index foods, overeating, and obesity. *Pediatrics.* 1999;103:e261–e266.

78. Jalilolghadr S, Afaghi A, O'Connor H, Chow CM. Effect of low and high glycaemic index drink on sleep pattern in children. *J Pak Med Assoc.* 2011 Jun;61(6):533–536.

79. Hallböök T, Lundgren J, Rosén I. Ketogenic diet improves sleep quality in children with therapy-resistant epilepsy. *Epilepsia.* 2007 Jan;48(1):59–65.

80. Schmidt M, Pfetzer N, Schwab M, Strauss I, Kämmerer U. Effects of a ketogenic diet on the quality of life in 16 patients with advanced cancer: A pilot trial. *Nutr Metab (Lond).* 2011 Jul 27;8(1):54. doi:10.1186/1743-7075-8-54.

81. Afaghi A, O'Connor H, Chow CM. Acute effects of the very low carbohydrate diet on sleep indices. *Nutr Neurosci.* 2008;11(4):146–154.

82. Husain AM, Yancy WS Jr, Carwile ST, Miller PP, Westman EC. Diet therapy for narcolepsy. *Neurology.* 2004;62:2300–2302.

83. Alaia SL. Life effects of narcolepsy: Measures of negative impact, social support, and psychological well-being. *Loss Grief Care.* 1992;5:1–22.

84. Neikrug AB, Crawford MR, Ong JC. Behavioral sleep medicine services for hypersomnia disorders: A survey study. *Behav Sleep Med.* 2017;15(2):158–171.

85. González JA, Jensen LT, Fugger L, Burdakov D. Metabolism-independent sugar sensing in central orexin neurons. *Diabetes.* 2008;57(10):2569–2576. doi:10.2337/db08-0548.

86. Cui Y, Niu K, Huang C, et al. Relationship between daily isoflavone intake and sleep in Japanese adults: A cross-sectional study. *Nutr J.* 2015;14:127. doi:10.1186/s12937-015-0117-x.

87. Hansen AL, Dahl L, Olson G, et al. Fish consumption, sleep, daily functioning, and heart rate variability. *J Clin Sleep Med.* 2014;10(5):567–575. doi:10.5664/jcsm.3714.

88. Peuhkuri K, Sihvola N, Korpela R. Dietary factors and fluctuating levels of melatonin. *Food Nutr Res.* 2012;56:10.3402/fnr.v56i0.17252.

89. Howatson G, Bell PG, Tallent J, Middleton B, McHugh MP, Ellis J. Effect of tart cherry juice (Prunus cerasus) on melatonin levels and enhanced sleep quality. *Eur J Nutr.* 2012 Dec;51(8):909–916.

90. Pigeon WR, Carr M, Gorman C, Perlis ML. Effects of a tart cherry juice beverage on the sleep of older adults with insomnia: A pilot study. *J Med Food.* 2010 Jun;13(3):579–583.

91. Campanini MZ, Guallar-Castillón P, Rodríguez-Artalejo F, Lopez-Garcia E. Mediterranean Diet and changes in sleep duration and indicators of sleep quality in older adults. *Sleep.* 2017 Mar 1;40(3). doi:10.1093/sleep/zsw083. PMID: 28364422.

11

Mind–Body Interventions and Sleep: Dealing with Stress and Improving Emotional Wellness

SOPHIE VON GARNIER, SHAUNA L. SHAPIRO, AND JASON C. ONG

Introduction

Research has shown that sleep is essential to our physical and mental well-being. In this chapter, we discuss the relationships between psychological functioning, stress, and sleep, demonstrating that sleep plays a key role in cognitive and emotional processes and mental health. We also illustrate how various psychological factors contribute to sleep disturbance and explore different relaxation techniques shown to improve sleep quality, including deep breathing, guided imagery, progressive muscle relaxation (PMR), and mindfulness meditation. Finally, we examine Mindfulness-Based Therapy for Insomnia, a pioneering intervention that integrates cognitive-behavioral therapy (CBT) and mindfulness training.

Mental Health, Stress, and Sleep

While we all intuitively know that a good night's sleep makes us feel better and less vulnerable to the myriad stressors we encounter each day, it is difficult to overstate just how important sleep is for our cognitive functioning, emotional and interpersonal lives, and mental health. In the following section, we provide a brief overview of how powerfully sleep influences each of our central life domains.

SLEEP'S IMPACT ON COGNITIVE FUNCTIONING

Sleep is essential in processing the constant flow of information we receive. If we do not get adequate sleep, our cognitive functions suffer. We are less likely to properly attend to important details, form new memories, and perform minor and major cognitive tasks well—all crucial in navigating our personal and professional lives successfully. In a meta-analysis of the impact of short-term sleep deprivation, Lim and Dinges[1] found that almost all cognitive processes were affected negatively, including short-term memory, processing speed, working memory, and complex attention tasks. The strongest negative correlations were found between sleep and reaction time, as well as lapses in simple attention tasks concerned with the detection of auditory or visual cues. Given how much in life depends on us being able to notice small details, such as at work, in our social lives, or during our commute, these correlations are alarming. In a study across 35 independent samples with close to 100,000 participants, Lo et al.[2] compared cognitive functioning between older adults (≥55 years) and found that those who reported "extreme" sleeping patterns (sleeping <5 or >9 hours) displayed poorer functioning in verbal memory, working memory, and executive functions, with short sleepers being 1.4 times more likely than normal sleepers to have poor overall cognitive functioning.

SLEEP'S IMPACT ON OUR EMOTIONAL AND INTERPERSONAL LIVES

The detrimental effects of too little sleep also extend to the way we process emotional experiences. Walker and van der Helm[3] reviewed studies that investigated the neurocognitive mechanisms of emotion regulation. They found that sleep, especially rapid eye movement (REM) sleep, is of fundamental importance to adequately process the emotional contents of the previous day.[3] As Walker[4] puts it, "Dream [REM] sleep appears to reset the magnetic north of our emotional compass." Furthermore, as Lim and Dinges[1] observed in their meta-analysis, a lack of sleep can result in missed informational cues that could be crucial not only to our own safety and well-being but to that of others as well. Similarly, Goldstein-Piekarski and colleagues[5] found that when study participants had a good night's sleep, they both read facial expressions and distinguished friendly faces from neutral or threatening faces with greater accuracy. Participants who lacked sleep overestimated the prevalence of threatening faces.[5]

Sleep is not only important to how well we can read emotions in others; it also plays a role in our own emotional expressivity as well. Minkel et al.[6] found that sleep-deprived participants displayed less positivity in their faces while seeing amusing stimuli compared to those who slept well the night before. We can conclude that social interactions might become more difficult when sleep-deprived, given that people are very attuned to others' faces when evaluating relationships and actions.[7] Insufficient sleep also affects how well we can resolve interpersonal difficulties. Gordon and Chen,[8] who investigated the effects of sleep deprivation on romantic couples' conflict behavior, found that even just one partner's lack of sleep negatively impacted both partner's empathic accuracy during conflict and increased the ratio of negative to positive affect. Consistent with the researchers' predictions, the best conditions for successful conflict resolution occurred when both partners were well rested.[8]

Furthermore, that affective variability and irritability are also associated with a lack of sleep[9] provides further support to the notion that sleep deprivation can negatively affect our interpersonal relationships. Considering how closely emotional states are linked to sleep, it should come as no surprise that the vast majority of anxiety and mood disorders are linked, often bidirectionally, to poor sleep quality.[10]

SLEEP AND VULNERABILITY TO MENTAL DISORDERS

As early as childhood, sleep disturbances are closely connected to our emotional states and mental health. In a large randomly selected population sample of children (4–12 years old), Maasalo and colleagues[11] found strong associations between sleep difficulties and both low mood and emotional problems. These and related findings highlight the importance of intervening early once dysregulated sleeping patterns are discovered in children.

Overall, the relationship between psychological disorders and decreased sleep quality and quantity has received significant research attention. For example, the link between depression and insomnia is well established.[12] Furthermore, not only have depression and anxiety been shown to increase the prevalence of insomnia, but there also exist bidirectional relationships between them.[13] A meta-analysis by Baglioni and colleagues[14] showed that non-depressed individuals who suffered from insomnia had double the risk of becoming depressed compared to people who did not report difficulties sleeping. And a longitudinal epidemiological study of young adults demonstrated that previous insomnia significantly predicted the onset of a depressive episode later in life.[15] Sleep disturbances have also been associated with an increased risk of suicidal behavior in people with psychiatric conditions.[16] In contrast to other risk factors for suicidality that are fixed (e.g., family history of suicide attempts), sleep is a modifiable risk factor that provides an avenue of hope for preventing suicidal behavior.

SLEEP AND LIFE STRESSORS

As we have seen, sleep is closely related to cognitive and emotional functioning as well as to mental health. Next, we examine life stress, which has bidirectional relationships with all of the previously mentioned components of well-being. Poor sleep quality leads to vulnerability to stress. And, at the same time, a variety of life stressors, both large and small, impact our sleep. Minkel and colleagues[17] found that sleep-deprived individuals were more reactive to mild stressors than were those who had slept well the night before. Following a battery of low-stress cognitive tasks, participants who lacked a good night's sleep reported feeling more angry, anxious, and stressed compared to the normal sleep group. The researchers suggest that this supports the notion that our threshold for what we perceive as stressful in the cognitive domain might be lowered by inadequate sleep.[17]

While lack of sleep can lower our tolerance to stress and thus increase our likelihood to experience it, stress from a multitude of life events, including interpersonal conflict,[18,19] trauma,[19–22] or financial woes,[18,23] can lead to poor sleep quality. For example, not only does intimate partner violence predict higher risk of depression and posttraumatic stress disorder (PTSD) symptomatology (which are associated with poor sleep),[20] it has also been directly linked to sleep difficulties.[19] There also seems to be a link between insomnia and adverse childhood experiences (ACEs). In a clinical sample, 46% of insomnia patients reported having experienced moderate or severe ACEs including abuse and neglect.[21] These individuals displayed different sleeping patterns (such as more frequent awakenings) than the other patients in the sample who reported few or none of these events.[21] Furthermore, research indicates a significant relationship between ACEs such as verbal abuse and neglect and sleep problems in young adulthood.[22]

Beyond potentially traumatic stressors such as ACEs and intimate partner violence, other situations and life events are also associated with poorer sleep quality. For older adults, continuing financial worries contribute to difficulties falling asleep and to decreased sleep continuity.[23] Additionally, adults who report social isolation, experience low emotional support, and mention more social interactions that they perceive as negative experience more sleep difficulties than those who have fewer social stressors.[18] Interestingly, some of these adverse effects were mediated by positive emotions and eudaemonic well-being.[18] In other words, experiencing more overall positivity seemed to weaken the effect that life stressors had on sleep quality and thus potentially served as a buffer. While research suggesting a connection between positive emotional states and high sleep quality holds promise, more rigorous studies are needed to make stronger claims about the actual strength of this relationship and its clinical implications.[24]

Overall, sleep quality and duration are closely linked to cognitive and emotional processes, interpersonal functioning, mental health, and a myriad of life stressors. Fortunately, there are many empirically supported interventions and stress reduction techniques that create positive ripple effects across the whole system and ultimately benefit sleep.

Relaxation Techniques and the Relaxation Response

One overarching goal of relaxation techniques is to induce the "relaxation response" (RR), which brings about a physiological pattern contrary to the stress response or, as most of us know it, the "fight-or-flight" response.[25] In contrast to the stress response, the RR reduces respiratory and heart rates and lowers oxygen consumption.[25] All relaxation techniques that will be discussed in this chapter, including deep breathing techniques, PMR, guided imagery, and meditation, have been shown to bring about the RR.[25] Herbert Benson, who coined the term after observing the benefits of meditation on human physiology nearly 50 years ago, stated that

> it's important to remember that most diseases have many different possible causes and contributing factors, and the relaxation response targets only one: stress. . . . [However,] to the extent that any disorder is caused or made worse by stress, the relaxation response is useful.[25,p. 236]

A closer look at Chang et al.'s[26] RR intervention study is helpful in deepening our understanding of how regularly inducing the RR benefits novices and long-term practitioners of relaxation techniques on both psychological and physiological levels. In their study, the researchers designed an 8-week intervention to train individuals to elicit the RR in themselves through techniques including deep (diaphragmatic) breathing and mindfulness meditation. This intervention was administered to a participating group of novices but not to long-term practitioners of relaxation techniques who were also studied. To qualify for the latter group, individuals were required to have practiced an established relaxation technique such as meditation or yoga for at least 4 years multiple times per week. Both groups were invited into the laboratory to complete measures of psychological and physiological functioning before, during, and after an RR-eliciting audio recording exercise. In the laboratory, researchers measured stress-related hormones such as cortisol and norepinephrine as well as self-reported psychological distress and anxiety.[26]

At the outset of the study, the long-term practitioners reported significantly lower anxiety and distress levels than the novices. However, after the intervention, levels of psychological distress declined significantly for the novices over the 8-week training period, reaching the levels of the long-term practitioners. While these findings are promising when considering short-term interventions, the study results for long-term practitioners are perhaps even more encouraging: this group's psychological distress levels decreased more quickly than that of the novices during the exercise. Furthermore, decreases in self-reported anxiety and psychological distress were associated with decreased levels of cortisol, adrenocorticotropic hormone (ACTH), and norepinephrine. Considering that novice practitioners did not experience any hormonal changes related to the stress response during the RR exercise, the authors suggest that, in seasoned practitioners, RR techniques truly had cultivated a more productive mind–body stress response.[26] Connecting to and expanding on the current literature, this finding is consistent with numerous studies demonstrating that RR techniques modulate psychological[27] and physiological responses over time.[28]

In the following section, we explore several of these relaxation techniques before delving more deeply into mindfulness and its effectiveness in treating insomnia.

DEEP BREATHING

Slow and deep breathing is a key component of most relaxation techniques including mindful breath meditation,[29] pranayama (i.e., yogic breathing or breath control),[30,31] and PMR.[32] But while we rarely reflect on the importance of breathing, the etymological roots of pranayama remind us just how important it is. *Prana* in pranayama is directly translated as, not only "breath," but also "life force."[30] Yet not all breathing involves this life-giving quality to the same degree. There are two main types of breathing: chest breathing and diaphragmatic breathing (or deep breathing).[32] In chest breathing, which is shallower, we mainly feel our chest rise and expand. In diaphragmatic breathing, we breathe in more deeply, optimally through the nose, and contract the diaphragm muscle. As the diaphragm moves downward to allow for more air to fill the lungs, our stomach rises.[32] And while both provide us with oxygen, they result in different physiological responses. Shallow chest breathing is more likely to stimulate the sympathetic branch of the autonomic nervous system (ANS), the same system that is activated when we feel fearful. Conversely, diaphragmatic breathing stimulates the parasympathetic branch of the ANS, which also activates when we feel calm.[32] Thus, by breathing deeply, we initiate physiological changes that are antithetical to stress or anxiety.[33]

Furthermore, RR interventions centered around diaphragmatic or paced breathing have been shown to provide stress and symptom relief to individuals who suffer from a range of medical and psychological disorders including insomnia,[34] anxiety disorders,[35] and migraines,[36] but these exercises can benefit nonclinical populations as well.

In their 2004 study, Pal and colleagues[37] examined ANS activity in young adults randomly assigned to practice a slow breathing pattern (~18 second intervals for each breath), to practice a fast breathing pattern (quick and deep breathing for 1 minute followed by a 3-minute break, 8–10 cycles), or to a control condition. Both treatment groups were trained extensively, and participants practiced daily for half an hour in the mornings and half an hour in the evenings over a period of

3 months. In comparison to the fast breathing treatment group and the controls who showed no significant ANS changes on study completion, those in the slow breathing group showed a significant decrease in sympathetic activity and an increase in parasympathetic activity.[37]

While the participants in Pal et al.'s slow breathing treatment group took a little more than three breaths per minute,[37] many slow or paced breathing intervention studies work with a higher rate, typically using respiratory intervals of 10 seconds or 6 breaths per minute.[34,38]

It is worth pointing out that in heart rate variability biofeedback (HRV-BF), an increasingly popular intervention for various health issues,[39] a similar breath per minute ratio (~6 breaths/min) is used.[40] HRV-BF has shown promising results in the area of sleep promotion, including increased cardiorespiratory resting function[41] and better sleep quality in healthy adults.[42]

While not all mind–body interventions focus primarily on the breath, understanding the life- and health-giving force behind deep breathing provides further insight into one of the most central mechanisms underlying relaxation techniques as a whole.

PROGRESSIVE MUSCLE RELAXATION

PMR is a stress management technique that combines deliberate muscle tension and subsequent relief with deep breathing to achieve holistic mind and body relaxation. It functions on the premise that when we feel stressed or anxious, our bodies react by tensing up.[43] In PMR, clients learn to deeply relax their muscles and engage in diaphragmatic breathing.[32] This process elicits the body's RR, which in turn decreases anxious mental states.[43]

While the first version of PMR was developed by the physician Edmund Jacobson in the 1930s,[44] several clinicians have since adapted his work on muscle relaxation by shortening the original format and grouping Jacobson's extensive list of muscles into larger units to allow for easier practice.[32,45]

In its modern application, PMR is successfully utilized as a primary intervention[27] and as an adjunct to other therapeutic approaches, [46] often alongside CBT. The benefits to mental and physical health of both clinical approaches are numerous. PMR has been shown to improve clients' tension headaches[46]; decrease stress,[27,47] depression,[48] and anxiety symptomology[47,48,50]; increase mindfulness[27] and mental and physical relaxation[49]; and improve sleep quality.[50] Diverse clinical populations, including cancer patients[51] and elderly patients with a history of heart failure,[52] have reported an increase in quality of life following a PMR intervention. Physiological changes following PMR treatment include reductions in heart rate[47] and lower cortisol levels.[47,53]

While self-help training books or online resources can help familiarize clients with PMR, Carlson and Hoyle[54] found that clinical effect sizes were highest if PMR was taught one-on-one. Additionally, longer and more frequent clinical PMR sessions are associated with treatment success.[54] Goldfried and Davison[55] highlight several important advantages of conducting PMR in a clinical setting including discussing treatment rationale with the clients and modeling the procedure for them during the first session if deemed appropriate.

While individual PMR practices can vary, the methodology follows a relatively set structure. Bernstein and colleagues[32] suggest that, after the clients have found a comfortable position and have taken several deep breaths, the therapist should begin by asking clients to clench their dominant hand into a fist and then bend it back, bringing further tension to wrist and forearm. After holding this position for about 5–7 seconds, the clients are instructed to let go and pay attention to the sensation of deepening relaxation in their dominant hand and forearm. Following this general procedure, the therapist guides the client through a sequence of 16 different muscle groups, which include muscles in the arms, face, neck, torso, and legs.[32] After clients complete the sequence, the therapist encourages them to feel the deepened relaxation throughout their body and, if applicable, bring attention to muscle groups that still feel tense.[55] A good way to simplify the PMR homework for the clients is to record the session for them to use as a practice aid.[55] It is important for clinicians to discuss with clients how they can create time and space at home where they can practice in a relaxing environment, devoid of distractions, for half an hour.[55]

After clients have mastered the basic technique, they can use the tape of their recorded session or a shorter version of PMR (by combining certain muscle groups) to help release tension before going to sleep. While PMR is a technique with very few risks to clients, some have mentioned experiencing intrusive thoughts or reported fear of losing control.[56] Especially for those clients who worry about the latter, practicing with open eyes at first can build their confidence in the exercise and strengthen the therapeutic alliance.[55]

While focusing on the different muscle groups and the process of PMR can help many clients achieve deep relaxation, some clients prefer a more visually stimulating approach, even when the sensations are solely and willfully imaginative.

GUIDED IMAGERY

Guided imagery, also called *imagery-induced relaxation*, is a mind–body intervention that uses visualization techniques to induce a calm state of mind. Achtenberg and Lawlis defined guided imagery as the "internal experience of a perceptual event in the absence of the actual external stimuli."[57, p. 248] One factor underlying guided imagery's effectiveness as a relaxation technique is our shared difficulty in focusing on two opposing ideas simultaneously. When a client is focused on a peaceful and relaxing mental scene, worrying or ruminating is very difficult.[58] Given the negative effect that self-defeating thoughts can have on our mood and physiology, consciously creating a calm and peaceful mental state with the help of visualizations can help elicit the RR.[43]

As with other relaxation techniques, guided imagery can be used either as a main intervention[59] or as an adjunct[60] to other therapeutic approaches. It has multiple strengths, including its cost effectiveness,[61,62] the ease with which it can be applied by mental health care providers and medical personnel,[58,61,62] and the great variety of ways it can be administered, including one-on-one,[58] in a group format,[63] or by providing audio files[61,64] and written instructions to clients.[61] Another major strength is the flexibility of intervention location[62] and duration.[61,64] Although short-format guided imagery interventions have generated positive change for clients,[65] clinical effect sizes of the intervention tend to increase with the number of sessions.[66]

While there are many different variations of guided imagery, there is a common structure between individual practices. Before being led through the visualization, clients are encouraged to close their eyes and breathe deeply to start the RR. While the clients are being guided through their visualization, they are encouraged to use all of their senses to fully immerse themselves in the scene.[58,67] Therapists can help clients make their visualization more graphic by asking detailed questions about the scene along the way.[58] After about 10–15 minutes of guiding the clients through a visualization, therapists will ask them to slowly open their eyes again and to sit with their feelings of calm and stillness.[67]

While the sequence of treatment is consistent throughout many applications of guided imagery, the content often differs widely. In her meta-analysis of guided imagery studies, Van Kuiken[66] distinguished four main types of guided imagery. The first and perhaps most prominent type is *pleasant imagery*, which includes any scenario that provides a deep sense of relaxation and calm, including happy memories or a safe and idyllic place in nature. Second, Van Kuiken[66] identified *physiologically focused imagery*, where patients direct attention toward a body part that causes difficulties and is in need of healing; for example, a patient with cancer undergoing chemotherapy might imagine in great detail how cancer cells are being attacked and eliminated.[62] The third kind is called *mental rehearsal*[66] and is frequently used in CBT.[58] Clients are encouraged to visualize how they would master a challenge they currently face or go about a life change they are planning to make. Van Kuiken's[66] fourth type, *receptive imagery*, is more reflective in nature and includes scanning the body and being open to sensations, symbolic images, or words that come to mind.[68]

As with other relaxation techniques discussed, guided imagery has been shown to benefit healthy and clinical populations alike. For example, in pregnant women, guided imagery can lead to increases in relaxation[65] and self-reported well-being[61] and reductions in stress,[64] fatigue,[64] and heat rate.[65] In mothers of preterm infants, a guided imagery intervention resulted in better sleep quality.[69] Furthermore, studies investigating its use in medical populations found guided imagery to be an effective adjunct therapy to treat the anxiety and depressive symptoms that can accompany a wide variety of physiological ailments including arthritis[70] and inflammatory bowel disease,[71] as well as medical treatments, such as chemotherapy[72] and joint replacement surgery.[73] And while studies disagree on guided imagery's effectiveness in reducing actual physical pain,[72,73] guided imagery might increase self-efficacy in dealing with pain symptomatology.[74] The scarcity of randomized-controlled studies directly investigating guided imagery's effects on sleep quality and duration is surprising. Yet, knowing that guided imagery helps reduce stress, anxiety, and even depressive symptoms provides insight into how this relaxation technique might promote healthy sleep.

MEDITATION AND MINDFULNESS

Numerous meditation practices such as breathing meditations and Transcendental Meditation have been shown to have positive mental and physical health benefits, including serving as buffers against the effects of stress[75,76] and decreasing anxiety,[77] PTSD symptomology[78,79] and sleepiness.[76] While most meditation practices emphasize deep breathing, many such traditions integrate it with other components, such as learning to cultivate open attention,[80] loving-kindness,[81] or self-compassion.[82]

One of the most researched meditation practices in the West is mindfulness meditation.[29] Mindfulness is also a core element of several mind–body interventions and psychotherapeutic techniques such as Mindfulness-Based Stress Reduction (MBSR)[83] and Mindfulness-Based Therapy for Insomnia (MBTI).[84]

Mindfulness is a "consciousness discipline," a way of training the mind and body to be fully present with life in an open, kind, and discerning way. It involves bringing full awareness to each moment. Although often associated with mental training, mindfulness is much more than a mental exercise. Awareness of the body and somatic practices to help train this awareness have always been at the heart of mindfulness. Furthermore, although mindfulness can be trained through formal meditation practices, it is, more broadly, a way of being, practiced moment by moment during the experiences of everyday life. In the model developed by Shapiro, Carlson, Astin, and Freedman,[85] mindfulness comprises three core elements: intention, attention, and attitude. *Intention* is knowing why one does things—the ultimate aims, visions, and aspirations a person holds for oneself and the world around one. *Attention* involves fully focusing on the inner and outer experiences of the present moment. *Attitude* refers to the open, kind, and curious attitude an individual should bring to his or her attention. These three elements, intention, attention, and attitude (IAA), are interwoven, each informing and feeding back into the others. Mindfulness, then, is the awareness that arises when intentionally attending to the present moment with kindness and curiosity.

The first core component of mindfulness, *intention*, requires conscious reflection on what one values. Yet achieving a sense of deep-seated intention can be challenging. Doing so requires individuals to make an honest inquiry about their hopes, desires, and aspirations, allowing the answers to arise organically. This inquiry results in increased awareness of unconscious values and helps them decide whether they are worth pursuing. Mindful intention can also be a powerful force in psychotherapy. When applying this element of the IAA model, the therapist should cultivate an environment where intentions can develop at their client's own pace.

Intention, in the context of mindfulness, is not striving or grasping for particular outcomes: it is about the process. For example, those who have practiced a form of mindful movement such as yoga might recognize intention as the conversation between the ideal that any one pose represents and the embodiment of that pose in a person's unique body. As Jack Kornfield puts it, "Intention is a direction, not a destination" (oral communication, 2012).

According to our model,[85] the second fundamental component of mindfulness is *attention*. Paying attention involves observing and experiencing our moment-to-moment experience. And yet research demonstrates just how difficult this is: Killingsworth and Gilbert[86] estimate that our mind wanders approximately 47% of the time. These findings substantiate the Buddhist analogy of the human mind as a "monkey mind," swinging from thought to thought as a monkey swings from limb to limb.[87]

Mindfulness is a tool that helps people tame and train their mind so that their attention becomes more stable and focused. In formal meditation practice, the breath is often treated as the anchor to human attention: when the mind wanders off, meditators attend to their breath in order to regain focus on the present moment. Whatever the focus of one's attention, it is essential that the mind remains in a state of "relaxed alertness." Often, when meditators try to too hard to pay attention, they become tense and contracted. This is because they mistakenly believe that being hypervigilant toward their thinking will lead to present-minded focus and attention. However, most, if not all, meditation traditions teach students a different kind of attention, one involving clarity and precision without stress or rigorous effort.[88] In addition to these qualities, mindful attention is also supposed to be deep and penetrating; as Bhikkhu Bodhi notes, "Whereas a mind without mindfulness 'floats' on the surface of its object the way a gourd floats on water, mindfulness sinks into its object the way a stone placed on the surface of water sinks to the bottom."[88, p. 7]

Attitude, the third core component of mindfulness, becomes relevant once individuals have learned to intentionally attend to the present moment. Once the stepping stone of mindful attention has been achieved, the individual begins to see that that the human mind is constantly judging. For example, attention can have a cold, critical quality or an openhearted, compassionate quality. In fact, the Japanese symbol for mindfulness combines the symbol for presence with a symbol that can mean mind, spirit, or heart depending on the context[89]—in other words, to be mindful is also to have presence of heart.[80]

The transformation from mind*less* to mind*ful* is catalyzed not just by the quantity but also the quality of one's practice. Thus, mindfulness requires not simply paying attention, but attending with the attitudes of kindness and curiosity. Attending to the present moment without utilizing the attitudinal qualities of curiosity, openness, acceptance, and love (COAL)[90] may result in an attention that is condemning or shaming of inner (or outer) experience. This may well have consequences contrary to the intentions of the practice; for example, clients and therapists alike may end up cultivating patterns of criticism and striving instead of equanimity and acceptance.

These attitudes of mindfulness do not have to alter an individual's experience but can simply contain it. For example, if during the meditation practice feelings of impatience arise, they can be simply noted before bringing acceptance and kindness to the impatience. These COAL attitudes are not meant to serve as substitutes for the impatience or means to make it disappear. They are not an attempt to make experiences be a certain way, but instead an attempt to relate to whatever *is* in a certain way. By teaching clients to intentionally bring the attitudes of COAL to the awareness of their experiences, clinicians can help them relinquish the habits of striving for pleasant experiences and pushing aversive experiences away. Instead, they learn to attend to whatever is happening in the present moment.

Mindfulness-Based Stress Reduction

Despite mindfulness' long-standing importance within Buddhist traditions and its kinship to Western thought as far back as ancient Greece,[91] it was John Kabat-Zinn's MBSR[83] that reintroduced mindfulness to Western scientific research and therapeutic practice. MBSR is a 2-month program during which clients meet weekly to learn relaxation techniques, including sitting meditation, gentle yoga, body scans, and walking meditation in a supportive group environment.[92] Other key elements of the MBSR intervention are a day-long meditation retreat toward the end of the course, where participants can deepen their practice, as well as daily homework assignments that allow participants to begin a meditation routine that helps sustain MBSR's benefits long after the intervention has ended.[92]

Additionally, MBSR has inspired other mindfulness-based interventions including Mindfulness-Based Cognitive Therapy (MBCT),[93] which was specifically developed to reduce relapse rates in patients suffering from depressive disorders and MBTI, [84] which we discuss later in more detail.

Benefits of Mindfulness-Based Interventions

Meta-analytic research on MBSR and related mindfulness interventions shows that they are most effective in treating chronic pain, anxiety, and depression.[94] However, these interventions have also shown promise in treating the symptoms of a wide variety of other psychological and physical disorders, including the negative psychological effects associated with acute and chronic medical disorders. For example, clients with cancer,[95] diabetes,[96] fibromyalgia,[97] and vascular disease[98] have reported decreases in anxiety and depressive symptoms following mindfulness-based interventions.

In addition to those struggling with anxiety and depression,[94] clients with other psychological disorders also tend to respond well to mindfulness-based interventions. There is increasing support for adding mindfulness components to the treatment of binge-eating disorder,[99] borderline personality disorder,[100] PTSD,[100] and substance use disorder.[101]

Yet mindfulness interventions are not only valuable in the clinical realm. Intervention studies examining nonclinical populations across various age groups have repeatedly shown that practicing mindfulness helps decrease stress,[102,103] rumination,[104] anxiety,[102,103] and depressive symptoms[103] as well as increases trait or dispositional mindfulness.[102]

It should come as no surprise that dispositional mindfulness is related to sleep quality.[105] In a recent study of young adults, researchers found that higher levels of self-reported trait mindfulness were positively correlated with better sleep quality, including longer sleep duration and fewer sleep disturbances, with lower levels of anxiety and depression mediating these relationships.[105] Furthering our understanding of these relationships, dispositional mindfulness and poor sleep quality have been shown to be inversely correlated in a large adolescent sample, with rumination serving as a mediator between them.[106]

Being more mindful might even positively affect one's dreams. Simor and colleagues[107] found that students who rated themselves as more mindful reported less negative dream quality. Furthermore, those who scored higher in mindfulness were less worried about having bad dreams, with lower scores in overall anxiety serving as a moderator.[107]

Finally, dispositional mindfulness is a powerful predictor of sleep quality later in life. In a study of older adults, higher scores in trait mindfulness were associated with higher subjective vitality.[108] This correlation was partially mediated by sleep efficiency and levels of daytime functioning associated with sleep quality. The study's authors[108] hypothesized that many of the benefits related to mindfulness, such as the ability to better calm one's mind or practice attending to the present moment, not only allow individuals to fall asleep more quickly and sleep more soundly, but also help them to be more alert during everyday activities even after a poor night's sleep.

While these studies have primarily examined individuals with relatively normal sleeping patterns, researchers have begun to study potential inverse relationships between mindfulness and chronic sleeplessness.

Mindfulness-Based Therapy for Insomnia

MBTI is a relatively new integrative intervention for sleep that has received a great deal of empirical support.[84] This intervention integrates traditional mindfulness training with established behavioral techniques for treating insomnia. MBTI is a meditation-based program tailored for people with chronic insomnia disorder that integrates components of MBSR, MBCT, and CBT for Insomnia (CBT-I).[109] Similar to other mindfulness-based interventions, MBTI is delivered in groups and consists of 8 weekly sessions plus an optional meditation retreat that is typically held between the sessions 6 and 7. Each session consists of three parts: guided formal meditations, a period of inquiry where personal experiences with mindfulness principles are discussed among group members, and insomnia-related activities and education. Between sessions, participants are asked to establish a meditation practice at home and follow specific behavioral sleep recommendations. Both guided and home meditation practices consist of quiet (e.g., breathing meditation, body scan) and movement meditations (e.g., hatha yoga, walking meditation) along with informal meditations. The MBTI program can be roughly divided into three phases: (1) acquiring fundamentals of mindfulness and insomnia, (2) synchronizing sleep behaviors with signals from the brain, and (3) taking a mindful stance in working with symptoms of insomnia.

MBTI uses the principles and practices of mindfulness meditation to improve sleep by teaching people with insomnia how to make metacognitive shifts in relating to the experience of sleeplessness. For example, people with insomnia often have cognitive distortions about the consequences of insufficient sleep or hold on to very rigid beliefs about the amount of sleep needed each night. Over time, persistence of these beliefs and attitudes can lead to absorption of the sleep problem or an attachment to immediate sleep needs. Through mindfulness meditation practice, MBTI teaches people with insomnia to allow the thoughts, feelings, and sensations occurring in the present moment to guide thoughtful actions that are compatible with their current state rather than the attachment to their sleep needs or goals. Particular emphasis is placed on cultivating awareness of the state of sleepiness since that is an important state which signals that the brain is ready for sleep. This is in contrast to the typical "mindless" behavior of forcing sleep to occur based on the time, previous sleep experience, or predictions about the next day's functioning. By practicing mindfulness meditation, patients can see the problem of insomnia from a different perspective rather than repeatedly trying harder to sleep, thus creating the space that is needed to allow sleep to occur effortlessly.

A series of research studies have been conducted that provide promising evidence of MBTI's effectiveness. Our first study[84] evaluated a 6-week version of MBTI on 30 people with chronic insomnia and revealed significant pre- to posttreatment improvements on several sleep parameters, significant decreases in maladaptive thoughts about sleep, and a significant decrease in sleep-related arousal. Subsequently, we revised the MBTI program to an 8-week program by enhancing the integration between mindfulness principles and the behavioral components for insomnia by connecting the concepts of awareness with the instructions for stimulus control and sleep restriction. We conducted a randomized controlled trial with 54 adults with chronic insomnia who were assigned to MBTI, MBSR, or a self-monitoring control using daily sleep diaries.[110] Both the MBTI and MBSR groups reported significantly greater reductions from baseline to posttreatment on the Insomnia Severity Index when compared to the control group. MBTI was also associated with a greater reduction in insomnia symptom severity from baseline to the 6-month follow-up compared to MBSR. In terms of clinical significance, MBTI had remission rates rising from 33.3% at posttreatment to 50% at 6-month follow-up and response rates increased from 60% at posttreatment to 78.6% at 6-month follow-up in MBTI. MBSR had remission rates of 46.2% at posttreatment, 38.5% at 3 months, and 41.7% at 6 months, and response rates of between 38.5% and 41.7%. Collectively, the findings from these studies indicate that mindfulness-based interventions can be effective for reducing symptoms of chronic insomnia, with some indication that MBTI might have long-term advantages over MBSR.

Future Directions and Implications

As demonstrated, there are numerous mind–body interventions that can positively impact sleep. In particular, the pioneering MBTI intervention shows great promise for treating insomnia. Thus far, MBTI has only been investigated in people with chronic insomnia who were not taking sleep medications and did not have significant co-occurring medical or psychiatric conditions. Therefore, future research should explore MBTI's effectiveness for patients who are prescribed sleep medications as a first-line treatment and present with comorbid conditions such as depression or chronic pain.

For research to continue to refine and expand our knowledge of mind–body interventions for sleep, the following topics should be further explored.

1. *Differentiation between types of meditation-based interventions.* There are many different types of meditation practice, yet researchers and therapists often assume that different meditation techniques have equivalent effects. While most meditation styles do have overlapping benefits, such as increases in psychological well-being, individual practices differ widely in their specific effects. Therefore, we need more extensive research into which meditations are the most beneficial for sleep.

2. *Temporal elements of relaxation techniques.* Further emphasis should be placed on understanding the relationships between overall practice duration, individual session length, and practice frequency of various relaxation techniques and sleep quality.

3. *Qualitative data.* Measuring the effects of mind–body practices on sleep with quantitative measures alone can be limiting. By placing a stronger focus on obtaining qualitative data in addition to quantitative data, we can achieve a more comprehensive understanding of the effectiveness of specific relaxation techniques.

4. *Component analysis.* The interventions reviewed in this chapter are complex processes with multiple effective components. Future research should further investigate which specific elements of mind–body interventions most strongly account for the positive psychological and physiological effects related to their use. For example, because MBTI contains both mindfulness meditation practices and established behavioral techniques for treating insomnia, future studies comparing MBTI and CBT-I using dismantling designs could help to clarify the relative effects of each component.

Conclusion

Over the past decades, research has shown that mind–body practices and their significant psychological and physiological benefits can help improve sleep quality. Given the close relationship between stress and sleep and the high stress levels accompanying our fast-paced lives, future research should continue to explore optimal ways in which cultivating mind–body practices can help individuals not only to enhance emotional wellness but also enjoy more restful sleep.

REFERENCES

1. Lim J, Dinges DF. A meta-analysis of the impact of short-term sleep deprivation on cognitive variables. *Psychol Bull.* 2010;136(3):375–389.
2. Lo JC, Groeger JA, Cheng GH, Dijk DJ, Chee MWL. Self-reported sleep duration and cognitive performance in older adults: A systematic review and meta-analysis. *Sleep Med.* 2016;17:87–98.
3. Walker MP, Van der Helm E. Overnight therapy? The role of sleep in emotional brain processing. *Psychol Bull.* 2009;135(5):731–748.
4. Anwar Y. The sleep-deprived brain can mistake friends for foes. 2015. https://vcresearch.berkeley.edu/news/sleep-deprived-brain-can-mistake-friends-foes
5. Goldstein-Piekarski AN, Greer SM, Saletin JM, Walker MP. Sleep deprivation impairs the human central and peripheral nervous system discrimination of social threat. *J Neurosci.* 2015;35(28):10135–10145.

6. Minkel J, Htaik O, Banks S, Dinges D. Emotional expressiveness in sleep-deprived healthy adults. *Behav Sleep Med.* 2011;9(1):5–14.

7. Ekman P. *Emotions revealed: Recognizing faces and feelings to improve communication and emotional life.* New York: Owl Books; 2003.

8. Gordon AM, Chen S. The role of sleep in interpersonal conflict: Do sleepless nights mean worse fights? *Soc Psychol Personal Sci.* 2014;5(2):168–175.

9. Horne, J. A. Sleep function, with particular reference to sleep deprivation. *Ann Clin Res.* 1985;17(5):199–208.

10. Goldstein AN, Walker MP. The role of sleep in emotional brain function. *Annu Rev Clin Psychol.* 2014;10:679–708.

11. Maasalo K, Fontell T, Wessman J, Aronen ET. Sleep and behavioral problems associate with low mood in Finish children aged 4-12 years: An epidemiological study. *Child Adolesc Psychiatry Ment Health.* 2016;10:37. doi:10.1186/s13034-016-0125-4

12. Lustberg L, Reynolds III CF. Depression and insomnia: Questions of cause and effect. *Sleep Med Rev.* 2000;4(3):253–262.

13. Jansson-Fröjmark M, Lindblom K. A bidirectional relationship between anxiety and depression, and insomnia? A prospective study in the general population. *J Psychosom Res.* 2008;64(4):443–449.

14. Baglioni C, Battagliese G, Feige B, et al. Insomnia as a predictor of depression: A meta-analytic evaluation of longitudinal epidemiological studies. *J Affect Disord.* 2011;135(1–3):10–19.

15. Breslau N, Roth T, Rosenthal L, Andreski P. Sleep disturbance and psychiatric disorders: A longitudinal epidemiological study of young adults. *Biol Psychiatry.* 1996;39(6):411–418.

16. Malik S, Kanwar A, Sim LA, et al. The association between sleep disturbances and suicidal behaviors in patients with psychiatric diagnoses: A systematic review and meta-analysis. *Syst Rev.* 2014;3:18 doi:10.1186/2046-4046-4053-3-18

17. Minkel JD, Banks S, Htaik O, et al. Sleep deprivation and stressors: Evidence for elevated negative affect in response to mild stressors when sleep deprived. *Emotion.* 2012;12(5):1015–1020.

18. Steptoe A, O'Donnell K, Marmot M, Wardle J. Positive affect, psychological well-being, and good sleep. *J Psychosom Res.* 2008;64:409–415.

19. Miller-Graff LE, Cheng P. Consequences of violence across the lifespan: Mental health and sleep quality in pregnant women. *Psychol Trauma.* 2017;9(5):587–595.

20. O'Campo P, Kub J, Woods, A, et al. Depression, PTSD, and comorbidity related to intimate partner violence in civilian and military women. *Brief Treat Crisis Interv.* 2006;6(2):99–110.

21. Bader K, Schäfer V, Schenkel M, Nissen L, Schwander J. Adverse childhood experiences associated with sleep in primary insomnia. *J Sleep Res.* 2007;16(3):258–296.

22. Miller-Graff LE, Cater ÅK, Howell KH, Graham-Bermann SA. Victimization in childhood: General and specific associations with physical health problems in young adulthood. *J Psychosom Res.* 2015;79(4):265–271.

23. Hall M, Buysse DJ, Nofzinger EA, et al. Financial strain is a significant correlate of sleep continuity disturbances in late-life. *Biol Psychol.* 2008;77(2):217–222.

24. Ong AD, Kim S, Young S, Steptoe A. Positive affect and sleep: A systematic review. *Sleep Med Rev.* 2017;35:21–32.

25. Benson H. The relaxation response. In Goleman D, Gurin J, eds. *Mind body medicine: How to use your mind for better health.* New York: Consumer Reports Book; 1993: 233–257.

26. Chang BH, Dusek JA, Benson H. Psychobiological changes from relaxation response elicitation: Long-term practitioners vs. novices. *Psychosomatics.* 2011;52(6):550–559.

27. Gao L, Curtiss J, Liu X, Hofmann SG. Differential treatment mechanisms in mindfulness meditation and progressive muscle relaxation. *Mindfulness (N Y).* 2017. doi:10.1007/s12671-017-0869-9

28. Krajewski J, Sauerland M, Wieland R. Relaxation-induced cortisol changes within lunch breaks: An experimental longitudinal worksite field study. *J Occup Organ Psychol.* 2011;84(2):382–394.

29. Germer CK. What is it? What does it? In Germer GK, Siegel RD, eds. *Mindfulness and psychotherapy,* 2nd ed. New York: Guilford; 2016: 3–35.

30. Feuerstein, G. *The Shambhala encyclopedia of yoga.* Boston, MA: Shambhala; 1997.

31. Rosen R. *Prananyama beyond the fundamentals: An in-depth guide to yogic breathing with instructional CD.* Boston, MA: Shambhala; 2006.

32. Bernstein DA, Borkovec TD, Hazlett-Stevens H. *New directions in progressive relaxation training: A guidebook for helping professionals.* Westport, CT: Praeger; 2000.

33. Hazlett-Stevens H, Craske MG. Breathing retraining and diaphragmatic breathing techniques. In O'Donohue WT, Fisher JE, eds. *General principles and empirically supported techniques of cognitive behavior therapy.* Hoboken, NJ: Wiley; 2009: 167–172.

34. Tsai HJ, Kuo TB, Lee GS, Yang CCH. Efficacy of paced breathing for insomnia: Enhances vagal tone and improves sleep quality. *Psychophysiol.* 2015;52(3):388–396.

35. Chen YF, Huang XY, Chien CH, Cheng JF. The effectiveness of diaphragmatic breathing relaxation training for reducing anxiety. *Perspect Psychiatr Care.* 2016;53(4):329–336.

36. Kaushik R, Kaushik RM, Mahajan SK, Rajesh V. Biofeedback assisted diaphragmatic breathing and systematic relaxation versus propranolol in long term prophylaxis of migraine. *Complement Ther Med.* 2005;13(3):165–174.

37. Pal GK, Velkumary S, Madanmohan. Effect of short-term practice of breathing exercises on automatic functions in normal human volunteers. *Indian J Med Res.* 2004;120(2):115–121.

38. Kaushik RM, Kaushik R, Mahajan SK, Rajesh V. Effects of mental relaxation and slow breathing in essential hypertension. *Complement Ther Med.* 2006;14(2):120–126.

39. Wheat AL, Larkin, KT. Biofeedback of heart rate variability and relayed physiology: A critical review. *Appl Psychophyisiol Biofeedback.* 2010;35(3):229–242.

40. Meule A, Kübler A. A pilot study on the effects of slow paced breathing on current food cravings. *Appl Psychophysiol Biofeedback*. 2017;42(1):59–68.

41. Sakakibara M, Hayano J, Oikawa LO, Katsamanis M, Lehrer P. Heart rate variability biofeedback improves cardiorespiratory resting function during sleep. *Appl Psychophysiol Biofeedback*. 2013;38(4):265–271.

42. Ebben MR, Kurbatov V, Pollak CP. Moderating laboratory adaption with the use of a heart-rate variability biofeedback device (StressEraser). *Appl Psychophysiol Biofeedback*. 2009;34:245. doi:10.1007/s10484-009-9086-1

43. Park ER, Traeger L, Vranceanu, AM. The development of a patient-centered program based on the relaxation response: The relaxation response resiliency program (3RP). *Psychosomatics*. 2013;54(2):165–174.

44. Jacobson E. *Progressive relaxation*. Chicago, IL: University of Chicago Press; 1938.

45. Wolpe J. *Psychotherapy by reciprocal inhibition*. Stanford, CA: Stanford University Press; 1958.

46. Blanchard EB, Appelbaum KA, Radnitz CL, et al. Placebo-controlled evaluation of abbreviated progressive muscle relaxation and of relaxation combined with cognitive therapy in the treatment of tension headache. *J Consult Clin Psychol*. 1990;58(2):210–215.

47. Pawlow, LA, Jones, GE. The impact of abbreviated progressive muscle relaxation on salivary cortisol and salivary immunoglobulin A (sIgA). *Appl Psychophysiol Biofeedback*. 2005;30(4):375–387.

48. Zhao L, Wu H, Zhou X, Wang Q, Weiwei Z, Jindon C. Effects of progressive muscle relaxation training on anxiety, depression, and quality of life in endometriosis patients under gonadotrophin-releasing hormone agonist therapy. *Eur J Obstet Gynecol Reprod Biol*. 2012;162(2):211–215.

49. Dolbier CL, Rush TE. Efficacy of abbreviated progressive muscle relaxation in a high-stress college sample. *Int J Stress Manag*. 2012;19(1):48–68.

50. Neeru; Khakha DC, Satapathy S, Dey AB. Impact of Jacobson progressive muscle relaxation (JPMR) and deep breathing exercises on anxiety, psychological distress, and quality of sleep of hospitalized older adults. *J Psychosom Res*. 2015;10(2):211–223.

51. Cheung YL, Molassiotis A, Chang AM. The effects of progressive muscle relaxation training on anxiety an quality of life after stoma surgery in colorectal cancer patients. *Psychooncology*. 2003;12(3):254–266.

52. Yu DSF, Lee DTF, Woo J, Hui E. Non-pharmacological interventions in older people with heart failure: Effects of exercise training and relaxation training. *Gerontology*. 2007;53(2):74–81.

53. Krajewski J, Sauerland M, Wieland R. Relaxation-induced cortisol changes within lunch breaks: An experimental longitudinal worksite field study. *J Occup Organ Psychol*. 2011;84(2):382–394.

54. Carlson CR, Hoyle, RH. Efficacy of abbreviated progressive muscle relaxation training: A quantitative review of behavioral medicine research. *J Consult Clin Psychol*. 1993;61(6):1059–1067.

55. Goldfried MR, Davison GC, eds. *Clinical and behavior therapy*, Exp ed. New York: Wiley; 1994.

56. Edinger JD, Jacobson R. Incidence and significance of relaxation treatment side effects. *Behav Ther (N Y N Y)*. 1982;5(4):137–138.

57. Achterberg J, Lawlis, GF. *Bridges of the bodymind*. Champaign, IL: IPAT; 1980. Cited by: Rider MS, Achterberg J. Effects of music-assisted imagery on neutrophils and lymphocytes. *Biofeedback Self Regul*. 1989;14(3):247–257.

58. Cormier S, Nurius PS, Osborn CJ, eds. *Interviewing and change strategies for helpers*, 5th ed. New York: Brooks Cole; 2002.

59. Menzies V, Lyon DE, Elswick Jr. RK, McCain NL, Gray DP. Effects of guided imagery on biobehavioral factors in women with fibromyalgia. *J Behav Med*. 2014;37(1):70–80.

60. Kwekkeboom, KL, Hau H, Wanta B, Bumpus M. Patients' perceptions of the effectiveness of guided imagery and progressive muscle relaxation interventions used for cancer pain. *Complement Ther Clin Pract*. 2008;14(3):185–194.

61. Gedde-Dahl M, Fors EA. Impact of self-administered relaxation and guided imagery techniques during final trimester and birth. *Complement Ther Clin Pract*. 2012;18(1):60–65.

62. Hart J. Guided imagery. *Altern Complement Ther*. 2008;14(6):295–299.

63. Schwartz AE. *Guided imagery for groups: Fifty visualizations that promote relaxation, problem-solving, creativity, and well-being*. Duluth, MN: Whole Person Associates Inc.; 1995.

64. Jallo N, Ruiz RJ, Elswick Jr. RK, French E. Guided imagery for stress and symptom management in pregnant African American women. *Evi Based Complement Alternat Med*. 2014. doi:http://dx.doi.org/10.1155/2014/840923.

65. Urech C, Fink NS, Hoesli I, Wilhelm FH, Bitzer J, Alder J. Effects of relaxation on psychobiological wellbeing during pregnancy: A randomized controlled trial. *Psychoneuroendocrinology*. 2010;35(9):1348–1355.

66. Van Kuiken D. A meta-analysis of the effect of guided imagery practice on outcomes. *J Holist Nurs*. 2004;22(2):164–179.

67. Kryger M. *The mystery of sleep: Why a good night's rest is vital to a better, healthier life*. New Haven, CT: Yale University Press; 2017.

68. Dossey, B. Complementary modalities/part 3: Using imagery to help your patient heal. *Am J Nurs*. 1995;95(6):40–47.

69. Schaffer L, Jallo N, Howland L, James K, Glaser D, Arnell K. Guided imagery: An innovative approach to improving maternal sleep quality. *J Perinat Neonat Nurs*. 2013;27(2):151–159.

70. Giacobbi PR, Stabler ME, Stewart J, Jaeschke AM, Siebert JL, Kelley GA. Guided imagery for arthritis and other rheumatic diseases: A systematic review of randomized controlled trials. *Pain Manag Nurs*. 2015;16(5):792–803.

71. Mizrahi MC, Reicher-Atir R, Levy S, Haramati S, Wengrower D, Israeli E, Goldin, E. Effects of guided imagery with relaxation training on anxiety and quality of life among patients with inflammatory bowel disease. *Psychol Health*. 2012;27(12):1463–1479.

72. Roffe L, Schmidt K, Ernst E. A systematic review of guided imagery as an adjuvant cancer therapy. *Psychooncology*. 2005;14(8):607–617.

73. Lin PC. An evaluation of the effectiveness of relaxation therapy patients receiving joint replacement surgery. *J Clin Nurs.* 2010;21(5–6):601–608.

74. Menzies V, Taylor AG, Bourguignon C. Effects of guided imagery on outcomes of pain, functional status, and self-efficacy in persons diagnosed with fibromyalgia. *J Altern Complement Med.* 2006;12(1):23–30.

75. Paul G, Elam B, Verhulst SJ. A longitudinal study of students' perceptions of using deep breathing meditation to reduce testing stresses. *Teach Learn Med.* 2007;19(3):287–292.

76. Travis F, Haaga DAF, Hagelin J, et al. Effects of Transcendental Meditation practice on brain functioning and stress reactivity in college students. *Int J Psychophysiol.* 2009;71(2):170–176.

77. Orme-Johnson DW, Barnes VA. Effects of transcendental meditation technique on trait anxiety: A meta-analysis of randomized controlled trials. *J Altern Complement Med.* 2014;20(5):330–341.

78. Seppälä, EM, Nitschke JB, Tudorascu DL, et al. Breathing-based meditation decreases posttraumatic stress disorders symptoms in U.S. military veterans: A randomized controlled longitudinal study. *J Trauma Stress.* 2014;27(4):397–405.

79. Barnes VA, Monto A, Williams JJ, Rigg JL. Impact of transcendental meditation on psychotropic medication use among active duty military service members with anxiety and PTSD. *Mil Med.* 2016;181(1):56–63.

80. Shapiro SL, Carlson LE. *The art and science of mindfulness: Integrating mindfulness into psychology and the helping professions*, 2nd ed. Washington, DC: American Psychological Association; 2017.

81. Fredrickson BL, Cohn MA, Coffey KA, Pek J, Finkel SM. Open hearts build lives: Positive emotions, induced through loving-kindness meditation, build consequential personal resources. *J Pers Soc Psychol.* 2008;95(5):1045–1062.

82. Germer CK, Neff KD. Self-compassion in clinical practice. *J Clin Psychol.* 2013;69(8):856–867.

83. Kabat-Zinn J. An outpatient program in behavioral medicine for chronic pain patients based on the practice of mindfulness meditation: Theoretical considerations and preliminary results. *Gen Hosp Psychiatry.* 1982;4(1):33–47.

84. Ong JC, Shapiro SL, Manber R. Combining mindfulness meditation with cognitive-behavior therapy for insomnia: A treatment-development study. *Behav Ther.* 2008;39(2):171–182.

85. Shapiro SL, Carlson LE, Astin JA, Freedman B. Mechanisms of mindfulness. *J Clin Psychol.* 2006;62(3):373–386.

86. Killingsworth, MA, Gilbert DT. A wandering mind is an unhappy mind. *Science.* 2010;330:932. doi:10.1126/science.1192439

87. Ricard M. *Why meditate: Working with thoughts and emotions.* Carlsbad, CA: Hay House; 2010.

88. Wallace AB, Bodhi B. The *nature of mindfulness and its role in Buddhist meditation: A correspondence between B. Alan Wallace and the Venerable Bikkhu Bodhi.* Santa Barbara, CA: Santa Barbara Institute for Consciousness Studies; 2006. http://shamatha.org/sites/default/files/Bhikkhu_Bodhi_Correspondence.pdf

89. Santorelli S. *Heal thy self: Lessons on mindfulness in medicine.* New York: Random House; 1999.
90. Siegel D. *The mindful brain: Reflection and attunement in the cultivation of well-being.* New York: Norton; 2007.
91. Brown KW, Ryan RM, Creswell JD. Mindfulness: Theoretical foundations and evidence for its salutary effects. *Psychol Inq.* 2007;18(4):211–237.
92. Kabat-Zinn J. *Full catastrophe living: Using the wisdom of your body and mind to face stress, pain, and illness.* New York: Delacorte Press; 1990.
93. Segal ZV, Williams MG, Teasdale JD. (2002). *Mindfulness-based cognitive therapy for depression: A new approach to preventing relapse.* New York: Guilford Press; 2002.
94. Goyal M, Singh S, Sibinga EMS, et al. Meditation programs for psychological stress and well-being: A systematic review and meta-analysis. *JAMA Intern Med.* 2014;174(3):357–368.
95. Piet J, Würtzen H, Zachariae R. The effect of mindfulness-based therapy on symptoms of anxiety and depression in adult cancer patients and survivors: A systematic review and meta-analysis. *J Consult Clin Psychol.* 2012;80(6):1007–1020.
96. Van Son J, Nyklíček I, Pop VJ, Blonk, MC, Erdtsieck RJ, Pouwer F. Mindfulness-based cognitive therapy for people with diabetes and emotional problems: Long-term follow-up findings from the DiaMind randomized controlled trial. *J Psychosom Res.* 2014;77(1):81–84.
97. Lauche R, Cramer H, Dobos G, Langhorst J, Schmidt S. A systematic review and meta-analysis of mindfulness-based stress reduction for the fibromyalgia syndrome. *J Psychosom Res.* 2013;75(6):500–510.
98. Abbott RA, Whear R, Rodgers LR, et al. Effectiveness of mindfulness-based stress reduction and mindfulness based cognitive therapy in vascular disease: A systematic review and meta-analysis of randomised controlled trials. *J Psychosom Res.* 2014;76(5):341–351.
99. Kristeller J, Wolever RQ, Sheets V. Mindfulness-based eating awareness training (MB-EAT) for binge eating: A randomized clinical trial. *Mindfulness (N Y).* 2014;5(3):282–297.
100. Meyers L, Vollner EK, McCallum EB, Thuras P, Shallcross S. Velasquez T, Meis L. Treating veterans with PTSD and borderline personality symptoms in a 12-week intensive outpatient setting: Findings from a pilot program. *J Trauma Stress.* 2017;30(2):178–181.
101. Chiesa A, Serretti A. Are mindfulness-based interventions effective for substance use disorders? A systematic review of the evidence. *Subst Use Misuse.* 2014);49(5):492–512.
102. Bamber MD, Schneider JK. Mindfulness-based meditation to decrease stress and anxiety in college students: A narrative synthesis of the research. *Educ Res Rev.* 2016;18:1–32.
103. Khoury B, Sharma M, Rush SE, Fournier C. Mindfulness-based stress reduction for healthy individuals: A meta-analysis. *J Psychosom Res.* 2015;78(6):519–528.

104. Mendelson T, Greenberg MT, Dariotis JK, Gould LF, Rhoades BL, Leaf PJ. Feasibility and preliminary outcomes of a school-based mindfulness intervention for urban youth. *J Abnorm Child Psychol.* 2010;38(7):985–994.

105. Bogusch LM, Fekete EM, Skinta MD. Anxiety and depressive symptoms as mediators of trait mindfulness and sleep quality in emerging adults. *Mindfulness (N Y).* 2016;7(4):962–970.

106. Liu QQ, Zhou ZK, Yang XJ, Kong FC, Sun XJ, Fan CY. Mindfulness and sleep quality in adolescents: Analysis of rumination as a mediator and self-control as a moderator. *Pers Individ Dif.* 2018;122(1):171–176.

107. Simor P, Köteles F, Sándor P, Petke Z, Bódizs R. Mindfulness and dream quality: The inverse relationship between mindfulness and negative dream affect. *Scand J Psychol.* 2011;52(4):369–375.

108. Visser PL, Hirsch JK, Brown KW, Ryan R, Moynihan JA. Components of sleep quality as mediators of the relation between mindfulness and subjective vitality among older adults. *Mindfulness (N Y).* 2015;6(4):723–731.

109. Ong JC. *Mindfulness-based therapy for insomnia.* Washington, DC: American Psychological Association; 2017.

110. Ong JC, Manber R, Segal Z, Xia Y, Shapiro S, Wyatt JK. Randomized controlled trial of mindfulness meditation for chronic insomnia. *Sleep.* 2014;37(9):1553–1566. doi:10.5665/sleep.4010.

12

Toward a Positive Psychology of Sleep

EMERSON M. WICKWIRE

The historical focus of Western medicine has been the treatment of disease and alleviation of suffering. However, over the past several decades, healthcare providers have begun to move beyond this narrow conceptualization of health as the absence of disease to focus on a "whole person" approach to medical care. Indeed, patients, providers, and multiple stakeholders increasingly recognize enhanced quality of life as a central purpose and key outcome of medical treatment. Because sleep and wake disorders incorporate all phases of the 24-hour day, sleep specialists are ideally positioned to move beyond simply alleviating disease toward leveraging sleep to increase positive life experiences and overall well-being.

Positive psychology is the domain of mental health research and practice that seeks to enhance such well-being and positive functioning by increasing positive emotion. Because sleep and positive emotion share neurological and behavioral underpinnings and demonstrate bidirectional relationships, positive psychology approaches hold great promise for enhancing outcomes among sleep disorders patients. Although sleep-specific treatment studies are only beginning to emerge in the literature, in other domains of medicine positive psychology interventions have shown promising if preliminary results. Furthermore, clinical experience suggests that adopting a positive psychology framework and integrating positive psychology interventions can enhance outcomes and adherence among sleep disorders patients.

The purpose of this chapter is to introduce a positive psychology framework to guide sleep medicine care. First, the scientific evidence relating sleep and positive emotion will be reviewed. Next, several core principles of positive psychology will be introduced. Finally, clinical recommendations will be provided to incorporate principles and intervention exercises into routine sleep medicine care.

The Emerging Science of Sleep and Positive Mood

In terms of emotional health, traditional medical models have focused on negative emotions such as anger, sadness, loneliness, boredom, and anhedonia. Consistent with this tradition, the vast majority of sleep-specific research to date has focused on the relationship between sleep and depressed mood. As reviewed elsewhere in this volume, hundreds of epidemiologic, clinical, and experimental studies have demonstrated a robust, bidirectional relationship between insufficient and disturbed sleep and negative emotion as well as depressive disorders.

However, emotion is not a unipolar construct. Equal and opposite to negative mood states, distinct positive mood states such as joy, happiness, contentment, and connection are the focus of positive psychology. Notably, one common misconception is that positive psychology is concerned primarily with "happiness." Instead, positive psychology research and practice focuses on the full range of positive emotions occurring throughout the life span and in multiple domains.

Within the past decade, a number of studies have sought to build on past literature examining sleep and depression to explore the relationship between sleep and positive mood.

For example, a correlational study found trait gratitude to be associated with self-reported sleep quality as measured by the Pittsburgh Sleep Quality Index.[1] Importantly, changes in pre-sleep cognitions were found to mediate the relationship between gratitude and enhanced sleep quality.[1] Although a comprehensive review is beyond the scope of this introductory chapter, Table 12.1 highlights key findings from many of these studies. Furthermore, a detailed consideration of two studies provides a helpful overview of key issues.

One of the earliest studies into sleep and positive mood is an unpublished report. Walker and Stickgold[2] recruited healthy undergraduate volunteers into a study examining sleep loss and subsequent memory formation. Prior to a memory encoding session, participants were randomized to two nights of self-administered sleep deprivation (i.e., 36 hours sleep loss) or normal sleep. Then, participants completed a straightforward memory task to memorize words from a list. However, surreptitiously, this list included words with positive, negative, and neutral emotional valence. Following completion of the memory task, participants were instructed to sleep normally. Two days later, participants returned for an unexpected follow-up assessment and were asked to recall as many words as they could. Overall, compared to the normal sleep controls, sleep-deprived participants recalled 40% fewer words. These results highlight the negative impact of sleep loss on subsequent memory formation, which is essential for learning and cognitive

Table 12.1 Summary of selected studies exploring sleep and positive emotion

Author	N	Design	Measures	Key findings
Blaxton et al.[13]	552 (307 midlife age 33–64; 245 later-life age 62–91)	Prospective cohort study: 56-day consecutive diary monitoring including self-reported sleep quality in morning; perceived daily stress, PA, NA in evening	sleep diary, PANAS, PSS	Good sleep quality and higher PA buffered impact of stress on NA. Age-related differences were observed, suggesting changes across adulthood.
Bower et al.[14]	96 (35 major depression, 25 minor depression, 36 healthy controls)	Micro-longitudinal study: Participants self-rated affect up to 10×/day over 3 days via ESM	PSQI, PA and NA adjective lists administered via ESM	No between-groups differences in PA were observed. NA was elevated in BD and insomnia.
Finan et al.[4]	62 healthy good sleeping adults	RCT: forced nocturnal awakenings, normal sleep (8h TIB), restricted sleep opportunity. All participants completed laboratory measures over 3 consecutive days.	PSG, POMS bipolar	Compared to uninterrupted and restricted sleep, fragmented sleep was associated w/reduced SWS after night 1 and reduced next-day PA after night 2.
Finan et al.[3]	45 healthy good sleeping adults	Randomized crossover study: participants completed 1 night forced awakenings and 1 night undisturbed sleep, followed by in-lab assessment of PA/NA, pain sensitivity, and neurocognitive performance	PSG, PANAS-X, laboratory pain testing measures	Compared to uninterrupted sleep, disrupted sleep diminished SWS, which in turn diminished multiple PA systems including inhibition of pain by PA. Disrupted sleep had no impact on NA systems.

(continued)

Table 12.1 Continued

Author	N	Design	Measures	Key findings
Fredman et al.[15]	229 (92 caregivers of friend/family w AD and 137 noncaregivers age >60 y)	Cross-sectional study: In-person interviews and questionnaires administered	PSQI, CES-D	Compared to caregivers w/low PA, caregivers w/high PA had fewer sleep problems. Caregivers w/depressive symptoms had more sleep problems. Among non-caregivers, PA was unrelated to sleep problems.
Hasler et al.[16]	100 insomnia (55 women)	Micro-longitudinal design: Participants completed daily sleep diaries and 4× daily mood diaries for 4–15 days, as well as laboratory PET imaging	CSM, Sleep diaries, PANAS, PET	Chronotype was significantly associated with diurnal patterns of affect. Compared to morning types, evening types demonstrated phase delay and lower amplitude of PA. Diurnal variation of metabolism was also reduced in metabolism of medial prefrontal cortex and striatum.
Levitt et al.[17]	7 insomnia, 8 matched controls	Micro-longitudinal design: Participants completed sleep diaries and 4× daily mood diaries for 1 week	Sleep diary; Mood diary	Compared to controls, insomnia group demonstrated greater variability in daytime symptoms.
Pilcher et al.[18]	59 (28 partial SD, 31 total SD)	Within-subject experiment: Participants rated emotional valence and arousal to +/− pictures during day (partial SD) or at night (total SD)	Actigraphy, IAPS International Affective Picture System	Sleep-deprived individuals responded less to positive pictures than they responded to negative pictures.

Study	Sample	Design	Measures	Findings
Talbot et al.[19]	49 bipolar disorder, 34 insomnia, 52 no psyc hx	Micro-longitudinal design: Participants completed sleep diaries and 2× daily mood measures for 1 week	Sleep diary, POMS-SF	Bipolar and insomnia groups reported greater morning and evening NA than controls. Among those with bipolar disorder but not insomnia, poor sleep quality predicted greater morning NA.
Walker et al.[2]	Undergraduates (unpublished)	RCT: 36h sleep loss or normal sleep prior to memory encoding session. All participants were asked to memorize a list of positive, negative, and neutral words. Following two subsequent nights of sleep, participants returned for an unannounced repeat administration/recognition task	Adjective list	Compared to normal sleep, 36h sleep loss was associated with 40% overall reduction in word recall. Significant differences were observed between groups in recall of PA but not NA or neutral words.
Wild-Hartmann et al.[20]	553 women	Micro-longitudinal design: Participants completed a 5-day baseline ESM assessment, then 4× serial assessments for depression over 1 year	Sleep diary, Likert affect scale administered via ESM, SCID-I, SCL-90-R	Prior night sleep predicted next day affect, especially PA. Daytime NA did not predict subsequent sleep. Baseline sleep predicted depressive symptoms.

(continued)

Table 12.1 Continued

Author	N	Design	Measures	Key findings
Winzeler et al.[21]	145 healthy young women	Micro-longitudinal design: participants completed 14 days of sleep diaries in morning and stress and pre-sleep measures each evening	Sleep diary, actigraphy, PSQI, Daily Stress Inventory (DSI)	Stress was positively associated with cognitive and somatic arousal. Somatic arousal mediated sleep quality between participants; cognitive arousal mediated sleep quality within participants.
Wood et al.[1]	401	Cross-sectional, questionnaire-based study	PSQI, GQ-6, Self-statement test	Gratitude was positively associated w/SQ, TST, and negatively associated with daytime dysfunction. Gratitude was also associated with less pre-sleep worry and more positive pre-sleep thoughts, which was in turn associated with higher sleep quality.

AD, Alzheimer's disease; CES-D, Center Epidemiological – Depression; DSI, Daily Stress Inventory; ESM, Ecological momentary sampling; GQ-6, Gratitude Questionnaire (6-item); IAPS International Affective Picture System; NA, negative affect; PA, positive affect; PANAS, Positive and Negative Affect Scale; POMS, Profile of Mood States; PSG, polysomnogram; PSQI, Pittsburgh Sleep Quality Index; PSS, Perceived Stress Scale; PSYC, psychiatric; RCT, randomized controlled trial; SCL-90-R; SD, sleep deprivation.

development. More impressively, although there was no difference between groups in recall for negative words, sleep-deprived participants recalled fewer than half (i.e., 59% fewer) of the positive words recalled by the normal sleep controls. The striking deficiency in recall of positive emotional words explained the majority of overall differences between groups.[2]

More recently, a series of highly controlled experimental studies was conducted to examine the impact of sleep on positive affect.[3,4] As part of a multinight protocol, healthy volunteers were randomized to a normal sleep control condition (i.e., 8 hours uninterrupted time in bed), simulated insomnia (i.e., experimental sleep fragmentation in which patients were awakened intermittently throughout the night), or a restricted sleep opportunity condition in which participants slept uninterrupted for several hours. After one night and compared to both normal sleep control and restricted sleep opportunity, participants in the simulated insomnia condition demonstrated decreased slow wave N3 sleep, as was expected. However, after a second night of experimental sleep fragmentation, participants in the simulated insomnia condition also reported diminished positive affect, with decreases in slow wave sleep mediating between groups differences in positive affect. In other words, simulated insomnia reduced positive affect even after controlling for sleep loss, and reductions in slow wave sleep mediated this process.[4]

Positive Psychology: A Very Brief Overview

DEFINING "THE GOOD LIFE"

An integrative approach to sleep disorders medicine requires attention and clinical care oriented toward the whole patient, including not only sleep and disease characteristics but also myriad aspects of daytime functioning, life satisfaction, and human development. Eminent psychologist Martin Seligman has characterized this "good life" as including positive emotion, engagement, relationships, meaning, achievement, and others (i.e., PERMA).[5] More broadly, a positive psychology approach to patient care focuses on positive feelings (i.e., emotion, affect) and positive functioning (i.e., maximizing strengths and contribution).[6] This simple framework can provide especially helpful guidance to nonbehavioral sleep medicine clinicians who have adopted an integrative approach to patient care. For example, when working with patients to develop collaborative treatment plans, sleep medicine providers should incorporate one or more affective and one or more functional outcomes at each treatment interval.

A STRENGTHS-BASED APPROACH

As anyone who has ever sought to learn a new skill (e.g., sports, theater, hobby, or profession) understands, superior performance is driven by leveraging strengths not eliminating weaknesses. Within a positive psychology framework, this same premise holds true of fulfillment, meaning, and life satisfaction—individuals possess unique strengths, which should be recognized, nurtured, and grown. This fundamental belief was first popularized by Donald O. Clifton, a pioneer in strengths-based thinking.[7] Clifton's strengths theory purports that greatness is achieved by developing personal strengths, which should be advanced and expanded. Conversely, weaknesses should only be managed to the extent that they do not impede strengths-based performance.

Unfortunately, as Clifton observed, the overall focus of modern American culture (as evidenced by parents, teachers, employers, healthcare providers, and others) generally remains on identifying weaknesses. Although elimination of weaknesses might be possible in some instances, the price of intensive effort required is not worth it; these resources would provide a better return on effort by focusing on strengths.

From a sleep medicine perspective, a strengths-based approach can serve as a cornerstone of an integrated, holistic approach to treatment planning and patient care. Sleep medicine treatments universally involve behavioral modification ranging from sleep scheduling to medication adherence, which must be sustained over time. Thus, identifying and leveraging patient strengths and interests, including past efforts at behavior change, can reduce perceived burden and increase patient confidence regarding behavioral treatment recommendations, such as stimulus control therapy or sleep restriction/sleep compression therapy.

BROADENING AND BUILDING POSITIVE EMOTION

In addition to recognizing and building on strengths, a core tenet of a positive psychology approach to sleep is building, broadening, and deepening experience of positive emotion. According to the broaden-and-build theory of positive emotion,[8] even brief experiences of positive emotion can expand an individual's cognitive, behavioral, and emotional repertoire. Psychologist Barbara Fredrickson has postulated that positive emotions briefly broaden thought–action repertoires, which can thus be developed into new resources.[9] In turn, these new resources can be supported and built on in support of personal growth and development. In other words, when it comes to increasing positive affect, small experiences of "feeling good" are like seeds that, properly nurtured, can blossom and provide nourishing fruits.

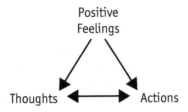

FIGURE 12.1 Thoughts, feelings, and actions are mutually influential. The broaden and build theory of positive emotion posits that even brief experiences of positive feeling will expand thought–action repertoires, thus leading to change. This humanistic view does not discount the substantial influences of genetics, biology, life circumstance, physical environment, and other factors in shaping human experience. Image © Emerson M. Wickwire, PhD. Used with permission.

Although often unstated, flexibility is central to the broaden-and-build theory of positive emotion. Sleep disorders and negative emotion are both defined in part by a loss of flexibility—a restricted range of experience. For example, many patients with sleep complaints describe a state of hyperarousal such that, during the day, they feel "tired but wired" and unable to fully engage. At the same time, during the night, these patients experience overly active minds or restless bodies such that they are unable to disengage fully. Similarly, mental health conditions such as depression and anxiety are characterized by a restricted range of negative feelings and thoughts, respectively. As another example, patients with chronic pain experience a loss of physical flexibility and, as a result, exercise less. Of course, regaining flexibility and safely increasing physical activity are core tenets of many chronic pain management protocols (Figure 12.1).

FURTHER BENEFITS OF POSITIVE EMOTION: UNDOING AND RESILIENCE

Building on her pioneering work in "broaden and building" positive emotions, Fredrickson has also demonstrated that positive emotion can undo the adverse effects of negative emotion. In a series of experiments, Fredrickson and colleagues found that experimentally induced positive emotions undid the adverse physiological effects of negative emotion, including lowering heart rate, blood pressure, and vasoconstriction.[10,11] Beyond undoing, Fredrickson has also demonstrated that positive emotion is a core component of resilience, including resilience to the trauma of the September 11, 2001, terrorist attacks in New York City.[12] Relatedly, sleep health is increasingly recognized as a core component of resilience in corporate, athletic, and military operational applications.

POSITIVE PSYCHOLOGY INTERVENTIONS

Unfortunately, despite the clear scientific linkages between sleep and positive mood, as well as the theoretical and practical consistencies between positive psychology approaches and enhanced patient quality of life, few studies have evaluated the beneficial impact of positive psychology interventions on sleep outcomes. As discussed in Chapter 11 of this volume, one notable exception is mindfulness training, which has seen an explosion in research interest over the past decade. Overall, mindfulness is associated with improvements in sleep quality, although the mechanisms remain incompletely understood. Nonetheless, despite scant clinical research, sleep medicine providers need practical tools to enhance positive feelings among their patients. Table 12.2 presents a nonexhaustive summary of common positive psychology interventions with applicability to sleep. Each is amenable for integration into routine clinical care.

Clinical Recommendations

Despite the lag in clinical trials, behavioral sleep specialists and integrated sleep medicine physicians have successfully integrated positive psychology interventions into routine sleep medicine care for decades. For example, behavioral activation, mindfulness, and gratitude can seamlessly be incorporated into all aspects of sleep medicine care, regardless of presenting sleep complaint. One reason is that these promising and patient-centered interventions have virtually no adverse side effects. Furthermore, clinical experience suggests that positive psychology approaches demonstrate a strong and consistent beneficial impact on patient quality of life, treatment adherence, and overall satisfaction. Positive psychology exercises build core behavioral and self-management skills that are highly transferrable to other domains of life. Finally, from an educational perspective, it is worth noting that sleep medicine fellows and other trainees routinely report great benefit from learning a strengths-based approach to patient care and from knowing how to augment traditional sleep medicine care with positive psychology approaches.

The following clinical recommendations are based on nearly 15 years of clinical experience treating sleep patients and substantial experience as a sleep medicine educator. Thus, they must not be interpreted as evidence-based medicine, which should of course remain the cornerstone of sleep medicine care. Nonetheless, to adopt a positive psychology approach, clinicians are advised to experiment with the exercises outlined in Table 12.2 and experience personally the benefits. Then, clinicians can begin by selecting one or a small number of exercises to recommend to their patients. Further guidance is presented in the next sections.

Table 12.2 Summary of select positive psychology interventions for sleep

Intervention	Application	Clinical approaches/Patient instructions
Behavioral activation[22]	Increase recreational activity Break a behavioral rut	Engage in a purposeful, recreational activity: Do something fun for yourself, no strings attached.
Gratitude	Counterbalance worry Recognize and savor what is good	Write a letter of gratitude.[23] Count your blessings.[24] Conclude a pre-sleep journal with a list of 3–5 things for which you are grateful.
Hope	Recognize that good results are possible and can be achieved	Clarify the objective. Brainstorm alternative pathways to achieve the objective.
Mindfulness	Reduce anxiety, worry, or restlessness Target physiologic hyperarousal Strengthen the relaxation muscles	Mindfulness training should be framed as learning to focus on "what is" rather than "what if." In-person trainings take place in professional settings, churches, and senior centers in every community. Mobile apps, CDs, and other self-study materials by John Kabat Zinn, Rubin Naiman, Belleruth Naparstek, and others receive positive reviews from patients.
Optimism	Recognize and overcome catastrophizing Replace negative expectations with positive ones	Best possible self.[25] Imagine that everything has gone as well as it possibly could. Write about this for 20 minutes per day.
Signature strengths	Recognize unique personal strengths	What is your superpower? Name your unique strength. How can this strength be used in the current situation?

ASSESSMENT

From a positive sleep perspective, the overarching goal of clinical assessment is to clarify patient goals for treatment and identify patient strengths that can be leveraged to help achieve these objectives. Thus, prior to initiating a clinical sleep history or physical examination, clinicians should ask patients the "magic wand" question to open dialogue regarding patient goals for enhanced quality of life: "If I had a magic wand and could change anything about your sleep, what would you want that to be?" As depicted in Figure 12.2, following general answers such as "I want more sleep" or "I'd like to sleep through the night," clinicians should seek

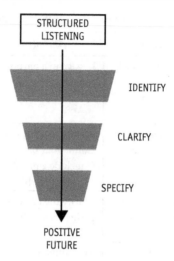

FIGURE 12.2 The Wickwire Funnel Framework as applied to sleep disorders assessment.
Image © Emerson M. Wickwire, PhD. Used with permission.

to clarify how this result would change the patient's life. For example, a helpful clarifying question is "If we were to accomplish that, how would your life be different?" Typically, patients will report that enhanced sleep will result in increased energy levels, decreased fatigue, or some other positive improvement. At this time, clinicians should seek to specify what this change would look like in behavioral terms, for example, by asking "And if your energy levels were increased, what would you do differently?" These specific behavioral objectives (e.g., return to exercise program, socialize with friends, increase leisure activity, etc) are then included as concrete, measurable patient-centered outcomes in the comprehensive, integrated treatment plan.

TAILORING INTERVENTIONS

Once patient goals for treatment have been collaboratively identified and refined, the sleep history and other examination should be conducted. Next, prior to composing an initial treatment plan, it is vital for a positive psychology approach to identify patient strengths and interests so that these can be nurtured and grown to support positive behavioral change. For example, when identifying possible recreational or physical exercise activities, clinicians should inquire regarding past experiences and particularly successes: "What kind of exercise have you enjoyed in the past?" "What were the factors that contributed to your success?" "How were you able to overcome any barriers?" "How did you benefit from

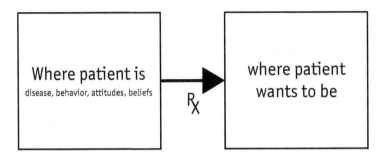

FIGURE 12.3 The central role of the sleep clinician is to help move patients from where they are to where they want to be. To maximize outcomes, integrated treatment plans must not only address biomedical concerns but also incorporate specific behavioral objectives to leverage sleep and enhance quality of life. Clinical experience suggests that positive psychology approaches can help.
Image © Emerson M. Wickwire, PhD. Used with permission.

the support of others?" "What name would you give that strength of yours?" These specific individual-level characteristics should be used to guide specific behavioral recommendations based on patient strengths and interests (Figure 12.3).

Measuring Outcomes

Just as sleep specialists monitor patient adherence to biomedical treatments for sleep disorders (e.g., objective adherence to positive airway pressure therapies for obstructive sleep apnea) as well as subjective treatment response (e.g., reduced daytime sleepiness, enhanced cognition), clinicians must evaluate adherence and effectiveness of positive psychology interventions delivered in a sleep medicine context. From a positive sleep perspective, these outcomes are integral to patient care and warrant the same care, attention, and commitment as other typically biomedical components of the treatment plan. Steps toward positive sleep must be discussed during treatment encounters, such discussion must be included in the patient chart, instructions must be provided during discharge, and follow-up visits must seek to adapt and adjust the clinical approach based on patient response.

Case Study: Positive Sleep in Action

Susan was a 37-year-old married mother of two young children. She reported for insomnia consultation in order to sleep through the night, which would make it easier to arise each morning as well as increase her daytime energy levels. With increased energy, Susan hoped to resume more regular exercise and increase her social activities.

During initial consultation, Susan reported severe insomnia (Insomnia Severity Index [ISI]: 23/28) and mild depressive symptomatology (Beck-Depression Inventory-2 [BDI-2]: 16/68). Baseline sleep diaries revealed a highly variable sleep–wake schedule, with bedtimes ranging from 8:45 PM to 1:30 AM, sleep latency mean of 60 minutes, number of awakenings of three, wake after sleep onset mean of 45 minutes, and wake times ranging from 4:30 to 8:30 AM.

Behavioral and pharmacologic treatment options were discussed, and Susan elected to proceed with cognitive-behavioral therapy for insomnia (CBT-I). In our center, CBT-I is delivered within an integrated care model, typically involving monthly encounters with a sleep-trained clinical psychologist who oversees sleep-related care, as well as a physician who provides E/M service for non-sleep medical comorbidities. Because Susan's verbal report of anhedonia and increasing social isolation was consistent with mild depression, it was agreed to closely monitor her mood symptoms and refer for specialty mental health care if needed.

Over the course of nine treatment encounters, Susan benefited from stimulus control therapy, restriction of time in bed, and mindfulness training. Positive sleep approaches were incorporated throughout. In terms of stimulus control, Susan was guided to establish a structured pre-sleep wind-down ritual, which included a gratitude list. Efforts at sleep restriction and sleep scheduling were enhanced by incorporating positive self-reward for getting out of bed each morning, ranging from enjoying her favorite toast and jam to savoring a few moments on her back porch. Throughout the course of her mindfulness practice, Susan was encouraged to focus on the positive, including both physical and emotional sensations. Finally, a behavioral activation approach was adopted to increase social and recreational engagement.

At the conclusion of treatment, Susan's score on the ISI had been reduced to 12/28, representing mild or subthreshold insomnia, and her score on the BDI-2 was 9/68, which is within normal limits. Her sleep schedule was stable, and her clinical sleep parameters had dramatically improved (sleep onset latency mean of 30 minutes and wake after sleep onset mean of 30 minutes). Perhaps most important, Susan was pleased with her progress toward her two stated objectives for seeking sleep specialty care: increased physical activity and social engagement.

Conclusion and Future Directions

The need for sleep medicine services has never been greater. In the United States and worldwide, we face an epidemic of insufficient and disordered sleep, with substantial adverse impact on health, safety, and quality of life. At the same time, the landscape of sleep medicine is changing. Patients, providers, and other stakeholders have become increasingly focused on patient quality of life as a key health metric and core, measurable outcome from patient-centered clinical care. There has been a parallel increase among the lay public in the impact of sleep on optimal human function and life satisfaction. By nurturing and growing positive affect, positive psychology provides a theoretical and practical framework to enhance patient-centered outcomes among sleep-disordered patients. Much work remains to be done, including conducting randomized controlled trials of positive psychology interventions in sleep-disordered populations, advancing the understanding of positive psychology interventions on sleep-related outcomes, and determining how to optimize positive psychology interventions. In the meantime, given their low risk and based on clinical experience, sleep medicine providers committed to an integrated approach should seek to incorporate a positive psychology approach into routine sleep medicine care.

REFERENCES

1. Wood AM, Joseph S, Lloyd J, Atkins S. Gratitude influences sleep through the mechanism of pre-sleep cognitions. *J Psychosom Res.* 2009;66(1):43–48.
2. Walker MP, Stickgold R. Sleep, memory, and plasticity. *Ann Rev Psychol.* 2006;57:139–166.
3. Finan PH, Quartana PJ, Remeniuk B, Garland EL, Rhudy JL, Hand M, Irwin MR, Smith MT. Partial sleep deprivation attenuates the positive affective system: Effects across multiple measurement modalities. *Sleep.* 2017 Jan 1;40(1):zsw017. doi:10.1093/sleep/zsw017. PMID: 28364467; PMCID: PMC6084750.
4. Finan PH, Quartana PJ, Smith MT. The effects of sleep continuity disruption on positive mood and sleep architecture in healthy adults. *Sleep.* 2015;38(11):1735–1742.
5. Seligman MEP. *Flourish: A visionary new understanding of happiness and well-being.* New York: Free Press; 2011.
6. Magyar-Moe JL, Owens RL, Conoley CW. Positive psychological interventions in counseling: What every counseling psychologist should know. *Counseling Psychologist.* 2015;43(4):508–557.
7. Clifton DO. Guiding principles for growing a company. *Psychologist-Manager J.* 1999;3(1):49–56.
8. Fredrickson BL. The role of positive emotions in positive psychology: The broaden-and-build theory of positive emotions. *Am Psychologist.* 2001;56(3):218–226.
9. Fredrickson BL, Branigan C. Positive emotions broaden the scope of attention and thought-action repertoires. *Cognition Emotion.* 2005;19(3):313–332.
10. Fredrickson BL, Levenson RW. Positive emotions speed recovery from the cardiovascular sequelae of negative emotions. *Cognition Emotion.* 1998;12(2):191–220.
11. Fredrickson BL, Mancuso RA, Branigan C, Tugade MM. The undoing effect of positive emotions. *Motivation Emotion.* 2000;24(4):237–258.

12. Fredrickson BL, Tugade MM, Waugh CE, Larkin GR. What good are positive emotions in crisis? A prospective study of resilience and emotions following the terrorist attacks on the United States on September 11th, 2001. *J Personality Soc Psychol.* 2003;84(2):365–376.

13. Blaxton JM, Bergeman CS, Whitehead BR, Braun ME, Payne JD. Relationships Among Nightly Sleep Quality, Daily Stress, and Daily Affect. *J Gerontol B Psychol Sci Soc Sci.* 2017;72(3):363–372.

14. Bower B, Bylsma LM, Morris BH, Rottenberg J. Poor reported sleep quality predicts low positive affect in daily life among healthy and mood-disordered persons. *J Sleep Res.* 2010;19(2):323–332.

15. Fredman L, Gordon SA, Heeren T, Stuver SO. Positive affect is associated with fewer sleep problems in older caregivers but not noncaregivers. *Gerontologist.* 2014;54(4):559–569.

16. Hasler BP, Germain A, Nofzinger EA, Kupfer DJ, Krafty RT, Rothenberger SD, et al. Chronotype and diurnal patterns of positive affect and affective neural circuitry in primary insomnia. *J Sleep Res.* 2012;21(5):515–526.

17. Levitt H, Wood A, Moul DE, Hall M, Germain A, Kupfer DJ, et al. A pilot study of subjective daytime alertness and mood in primary insomnia participants using ecological momentary assessment. *Behav Sleep Med.* 2004;2(2):113–131.

18. Pilcher JJ, Callan C, Posey JL. Sleep deprivation affects reactivity to positive but not negative stimuli. *J Psychosom Res.* 2015;79(6):657–662.

19. Talbot LS, Stone S, Gruber J, Hairston IS, Eidelman P, Harvey AG. A test of the bi-directional association between sleep and mood in bipolar disorder and insomnia. *J Abnorm Psychol.* 2012;121(1):39–50.

20. de Wild-Hartmann JA, Wichers M, van Bemmel AL, Derom C, Thiery E, Jacobs N, et al. Day-to-day associations between subjective sleep and affect in regard to future depression in a female population-based sample. *Br J Psychiatry.* 2013;202:407–412.

21. Winzeler K, Voellmin A, Schafer V, Meyer AH, Cajochen C, Wilhelm FH, et al. Daily stress, pre-sleep arousal, and sleep in healthy young women: A daily life computerized sleep diary and actigraphy study. *Sleep Med.* 2014;15(3):359–366.

22. Jacobson NS, Martell CR, Dimidjian S. Behavioral activation treatment for depression: Returning to contextual roots. *Clin Psychol Sci Pract.* 2001;8(3):255–270.

23. Seligman MEP, Steen TA, Park N, Peterson C. Positive psychology progress: Empirical validation of interventions. *Tidsskrift for Norsk Psykologforening.* 2005;42(10):874–884.

24. Emmons RA, McCullough ME. Counting blessings versus burdens: An experimental investigation of gratitude and subjective well-being in daily life. *J Personality Soc Psychol.* 2003;84(2):377–389.

25. King LA. The health benefits of writing about life goals. *Personality Soc Psychol Bull.* 2001;27(7):798–807.

13

Integrative Dream Medicine

RUBIN NAIMAN

Introduction

Widely acknowledged as the roots of modern medicine, ancient Greek Asklepian practices emphasized the role of dreams in healing. Conventional medicine has, in contrast, shown limited interest in clinical aspects of rapid eye movement (REM) sleep and even less in dreaming. REM sleep has been subsumed under the general rubric of sleep, relegating it to a stepchild-like status in sleep medicine, and dreaming has been largely dismissed as a meaningless artifact of REM sleep neurophysiology. Today, healthcare providers routinely ask patients about their sleep but not their dreams. Even psychotherapists, who traditionally viewed dreams as "the royal road to the unconscious," have shown considerably less interest in dreamwork over recent years.[1]

This chapter provides an overview of an integrative approach to REM sleep and dreams, which highlights their key role in neurological and mental health. The challenge in doing so involves integrating two largely independent streams of literature historically segregated along the classic mind–body rift. REM sleep has been understood primarily as a physiological process, while dreaming has been viewed as a phenomenological experience. As we will see, there is a critical interplay between body and mind that is essential in understanding REM/ dreaming (Although REM sleep and dreaming are generally viewed as independent constructs, this chapter uses the terms REM/dream(s) and REM/dreaming to refer to their overlay.)

While sleep and dream disorders are clearly medical issues, sleep and dreams, per se, are not; they are personal experiences. Reducing dreaming to REM sleep physiology unnecessarily medicalizes a ubiquitous and meaningful life experience, discouraging patients and clinicians alike from adequately attending to it. Intense dream experiences, such as hypnagogic hallucinations, sleep paralysis, and recurrent nightmares, are, furthermore, overly pathologized and widely presumed to be personally meaningless. Overly medicalizing and pathologizing even challenging dreams can contribute to an erosion of trust in one's unconscious. An integrative approach recognizes REM/dreaming, even when it has gone awry, as a natural, endogenous healing process.

The purpose of this chapter is to review the current understanding of REM/dreaming as a foundation and rationale for addressing related clinical issues in primary and secondary care. It includes discussions of the neurophysiology of REM sleep, the phenomenology of dreaming, the functions of REM/dreaming, the silent epidemic of REM/dream loss, and recommendations for health professionals.

The Physiology of REM Sleep

REM sleep, unique to mammals and birds, was first observed and described by Aserinsky and Kleitman in the 1950s.[2] Subsequent findings revealed the critical influence of chronobiology or rhythmic processes on sleep, dreams, and waking consciousness.[3]

In addition to 24-hour circadian rhythms, 90-minute ultradian rhythms provide a fundamental temporal structure for brain and body physiology during waking and sleep. Ultradian rhythms include oscillations of activity and rest by day that transpose to sleep and dreams by night, reflecting a critical continuity of consciousness.[4] Composed primarily of non–REM (NREM) sleep, including slow wave sleep (SWS), the first two sleep cycles also include initial brief periods of REM sleep. Subsequently, SWS sleep decreases while REM sleep increases through the night, positioning our most protracted REM periods in the early morning hours. The reciprocal-interaction model of REM and NREM sleep proposes they are structurally linked through ultradian rhythms.[5] The quality of our sleep, then, is inextricably linked to the quality of REM sleep.

Brain regions activated during REM sleep are essentially the inverse of those activated during NREM sleep.[6] Positron emission tomography (PET) studies suggest REM sleep is characterized by activation of the brainstem as well as the limbic and paralimbic systems.[7] The anterior paralimbic REM activation area is specifically associated with emotion, memory, fear, and sex.[8] In contrast to SWS, REM sleep hippocampal activity is not linked to the prefrontal cortex,[9] disengaging it from executive function. In contrast to NREM sleep and waking, REM sleep is also characterized by an unusual suspension of centrally mediated homeostasis.[10]

From an electroencephalographic (EEG) perspective, REM, or *paradoxical sleep*, is a hybrid of sleep and waking states marked by alternations of distinct tonic and phasic components. *Tonic REM sleep* is parasympathetically driven and associated with relaxed eyes and theta waves. *Phasic REM* is sympathetically driven and defined by beta and gamma waves, bursts of rapid eye movements, muscle twitching, and irregular respiration.[11]

Phasic REM sleep is also associated with "autonomic nervous system (ANS) storms"—intense emotional and somatic reactions that include increased heart rate and blood pressure as well as heightened risk of hypoxia, plaque rupture, and coronary arterial spasm. As periods of REM sleep increase through the night, ANS storms escalate, leaving cardiovascular disease patients more likely to die then than at any other time of day.[12] (*Dying in one's sleep* may more accurately be about dying in one's dreams.) It's important to note that REM/dreaming appears to impact the body and mind in much the same way as waking experiences do, and we generally are in denial about this.

Somatic features of REM sleep include suppression of sensory processing and REM atonia—a loss of skeletal muscle tone resulting from centrally mediated motor neuron inhibition. Commonly referred to as *sleep paralysis*, REM atonia precludes the acting out of dream narratives. REM sleep is also associated with involuntary sexual arousal in males, who experience penile erections, and females, who experience clitoral tumescence and transudation. These responses occur independently of sexual dream content.[13]

Neurochemically, REM sleep is generally mediated by central nervous system decreases in monoamine neurotransmitters and increases in acetylcholine. The activation-synthesis hypothesis of REM sleep regulation[14] proposes that cholinergic "REM-on" neurons and aminergic "REM off" neurons regulate cycling between REM and NREM sleep.

Although best understood in terms of its regulation of circadian rhythms, melatonin (MT) also plays a key role in mediating REM sleep. With continued exposure to dim light and darkness, MT levels gradually rise through the night, encouraging peripheral vascular dilation to decrease core body temperature. As MT levels peak in early morning hours, core body temperature reaches its nadir (Core T_{min}), and REM sleep periods become most protracted. Exogenous MT has been shown to increase diminished REM sleep in humans.[15]

A recent comprehensive review of REM sleep physiology concluded that "the adaptive role of rapid eye movement (REM) sleep remains a complete mystery."[16] Could this perspective stem from an inadequate consideration of REM sleep's role in the phenomenology of dreaming?

The Phenomenology of Dreaming

In a recent "Manifesto for a Post-Materialist Science,"[17] a group of internationally renowned scientists concluded that the nearly absolute dominance of materialism in the academic world has seriously constricted the sciences and hampered the development of the scientific study of mind and spirituality. Faith in this ideology, as an exclusive explanatory framework for reality, has compelled scientists to neglect the subjective dimension of human experience. This has led to a severely distorted and impoverished understanding of ourselves and our place in nature.

Similar themes have echoed through the work of notable philosophers, psychologists, physicians, and spiritual teachers across time. For example, Andrew Weil's first book, *The Natural Mind*,[18] emphasizes the innate human need to transcend ordinary waking consciousness, a need too often neglected or subverted with drugs or substances. Whatever ever else it does, dreaming provides a daily opportunity to directly experience such transcendence.

It does so by liberating consciousness from somatic constraints. The suppression of normal sensory and motor processes in REM sleep suggests that dreaming is mediated by a functional *disembodiment* or out-of-body experience (OBE), reminiscent of the ubiquitous spiritual notion that the soul leaves the body during sleep. Having done so, the mind is free to transcend waking consciousness—to fly, time travel, observe itself, or morph into other beings. The suspension of communication between prefrontal executive function and limbic-mediated emotionality further explains the dream's fantasy, mystery, and numinosity, which cannot be navigated with maps of everyday waking life.

Decades of phenomenological dream research has been devoted to exploring and mapping the world of dream consciousness. Different kinds of dreams occur in association with different sleep states. *Liminal dreams* include those occurring in hypnagogic and hypnopompic or sleep onset and sleep offset processes, respectively. These hybrid dream–wake states are characterized by a rapid kaleidoscopic flow of imagery lacking any cohesive narrative. Although first observed shortly after the discovery of REM/dreams, NREM dreams have received considerably less attention. They are generally short, fragmented, thought-like, and mundane in comparison to REM dreams, which are usually longer, more elaborate, vivid, emotional, and bizarre.[19,20] If REM dreams are depicted as bold and bright cumulus billows, NREM dreams would be wispy upper-atmosphere cirrus clouds.

Phenomenological investigations of dreams began more than a century ago. In recent years, digitized dream databases that include tens of thousands of dreams have encouraged rigorous empirical investigations of dream content and process.[21,22] Dream research findings have been used to support a broad range of impersonal neurological, personal psychological, and transpersonal spiritual theories about the meaning of dreams.

Strict neurophysiological perspectives, such as the classic activation-synthesis hypothesis[14] mentioned earlier, presume that dreams arise from the brain's attempt to make sense of neural activation during sleep and are inherently meaningless. This position is virtually universal among REM sleep neuroscientists and most striking in studies that reduce profound religious, spiritual, or transpersonal dream experiences to neural activity.[23] Because we cannot prove a negative, however, asserting that dreams are meaningless is a personal belief, not a scientific conclusion. Disguising such beliefs as science may discourage individuals from attending to, let alone relying on, dreams to inform their lives. Additionally, denying the meaning of dreams should not be confused with denying the meaningfulness of dreams. As is the case with good fiction, films, or mythic tales, one can believe that dreams have no personal meaning but still recognize that they impact us in most meaningful ways.

Neuroscientific views of transcendent, spiritual, or religious experiences can be used to better understand rather than negate them. Bulkeley's extensive exploration of the role of REM/dreaming in the evolution of world religions is an outstanding example of this.[24]

A recent investigation found that 56% of Americans reported believing dreams were personally meaningful.[25] Different psychological theories employ distinct methods of framing, analyzing, and ascribing personal meaning to dreams. Freud presumed that dreams released psychological pressure arising from conflict between instinctual drives and social norms by cloaking unacceptable drives in socially acceptable images. He believed careful analysis could reveal the dream's latent content to help resolve developmental conflicts.[13] Jung saw dreaming as an endogenous healing processes that integrated conscious and unconscious aspects of the self, even independently of analysis.[26] Hall believed dreaming provided symbolic reflections of one's cognitive processes. Hall and Van De Castle developed a quantitative method of dream content analysis that has been used to establish a baseline for ongoing research.[27]

The most popular culture-wide approach to dream interpretation is the "dream dictionary," which presumes that dream images are personal but have standard meanings. Derived largely from an oversimplification of psychological approaches, dream dictionaries assign meaning to dream images in terms of their symbolic representations of waking world imagery. Dream dictionaries can provide a sense of comfort and control over disturbing dreams, but they obscure personal meaning and reduce dreaming to a subset of waking consciousness.[28]

Most personal, psychological, and popular approaches are *wake-centric*—that is, they view dreaming as subconscious and subservient to waking consciousness.[29] Like reflections in fun-house mirrors, dreams are seen as distorted representations of waking life that require corrective analysis. In contrast, transpersonal approaches suggest that dreaming is not simply a mirror but also a wonderland-like looking glass we might pass through to transcend our ordinary sense of self and access the literally unforgettable experiences Jung called *big dreams*.[30]

A recent comprehensive review revealed the central role of big dreams in the evolution of the world's major religious traditions.[23] Additionally, diverse transpersonal approaches, such as archetypal psychology, alchemy, and shamanism share an assumption that dreams can serve as a portal to the collective unconscious.[31] Jung, who believed the unconscious was both personal and transpersonal, wrote, "We are so captivated by and entangled in our subjective consciousness that we have forgotten the age-old fact that God speaks chiefly through dreams and visions."[32] Variations of the notion that "life is but a dream" is a common tenet in numerous sacred traditions. This highlights the critical question as to whether dreaming is a dissociative experience that draws us away from reality, a rapprochement with a deeper transcendent reality, or both.

"What dreaming does," said Carlos Castaneda, "is give us the fluidity to enter into other worlds by destroying our sense of knowing this world."[33] This deconstructive feature of dreaming may account for the fact that most of the emotional content of dreams is negative.[34] It might also help explain the healing potential of nightmares. Clinical responses to bad dreams and nightmares depend on whether they are viewed as symptoms of pathology or reflections of an endogenous healing process. Pathological views encourage symptom-suppressive medication, while healing views endorse various forms of dreamwork.

The Functions of REM/Dreaming

The continuity hypothesis of REM/dreaming, which views dream life as continuous with waking life, is the most common theoretical ground shared by REM/dream investigators ranging from classical Freudians to contemporary neuroscientists.[35,36] Although there are differing views of how wake–dreaming continuity functions, there is general agreement that REM/dreaming supports waking memory consolidation, mood regulation, and creativity. More specifically, REM/dreaming plays a critical role in the consolidation of procedural memories, the downregulation of depressed mood, and the transcendence of ordinary consciousness.

Despite long-standing controversy about the REM sleep's role in memory,[37] recent investigations confirm that memory consolidation is optimized via complex interactions between circadian,[38] NREM, and REM sleep[39] processes. More specifically, REM/dreaming appears to play a critical role in the consolidation of implicit procedural memory.[40] Further support comes from studies linking disruptions of REM/dreaming to memory difficulties,[39] dementia, and Alzheimer's disease.[41]

A substantial body of research suggests that, in conjunction with memory consolidation, REM/dreaming downregulates negative emotion by assimilating and integrating waking experiences into existing memory systems.[42,43] REM/dream mood regulation is essentially a psychological digestive process that sifts through, breaks down, and assimilates previously consumed waking life experiences. More specifically, the sequential hypothesis suggests waking experiences are processed in two distinct, complementary, and serial steps of SWS and REM sleep. SWS distinguishes memories to be retained from those to be downgraded or eliminated. Retained memories are then integrated into preexisting networks during REM sleep.[44,45] This process, which is symbolically represented in dream narratives,[46] downregulates negative emotion[47,48] and provides a refreshed sense of self upon awakening.[34]

Most waking life experiences do not need to be processed; some are readily digested and assimilated, and others may be more difficult to digest and assimilate, requiring repeated cycles through NREM and REM/dreaming through the night and over time. Hartman theorized that posttraumatic dream series, which are driven primarily by emotional concerns and serve to establish new neural connections that are integrated into the self, provide a model for the endogenous healing process inherent in all REM/dreaming.[49]

Impaired REM/dreaming is strongly linked to depression. A reduced REM latency, the hallmark of this impairment, is associated with an increased duration of poor-quality REM sleep and decreased SWS displaced by rebounding REM. Dreams of depressed patients are generally more difficult to recall, impoverished, passive, mundane, and unemotional.[50–52] Additionally, in contrast to healthy REM/dreaming, depressed patients exhibit excessive activation of limbic and paralimbic areas along with increased activity in the executive prefrontal region.[36] Might this suggest a failure to downregulate emotion resulting from excessive oversight by the rational waking self?

Studies of depressed patients' healthy relatives suggest REM sleep abnormalities may precede the onset of depression and predict risk, relapse, and recurrence.[53] Human and animal subjects who have had their REM sleep selectively deprived exhibit a rebound pattern with strikingly similar abnormalities to those seen in depression, lending support to the classic psychoanalytic notion that depression is a loss of one's dreams.[54] Given the normal mood management function of REM/dreaming, it is possible that the REM sleep rebound seen in reduced REM latencies is evidence of an endogenous healing response that has gone awry. If so, REM sleep–suppressive antidepressants reinforce this process.

Cartwright et al. found that depressed negative affect progressively diminished in dreams elicited from successive REM periods during a night's sleep.[48] She also observed a pattern in which negative affect present in early REM periods transitioned to positive affect in later REM/dreaming, eventually resulting in remission.[55] The cyclic pattern of brain deactivation in NREM and reactivation in REM may serve to regulate emotion via an extinction process.[56] Pace-Schott et al. concluded that emotional homeostasis resulted from a combination of selectively activated REM physiology along with the subjective experience of dreaming.[57]

In a longitudinal series of studies, Cartwright found that healthy dreamers, those whose REM dreams were rich and complex, recovered more quickly from depression associated with process of divorce.[36] In related work, Palagini et al. hypothesized that REM abnormalities may contribute to nocturnal consolidation of negatively toned emotional memories.[53]

In summary, depression can be understood in terms of impaired assimilation of challenging waking life experiences—a metaphoric psychological digestive disorder preventing individuals from extracting and assimilating emotionally nourishing experiences from daily life. Healthy REM/dreaming offers a form of endogenous psychotherapy that warrants active support.

Disrupted sleep and dreaming has long been recognized in the pathogenesis of PTSD.[58] Dysfunctional memory consolidation can exacerbate PTSD,[59] resulting in both nightmares and impaired waking regulation of emotion.[56] Many PTSD patients exhibit attenuated prefrontal executive function that may result in a maladaptive REM-dependent overconsolidation of learned fear following traumatic experiences.[60] Other investigations suggest that healthy REM/dreaming can reestablish prefrontal connectivity by decreasing amygdala activity and reducing brain and behavioral reactivity,[61] possibly contributing to preventing PTSD symptoms.

Theories of REM/dreaming generally presume that it functions as an underpinning of waking consciousness. Hobson proposed that "REM sleep may constitute a protoconscious state, providing a virtual reality model of the world that is of functional use to the development and maintenance of waking consciousness." In sharp contrast to waking, *protoconsciousness* is an altered state of primordial consciousness characterized by a focus on the present moment.[62]

Because it is untethered from considerations of the past or future, such a present-moment focus affords the dreamer an opportunity to process waking-life experiences in a new, expanded theater of consciousness that reframes and transforms memories as well as one's sense of self. Dreaming is, fundamentally, a creative process that supports problem-solving, healing, and transcendence.

The link between creativity and dreaming is supported by several studies as well as numerous anecdotal reports. REM sleep has been shown to facilitate insight[63]as well as promote cognitive flexibility[64] and creative problem-solving.[65] Well-known examples of anecdotal reports include dream-based inspiration for the invention of the sewing machine, the plot of *Dr. Jekyll and Mr. Hyde*, and Paul McCartney's song "Yesterday." The creative process involves varying degrees of transcendence ranging from "out of the box thinking" to life-changing insights and big dreams. Piaget's model of cognitive development suggests that ordinary dreams can be understood in terms of assimilative learning, while big dreams require accommodation—a fundamental transformation of the structure of self, involving the disintegration and recombination of existing mental schemas[66] to accommodate new experiences.

The Silent Epidemic of REM/Dream Loss

It is striking that, despite awareness of the importance of REM/dreaming, there has been little acknowledgment that we are in the midst of an epidemic of REM/dream loss. Addressed by the author in a recent review paper,[67] REM/dream loss results from several sets of factors that compromise the quality and/or the extent of REM/dreaming. These include (1) excessive consumption of commonly used substances, especially alcohol and cannabis; (2) the extensive reliance on REM/dream suppressive prescription and over-the-counter medications, such as anticholinergics, antidepressants, benzodiazepines, stimulants, opioids, and antihistamines; (3) the impact of major sleep disorders, including insufficient sleep syndrome, insomnia disorder, and obstructive sleep apnea (OSA); (4) and REM/dream-interfering lifestyle factors, such as overexposure to artificial light at night, which suppresses MT, and routine morning alarm-clock awakenings, which subvert the culmination of morning REM/dreams.

Despite its glaring prevalence, epidemiological research focused specifically on quantifying REM/dream loss is nonexistent. However, given population estimates of substance and medication use, prevalence data for sleep disorders, and the ubiquity of lifestyle factors impinging on sleep and REM/dreams, it is probable that tens of millions of people experience degrees of clinically significant REM/dream loss on a nightly basis.[66]

Given the widespread and critical health ramifications of REM/dream loss, this author believes that establishing a new diagnosis for it is warranted. Designating REM/dream deficiency as a medical disorder would encourage related documentation and treatment, as well as public health and research initiatives. Such a diagnosis would need to account for REM sleep as well as subjective dream loss.

Dream loss is not just a personal health issue. In his classic essay, *The Significance of Dreams in a Dream Deprived Society*, Ullman addresses the ramifications of dream loss on culture stating, "Dreams reveal the state of connectedness of the individual to his or her past, to others, and to the supports and constraints of the social order."[68] Epidemic REM/dream loss can potentially constrict collective consciousness to erode creativity, art, and spirituality.

Recommendations

In contrast to conventional medicine, alternative medical systems, such as homeopathy,[69] traditional Chinese medicine,[70] and Ayurvedic medicine[71] routinely utilize dreams to inform diagnosis and treatment. Although our understanding of its functions continue to evolve, clinicians should inform patients of the health benefits of REM/dreaming and incorporate related screening, treatment, and health promotion into their practices. Primary care providers, psychiatrists, neurologists, sleep specialists, and psychologists, in particular, need to be trained and encouraged to address REM/dream factors.

All patients should routinely be screened for REM/dream deficiencies. More specifically, the treatment of depression, dementia, sleep disorders, and PTSD should include evaluation and restoration of REM/dreaming. Restoring REM/dreaming is largely about disinhibiting a natural process that has inadvertently been suppressed by medications, substances, and lifestyle factors.

Integrative mental health interventions offer effective alternatives to conventional antidepressants[72] and other REM-suppressant psychiatric medications.[73] Because the brain prioritizes sleep over dreams, restoring healthy sleep is a prerequisite to REM/dream health.[74] In addition to sleep hygiene practices, it is essential to reduce excessive exposure to artificial light at night by dimming lights and using blue blocker technology[75] and to adhere to reasonable bedtimes to reduce dependence on alarm clocks.

Primary sleep disorders typically involve impaired REM/dreaming. Riemann et al.[76] address the largely unexamined but critical role of REM sleep in the pathophysiology of insomnia disorder. Because it is the most highly aroused state of sleep, individuals with persistent hyperarousal are prone to experience disrupted sleep during REM/dreams. Continuity theory further suggests that common pre-sleep anxieties of insomnia patients visibly intrude into dream content, fragmenting REM sleep and impacting memory formation and morning recall of the experience of poor sleep. Fragmented REM/dreaming can further compromise the downregulation of negative emotion, contributing to depression.

A recent novel investigation found insomnia patients were significantly more likely than good sleepers to report REM sleep as waking, suggesting that the subjective experience of insomnia might be coupled to the REM sleep state.[77] Given that most wake after sleep onset (WASO) is more accurately wake after dream onset (WADO), providing support for healthy REM/dreaming should be a routine part of managing insomnia disorder. Likewise, the common disruption of REM sleep in OSA, narcolepsy-hypersomnia, and both idiopathic and posttraumatic nightmares should be routinely evaluated and addressed in treatment.

REM/dreaming can be potentiated by several botanicals and nutraceuticals.[78] MT also potentiates REM/dreaming,[15] but there is limited informed guidance available for its appropriate use. Generally speaking, 0.3–1.0 mg of a time-released formulation is often effective. Nootropics that support the activity of acetylcholine, such as galantamine, ginkgo biloba, and vitamins B_1, B_6, and B_{12}, may also function as oneirogens, which are dream promoting substances.[79]

Dreamwork—psychological interpretation, analysis, and support for REM/dreaming—can be useful in treating depression.[55,80,81] Similarly, recurrent nightmares, which are commonly managed with REM-suppressive medications,[82] can also be effectively treated with psychological interventions.[83] One marked advantage of psychotherapeutic approaches stems from their view of disordered REM/dreaming as an endogenous healing process that has gone awry but can be corrected. Dreamwork generally involves practices that encourage trusting one's unconscious, which can enhance self-efficacy or, in more colloquial terms, faith in oneself.

Dreamwork is also commonly used for personal growth and for facilitating creativity and spiritual exploration. Dream journaling,[84] dream groups or circles,[85] sandplay therapy,[86] waking dream work,[87] shamanic journeying,[88] lucid dreaming,[89] liminal dreaming,[90] and dream yogas[91] are among a myriad of popular forms of dreamwork available. Studies of dream practices in indigenous cultures align with scientific investigation in confirming the value of sharing dreams with others through informal conversations or organized dream circles. Such *dream tending* can enhance feelings of depth and purpose, self-concept, and one's sense of community.[92–95]

Promoting REM/dream health will require concerted public health initiatives directed at the public as well as at health professionals and industries. Public education campaigns need to highlight the important role of REM/dreaming in health. Clinicians and the medical community at large need to be sensitized to common iatrogenic factors in REM/dream deficiency, especially the widespread use of REM-suppressant medications. The pharmaceutical industry should routinely evaluate and provide data about the impact of drugs on REM sleep. Patients should likewise be informed of REM-suppressant side effects of medications. Professional advocacy organizations that support sleep health should include an emphasis on REM/dream health. Sleep specialists, in particular, need to recognize that sleep medicine has inadvertently relegated dreaming to a stepchild status and be open to a greater focus on REM/dreaming. Sleep medicine should be sleep and dream medicine.

One of the main reasons we are losing our dreams is that we do not value them sufficiently. Restoring healthy REM/dreaming requires a transformation of social consciousness. Scientists and clinicians, in particular, need to be more respectful of dream phenomenology. Whether one believes dreams have inherent meaning or not, they impact us in meaningful ways. Attending to our own dreams is a helpful step in the needed social transformation. In doing so, we practice transcending ordinary waking consciousness to encounter the unconscious. Our relationship to REM/dreaming is fundamentally about our relationship with the unconscious.

REFERENCES

1. Pesant N, Zadra A. Working with dreams in therapy: What do we know and what should we do? *Clin Psychol Rev.* 2004;24(5):489–512.

2. Aserinsky E, Kleitman N. Regularly occurring periods of eye motility, and concomitant phenomena, during sleep. *Science.* 1953;118;3062:273–274.

3. Lack LC, Wright HR. Chronobiology of sleep in humans. *Cell Mol Life Sci.* 2007;64(10):1205.

4. Antrobus JS, Bertini M, editors. *The neuropsychology of sleep and dreaming.* New York: Psychology Press; 2013.

5. McCarley RW, Hobson JA. Neuronal excitability modulation over the sleep cycle: A structural and mathematical model. *Science.* 1975;189(4196):58–60.

6. Hobson JA, Pace-Schott EF, Stickgold R. Dreaming and the brain: Toward a cognitive neuroscience of conscious states. *Behav Brain Sci.* 2000;23(6):793–842.

7. Matarazzo L, Foret A, Mascetti L, Muto V, Shaffii A, Maquet P. A systems-level approach to human REM sleep. *REM Sleep Reg Funct.* 2011;14;8:71.

8. Pace-Schott EF. REM sleep and dreaming. *REM Sleep Reg Funct.* 2011;14:8–20.

9. Mölle M, Born J. Hippocampus whispering in deep sleep to prefrontal cortex—for good memories? *Neuron.* 2009;26;61(4):496–498.

10. Parmeggiani PL. Systemic homeostasis and poikilostasis in sleep: Is REM sleep a physiological paradox? *World Sci.* 2011. https://www.worldcat.org/title/systemic-homeostasis-and-poikilostasis-in-sleep-is-rem-sleep-a-physiological-paradox/oclc/963824239

11. Simor P, Gombos F, Blaskovich B, Bódizs R. Long-range alpha and beta and short-range gamma EEG synchronization distinguishes phasic and tonic REM periods. *Sleep.* 2018 Mar 1;41(3). doi:10.1093/sleep/zsx210. PMID: 29309685.

12. McNamara P. The very, very strange properties of REM sleep. *Psychology Today,* August 13, 2011. https://www.psychologytoday.com/blog/

13. Siegel JM. REM sleep. *Princip Pract Sleep Med.* 2005:120–135.

14. Hobson JA, McCarley RW. The brain as a dream state generator: An activation-synthesis hypothesis of the dream process. *Am J Psychiatry.*1977;134:1335–1348.

15. Kunz D, Mahlberg R, Müller C, Tilmann A, Bes F. Melatonin in patients with reduced REM sleep duration: Two randomized controlled trials. *J Clin Endocrinol Metabol.* 2004;89(1):128–134.

16. Siegel JM. REM sleep: A biological and psychological paradox. *Sleep Med Rev.* 2011;15(3):139–142.

17. Beauregard M, Schwartz GE, Miller L, Dossey L, et al. Manifesto for a post-materialist science. *Explore.* 2014;10(5):272–274.

18. Weil A, Crowell C. *The natural mind: A new way of looking at drugs and the higher consciousness.* Boston: Houghton Mifflin; 1972.

19. Carr M, Solomonova E. Dream recall and content in different stages of sleep and time-of-night effect. In Valli K, Hoss R, Gongloff R, eds. *Dreams: Biology, psychology, and culture.* Denver, CO: Greenwood Publishing Group; 2018: 167–172.

20. Suzuki H, Uchiyama M, Tagaya H, et al. Dreaming during non-rapid eye movement sleep in the absence of prior rapid eye movement sleep. *Sleep.* 2004;27(8):1486–1490.

21. Bulkeley K. A guide to the sleep and dream database. SDDb Research Papers 1. 2017. https://www.academia.edu/34960217/A_Guide_to_the_Sleep_and_Dream_Database.docx

22. Domhoff GW, Schneider A. Studying dream content using the archive and search engine on DreamBank. net. *Conscious Cognit.* 2008;17(4):1238–1247.

23. Alper M. *The "God" part of the brain: A scientific interpretation of human spirituality and God.* Naperville, IL: Sourcebooks, Inc.; 2008.

24. Bulkeley K. *Big dreams: The science of dreaming and the origins of religion.* New York: Oxford University Press; 2016.

25. Morewedge CK, Norton MI. When dreaming is believing: The (motivated) interpretation of dreams. *J Personal Soc Psychol.* 2009;96(2):249.

26. Jung CG. *Psychology and alchemy. Collected works.* New York: Routledge; 2014: 609–617.

27. Hall C, Van de Castle R. *The content analysis of dreams.* New York: Appleton-Century-Crofts; 1966.

28. Naiman RR. *Healing night: The science and spirit of sleeping, dreaming, and awakening.* Minneapolis, MN: Syren Book Company; 2006: 99–100.

29. Naiman R. Falling for sleep. Aeon. 2016. https://aeon.co/essays/the-cure-for-insomnia-is-to-fall-in-love-with-sleep-again

30. Jung CG. On the nature of dreams. In Read H, Fordham M, Adler G, eds. *The collected works of C.G. Jung.* London: Routledge. (Original work published 1948.); 1960c: Vol. 8, pp. 281–297).

31. Hunt HT. A collective unconscious reconsidered: Jung's archetypal imagination in the light of contemporary psychology and social science. *J Analytic Psychol.* 2012;57(1):76–98.

32. Jung CG. *The symbolic life: Miscellaneous writings.* New York: Routledge; 2014.

33. Castaneda C. *The art of dreaming.* New York: Harper Collins; 1993.

34. Valli K, Strandholm T, Sillanmäki L, Revonsuo A. Dreams are more negative than real life: Implications for the function of dreaming. *Cognition Emotion.* 2008;22(5):833–861.

35. Erdelyi MH. The continuity hypothesis. *Dreaming.* 2017;27(4):334.

36. Cartwright RD. *The twenty-four hour mind: The role of sleep and dreaming in our emotional lives.* New York: Oxford University Press; 2010.

37. Siegel JM. The REM sleep-memory consolidation hypothesis. *Science.* 2001;2(294):1058–1063.

38. Xia Z, Storm D. Role of circadian rhythm and REM sleep for memory consolidation. *Neurosci Res.* 2017 May 1;118:13–20.

39. Boyce R, Williams S, Adamantidis A. REM sleep and memory. *Curr Opin Neurobiol.* 2017;44:167–177.

40. Rasch B, Born J. About sleep's role in memory. *Physiol Rev.* 2013;93(2):681–766.

41. Petit D, Montplaisir J, Boeve BF. Alzheimer's disease and other dementias. In Kryger MH, et al., eds. *Principles and practice of sleep medicine,* 5th ed. New York: Elsevier Saunders; 2010: 1038–1047.

42. Cartwright R. Dreaming as a mood regulation system. Kryger MH, et al., eds. *Principles and practice of sleep medicine,* 4th ed. New York: Elsevier Saunders; 2005: 565–572.

43. Hartmann E. *The nature and functions of dreaming.* New York: Oxford University Press; 2007: 171–192.
44. Ribeiro S, Nicolelis MA. Reverberation, storage, and postsynaptic propagation of memories during sleep. *Learning Memory.* 2004;11(6):686–696.
45. Giuditta A, Mandile, Montagnese P, Piscopo S, Vescia S. The role of sleep in memory processing: The sequential hypothesis. *Sleep Brain Plast.* 2003;157–178.
46. Mutz J, Javadi AH. Exploring the neural correlates of dream phenomenology and altered states of consciousness during sleep. *Neurosci Conscious.* 2017;3(1):nix009.
47. Kramer M. *The dream experience: A systematic exploration.* New York: Routledge; 2013.
48. Cartwright R, Luten A, Young M, Mercer P, Bears M. Role of REM sleep and dream affect in overnight mood regulation: A study of normal volunteers. *Psychiatry Res.* 1998;19;81(1):1–8.
49. Hartmann E. Nightmare after trauma as paradigm for all dreams: A new approach to the nature and functions of dreaming. *Psychiatry.* 1998;61(3):223–238.
50. Schredl M, Engelhardt H. Dreaming and psychopathology: Dream recall and dream content of psychiatric inpatients. *Sleep Hypnosis.* 2001.
51. Zanasi M, Pecorella M, Chiaramonte C, Niolu C, Siracusano A. Dreams by persons with mood disorders. *Psychol Rep.* 2008;103(2):381–394.
52. McNamara P, Auerbach S, Johnson P, Harris E, Doros G. Impact of REM sleep on distortions of self-concept, mood and memory in depressed/anxious participants. *J Affec Dis.* 2010;122:198–207.
53. Palagini L, Baglioni C, Ciapparelli A, Gemignani A, Riemann D. REM sleep dysregulation in depression: State of the art. *Sleep Med Rev.* 2013;17(5):377–390.
54. Naiman R. Circadian rhythm and blues: The interface of depression with sleep and dreams. *PsychologyToday.com.* 2011.https://www.psychology today.com/blog/mindful-sleep-mindful-dreams/201103/ circadian-rhythm-and-blues
55. Cartwright R, Young MA, Mercer P, Bears M. Role of REM sleep and dream variables in the prediction of remission from depression. *Psychiatry Res.* 1998;80(3):249–255.
56. Levin R, Nielsen TA. Disturbed dreaming, posttraumatic stress disorder, and affect distress: A review and neurocognitive model. *Psychol Bull.* 2007;133(3):482.
57. Pace-Schott EF, Milad MR, Orr SP, Rauch SL, Stickgold R, Pitman RK. Sleep promotes generalization of extinction of conditioned fear. *Sleep.* 2009;32(1):19–26.
58. Ross RJ, Ball WA, Sullivan KA, Caroff SN. Sleep disturbance as the hallmark of posttraumatic stress disorder. *Am J Psychiatry.* 1989;1;146(6):697.
59. Germain A. Sleep disturbances as the hallmark of PTSD: Where are we now? *Am J Psychiatry.* 2013;170(4):372–382.
60. Murkar A, De Koninck J. Consolidative mechanisms of emotional processing in REM sleep and PTSD. *Sleep Med Rev.* 2018;41:173–184. doi: 10.1016/j.smrv.2018.03.001. Epub 2018 Mar 15. PMID: 29628334.
61. van der Helm E, Yao J, Dutt S, Rao V, Saletin JM, Walker MP. REM sleep depotentiates amygdala activity to previous emotional experiences. *Curr Biol.* 2011;21(23):2029–2032.

62. Hobson JA. REM sleep and dreaming: Towards a theory of protoconsciousness. *Nat Rev Neurosci.* 2009;10(11):803.

63. Wagner U, Gais S, Haider H, Verleger R, Born J. Sleep inspires insight. *Nature.* 2004;427(6972):352.

64. Walker MP, Liston C, Hobson JA, Stickgold R. Cognitive flexibility across the sleep-wake cycle: REM-sleep enhancement of anagram problem solving. *Cogn Brain Res.* 2002;14(3):317–324.

65. Cai DJ, Mednick SA, Harrison EM, Kanady JC, Mednick SC. REM, not incubation, improves creativity by priming associative networks. *Proc Natl Acad Sci.* 2009;106(25):10130–10134.

66. Landmann N, Kuhn M, Maier JG, et al. REM sleep and memory reorganization: Potential relevance for psychiatry and psychotherapy. *Neurobiol Learning Memory.* 2015;122:28–40.

67. Naiman R. Dreamless: The silent epidemic of REM sleep loss. *Ann NY Acad Sci.* 2017 Oct 1;1406(1):77–85.

68. Ullman M. The significance of dreams in a dream deprived society. 1996. http://siivola.org/monte/papers_grouped/uncopyrighted/Dreams/significance_of_dreams_in_a_dream_deprived_society.htm

69. Cicchetti J. *Dreams, symbols & homeopathy: Archetypal dimensions of healing.* Berkeley, CA: North Atlantic Books; 2004.

70. Montakab H. *Acupuncture for insomnia.* New York: Thieme Medical Publishers; 2012.

71. Lad V. *Textbook of ayurveda.* Albuqueque, NM: Ayurvedic Press;2002.

72. Weil A. *Spontaneous happiness: A new path to emotional well-being.* New York: Little, Brown; 2011.

73. Weil A. *Mind over meds: Know when drugs are necessary, when alternatives are better—and when to let your body heal on its own.* New York: Little, Brown; 2017.

74. Berger RJ, Oswald I. Effects of sleep deprivation on behaviour, subsequent sleep, and dreaming. *J Ment Sci.* 1962;108(455):457–465.

75. Burkhart K, Phelps JR. Amber lenses to block blue light and improve sleep: A randomized trial. *Chronobiology Int.* 2009;26:1602–1612.

76. Riemann D, Spiegelhalder K, Nissen C, Hirscher V, Baglioni C, Feige B. REM sleep instability: A new pathway for insomnia? *Pharmacopsychiatry.* 2012;45(05):167–176.

77. Feige B, Nanovska S, Baglioni C, et al. Insomnia: Perchance a dream? Results from a NREM/REM sleep awakening study in good sleepers and patients with insomnia. *Sleep.* 2018;8;41(5):zsy032.

78. Dumpert J. Meeting in the dream world: Oneirogens and tips for better dreaming. *Utne Reader,* 2013. https://www.utne.com/mind-and-body/oneirogens-zeoz1302zgar

79. Suliman NA, Mat Taib CN, Mohd Moklas MA, Adenan MI, Hidayat Baharuldin MT, Basir R. Establishing natural nootropics: Recent molecular enhancement influenced by natural nootropic. *Evid Based Complement Alternat Med.* 2016;2016:4391375. doi:10.1155/2016/4391375. Epub 2016 Aug 30. PMID: 27656235; PMCID: PMC5021479.

80. Sharpe EF. *Dream analysis: A practical handbook of psychoanalysis.* New York: Routledge; 2018.
81. Hill CE, Knox S. The use of dreams in modern psychotherapy. *Int Rev Neurobiol.* 2010;92:291–317.
82. George KC, Kebejian L, Ruth LJ, Miller CW, Himelhoch S. Meta-analysis of the efficacy and safety of prazosin versus placebo for the treatment of nightmares and sleep disturbances in adults with posttraumatic stress disorder. *J Trauma Dissociation.* 2016;17(4):494–510.
83. Davis JL. *Treating post-trauma nightmares: A cognitive behavioral approach.* New York: Springer; 2008.
84. Bulkeley K. *Transforming dreams: Learning spiritual lessons from the dreams you never forget.* New York: Wiley; 2000.
85. Castleman T. *Sacred dream circles: A guide to facilitating Jungian dream groups.* Einsiedeln, Switzerland: Daimon; 2009.
86. Kalff DM. *Sandplay: A psychotherapeutic approach to the psyche.* Santa Monica, CA: Sigo Press; 1980.
87. Watkins MM. *Waking dreams.* New York: Springer; 1998.
88. Ingerman S. *Shamanic journeying: A beginner's guide.* Louisville, CO: Sounds True; 2008.
89. Gackenbach J, LaBarge S, eds. *Conscious mind, sleeping brain: Perspectives on lucid dreaming.* New York: Springer Science & Business Media; 2012.
90. Dumpert J. *Liminal dreaming: Experiments with consciousness.* Berkeley, CA: North Atlantic Books;2019.
91. Rinpoche CN, Katz M. *Dream yoga and the practice of natural light.* Boulder, CO: Shambhala; 1992.
92. Aizenstat S. *Dream tending: Awakening to the healing power of dreams.* New Orleans, LA: Spring Journal; 2011.
93. Taylor J. *Where people fly and water runs uphill: Using dreams to tap the wisdom of the unconscious.* New York: Warner Books; 1992.
94. Van de Castle RL. *Our dreaming mind.* New York: Ballantine Books; 1994 May.
95. Mellick J. *The natural artistry of dreams: Creative ways to bring the wisdom of dreams to waking life.* Newburyport, MA: Conari Press; 1996.

14

Spirituality, Religion, and Sleep

FREDERIC C. CRAIGIE, JR.

S pirituality is a vital element of integrative health and well-being. In a letter to Greek chief physician Criton of Heraclea, first-century philosopher Apollonius of Tyana is quoted as saying

> Pythagoras said that the most divine art was that of healing. And if the healing art is most divine, it must occupy itself with the soul as well as with the body; for no creature can be sound so long as the higher part in it is sickly.[1]

As we now move along into the twenty-first century, there is a substantial and ever-growing body of evidence that this is true. Integrative health and well-being encompass not only what we eat and how we move; they encompass the sacred values, commitments, and activities that make our lives worth living.

The interface of spirituality with sleep, however, is an area of integrative medicine and health that is less well developed than others. In this chapter, we look at some literature and some clinical approaches to explore the following questions:

- What *is* spirituality? What is the relationship of spirituality with religion?
- How, broadly, does spirituality influence health?
- How does spirituality influence sleep? What can we glean from current descriptive and interventional research?
- What mechanisms might underlie associations of spirituality with sleep?
- If spirituality does indeed have a salutary effect on sleep, how might we support this clinically with our patients?

And we include a short section on spirituality and dreams.

Background

There is no consensus definition of spirituality. In my work, I often cite a fine, short, inclusive perspective on spirituality from former Surgeon General Dr. C. Everett Koop[2]:

The vital center of a person; that which is held sacred.

The idea of *vitality* (Latin *vitālis*, "of life, life-giving") has to do with aliveness and energetic engagement in life. The idea of *sacredness* conveys a depth of meaning that goes beyond "really important." For many people, for instance, being a productive worker is really important, but loving a partner or being faithful to deeply held personal values are sacred. In addition, the idea of sacredness is inclusive; it is not aligned with any particular spiritual or religious tradition and, indeed, may or may not involve a theistic perspective. Spirituality in your life has to do with what is sacred, *for you.*

OUTER AND INNER

Spirituality involves both "outer" and "inner" experience. The "outer" aspects of spirituality have to do with practices and relationships. One can practice meditation or prayer, or read sacred literature, or chant, or participate in an organized spiritual community. The "inner" aspects of spirituality have to do with the personal values, passions, and commitments that inform and energize the ways that people live.

A woman maintains a nighttime practice of keeping a gratitude journal and praying, and she finds that this focusing and calming practice helps her to sleep consistently well. During the day, she engages in activities, like exercise and responsible nutrition, that she knows will be associated with sleep quality by reminding herself that "the body is the temple of the Spirit." These are, respectively, outer and inner expressions of what is "vital and sacred" for her.

As we think about spirituality, this distinction matters. The field of integrative medicine is replete with particular practices that are associated with health and well-being. One can follow a walking program, take supplements, practice self-hypnosis, follow an anti-inflammatory diet, or carefully monitor environmental exposures. Spiritual well-being is indeed nurtured with practices like those we have mentioned, but it is more than that. Spiritual well-being in integrative medicine also is nurtured by exploring questions that frame the "inner" aspect of spirituality.

What is sacred for you?
What do you deeply care about?
What does it mean to you to live a good life?
When do you feel really alive?
What kind of person do you aspire to be?
What would you hope the legacy of your life would be?

SPIRITUALITY AND RELIGION

Spirituality and religion are related and also distinct. Some people express spirituality in particular religious traditions and communities, finding value in the doctrines, rituals and ceremonies, and relationships that religious communities offer. For other people, spirituality involves more of a personally charted journey in expressing the "vital and sacred" in ways that may draw on different traditions without specifically following any among them.

Research

SPIRITUALITY AND HEALTH

There is a very large and continually growing empirical literature that attests to the health benefits of spiritual beliefs and practices. A recent meta-analytic review summarizes this literature well. Citing more than 3,000 studies, Koenig[3] found substantially beneficial associations of spiritual beliefs and practices with mental health outcomes (such as depression, anxiety, substance abuse, coping with adversity, well-being and happiness, optimism, meaning and purpose, and hope), health behaviors (cigarette smoking, exercise, and diet), and physical health (heart disease, hypertension, and immune and endocrine function).

Increasingly, researchers have been exploring dimensions, or components, of spirituality. A particularly intriguing distinction has been the partitioning of "spiritual well-being" into the methodologically and empirically distinct components of "religious well-being" and "existential well-being." *Religious well-being* encompasses a variety of religious practices and often pertains to people's perceived relationships with God. *Existential well-being* pertains to a sense of satisfaction and life purpose. While both of these components are typically associated with health, existential well-being tends to be more robust.[4]

SPIRITUALITY AND SLEEP

The empirical literature on spirituality and sleep is a work in progress. There are, however, a number of intriguing reports in the past 10 years that generally point to salutary effects of spirituality with sleep that are in line with the literature on other health issues.

Descriptive Research: Spiritual Well-Being

Recent correlational research suggests that spiritual and religious factors (defined variously; in the interests of parsimony, we will use the term "spirituality") are beneficially related to sleep. Overall spiritual well-being has been found to be associated with sleep quality in studies with hemodialysis patients,[5] HIV-infected men,[6] and university students.[7] Exploration of mediating variables in these studies suggests that (a) existential well-being is more strongly associated with sleep quality than religious well-being, and (b) spiritual well-being serves as a protective factor in the face of personal distress and that lesser personal distress enables better sleep quality.

Some research has looked particularly at components of spiritual experience. Drawing on a national spirituality and health dataset, Krause and colleagues found that people who viewed the body as sacred and had a strong sense of partnership with God showed better dietary practices, exercise habits, and better sleep than those who did not.[8] Among church members and elders, Ellison and colleagues reported that religious doubts were inversely related to sleep quality and directly related to the frequency of sleep problems and the use of sleeping medications.[9] It was suggested that serious religious struggles and doubts might prompt existential and psychological distress which would, in turn, have a deleterious effect on sleep.

Cross-sectional correlational research, of course, always poses interpretive challenges. Two studies[10,11] found that particular strongly held spiritual beliefs were associated with *greater* sleep disturbances. It was proposed that observations of inverse relationships of spiritual well-being with sleep quality might have to do with poor sleepers turning to faith and spiritual support to cope with their sleep difficulties in a way that better sleepers need not do.

Descriptive Research: Ancillary Spiritual Qualities

In addition to research that looks at associations of sleep with expressly spiritual measures and variables, there are pertinent lines of research that look at spiritually informed qualities and practices that have typically been associated with health and well-being. Here, we touch on four.

Mindfulness has to do with the ability to be present to one's experience in a calm, accepting, and nonjudgmental way. In addition to a large empirical literature on health benefits of mindfulness, a number of recent studies have examined the relationship of mindfulness and sleep, finding that greater levels of mindfulness are associated with better sleep quality (again, with perceived stress being a potential mediating variable).[12,13]

A practice of *gratitude* or gratefulness has been associated with substantial health benefits overall.[14] Focusing particularly on sleep, greater levels of trait (or "dispositional") gratitude have been associated with better sleep quality.[15,16] Likely mediating variables include mood and pre-sleep cognition, whereby gratefulness improves mood, which diminishes distressing pre-sleep thought, which improves sleep quality.

Forgiveness is an ancient spiritual practice in all major world religions, with a substantial modern empirical literature.[17,18] Recent studies have reported associations of forgiveness with sleep quality, with spirituality and concomitant effects on negative affect and anger ruminations playing important roles in these relationships.[19,20]

The idea that forgiveness and gentleness extend to oneself has been the foundation of recent empirical work on *self-compassion*.[21,22] (Self-compassion, of course, pertains to anyone but arguably has a particular urgency for practitioners in the arena of health and healing.) Regarding sleep, Sirois, Kitner, and Hirsch[23] reported findings parallel to those just cited, that self-compassion is directly associated with self-care behaviors that promote healthy sleep.

Intervention Research

In addition to descriptive research, there have been a number of initiatives in applying spiritually related interventions to enhance sleep quality. Chief among them have been intervention programs related to mindfulness and mindfulness meditation practices. A mindful awareness practices intervention, for instance, was compared to a traditional sleep hygiene education intervention with older adults with moderate sleep disturbances.[24] The mindful practices group had significant improvement in sleep quality compared with the sleep hygiene group, and mindfulness training had additional benefits in depression symptoms and fatigue.

Similar salutary mindfulness interventions for sleep quality have been reported with breast cancer survivors,[25] with an Internet-based instructor-led mindfulness intervention in an occupational health setting,[26] and in programs of mindfulness-based intervention for insomnia.[27,28] We also note two helpful reviews of mindfulness-based interventions for sleep.[29,30] Other spiritually grounded interventions for sleep issues have been explored as well. Beneficial effects on sleep quality have been reported from gratitude interventions,[31,32] tai chi,[33] yoga,[34,35] and tai chi and yoga combined.[36]

Themes and Mechanisms

We may extract several themes from this modest body of research.

- Spirituality, variously measured, seems to be positively associated with sleep quality.
- A number of mechanisms have been proposed, among them
  - o Enhancement of mood and reduction of negative affect
  - o Support in management and coping with stress
  - o Calming
  - o Reduction in deleterious pre-sleep cognitions
  - o Salutary personal beliefs, such as "sacred body view," prompting health practices that support sleep quality
- Occasional outlying reports of an inverse association between spirituality and sleep quality are understood in terms of people who are especially distressed turning to spirituality for comfort.
- Intervention initiatives that have enhanced sleep quality have been based especially in mindfulness and mindfulness/meditative practices. Other initiatives have been organized around energy medicine (tai chi and yoga) and gratitude.

The mechanisms of spirituality–sleep associations that we see in this literature do not, of course, exhaust the possibilities. Readers who are interested in the scientific (and philosophical) question of why spirituality may influence health would enjoy an exquisite review from epidemiologist Jeff Levin.[37] Levin proposes five "pathways" of spirituality–health associations: biological, psychosocial, energy-based, nonlocal, and supernatural.

Overall, these data and the research on which they are based suggest that working with spiritual beliefs and practices can be a legitimate and beneficial aspect of integrative medicine care for overall health and for sleep.

Dreams

Thus far, we have looked at empirical literature about spiritual and religious beliefs and practices and sleep. Along with such data, any reflection on spirituality and sleep needs to touch on the ages-old spiritual and religious significance of dreams. Across time and cultures, dreams have been understood to provide a pathway of relationship between the Divine and humankind and may, historically, have played a seminal role in the development of religion itself.

Beliefs about the origins of dreams have arisen from and reflected the cosmologies of many cultural and religious groups. Some cultures have viewed dreams as a natural expression of the workings of the human mind. Other cultures have viewed dreams as messages from ancestors, and many cultures have viewed dreams as divine intercession into human consciousness.[38]

Regardless of cultural differences concerning the origins of dreams, there are a number of recurring, spiritually informed ways in which dreams have been understood to function in people's lives. These include:

- *Revelation and prophesy.* Foretelling of future events. In the Christian tradition, for instance, Joseph was warned in a dream to avoid the Slaughter of the Innocents by fleeing to Egypt.
- *Healing.* Dreams may provide both inspiration and direction for healing. A patient who was mired in bitterness and vengefulness after being badly mistreated began a new direction of healing when, in a dream, she heard a voice saying, "I don't want you to live like this." In our modern understanding, moreover, dreams may also have substantial, direct biological effects in eliciting innate healing responses.[39]
- *Communication with sacred and divine beings; wisdom, affirmation, and guidance for daily living.* Another patient was sustained through hard times by experiencing messages of affirmation and love from cherished grandparents long passed on. And other patients have reported being visited by divine beings or presences—angels, Jesus, warm light—with similar messages of love and comfort.

For these and other functions of dreams, the premise is that a continuity exists between the dreaming and waking worlds and that dreams and visions provide wisdom and direction to support wholeness and well-being in waking life. Sometimes, as most readers will recognize, dreams have obvious meaning. Other times, dreams come to us with complexities of symbols and allegories that defy easy interpretation and that, in some cultures, have spurred the development of professional dream interpreters. Regardless, it is clear that there is a deep human connection between religious experience and dreaming, and that, in our paradigm here, dreams provide a conduit to the "vital and sacred" in people's lives.

Working with Spirituality in Integrative Care

These are some modern empirical data, associated with and drawing on ancient spiritual traditions. What are the implications for integrative care practitioners? How might we incorporate spirituality and spiritual care into integrative approaches to sleep health?

Certainly, given the literature we have reviewed, supporting people's spiritual well-being might simply (and appropriately) consist of encouraging the specific spiritually informed practices that have been associated with sleep quality: mindfulness, mindfulness meditation, gratitude, tai chi, and yoga. As we have discussed, the spiritual journey does indeed consist of particular practices—these and countless others, like reading sacred texts, prayer, daily devotions, retreats and pilgrimages, ceremonies and rituals, and fellowship with other people who are fellow travelers.

Spiritual care in integrative medicine, however, encompasses more than encouraging specific practices and techniques. I have proposed a framework for working with spirituality in integrative, person-centered care that includes three arenas.[40] A *personal* arena has to do with our own spiritual groundedness, equanimity, and compassionate presence as clinicians and caregivers. A *clinical* arena has to do with the ways in which we understand and support that which is "vital and sacred" in the lives of our patients. An *organizational* arena has to do with organizational culture and "soul," the ways in which our healthcare organizations and teams can be affirming and empowering places for workers and patients alike. All three of these arenas need to work in concert, with spiritually grounded and "present" practitioners understanding, honoring, and supporting the sacred values of their patients in organizations that are welcoming and hospitable and "bring out the best" in everyone who walks through the door. Together, they provide pathways for supporting the spiritual well-being of the people with whom we work.

PERSONAL

The personal arena is foundational in providing good spiritual care. Our ability to be spiritually centered and genuinely present as we work is meaningful for our own well-being in the midst of the multiple challenges that we all face and has remarkable power to comfort and encourage other people, regardless of whatever specific clinical approaches we may choose.

How does one cultivate the inner qualities of centeredness, groundedness, and spiritual well-being that undergird our compassionate and healing presence with people? Four suggestions:

1. *Remember your calling.* Most clinicians go into healthcare out of a genuine calling to make a difference. This has energy. Remembering your calling has the ability to bring your attention and heart away from the daily ups and downs and back to what is sacred for you. Who are you, as a professional and as a human being? What matters most to you about the work you do? What qualities of living do you wish to express, no matter where you find yourself?

2. *Let go of what you can't control.* Patients don't always keep sleep diaries. Administrators may have outlandish requirements. Someone else on your team may be having a bad day. You may have—as I suspect is the case with most of us—a voice in your head that says that you're not really as effective or as smart as you should be. We can certainly do problem-solving around some such things, but often the external and internal challenges that we face can't easily be fixed or changed, and it is more a matter of mindfully accepting these things and not giving them power to keep you from being who you are. There are a number of approaches from psychological work and spiritual traditions that help with the process of letting go of uncontrollable challenges and putting energy and heart into what is most important. They include such things as acceptance, nonattachment, gratitude, forgiveness, mindfulness, and serenity.[41]

3. *Be healthy.* Do the things that are understood, in integrative medicine, to promote health and well-being. Nutrition. Exercise. Positive and meaningful relationships. Creative practices. Sources of laughter and joy.

4. *Be reflective.* Create some practices that help you to learn from your experience. Journaling. Prayer and contemplative practices. Retreats. Coffee and conversation with a trusted friend.

CLINICAL

Conversation

In addition to encouraging particular spiritual practices, spiritual care means making meaningful connections with people and helping them to understand and express what is "vital and sacred" in their lives. Essentially, the conversation is

- What matters to you and what are you going to do about it?
- What do you care deeply about, and how can you "give life" to this?
- What is sacred for you, and how can you best honor this?

I often quote organizational consultant Margaret Wheatley:

Real change begins with the simple act of people talking about what they care about.[42, p. 22]

This does not mean giving advice. It is not about fixing people's problems. It is not theological. Rather, it is providing people with the opportunity to give voice to what is vital and sacred to them—what it means to them to live a good life—and to begin to partner with them in moving in that direction.

There are many ways of structuring this conversation. I often suggest to our residents that the most important things they bring to conversations are curiosity and an open heart and that spiritually grounded conversations can begin with any manner of curious and open-hearted questions.

- What keeps you going?
- How do you hope to make your way through this?
- What do you want?
- What kind of person do you want to be, as you face these things?
- What's most important to you at this point?
- What have you learned in your life about what you need to keep focused on?

I do find, by the way, that it is often particularly meaningful to elicit stories. Stories—narratives—often have power and learning value that conceptual answers lack.

- When has there been a time when you've felt really alive?
- Tell me a story about you at your best.
- Describe something hard that you've made your way through.

Next Steps

Spiritual care conversations lead to change. Changes can be as substantial as stopping alcohol use or leaving an abusive relationship, or as subtle as looking for some concrete ways to embody a little more kindness at work or having a cup of passion flower tea before bed. In whatever directions they may lead, our conversations with people help them to take next steps in faithfulness to what is vital and sacred for them. We work with people to develop specific plans, grounded in their values, patient-centered, and realistic and manageable. Change is generative, and even small steps help to empower people toward greater levels of spiritual well-being.

ORGANIZATIONAL

Although it is beyond the scope of this chapter to explore this area in detail, I can mention that there is a (perhaps surprisingly) substantial literature about the beneficial effects in healthcare of what has variously been called organizational "soul," "spirit," "culture," or "atmosphere." Healthcare and other organizations that have a clear sense of mission, that have a spirit of community among staff (both in the sense of partnership of work responsibilities and in the sense of personal valuing and caring), and that have visionary and affirming/empowering leadership show significant benefits with outcomes like staff satisfaction and retention, patient satisfaction, and various process and outcome measures of quality care.[43,40]

SPIRITUAL CARE SPECIALISTS

The paradigm I am presenting here is oriented to clinicians in integrative care who are not spiritual care professionals. As you may see from this perspective, I think that physicians, nurses, counselors, and other healthcare professionals are often the front-line providers of spiritual care as we define it. There are, of course, issues that warrant—and substantially benefit from—the engagement of spiritual care professionals like chaplains, spiritual directors, and clergy. People dealing with existential issues around deep human suffering ("Why do little children die of cancer?" "Where was God in the Holocaust?") often find the wisdom and skill of these professionals comforting and meaningful.

Conclusion

Although somewhat less well formed than other areas of spirituality and health, literature suggests that spiritual beliefs, practices, and overall spiritual well-being have salutary effects on sleep quality. Integrative care clinicians can support the spiritual well-being of their patients by nurturing their own spiritual centeredness and presence by suggesting spiritually grounded practices such as mindfulness meditation and gratitude, by partnering with patients in understanding and giving expression to what is "vital and sacred" for them, and by contributing to the spirit and affirming culture of the healthcare organizations in which they practice.

REFERENCES

1. Mead GRS. *Apollonius of Tyana*. London: Theosophical Publishing Society; 1901.
2. Koop CE. Spirituality and health. Paper presented at the Thomas Nevola, MD Symposium on Spirituality and Health, June 8, Augusta, ME.
3. Koenig HG. Religion, spirituality, and health: The research and clinical implications. *ISRN Psychiatry*. doi:10.5402/2012/278730.
4. Tsuang MT, Simpson JC, Koenen KC, Kremen WS, Lyons MJ. Spiritual well-being and health. *J Nerv Ment Dis*. 2007;195(8):673–680.

5. Martínez BB, Custódio RP. Relationship between mental health and spiritual wellbeing among hemodialysis patients: A correlation study. *Sao Paulo Med J.* 2014;132(1):23–27.

6. Phillips KD, Mock KS, Bopp CM, Dudgeon WA, Hand GA. Spiritual well-being, sleep disturbance, and mental and physical health status in HIV-infected individuals. *Iss Ment Health Nurs.* 2006;27:125–139.

7. Knowlden AP, Shewmake ME, Burns M, Harcrow A. Sex-specific impact of spiritual beliefs and sleep quality on degree of psychological distress. *J Religion Health.* 2016 Dec 27. doi:10.1007/s10943-016-0342 4. [Epub ahead of print].

8. Krause N, Hill PC, Emmons R, Pargament KI, Ironson G. Assessing the relationship between religious involvement and health behaviors. *Health Edu Behav.* 2017;44(2):278–284.

9. Ellison CG, Bradshaw M, Storch J, Marcum JP, Hill TD. Religious doubts and sleep quality: Findings from a nationwide study of Presbyterians. *Rev Religious Res.* 2011;53(1):19–136.

10. Khoramirad A, Mousavi M, Dadkhahtehrani T, Pourmarzi D. Relationship between sleep quality and spiritual well-being/religious activities in Muslim women with breast cancer. *J Religion Health.* 2015;54:2276–2285.

11. Yang J, Huang J, Kao T, et al. Impact of spiritual and religious activity on quality of sleep in hemodialysis patients. *Blood Purification.* 2008;26:221–225.

12. Brisbon NM, Lachman ME. Dispositional mindfulness and memory problems: The role of perceived stress and sleep quality. *Mindfulness (NY).* 2017;8(2):379–386.

13. Kemper KJ, Mo X, Khayat R. Are mindfulness and self-compassion associated with sleep and resilience in health professionals? *J Alt Complement Med.* 2015;8:496–503.

14. Emmons RA, McCullough ME, eds. *The psychology of gratitude* (series in affective science). New York: Oxford University Press; 2004.

15. Alkozei A, Smith R, Kotzin MD, Waugaman DL, Killgore WDS. The association between trait gratitude and self-reported sleep quality Is mediated by depressive mood state. *Behavi Sleep Med.* 2017 Jan 27: 1–9.

16. Wood AM, Joseph S, Lloyd J, Atkins S. Gratitude influences sleep through the mechanism of pre-sleep cognitions. *J Psychosomatic Res.* 2009;66(1):43–48.

17. Enright RD. *The forgiving life: A pathway to overcoming resentment and creating a legacy of love.* Washington, DC: American Psychological Association; 2012.

18. Luskin F. *Forgive for good: A proven prescription for health and happiness.* San Francisco, CA: HarperOne; 2003.

19. Lawler KA, Younger JW, Piferi RL, Jobe RL, Edmondson KA, Jones WH. The unique effects of forgiveness on health: An exploration of pathways. *J Behav Med.* 2005;28(2):157–167.

20. Stoia-Caraballo R, Rye MS, Pan W, Brown Kirschman KJ, Lutz-Zois C, Lyons AM. Negative affect and anger rumination as mediators between forgiveness and sleep quality. *J Behav Med.* 2008;31(6):478–488.

21. Germer CK. *The mindful path to self-compassion.* New York: Guilford; 2009.

22. Neff K. *Self-compassion.* New York: William Morrow, 2010.

23. Sirois FM, Kitner R, Hirsch JK. Self-compassion, affect, and health-promoting behaviors. *Health Psychol.* 2015;34(6):661–669.

24. Black DS, O'Reilly GA, Olmstead R, Breen EC, Irwin MR. Mindfulness meditation and improvement in sleep quality and daytime impairment among older adults with sleep disturbances: A randomized clinical trial. *JAMA Intern Med.* 2015;175(4):494–501.

25. Yun MR, Song M, Jung K, Yu BJ, Lee KJ. The effects of mind subtraction meditation on breast cancer survivors' psychological and spiritual well-being and sleep quality. *Cancer Nurs.* 2017;40(5):377–385.

26. Querstret D, Cropley M, Fife-Schaw C. Internet-based instructor-led mindfulness for work-related rumination, fatigue, and sleep: Assessing facets of mindfulness as mechanisms of change. A randomized waitlist control trial. *J Occ Health Psychol.* 2017;22(2):153–169.

27. Ong JC, Manber R, Segal Z, Xia Y, Shapiro S, Wyatt JK. A randomized controlled trial of mindfulness meditation for chronic insomnia. *Sleep.* 2014;37(9):1553–1563.

28. Hubbling A, Reilly Spong M, Kreitzer MJ, Gross CR. How mindfulness changed my sleep: Focus groups with chronic insomnia patients. *BMC Comp Alt Med.* 2014;14:50.

29. Martires J, Zeidler M. The value of mindfulness meditation in the treatment of insomnia. *Curr Opin Pulmon Med.* 2015;21(6):547–552.

30. Winbush NY, Gross CR, Kreitzer MJ. The effects of mindfulness-based stress reduction on sleep disturbance: A systematic review. *Explore (NY).* 2007;3(6):585–591.

31. Jackowska M, Brown J, Ronaldson A, Steptoe A. The impact of a brief gratitude intervention on subjective well-being, biology and sleep. *J Health Psychol.* 2016;21(10):2207–2217.

32. Digdon N, Koble A. Effects of constructive worry, imagery distraction, and gratitude interventions on sleep quality: A pilot trial. *Appl Psych Health Well-Being.* 2011;3(2):193–206.

33. Li F, Fisher KJ, Harmer P, Irbe D, Tearse RG, Weimer C. Tai chi and self-rated quality of sleep and daytime sleepiness in older adults: A randomized controlled trial. *J Am Geriatr Soc.* 2004;52(6):892–900.

34. Halpern J, Cohen M, Kennedy G, Reece J, Cahan C, Baharav A. Yoga for improving sleep quality and quality of life for older adults. *Alt Ther Health Med.* 2014;20(3):37–46.

35. Taibi DM, Vitiello MV. A pilot study of gentle yoga for sleep disturbance in women with osteoarthritis. *Sleep Med.* 2011;12(5):512–517.

36. Field T, Diegoa M, Delgadoa J, Medinaa L. Tai chi/yoga reduces prenatal depression, anxiety and sleep disturbances. *Comp Ther Clin Pract.* 2013;19(1):6–10.

37. Levin J. Spiritual determinants of health and healing: An epidemiologic perspective on salutogenic perspectives. *Alt Ther.* 2003; 9(6):48–57.

38. Bulkeley K. *Dreaming in the world's religions.* New York: New York University Press; 2008.

39. Bulkeley K. *Big dreams: The science of dreaming and the origins of religion.* New York: Oxford University Press; 2016.
40. Craigie FC. *Positive spirituality in health care: Nine practical approaches to pursuing wholeness for clinicians, patients, and health care organizations.* Minneapolis, MN: Mill City Press; 2010.
41. Craigie FC. Three steps to make life count from here on. *Spirituality Health.* 2012 Jan/Feb: 66–71.
42. Wheatley M. *Turning to one another: Simple conversations to restore hope to the future.* San Francisco, CA: Berrett-Koehler; 2002.
43. Craigie FC, Hobbs RF. Exploring the organizational culture of exemplary community health center practices. *Fam Med.* 2004;36(10): 733–738.

15

Dietary and Herbal Supplements for Sleep

DAVID KIEFER

Introduction

Consider this scenario. It was a busy clinic day, and, as you complete your charting, you reflect on the fact that four patients asked you about dietary supplements (DS) that might be effective for their insomnia or other sleep perturbation. For example, a 40-year-old attorney mentioned delayed sleep latency, mild to moderate anxiety during the day, and the fact that an infusion of lavender before bed "didn't help." Another patient was a 5-year-old with a "nervous stomach" who gets "hyper" before bed, which is also almost always after her earned hour on the iPad; her parents are wondering which, if any, natural cures might be helpful. In addition, there was a 53-year-old with significantly delayed sleep latency ("my mind just keeps going") despite almost nightly alprazolam who wanted to continue taking a low-dose of the pharmaceutical in addition to a safe adjunctive herb. And you finished the day with a call from an assisted living facility about an 83-year-old man recovering from knee surgery who displayed "sundowning" behavior and seemed to be restless all night long.

Patient interest in and questions about DS are common and not unlike the hypothetical scenarios just outlined. DS are defined as a substance that is meant to supplement the diet (not take the place of food), is intended to be taken by mouth, and that includes such ingredients as vitamins, herbs, enzymes, minerals, and amino acids.[1,2] A variety of compounds can be considered DS, including vitamins, minerals, omega-3 fatty acids, amino acids, and herbal or botanical medicines. The latter plant-based compounds are variously defined as herbs, herbal medicines, plant medicines, botanicals, or botanical medicines.[3] Worldwide, the use of botanical medicines is extremely common, with estimates that 80% of people rely on traditional medicine, primarily botanical medicine, to meet their primary health-care needs.[4,5] Botanical medicines constitute a significant part of annual sales and use of DS in the United States.

There has been a significant amount of qualitative research undertaken to de-lineate which demographic groups have a higher tendency to ingest DS, as well as which DS are most commonly ingested and for which diagnoses. Teasing out trends from this research can be a challenge; some of the studies asked study participants about DS use, while others focused on non-vitamin, non-mineral DS or simply limited the research to the botanical medicine subset of DS. That said, most studies have found that approximately 20% of people in the United States regularly use DS.[6-8] The prevalence of herbal medicine use by some ethnic and cul-tural groups in the United States may be even higher: one meta-analysis found that 4–100% (mean 30%) of Latinos living in the United States regularly used herbal medicine.[9]

Out of these general trends, DS are also regularly turned to in order to aid sleep and treat insomnia.[10] For example, valerian (*Valeriana officinalis*, Family Valerianaceae) is one of the top-selling botanical medicines in one list,[11] while mel-atonin is commonly used, as per a nationwide DS use survey.[12]

This chapter explores the evidence for (and against) the use of DS for in-somnia and sleep. Specifically, the details behind the use of three commonly used nonbotanical DS and seven botanical medicines (see Table 15.1) will be described, including relevant meta-analyses and randomized controlled trials (RCTs), dosing, and adverse effects and/or safety concerns. Of note, numerous DS have anecdotal reports of benefits for insomnia but lack clinical trials or mechanistic support for this use. Examples are 5-hydroxytrypotphan (5-HTP), S-adenosylmethionine (SAMe), and skullcap (*Scuttelaria lateriflora*). These DS will not be discussed in this chapter.

Table 15.1 Dietary supplements with potential benefits for sleep disorders

Non-botanical dietary supplements	Botanical medicines
Melatonin	Valerian
Magnesium	Hops
	Chamomile
	Passionflower
	Lavender
	Lemon balm
	Kava kava
	L-theanine

Nonbotanical Dietary Supplements

MELATONIN

Melatonin, an endogenous hormone with physiologic activities relevant to the sleep–wake cycle, has also been used as a DS for circadian rhythm disorders and other sleep abnormalities.[13] Melatonin has many biological effects, including those relative to sleep; its production in the human body increases at night and decreases during the day.[14] For instance, it may regulate sleep by activating receptors MT_1 and MT_2, as well as changing the expression of "clock genes" and genes involved with serotonin production.[14] It does not appear to delay the onset of nor suppress rapid eye movement (REM) sleep.[15] These effects all combine to help improve sleep initiation, increase sleep duration, and change sleep architecture.

There have been numerous clinical trials examining the use of melatonin for sleep. Capturing these results are reviews and meta-analyses. One example is a meta-analysis of 12 clinical trials that found that melatonin reduces sleep latency compared to placebo in primary insomnia by 5.05 minutes (P = 0.004).[15] In this same analysis, melatonin was also found to reduce sleep latency by 22.05 minutes in delayed sleep phase syndrome (P <0.0001). Another meta-analysis looked at eight clinical trials published after 2002, five of which used sustained-release melatonin.[16] The authors of this analysis found evidence of benefit for several sleep parameters with the use of both immediate-release (5 mg/d for 8 weeks) and sustained-release (2 mg/d for 3 weeks) melatonin, with perhaps a more pronounced effect on sleep latency seen in people 55 years and older and with use of sustained-release formulations.

Yet another meta-analysis weighed in on some of the details with melatonin use.[17] Studies ($n = 19$) examining the use of melatonin for primary insomnia were reviewed, finding a reduction in sleep latency of 7.06 minutes (P <0.001), an increase in sleep time of 8.25 minutes (P = 0.013), and an improvement in sleep quality (P <0.001) compared to placebo groups. There seemed to be slightly more benefit with higher doses (doses used in the studies ranged from 0.3 to 5 mg) and when melatonin was used for longer periods of time (study duration ranged from 7 to 126 days), and it did not seem as if melatonin's effects waned with time even though these effects are less than would be seen with pharmaceuticals. Adverse effects were not detailed in this analysis. Despite the results of the above-mentioned meta-analyses and reviews, some experts have found evidence of benefit to be minimal, and both American and European guidelines do not officially recommend the use of melatonin.[18,19]

With respect to dosing, a range of doses have been used in clinical trials. One meta-analysis (nine randomized controlled trials, five case-series, and two open-label studies) of dosing in adults 55 years and older found a dose-dependent increase in serum melatonin levels after exogenous administration; even 0.5 mg induces an effect.[20] They found many variables that affect melatonin's effects on a particular individual and that the effective dose is still not definitively known. They cite data that show that lower doses may achieve more effective sleep effects without changing body core temperature or leading to increased serum levels over time; their recommendation was that "supplementation needs to be as low as possible."

The data related to the effect of immediate-release versus sustained-release melatonin continue to evolve. One meta-analysis of 16 studies in adults over the age of 55 years, which also followed melatonin levels (measured in several different ways), raised some concerns over sustained-release preparations in that there is the risk of prolonged elevated melatonin levels that could lead to adverse effects.[20] In contrast, another review analyzed eight studies that met their inclusion criteria for the use of over-the-counter preparations in primary insomnia, five of which used sustained-release melatonin preparations. The authors concluded that there is better evidence for the positive effects of sustained-release melatonin on insomnia, especially in adults older than 55 years, than for immediate-release preparations.[16] Other reviews did not differentiate between the type of melatonin preparations.[15,17]

Adverse effects with melatonin are mild (headache, drowsiness, nausea, dizziness), with no lingering effects the next day, no tolerance, and no dependence, and melatonin appears to be non-toxic with short-term use (doses up to 10 mg for 1 month).[15,16,19]

MAGNESIUM

The mineral magnesium may have soporific properties, as per mechanistic studies and some limited clinical trials. A divalent cation, magnesium in supplements or from dietary sources exists in a variety of forms, such as magnesium sulfate, magnesium oxide, magnesium glycinate, or magnesium citrate. It plays a role in many biochemical reactions, including those relevant to nervous system function, by antagonizing the N-methyl-D-aspartic acid (NMDA) receptor and serving as a gamma-aminobutyric acid (GABA) receptor agonist.[21] Some studies have pointed at an association between hypomagnesemia and poor quality sleep, though the details of that interaction are still being elucidated.[22]

Clinical trials in insomnia are few, though one placebo-controlled study in the elderly showed that 500 mg of elemental magnesium (form not specified) daily for 8 weeks improved various sleep parameters, including sleep time, sleep efficiency, and sleep onset latency.[21] Other clinical trials show that magnesium may improve symptoms that indirectly could improve sleep. For example, nocturnal leg cramps and restless leg syndrome have shown improvement with magnesium supplementation in some, but not all, clinical trials.[23,24] Also, for individuals withdrawing from alcohol use, magnesium supplementation may be beneficial, as per one small, open-label study.[25]

A limitation to the use of magnesium clinically is its laxative effect, which is usually dose-dependent and may be more pronounced with the oxide form of the supplement. It should be used with caution in patients with renal disease. In appropriately selected patients, a trial of magnesium supplementation is not unreasonable given its generally low side-effect profile.

Botanical Medicines

VALERIAN

Probably the most well-known botanical medicine for sleep is valerian. Made from the roots of the plant *Valeriana officinalis*, valerian has a long history of use as a sedative, sleep aid, and anxiolytic.[26] Its physiologic effects stem from 100–150 phytochemicals, including valerenic acid (an organic acid) and valeprotriates.[26–29] As with many other sedative substances, the effect of valerian seems to be mediated through the neurotransmitter GABA; studies have shown that valerian and/or its isolated phytochemicals possess a GABA reuptake inhibitory effect or induce stimulation of GABA release.[27,28,30,31] Valerian may also act as a serotonin and adenosine agonist.[30,31]

Valerian has been the subject of numerous clinical trials, meta-analyses, and reviews on various aspects of sleep and sleep disorders.[10,27,32] For example, one review of nine placebo-controlled trials and two non–placebo-controlled trials found a range of methodologies, including study duration (1 day to 6 weeks), valerian dose (200–900 mg), and form (ethanol or aqueous extractions). Results ranged from minimal to no effect to some benefit on at least one sleep parameter (i.e., sleep latency, sleep quality, night awakenings, etc). measured. A meta-analysis of five clinical trials found that only one showed marginally significant differences in sleep latency (0.27 on a 7-point scale; $P = 0.06$), and none of the five trials found a difference in sleep duration (-1.115 minutes; $P = 0.89$), sleep quality (0.29; $P = 0.48$), or sleep efficiency percentage (0.59; $P = 0.78$).[10]

A common combination product that has been subject to clinic trials is a blend of valerian with hops.[32] Out of four clinical trials reviewed, three found that the valerian-hops treatment group showed improvements in at least one sleep parameter.[32] Another blend combines valerian, hops, and passionflower in an extract called NSF-3. NSF-3 was studied in people with primary insomnia and showed short-term benefits in various sleep parameters after 2 weeks of use.[33]

A typical dose for valerian averages 300–600 mg of the dried root in tablet or capsule form,[28] though higher daily doses (2–3 g) are sometimes use.[30] Tinctures providing 2–4 mL of a daily dose are also available.[30]

Overall, valerian appears safe as per clinical trials and other literature reviews[26] even in supratherapeutic doses.[28] Valerian may have mild gastrointestinal side effects, and it may produce headache, drowsiness, or nervousness, but these are consider self-limiting and usually occur in rates similar to placebo groups in clinical trials.[30,31] A review on the use of valerian in the elderly mentions the possible risk of headache, drowsiness, and depression but likely not subsequent daytime sedation; this is all based few clinical trials in that demographic.[31] Valerian appears to have no effect on the common cytochrome detoxification enzymes, rendering it free of supplement–pharmaceutical interactions.[34,35] A general rule of thumb with sedative botanicals is to use with caution (or not at all) in combination with anxiolytic pharmaceuticals such as benzodiazepenes.[30]

HOPS

A popular beer preservative and flavoring, hops (*Humulus lupus*, plant Family Cannabaceae) is also a botanical medicine with a long history of use for a variety of health conditions including anxiety and insomnia. The medicine is derived from the seed cone, also called a strobile, and yields the resinous compounds humulone, lupulin, and lupulone, as well as terpenoids, volatile oils, tannins, and flavonoids.[27,36] Relevant to anxiety and insomnia, hops has activity on the GABAergic system, specifically $GABA_A$ receptor potentiation.[27]

Most of the hops research centers on its effect as an anxiolytic, though there are clinical trials exploring its sleep effects. Hops has also been studied as a combination product with magnesium, vitamin B_6, a milk extract, and the Chinese herb *Zizyphus*, though clinical research on this mixture has not shown significant sleep benefits.[37] Other clinical trials used a combination of hops and valerian. The effective dose varies based on the particular product or extract, but some sources recommend 500 mg of the dried herb or its equivalent, one to several times daily.[36] With respect to interactions, there is the potential for hops to increase the effect of coadministered melatonin or sedative pharmaceuticals and botanical medicines.[38,39]

LAVENDER

Lavender (*Lavandula augustifolia*) flowers have long history of cosmetic and medicinal use, ranging from acne and alopecia to anxiety and insomnia. Lavender has been prescribed for these various conditions in both oral and inhalation forms with varying degrees of proven efficacy. The flowers contain approximately 1.5% essential oils, the main ones being linalool, linalyl acetate, camphor, beta-ocimene, terpinen-4-ol, and 1,8-cineole.[28,36] The anxiolytic properties and presumed positive effects on sleep of lavender have been ascribed to numerous of the chemical constituents but appears to exert effects on $GABA_A$ receptors as well as on presynaptic calcium channels.[40]

For example, lavender aromatherapy in one randomized, controlled clinical trial improved the Chinese version of the Pittsburgh Sleep Quality Index Score (PSQI) after 12 weeks in 67 women with insomnia (P <0.001).[41] A control group who only received health education about sleep hygiene had no such improvement. The lavender was administered for 20 minutes twice weekly by mixing 0.25 mL of lavender essential oil in 50 mL of water and placing the solution in an ultrasonic ionizer aromatherapy diffuser next to the chair where the research participant was resting. Another study, this time a randomized, single-blind, cross-over study of lavender aromatherapy and almond oil as the control in 10 people with insomnia found a 2.5-point non-statistically significant improvement in the PSQI after 4 weeks (P = 0.07).[42] For the treatment arm of this study, 6–8 drops of lavender essential oil was placed in an aromatherapy cartridge by research volunteers, and then the research participants used the aromatherapy throughout the night while they were sleeping. The authors pointed out the sound methodology and the trend toward benefit, calling for larger studies to corroborate the results. A lavender essential oil patch (55 mg of lavender essential oil) was used in 79 college students with self-reported "sleep issues" and found to benefit sleep (P = 0.01), energy (P = 0.03), and vibrancy (P = 0.05) as per self-assessment after 5 consecutive nights.[43] A control group used a placebo patch, and both groups were instructed in sleep hygiene techniques.

Lavender aromatherapy has been used successfully in other demographics, including oncology patients suffering from insomnia.[44] In this 3-week, randomized, placebo-controlled, cross-over study, 50 patients admitted for chemotherapy to treat acute leukemia were offered one of three scents (lavender, peppermint, or chamomile) to be administered by aromatherapy (8 drops of essential oil via a diffuser for 8 hours at night). Various parameters were measured, including sleep quality (measured by the PSQI), anxiety, depression, drowsiness, and tiredness, among others. Lavender was the most common scent chosen (the exact numbers per essential oil were not specified), and overall aromatherapy improved the PSQI by 2.53 points versus placebo (p = 0.0001).

Alternatively, some studies have used lavender oil capsules. A case series in eight people with major depression and associated symptoms demonstrated improvement in sleep onset (*n* = 3) and sleep maintenance (*n* = 3) with the oral ingestion of a capsule of lavender oil.[45] The capsules, Lasea, are orally administered via an 80 mg immediate-release soft gelatin capsule. The patented extract Silexan, which is the active substance of Lasea, is oil produced from lavender flowers through the process of steam distillation. The main constituents of the extracted lavender oil are linalool, linalyl acetate, 1.8-cineole, beta-ocimene, terpinen-4-ol, and camphor.

A randomized, placebo-controlled trial looked at Silexan for "restlessness" and related sleep disturbances in 170 people.[46] The research participants received 80 mg Silexan or placebo once daily for 10 weeks. After the study period, the Hamilton Anxiety Scale decreased 12 and 9 points in the treatment and placebo groups, respectively ($P = 0.03$). The researchers monitored numerous other parameters, including sleep impairment. Sleep impairment at the study conclusion was verbally rated on a 4-point scale, and 55% of the people in the treatment groups versus 45% in the placebo group claimed that they "never, seldom, or sometimes" suffered from disturbed sleep (no P value given). Overall, adverse effects in this trial were similar between the two groups, though more people in the Silexan group experienced eructation ($n = 6$ vs. $n = 0$) and other gastrointestinal side effects. Of note, Silexan has also been studied for generalized anxiety disorder, usually in doses of 160 mg/d.[47]

Lavender is generally considered safe to use.[36] Unlike some other sleep aids, it appears that lavender does not cause withdrawal symptoms even when abruptly discontinued.[48]

LEMON BALM

Lemon balm (*Melissa officinalis*) is a plant in the mint family (Family Lamiaceae), the leaves of which contain essential oils and other phytochemicals that may have sedative effects.[37] It has a long-standing traditional use as a medicine, and it seems to increase GABA levels through inhibition of the transporter $GABA_T$ and binding to the $GABA_A$-benzodiazepine receptor.[27]

There is a dearth of clinical trials corroborating its traditional use, especially for botanical monotherapy. One study using a combination of valerian with lemon balm demonstrated an improvement in the PSQI score in 100 menopausal women with sleep disorders.[49] Study participants were blinded to whether they were taking two capsules of the valerian and lemon balm mixture (160 mg valerian/ 80 mg lemon balm) or placebo. After 1 month of the treatments daily, 36% of the botanical medicine group had an improvement in sleep versus only 8% in the placebo group. Sleep scores in the botanical group improved by 5 points ($P = 0.0001$).

Lemon balm may have anxiolytic effects as per human clinical trials[27] and has been used in a combination product with *Bacopa monieri* and other plants for attention deficit hyperactivity disorder.[50]

It is usually dosed as an infusion of fresh (1 Tb) or dried (1 tsp) leaves in a cup of hot water, covered, and steeped for 3–5 minutes. This solution is then cooled to a comfortable temperature, strained, and ingested. Tinctures are also used; one dropperful of an alcohol or glycerin tincture can be used 1–4 times daily as needed for anxiety or to promote sleep. Moreover, more often than not, lemon balm is used in combination with other herbs including hops. All botanical sedatives may have additive effects with other centrally depressing substances, including pharmaceuticals and botanical. It is possible that lemon balm could worsen glaucoma, prostatic hypertrophy, and hypothyroidism.[39]

CHAMOMILE

Chamomile (*Matricaria recutita, M. chamomilla*; Family Asteraceae) flowers are a popular sleep aid[10] and have been found to have mild anxiolytic and sleep-promoting effects, with clinical data having mixed results to corroborate long-standing traditional use.[27,51] There are two species of chamomile, German chamomile (*Matricaria recutita*) and wild chamomile (*Matricaria chamomila*), though German chamomile is discussed more often in the scientific literature. There are numerous phytochemicals in chamomile, some of which fall into the class of flavonoids.[36] One flavonoid, apigenin, is thought to account for some of chamomile's sedative effects, affecting the benzodiazepine site in the brain,[28] which, as per animal research, leads to depressed central nervous system activity.[28] The benzodiazepine effects may be moderated by GABA receptor changes.[27]

Recent reviews on botanical medicines for sleep have centered on one clinical trial from 2011 using an extract of German chamomile standardized to the phytochemicals bisabolol and apigenin[10,27]; no statistically significant difference in sleep outcomes or adverse effects was seen between the treatment and placebo groups. There is a more extensive literature on chamomile's anxiolytic effects,[27] which could potentially be extrapolated to overall calming effects benefitting sleep. For example, 8 weeks of daily ingestion of a chamomile extract led to improvements in the anxiety and well-being scores in 179 people with general anxiety disorder, a response similar to what might be expected from pharmaceuticals.[52] Long-term follow-up of a subset of these patients found chamomile to be safe.[53]

Chamomile is most often used as an infusion made by pouring hot water over fresh or dried flowers. A typical dose is 1 cup of hot water poured over 1–2 teaspoons of fresh or dried chamomile flowers and steeped for 5–10 minutes. One to several cups of this infusion can be used daily.[51] Alternatively, chamomile tinctures exist, dosed at 1–4 mL/d.[51] Extracts of various strengths exist, though there is little reason to use such formulations due to the wide availability and effectiveness of the raw, unprocessed plant material.

As alluded to earlier, chamomile has a favorable safety profile. There is some concern about an allergic cross-reactivity between chamomile and other plants in the daisy family (Family Asteraceae) including anaphylaxis, so caution is advised in people with such allergies.[39] This risk is considered to be overall quite low, and, given the paucity of pharmaceutical interactions and other side effects, chamomile is overall considered to be a safe choice as a mild sedative and sleep aid.[36,51]

PASSIONFLOWER

The above-ground parts (dried flowers, stems, and leaves) of passionflower (*Passiflora incarnata*) have worldwide folkloric use as a sedative and sleep aid.[27,54,55] The primary phytochemicals in passionflower are flavonoids, alkaloids, and phenolic compounds.[27,36] As with many of the sedative plants, passionflower affects the GABA-nergic system, through $GABA_A$ and $GABA_B$ receptor binding and GABA uptake inhibition.[27] There are some clinical trials showing anxiolytic effects,[27] but, with respect to sleep, the research is more sparse. One clinical trial used 1 cup of passionflower tea daily in 41 adults and analyzed their sleep diaries, finding an improvement in sleep quality versus placebo (parsley tea) ($P < 0.01$).[56] The passionflower tea was made from 2 g of dried leaves, stems, seeds, and flowers.

It may have mild adverse effects, such as drowsiness, dizziness, and confusion.[54] Coexisting depression is considered a contraindication due to its sedation, and it may have additive blood-thinning effects with warfarin.[39] In addition, there is one case report of cardiac rhythm abnormalities possibly correlated with the use of passionflower; caution is advised in people with underlying arrhythmias.[55]

KAVA KAVA

Kava kava (*Piper methysticum*, Family Piperaceae) rhizomes contain active compounds, kavalactones, responsible for anxiolytic and soporific effects, and it has a long history of traditional and ceremonial use centered on Polynesia.[27,30,54,57] Kavalactones appear to bind to GABA, serotonin, and dopamine receptors.[27,30,54] Most of kava's clinical benefits appear to be on anxiety.[57] For example, a recent review of six studies found that four of them supported the use of kava for anxiety (Cohen's d = 1.1).[58]

There have been mixed clinical data to support the use of kava kava for sleep.[30] One pilot, non–placebo-controlled study in 24 adults with "stress induced insomnia" followed sleep parameters for 6 weeks using 120 mg of "standardized" kava (no details given) daily.[28] After 6 weeks of kava, the total insomnia score (maximum score possible was 300) fell to 107.1 from 138.0 ($P < 0.05$). Two study participants each complained of dry mouth, "gastric disturbances," and diarrhea, while three complained of dizziness. Without a placebo control, it is difficult to draw firm conclusions from either the efficacy or adverse effects. Another review detailed a clinical trial using a kava extract providing 100 mg of kavalactones three times daily and found no significant changes in insomnia severity, sleep onset latency, and nocturnal awakenings for the kava group compared to comparison placebo and valerian groups.[10] In contrast, a 4-week study found benefits on sleep quality (P = 0.007) and recuperative effect after sleep (P = 0.018) using 200 mg/d of an extract of the dried root of kava (WS 1490, standardized to 70% kava).[59] The study population (n = 61) was adults with sleep disturbances considered secondary to anxiety, and the treatment was considered safe (no changes in laboratory parameters and only one gastrointestinal adverse effect in the placebo group).

Dosing of kava varies with the formulation, but most clinical trials have used between 100 and 200 mg of kavalactones daily.[60] Kava extracts may be a source of concern, especially due to reports of hepatotoxicity.[30,57,60] It is possible that the method of preparation, plant parts used, and solvent used in the extractions are important variables that determine safety or toxicity[30,57]; for example, it may be that water-based preparations are safer.[57] Kava may interact adversely with acetaminophen and other liver-metabolized substances, including alcohol.[57,60,61] There may also be additive effects if combined with sedating pharmaceuticals.[60] Some experts caution against using high doses of kava when operating heavy machinery or while driving, and suggest that liver function be monitored during long-term use.[58]

L-THEANINE

One of the compounds in tea (Camellia sinensis) is L-theanine, a non-protein amino acid which may have calming effects.[62-64] The compound affects the central nervous system and is mediated by glutamate, dopamine, GABA, and glycine.[62-65] Much of the L-theanine research has focused on its benefits in anxiety,[62,64,65] stress,[63,64,66] and cognitive performance.[66,67] Some benefits on sleep have also been noted in clinical trials, though at least one author's hypothesis was that the sleep benefits were achieved through improving anxiety.[65] That said, in one clinical trial, 30 adults took 200 mg/d of L-theanine for 4 weeks in order to examine its effects on stress and cognition. Improvements in sleep were noted as per PSQI testing, especially for latency, disturbance, and medication use.[66] In another study of 46 participants with general anxiety disorder, 225 mg of L-theanine twice daily over an 8-week placebo-controlled period showed benefits in sleep satisfaction though there was no benefit on the overall Insomnia Severity Index.[62] In this study, there were no differences in adverse effects between placebo and treatment groups. Other studies have found sleep benefits using L-theanine in people with diagnoses such as attention deficit hyperactivity disorder[68] and schizophrenia.[69]

Doses of L-theanine range from 15 to 900 mg, though more commonly 200–400 mg is used daily[65]; it is not recommended that more than 1,200 mg/d are ingested.[63] Overall, L-theanine appears to have a good safety profile, with clinical trials showing adverse effect rates similar to those in placebo groups and reassurances for short-term use (less than 8 weeks).[64,65]

Conclusion

This chapter detailed some of the recent evidence for the efficacy and safety of nonbotanical and botanical DS with effects on sleep. Clinically, there may be an individuality to the response to these treatments, affected, of course, by a person's particular health history, including concomitant use of pharmaceuticals. With the use of any DS, it is imperative to review a patient's pharmaceutical and DS list and assure that there are no clinically relevant interactions.

REFERENCES

1. National Institutes of Health Office of Dietary Supplements (NIH ODS). What is a dietary supplement? https://ods.od.nih.gov/factsheets/DietarySupplements-HealthProfessional/

2. US Food and Drug Administration. Dietary supplements: What you need to know. https://www.fda.gov/Food/DietarySupplements/UsingDietarySupplements/ucm109760.htm

3. National Center for Complementary and Integrative Health (NCCIH). What is complementary and alternative medicine? June 2016. http://nccam.nih.gov/health/whatiscam

4. Farnsworth NR, Akerele O, Bingel AS, Soejarto DD, Zhengang G. Medicinal plants in therapy. *Bull WHO.* 1985;63(6):965–981.

5. World Health Organization (WHO). Essential medicines and health information portal. Traditional medicine. Herbal medicines. http://apps.who.int/medicinedocs/en/cl/CL10.1.1.2.4/clmd,50.html#hlCL10_1_1_2_4

6. Wu CH, Wang CC, Tsai MT, et al. Trend and pattern of herb and supplement use in the United States: Results from the 2002, 2007, and 2012 National Health Interview Surveys. *Evidence-Based Compl Alt Med.* 2014;7.

7. Peregoy JA, Clarke TC, Jones LI, et al. Regional variation in use of complementary health approaches by US adults. *NCHS Data Brief No.* 146. April 2014.

8. Barnes PM, Bloom B, Nahin RL. Complementary and alternative medicine use among adults and children: United States, 2007. *Natl Health Stat Rep.* 2008;12:1–23.

9. Gardiner P, Whelan J, White LF, Filippelli AC, Bharmal N, Kaptchuk TJ. A systematic review of the prevalence of herb usage among racial/ethnic minorities in the United States. *J Immigr Minor Health.* 2013;15(4)817–828.

10. Leach MJ, Page AT. Herbal medicine for insomnia: A systematic review and meta-analysis. *Sleep Med Rev.* 2015;24:1–12.

11. Tyler Smith MEL, Johnson J, Kawa K, Bauman H, Blumenthal M. Herbal dietary supplement sales in US increase 6.8% in 2014. *HerbalGram*. American Botanical Council; 2015; 52–59.

12. National Center for Complementary and Integrative Health (NCCIH). Use of complementary health approaches in the US National Health Interview Survey (NHIS). 2012. https://nccih.nih.gov/research/statistics/NHIS/2012

13. Matheson E, Hainer BL. Insomnia: Pharmacologic therapy. *Am Fam Physician*. 2017 Jul 1;96(1):29–35.

14. Meng X, Li Y, Li S, Zhou Y, Gan RY, Xu DP, Li HB. Dietary sources and bioactivities of melatonin. *Nutrients*. 2017 Apr 7;9(4):367.

15. Auld F, Maschauer EL, Morrison I, Skene DJ, Riha RL. Evidence for the efficacy of melatonin in the treatment of primary adult sleep disorders. *Sleep Med Rev*. 2017 Aug;34:10–22.

16. Culpepper L, Wingertzahn MA. Over-the-counter agents for the treatment of occasional disturbed sleep or transient insomnia: A systematic review of efficacy and safety. *Prim Care Companion CNS Dis*. 2015 Dec 31;17(6).

17. Ferracioli-Oda E, Qawasmi A, Bloch MH. Meta-analysis: Melatonin for the treatment of primary sleep disorders. *PLoS One*. 2013 May 17;8(5):e63773.

18. Sateia MJ, Buysse DJ, Krystal AD, Neubauer DN, Heald JL. Clinical Practice Guideline for the Pharmacologic Treatment of Chronic Insomnia in Adults: An American Academy of Sleep Medicine Clinical Practice Guideline. *J Clin Sleep Med*. 2017 Feb 15;13(2):307–349.

19. Riemann D, Baglioni C, Bassetti C, et al. European guideline for the diagnosis and treatment of insomnia. *J Sleep Res*. 2017 Dec;26(6):675–700.

20. Vural EM, van Munster BC, de Rooij SE. Optimal dosages for melatonin supplementation therapy in older adults: A systematic review of current literature. *Drugs Aging*. 2014 Jun;31(6):441–451.

21. Abbasi B, Kimiagar M, Sadeghniiat K, Shirazi MM, Hedayati M, Rashidkhani B. The effect of magnesium supplementation on primary insomnia in elderly: A double-blind placebo-controlled clinical trial. *J Res Med Sci*. 2012 Dec;17(12):1161–1169.

22. Nielsen FH, Johnson LK, Zeng H. Magnesium supplementation improves indicators of low magnesium status and inflammatory stress in adults older than 51 years with poor quality sleep. *Magnes Res*. 2010 Dec;23(4):158–168.

23. Allen RE, Kirby KA. Nocturnal leg cramps. *Am Fam Physician*. 2012 Aug 15;86(4):350–355.

24. Sebo P, Cerutti B, Haller DM. Effect of magnesium therapy on nocturnal leg cramps: A systematic review of randomized controlled trials with meta-analysis using simulations. *Fam Pract*. 2014 Feb;31(1):7–19.

25. Kolla BP, Mansukhani MP, Schneekloth T. Pharmacological treatment of insomnia in alcohol recovery: A systematic review. *Alcohol Alcohol*. 2011 Sep-Oct;46(5):578–585.

26. Dietz BM, Mahady GB, Pauli GF, Farnsworth NR. Valerian extract and valerenic acid are partial agonists of the 5-HT5a receptor in vitro. *Brain Res Mol Brain Res*. 2005 Aug 18;138(2):191–197.

27. Savage K, Firth J, Stough C, Sarris J. GABA-modulating phytomedicines for anxiety: A systematic review of preclinical and clinical evidence. *Phytother Res.* 2018 Jan;32(1):3–18.

28. Wheatley D. Kava and valerian in the treatment of stress-induced insomnia. *Phytother Res.* 2001 Sep;15(6):549–551.

29. Jarema M. Herbal drug treatment. *Neuroendocrinol Lett.* 2008;29 (Suppl 1):93–104.

30. Yurcheshen M, Seehuus M, Pigeon W. Updates on nutraceutical sleep therapeutics and investigational research. *Evid Based Compl Alt Med.* 2015;2015:105256. doi:10.1155/2015/105256. Epub 2015 Jul 21.

31. Schroeck JL, Ford J, Conway EL, Kurtzhalts KE, Gee ME, Vollmer KA, Mergenhagen KA. Review of safety and efficacy of sleep medicines in older adults. *Clin Ther.* 2016 Nov;38(11):2340–2372.

32. Salter S, Brownie S. Treating primary insomnia—the efficacy of valerian and hops. *Aust Fam Physician.* 2010 Jun;39(6):433–437.

33. Maroo N, Hazra A, Das T. Efficacy and safety of a polyherbal sedative-hypnotic formulation NSF-3 in primary insomnia in comparison to zolpidem: A randomized controlled trial. *Indian J Pharmacol.* 2013 Jan-Feb;45(1):34–39.

34. Asher GN, Corbett AH, Hawke RL. Common herbal dietary supplement-drug interactions. *Am Fam Physician.* 2017 Jul 15;96(2):101–107.

35. Kelber O, Nieber K, Kraft K. Valerian: No evidence for clinically relevant interactions. *Evid Based Compl Alt Med.* 2014;2014:879396.

36. Schulz V, Hansel R, Blumenthal M. Tyler VE. *Rational phytotherapy: A reference guide for physicians and pharmacists.* Berlin: Springer-Verlag; 2004.

37. Scholey A, Benson S, Gibbs A, Perry N, Sarris J, Murray G. Exploring the effect of Lactium™ and zizyphus complex on sleep quality: A double-blind, randomized placebo-controlled trial. *Nutrients.* 2017 Feb 17;9(2):154.

38. Stargrove MB, Treasure J, McKee DL. *Herb, nutrient, and drug interactions.* St. Louis, MO: Mosby Elsevier; 2008.

39. Brinker F. *Herb contraindications and drug interactions plus herbal adjuncts with medicines*, 4th ed. Sandy, OR: Eclectic Medical Productions; 2010.

40. Generoso MB, Soares A, Taiar IT, et al. Lavender oil preparation (Silexan) for treating anxiety: An updated meta-analysis. *J Clin Psychopharmacol.* 2017;37(1):115–117.

41. Chien LW, Cheng SL, Liu CF. The effect of lavender aromatherapy on autonomic nervous system in midlife women with insomnia. *Evid Based Compl Alt Med.* 2012;2012:740813.

42. Lewith GT, Godfrey AD, Prescott P. A single-blinded, randomized pilot study evaluating the aroma of Lavandula augustifolia as a treatment for mild insomnia. *J Alt Compl Med.* 2005 Aug;11(4):631–637.

43. Lillehei AS, Halcón L, Gross CR, Savik K, Reis R. Well-being and self-assessment of change: Secondary analysis of an RCT that demonstrated benefit of inhaled lavender and sleep hygiene in college students with sleep problems. *Explore (NY).* 2016 Nov–Dec;12(6):427–435.

44. Blackburn L, Achor S, Allen B, et al. The effect of aromatherapy on insomnia and other common symptoms among patients with acute leukemia. *Oncol Nurs Forum.* 2017 Jul 1;44(4):E185–E193.

45. Fißler M, Quante A. A case series on the use of lavendula oil capsules in patients suffering from major depressive disorder and symptoms of psychomotor agitation, insomnia and anxiety. *Complement Ther Med.* 2014 Feb;22(1):63–69.

46. Kasper S, Anghelescu I, Dienel A. Efficacy of orally administered Silexan in patients with anxiety-related restlessness and disturbed sleep: A randomized, placebo-controlled trial. *Eur Neuropsychopharmacol.* 2015 Nov;25(11):1960–1967.

47. Kasper S, Moller HJ, Volz HP, Schläfke S, Dienel A. Silexan in generalized anxiety disorder: Investigation of the therapeutic dosage range in a pooled data set. *Int J Psychiatry Clin Pract.* 2017;32(4):195–204.

48. Gastpar M, Muller WE, Volz HP, et al. Silexan does not cause withdrawal symptoms even when abruptly discontinued. *Int J Psychiatry Clin Pract.* 2017;20:1–4.

49. Taavoni S, Nazem Ekbatani N, Haghani H. Valerian/lemon balm use for sleep disorders during menopause. *Complement Ther Clin Pract.* 2013 Nov;19(4):193–196.

50. Anheyer D, Lauche R, Schumann D, Dobos G, Cramer H. Herbal medicines in children with attention deficit hyperactivity disorder (ADHD): A systematic review. *Complement Ther Med.* 2017 Feb;30:14–23.

51. Zhou ES, Gardiner P, Bertisch SM. Integrative Medicine for Insomnia. *Med Clin North Am.* 2017 Sep;101(5):865–879. doi:10.1016/j.mcna.2017.04.005. Epub 2017 Jun 20. PMID: 28802468.

52. Keefe JR, Mao JJ, Soeller I, Li QS, Amsterdam JD. Short-term open-label chamomile (Matricaria chamomilla L.) therapy of moderate to severe generalized anxiety disorder. *Phytomedicine.* 2016 Dec 15;23(14):1699–1705.

53. Mao JJ, Xie SX, Keefe JR, Soeller I, Li QS, Amsterdam JD. Long-term chamomile (Matricaria chamomilla L.) treatment for generalized anxiety disorder: A randomized clinical trial. *Phytomedicine.* 2016 Dec 15;23(14):1735–1742.

54. Lakhan SE, Vieira KF. Nutritional and herbal supplements for anxiety and anxiety-related disorders: Systematic review. *Nutr J.* 2010 Oct 7;9:42.

55. Modabbernia A, Akhondzadeh S. Saffron, passionflower, valerian and sage for mental health. *Psychiatric Clin North Am.* 2013 Mar;36(1):85–91.

56. Ngan A, Conduit R. A double-blind, placebo-controlled investigation of the effects of Passiflora incarnata (passionflower) herbal tea on subjective sleep quality. *Phytother Res* 2011;25(8):1153–1159.

57. Ross SM. Psychophytomedicine: An overview of clinical efficacy and phytopharmacology for treatment of depression, anxiety and insomnia. *Holist Nurs Pract.* 2014 Jul-Aug;28(4):275–280.

58. Sarris J, Byrne GJ. A systematic review of insomnia and complementary medicine. *Sleep Med Rev.* 2011;15:99–106.

59. Lehrl S. Clinical efficacy of kava extract WS 1490 in sleep disturbances associated with anxiety disorders. Results of a multicenter, randomized, placebo-controlled, double-blind clinical trial. *J Affect Disord.* 2004 Feb;78(2):101–110.

60. Bressler R. Herb-drug interactions: Interactions between kava and prescription medications. *Geriatrics*. 2005 Sep;60(9):24–25.

61. Yang X, Salminen WF. Kava extract, an herbal alternative for anxiety relief, potentiates acetaminophen-induced cytotoxicity in rat hepatic cells. *Phytomedicine*. 2011 May 15;18(7):592–600.

62. Sarris J, Byrne GJ, Cribb L, et al. L-theanine in the adjunctive treatment of generalized anxiety disorder: A double-blind, randomised, placebo-controlled trial. *J Psychiatr Res*. 2019 Mar;110:31–37.

63. Türközü D, Şanlier N. L-theanine, unique amino acid of tea, and its metabolism, health effects, and safety. *Crit Rev Food Sci Nutr*. 2017 May 24;57(8):1681–1687.

64. Williams JL, Everett JM, D'Cunha NM, et al. The effects of green tea amino acid l-theanine consumption on the ability to manage stress and anxiety levels: A systematic review. *Plant Foods Hum Nutr*. 2020 Mar;75(1):12–23.

65. Lopes Sakamoto F, Metzker Pereira Ribeiro R, Amador Bueno A, Oliveira Santos H. Psychotropic effects of (L)-theanine and its clinical properties: From the management of anxiety and stress to a potential use in schizophrenia. *Pharmacol Res*. 2019 Sep;147:104395.

66. Hidese S, Ogawa S, Ota M, Ishida I, Yasukawa Z, Ozeki M, Kunugi H. Effects of l-theanine administration on stress-related symptoms and cognitive functions in healthy adults: A randomized controlled trial. *Nutrients*. 2019 Oct 3;11(10):2362.

67. Camfield DA, Stough C, Farrimond J, Scholey AB. Acute effects of tea constituents L-theanine, caffeine, and epigallocatechin gallate on cognitive function and mood: A systematic review and meta-analysis. *Nutr Rev*. 2014 Aug;72(8):507–522.

68. Lyon MR, Kapoor MP, Juneja LR. The effects of l-theanine (Suntheanine) on objective sleep quality in boys with attention deficit hyperactivity disorder (ADHD): A randomized, double-blind, placebo-controlled clinical trial. *Altern Med Rev*. 2011 Dec;16(4):348–354.

69. Ota M, Wakabayashi C, Sato N, et al. Effect of L-theanine on glutamatergic function in patients with schizophrenia. *Acta Neuropsychiatr*. 2015 Oct;27(5):291–296.

16

Sleep and Cannabis

PARAM DEDHIA AND ALISON KOLE

Introduction

Whether a provider agrees or disagrees with cannabis use, a growing number of patients are asking questions about it. Cannabis has moved from the margins to the mainstream. The science of cannabis has been outpaced by its marketplace. Cannabis usage has been on the rise in the United States, with more support as legalization grows. A 2018 Gallup poll showed that 66% of Americans favor legalization.[1] Legal cannabis sales have increased to $15 billion in 2019.[2] As of January 2020, 33 states and the District of Columbia have legalized cannabis for medical conditions despite the federal government classifying it as a drug with no acceptable medical use.[69] This highlights both the controversy and the curiosity regarding cannabis as a medicine.

The only thing growing faster than the cannabis industry is the confusion on its medical indications and usage. Cannabis is being marketed as a cure-all for a wide-ranging set of conditions—including sleep difficulties.

More frequently, the term *medicinal cannabis* is being used. This has led to the belief that people can speak to their healthcare provider about cannabis, yet most medical professionals do not feel equipped to talk about cannabis with their patients.[3] As a result, patients are consulting sources without medical training. Patients are seeking out medicinal cannabis for pain, anxiety, and sleep.

With regard to sleep issues, the research is growing yet notably limited. Health practitioners who have experience with cannabis suggest that cannabis works on the symptoms disrupting sleep as opposed to acting like a hypnotic that induces sleep. Much work is needed to truly know how cannabis may help sleep. This chapter will help the healthcare provider understand cannabis, its impact on sleep health, and its use as integrative therapy for sleep conditions.

NOMENCLATURE

The terms *cannabis, marijuana,* and *hemp* are often used interchangeably, but there is a distinction between them. *Cannabis* is the medical term,[4] and thus it is the one used in this chapter. The use of the word *marijuana* stems from a political history connected to the 1937 Marihuana Tax Act.[5] *Hemp* classifies strains of cannabis that contain 0.3% or less delta-9-tetrahydrocannabinol (THC). The primary focus has been on the two cannabinoids within cannabis: THC, which is popularly known for its euphoric effects, and cannabidiol, which is nonimpairing and is more easily referred to as CBD.

HISTORY OF CANNABIS AND THE RISING INTEREST IN CANNABIS AS A MEDICINE

The medical use of cannabis is not new. It was used in ancient Asia for a wide range of medical conditions. Throughout the nineteenth century, the concept of cannabis as a medicine steadily moved west. In the late 1800s and early 1900s, cannabis was seen as a medicine in the United States. Eli Lilly, Parke-Davis (now owned by Pfizer), and Squibb of Bristol-Myers Squibb all sold medical cannabis to treat migraines, rheumatism, and insomnia.[6]

Medicinal cannabis fell out of common use with the passing of the politically charged Marihuana Tax Act of 1937. Cannabis was officially outlawed in 1970 for any use with the passage of the Controlled Substances Act (CSA).[7]

California was the first state to go against the federal ban and legalize medical cannabis in 1996.[8] This sparked a trend across the United States, with many states approving cannabis for medicinal use. Interest in cannabinoids increased following a patent issued by the US government for CBD and "nonpsychoactive" cannabinoids that excluded THC. Another big shift in cannabis medicine followed the passage of the US Farm Bill in 2018, which legalized hemp cultivation.[9] Because hemp has a very limited amount of THC, it has robust levels of CBD. This allows for the wide availability of CBD products and explains why it is now seemingly available everywhere. Yet again, the marketplace has grown faster than the medical science of cannabis.

RESEARCH ON CANNABIS

Regrettably, there has been very little research on medicinal cannabis. In the United States, cannabis is federally illegal. Cannabis is listed as a Schedule 1 drug, meaning that it is deemed to have no medical benefit and a high risk for abuse.

As a result, clinical research has been limited. In the United States, cannabis for research purposes is available only through the National Institute of Drug Abuse[10] and is sourced solely from one cultivator since 1968. The cannabis from this farm has not been of comparable potency and genetics to what patients obtain at their dispensaries.[11-13] This makes both the validity and generalizability of previous research findings questionable.

Beyond federal research, pharmaceutical companies have studied extracts of cannabis isolates or have created synthetic cannabis medicines. These have been listed as Schedule 2 or 3 compounds and thus are acknowledged as having medical benefit. These federally legal medicines have paved a way for cannabis to be researched by focusing on standardized components within cannabis as opposed to the whole flower or full-extract cannabis oil.

The Chemistry of Cannabis: Strains and Chemovars

Cannabis is highly complex. To date, it has been found to have more than 500 distinct compounds, including more than 100 cannabinoids and more than 200 terpenes along with flavonoids and omega fatty acids. Cannabis has been discussed with different strains in mind. Traditionally, *Cannabis sativa* is known for its uplifting qualities and *Cannabis indica* is characterized by its soothing effects. However, in recent years, this has been a less helpful way to categorize cannabis due to breeding techniques leading to a shift in the plant's chemistry. As a result, there has been a move to speak to its chemical varieties, or *chemovars*.[14] Chemovars distinguish varieties and strains from one another based on their chemistry. This method allows for the scientific approach to how a certain variety may affect a given patient.

CANNABINOIDS

Cannabinoids are the abundant compounds within the cannabis plant. They are also found within the human body, where they have a wide range of activity. When found in plants, they are called *phyto*cannabinoids and when noted in the body they are referred to as *endo*cannabinoids. Manufactured versions from pharmaceutical companies are categorized as synthetic cannabinoids.

The two most studied cannabinoids are THC and CBD. This chapter focuses primarily on THC and CBD, but it is important to appreciate that other cannabinoids such as cannabinol (CBN), cannabichromene (CBC), and cannabigerolic acid (CBGA) have recently been isolated and may have a more direct role in sleep medicine in the future.

DELTA-9-TETRAHYDROCANNABINOL

THC is the most famous of the cannabinoids and is responsible for the "high" of cannabis. It affects perception, mood, emotion, memory, cognition, and motor function. When THC binds to receptors in the brain, it stimulates the increased release of dopamine, which activates the brain's reward system and contributes to cannabis's pleasurable effects. THC has many medicinal effects beyond euphoria. These include the relief of pain, inflammation, spasticity, nausea, anxiety, itching, and seizures. This highlights how cannabis may promote sleep by reducing pain, anxiety, or excessive mental activity.

CANNABIDIOL

CBD has become a focus of medical research with its recent federal legalization. Noted for its application as an antiepileptic for Dravet and Lennox-Gastaut syndromes,[15] CBD has also been found to have many other medicinal properties: neuroprotective, anxiolytic, antipsychotic, analgesic, anti-inflammatory, anti-asthmatic, and antitumor.[16–18] Although many of these effects may promote sleep, the focus has been on the potential to reduce anxiety and ease pain.

The safety of CBD as an extract from cannabis was stated in a 2018 World Health Organization (WHO) report. The WHO noted that CBD is safe, well-tolerated, and unlikely to cause physical dependence or abuse.[19] Even so, the most commonly reported side effects were fatigue, diarrhea, and changes of appetite/weight. Moreover, increased liver enzymes (AST, ALT, and bilirubin) have been noted when taken at high doses.[20]

TERPENOIDS

Beyond the cannabinoids, there is a focus on select terpenoids and their soporific potential to quickly penetrate the central nervous system and induce relaxation.[21] Terpenoids are volatile oils found in some flowering plants and are responsible for the aroma or odor of cannabis.[22] They also have medical properties and are generally recognized as safe by the US Food and Drug Administration (FDA).

THE ENTOURAGE EFFECT

Some cannabis experts do not recommend the use of isolated cannabis components. Instead they encourage the benefits from the "entourage effect" by using full-spectrum cannabis extract or flower. The "entourage effect" is a proposed mechanism by which combining cannabis compounds creates an effect and synergy that differs from any single compound on its own.[22] This is based on anecdotes about different strains of cannabis affecting people in different ways—one may improve sleep whereas another may reduce pain.

The entourage effect is highlighted by the impact that CBD has on THC when used together. Separately, THC can be impairing while CBD is non-impairing. But when used together, CBD blocks or reduces many of the undesirable effects of THC: intoxication, sedation, increased appetite, and rapid heart rate.[22] The balancing of CBD-to-THC ratios can allow for beneficial effects while reducing untoward ones.

It is suggested that other cannabinoids, terpenoids, and flavonoids may be a part of the "entourage effect" and can be used to fine-tune the recommendations of chemovars to fit individual needs. Again, additional study is needed to confirm this concept.

Cannabis Formulations Approved by the FDA

Current commercially available synthetic formulations of either THC or THC/ CBD include dronabinol, nabilone, and nabiximols. Dronabinol is a THC isomer, nabilone is a THC analog, and nabiximols contain THC and CBD in a 1:1 ratio. Both dronabinol and nabilone are FDA approved for refractory nausea and vomiting in cancer patients. Nabiximols is used in Europe for spasticity due to multiple sclerosis but not yet approved in the United States. None of these medicines has been approved for pain, anxiety, or sleep.

The Endocannabinoid System

The interest in cannabis as a medicinal increased with the discovery and emerging role of the endocannabinoid system (ECS). The human body creates a chemistry similar to plant cannabinoids and has its own vast and intricate cannabinoid system. The ECS is a complex signaling system involved in regulating the central nervous system at the synaptic level and adjusting a variety of functions in the peripheral body.[23] In summarizing the current understanding of the ECS, its main function is to maintain homeostasis in response to changes in the environment.[24]

The ECS is made up of three main components throughout the entire body: endocannabinoids, the enzymes that break them down, and the endocannabinoid receptors. The two main receptors are CB_1 and CB_2. A majority of the CB_1 cannabinoid receptors are expressed in the central nervous system and influence sleep, mood, cognition, and the reward center. CB_2 receptors are expressed in the peripheral nervous, immune, and gastrointestinal systems, and they have been an area of increasing interest in understanding inflammation.[25] It is thought that this action may provide an indirect pathway of reducing conditions that would otherwise disrupt sleep.

MECHANISMS OF ACTION OF CANNABINOIDS TO PROMOTE SEDATION AND POTENTIALLY SLEEP

The current thought is that cannabis promotes sleep by decreasing symptoms of the comorbid conditions known to challenge or fragment sleep. At this point, cannabis has not been found to act as a hypnotic at low or moderate doses. Research from animal models suggests that cannabis may mimic endogenous cannabinoids by increasing levels of adenosine,[26] which is sleep promoting.

The psychoactive component THC initially may have a stimulating effect followed by a sedating effect. Both of these effects may be attenuated in the presence of CBD.[27] By itself CBD is noted to be mildly potential-alerting in some people; but the majority of people find no interference in their sleep from CBD.

CANNABINOIDS AND CIRCADIAN RHYTHM

Cannabinoids have been found to have a direct impact on circadian rhythms. Circadian disruption is known to impact the sleep–wake cycle, motor disability, and the autonomic nervous system. Endocannabinoids connect the output of the central circadian pacemaker in the suprachiasmatic nucleus (SCN) with appetite, feeding, peripheral metabolism, anxiety, and depression. Healthy humans have endocannabinoid blood levels that follow a circadian rhythm and are three times higher on waking than just before sleep.[28] The intake of cannabis reduces the ability of the circadian clock to entrain to light and thereby creates a disorientation to time.[29] Cannabinoid receptor signaling has been pharmacologically manipulated to affect sleep–wake cycles, temperature regulation, food consumption, fat storage, central nervous system regulation of autonomic and endocrine functions, reward-driven behavior, gastrointestinal function, mood, and sensory perception.[30] Many of these effects can have a direct or indirect influence on sleep.

Polysomnographic Effects of Cannabis on Sleep

Current data regarding the effects of cannabis consumption on sleep architecture is limited as most studies were completed in the 1970s and the results were mixed.[31–35] The general consensus from these studies is that short-term use of cannabis causes an increase in slow wave sleep (SWS), a decrease in sleep onset latency (SOL), a decrease in wake after sleep onset (WASO), and a decrease in rapid eye movement (REM) sleep. However, with consistent cannabis use extending past a month, the research notes diminished quality of sleep. Chronic and heavy use of cannabis is associated with habituation to the sleep-inducing and SWS-enhancing properties, resulting in a reduction in SWS, inconsistent REM sleep patterns, and increased sleep fragmentation. Ultimately, chronic consumption poses the potential risk in some users of evolving into a self-perpetuating negative cycle of using cannabis for sleep, habituation, progressive increase in intake, and increased sleep disruption.[36,37]

What is missing from these studies is the opportunity to change the dosing of CBD and THC if a patient uses cannabis long term for sleep. With consistent cannabis use, new users of cannabis will likely experience a shift in their endocannabinoid system. Once the system and receptors are saturated, there may be a need for a reduction in dosing. This is counterintuitive to most providers—when a person experiences less of an effect of a substance, they assume a tolerance. As a result, they would increase the dose. In regard to cannabis, the helpful next step may be to reduce the dose.

It is important to note the impact of discontinuing cannabis use after habituation in some chronic and heavy users who may experience adverse withdrawal symptoms including strange dreams, insomnia, and poor sleep quality. It has been shown that this may occur in 36–76% of persons.[38] Bolla et al. demonstrated that abstinence for 14 days in chronic cannabis users led to reduced total sleep time, sleep efficiency, and total REM sleep, while WASO and periodic limb movements increased. SWS showed a small but not significant improvement over the same time frame.[39] Ultimately, the concern is that sleep fragmentation from abstinence may lead to relapse in those seeking abstinence. Chronic, heavy users may lessen or avoid the withdrawal symptoms by tapering their cannabis use over a period of 2–4 weeks.

Another concern is the potential for daytime impairment and excessive daytime sleepiness with cannabis use. In 2015, Dzodzomenyo and colleagues published a retrospective review of multiple sleep latency test (MSLT) results from 383 pediatric patients with a mean age of 13 (±3 years) who were evaluated for excessive daytime somnolence.[40] Patients who tested positive for THC on drug screening were found to have a higher likelihood of having two sleep onset REM periods, which is one of the MSLT criteria for narcolepsy. Forty-three percent of these patients would have been diagnosed inappropriately with narcolepsy. This highlights the need to assess for cannabis use in patients with excessive daytime sleepiness as cannabis use may cause untoward effects both at night and during the day.

Cannabis and Sleep Conditions

CANNABIS, SLEEP QUALITY, AND INSOMNIA

There is minimal data on the efficacy of cannabis for clinically diagnosed insomnia. However, self-reported insomnia in regular cannabis users was retrospectively analyzed using data from two cannabis clinics.[41] Among 166 subjects who initially reported "trouble sleeping," 79% noted that cannabis use improved sleep quality, with a statistically significant reduction in SOL. Significant limitations of these data include varying durations of use and variations in dose and times of use during the day, as well as differing routes of administration (mainly inhalation and oral consumption).

Addressing some of these limitations, Vigil et al., in 2018, used a mobile device powered with a data collection software application.[42] These investigators reviewed data from 409 people who smoked cannabis and had a reported diagnosis of insomnia. It is not clear if this was self-diagnosed or formally diagnosed by a medical professional. The participants recorded THC and CBD dose as well as route of administration. THC and CBD were reported as the amount of cannabinoids relative to the total dry weight of the cannabis flower smoked. The authors omitted observations from subjects involving THC potencies of greater than 35% or CBD potencies of greater than 30%, as these are not naturally occurring. The route of administration was all inhalational: vape (49%), pipe (38%), or joint (13%). There were 461 strains of cannabis used per subject reports. The most frequent strains consumed were THC-dominant with low CBD-to-THC ratios (4–7% CBD and 20% THC). General insomnia symptom improvement was noted overall and was associated with higher THC and lower CBD levels. Pipes and vaporizers were preferred, as they were associated with greater symptom relief and lower side effects compared with joints.

Insomnia is one of the most common sleep complaints in adults, and it is also a common reason that people seek out cannabis. While self-reported benefits for insomnia are noted, rigorous studies are lacking and are needed. Although users of cannabis tout the benefits for getting to sleep and staying asleep, research in the medical literature offers little guidance to the healthcare provider on cannabis use for insomnia.

OBSTRUCTIVE SLEEP APNEA AND DRONABINOL

Recent research has looked at cannabis for obstructive sleep apnea (OSA). The prevalence of OSA continues to increase, and although positive airway pressure therapy is often effective, compliance with its use is poor. As a result, there has been ongoing interest in finding additional therapeutic approaches. There have been no approved pharmaceutical approaches to improving OSA. However, early research suggests that cannabis may be helpful in some individuals.

Based on rat model data suggesting that cannabinoid agonists improve respiratory stability via a mechanism that involves peripheral serotonergic antagonism, Prasad et al. conducted a proof-of-concept trial in 17 patients using dronabinol (THC isomer) for the treatment of OSA.[43] Improvement in the apnea-hypopnea-index (AHI) was statistically significant, with a decrease of 14.1 ± 17.5 events/hour (p = 0.007), but results were highly variable, and three patients had no improvement or worsening of AHI. A larger follow-up study of dronabinol in 73 moderate to severe OSA patients showed similar results.[44] Dronabinol dose-dependently reduced AHI by 10.7 ± 4.4 (p = .02) and 12.9 ± 4.3 (p = .003) events/hour at doses of 2.5 and 10 mg/d, respectively. However, the treatment group did not demonstrate any improvements in sleep architecture, maintenance of wakefulness test sleep latencies, or overnight oxygenation parameters, and the placebo group had a worsening of OSA. These findings could not be readily explained.

A position statement from the American Academy of Sleep Medicine recommends that "medical cannabis and/or its synthetic extracts should not be used for the treatment of OSA due to unreliable delivery methods and insufficient evidence of effectiveness, tolerability, and safety. OSA should be excluded from the list of chronic medical conditions for state medical cannabis programs."[45] Therefore, although the use of dronabinol demonstrated statistical benefit in recent research, the subanalysis showed clinical meaningful improvement was only found in a small subset of responders (6 out of 39). Therefore, much more research needs to be performed before cannabis can be reliably recommended for OSA.

CANNABIS AND RESTLESS LEG SYNDROME

Cannabis has been used for restless legs syndrome (RLS) with anecdotal reports of benefit, but studies are very limited. The treatment of RLS can be challenging. Treatment failures are known to every sleep clinic. Moreover, worsening of RLS symptoms can occur despite previously effective treatment. In an intriguing paper, Megelin reported on six patients with RLS refractory to conventional treatment including dopamine agonists, opiates, or gabapentin. These patients endorsed subjective improvement and total remission of RLS symptoms following cannabis use.[46] Five patients smoked cannabis, and one patient used sublingual cannabis. Although these results are encouraging, the small sample size limits the ability to recommend cannabis for the treatment of RLS.

CBD AND REM BEHAVIOR DISORDER

Positive benefits from cannabis usage have been reported in a small number of patients with REM behavior disorder (RBD), which is a dream enactment disorder. First-line therapy includes the use of clonazepam or melatonin, but it should be emphasized that benzodiazepines have adverse side effects and may not be appropriate for some individuals.

Chagas et al. published a case series of four patients who had evidence of RBD.[47] All of them had a diagnosis of Parkinson's disease and manifested complex sleep behaviors at least twice per week. Three patients received a dose of 75 mg CBD, and one patient took 300 mg CBD. There were no matched placebo patients. All patients experienced an improvement in symptoms immediately and throughout the 6 weeks of treatment. These findings were explained by the role that cholinergic REM-active neurons play in REM sleep initiation and control over motor atonia. The proposed mechanism for the positive effect was that the activity at the CB_1 receptor stimulated cholinergic neurons to release acetylcholine, leading to improvement in symptoms.[48] Although the early results are encouraging, additional research on cannabis for RBD is needed as the small sample size limits the generalizability these findings.

POSTTRAUMATIC STRESS DISORDER AND NABILONE

Early studies of cannabis for posttraumatic stress disorder (PTSD) have shown benefit in reducing nightmares. Sleep symptoms are routinely found in patients with PTSD, and patients commonly report insomnia and nightmares. Standard treatments can yield mixed results, which is especially true for the nightmares related to PTSD. Hence, there is continued interest in seeking effective therapies. Fraser used nabilone (a THC analog) to treat 47 patients with self-reported, persistent nightmares despite conventional antidepressant and hypnotic therapies.[49] The average effective dose of nabilone was 0.5 mg one hour before bedtime, with dosages ranging from 0.2 mg to 4 mg. Thirty-four (72%) patients experienced total cessation or lessening of the severity of their nightmares, 28 patients had a total cessation of nightmares, and 6 had a satisfactory reduction. The discontinuation of medication was successful in four patients following 4–12 months of nabilone therapy. In these patients, nightmares did not return or returned at a reduced level which did not require further medication control. In other patients, there was a recurrence of nightmares within the first 2 nights after nabilone withdrawal. These patients experienced control of nightmares once nabilone treatment was restarted. In some cases, the benefits of treatment included a subjective improvement in sleep time and a reduction of daytime flashbacks. Thirteen (28%) patients experienced mild to moderate side effects including lightheadedness, forgetfulness, dizziness, and headache. These adverse effects occurred shortly following nabilone initiation and often led to discontinuation of nabilone therapy. Cameron et al. reported similar findings, including improved sleep duration, reduced nightmare frequency, and reduced PTSD symptoms when nabilone was used to manage PTSD in 104 correctional facility inmates with serious comorbid mental illness.[50]

Cannabis has garnered increased interest as a potential treatment for nightmares in PTSD patients. It is not yet recommended for routine use until the risks and benefits are better characterized through additional research.

CANNABIS USE IN CHRONIC PAIN

Pain is a common disruptor of sleep and a common reason for cannabis use. In a systematic review of 18 randomized controlled trials involving a total of 766 participants, researchers examined cannabinoids in the treatment of chronic noncancer pain.[51] These trials included various modalities of cannabis consumption with varying degrees of THC and CBD content. Fifteen of the eighteen trials demonstrated significant analgesic effect compared with placebo. Adverse effects of treatment were generally mild to moderate and well tolerated. These included sedation, dizziness, dry mouth, nausea, and difficulty with concentration.

In another review, the effects of cannabinoids on pain and sleep were studied in the context of medical treatment of neuropathic pain and symptoms of multiple sclerosis.[52] The research focused on oromucosal cannabis-based medicines containing primarily CBD, THC, or a 1:1 CBD-to-THC combination (Sativex). Experience with 1:1 CBD:THC on 2,000 subjects with 1,000 patient years of exposure demonstrated an improvement in subjective sleep parameters in a wide variety of pain conditions including multiple sclerosis, peripheral neuropathic pain, intractable cancer pain, and rheumatoid arthritis, with a minimal adverse event profile. There was neither tolerance to the benefit of 1:1 CBD:THC on pain or sleep, nor a need for dosage increases over a 4-year period. About 40–50% of subjects attained good or very good sleep quality.

These reviews support the possible benefits of cannabis for people who have disrupted sleep because of pain. As equal dosing of CBD and THC has been shown to be helpful for these patients, future research can build on this information to develop dosing recommendations.

Concerns about Cannabis and Inadequate Regulation

Despite the growth of medicinal cannabis research, studies are very limited. A primary set of challenges is the lack of standards in place for producing, labeling, or testing cannabis and CBD products. Penn Medicine researchers found that nearly 70% of CBD products purchased from the Internet contained either more or less CBD than the label indicated, which could negate any potential benefits.[53,54] Many products also contained significant amounts of THC. Contaminants such as residual solvents, pesticides, heavy metals, and mycotoxins are also a concern. Without reliable products and safety testing, the ability to study medical cannabis will continue to slow the discussion between healthcare providers and patients.

Risks of Cannabis

In 2017, an expert committee of the National Academies of Sciences, Engineering, and Medicine reviewed the available data on the therapeutic and side effects of cannabis and cannabinoids.[55] The committee provided recommendations based on evidence ranging from conclusive to insufficient evidence. There is moderate evidence to suggest that acute use of cannabis is associated with impairment in learning, memory, and attention, and this occurs within several hours after administration. With prolonged use, there is a risk of dependence and abuse which may result in cannabis use disorder. Also, frequent users were at an increased risk for the development of schizophrenia and other psychoses in those with a personal or family history of schizophrenia. Maternal cannabis smoking is substantially associated with decreased birth weight in infants. There is an increased risk of motor vehicle accidents if cannabis is used within a few hours prior to driving.

Tobacco use combined with chronic cannabis smoking increases the likelihood of symptoms of chronic bronchitis.[56] There are limited data for the risk of chronic obstructive pulmonary disease or emphysema in cannabis smokers. Interestingly, analysis of four longitudinal studies has not found substantial decline in forced expiratory volume (FEV_1) over time in cannabis smokers versus nonsmokers compared with tobacco smokers.[57-61] However, variations in the amount smoked and age of smokers limits the generalizability of these findings. There is moderate evidence for no association between cannabis and lung cancer, as well as head and neck cancers.[62] THC and other cannabinoids have demonstrated a tumor suppressive effect via decrease in inflammatory cytokines.[63]

Although cannabinoids have been shown to act as anti-inflammatory agents in a wide range of immune-mediated diseases, this may produce an exaggerated response in some individuals at higher doses and thus may result in an immunosuppressive effect that could impair the bactericidal and fungicidal activity of alveolar macrophages. A growing concern is that cannabis has also been shown to be frequently contaminated with mold, such as *Aspergillus fumigatus,* and/or with pathogenic gram-negative bacteria.[64] A potential increased risk of pneumonia with inhalational cannabis use has not been excluded.[65]

Dosing, Therapeutic Window, and Biphasic Response

In reviewing clinical use of cannabis for pain, anxiety, or sleep, people report therapeutic benefits at a wide range of doses. Different people will note medicinal benefits to a particular cannabis strain or product between a range from as low as 0.1 to 2.0 mg/kg/d (with the milligrams referencing the active constituents of THC or CBD). This is rather different from conventional medicines, which have recommend start dosages and established therapeutic dosing ranges.

It is classically observed that people who have not used cannabis are more likely to experience negative side effects than regular users. This may be due to the brain and tissues in the body experiencing tolerance to THC at different rates. The therapeutic effects of THC, such as pain control, are more resistant to tolerance-building than to the unwanted effects such as unsteadiness or loss of balance. The *therapeutic window* is a crucial topic in cannabis dosing. With initial use, this window is very narrow. The unwanted side effects are more likely to occur with increasing dosages when an individual starts using cannabis. The therapeutic window for THC can be widened by starting at a low dose then increasing the dose gradually to allow tolerance to unwanted side effects. For these reasons, it has been recommended to follow the adage of "start low and go slow."

The dose response to cannabis does not follow a traditional pattern. Most medicines have a monophasic response to use, with a direct relationship between dose and effect. Cannabis has a biphasic response. This means an increased dose of cannabis correlates with increased effects, but, after a certain threshold, increasing the dose may result in diminished effects. Then, after increasing to higher doses, therapeutic effects may begin to increase again.[66,67]

Administration Routes

After selecting a cannabis chemovar, it is then most important to consider the delivery method (Table 16.1). Depending on the desired onset of action and duration of activity, patients may be directed toward one route of administration over another. For example, a patient seeking assistance with sleep onset may choose the inhalational or oromucosal route for faster onset over ingestion. However, if a longer duration of activity is more important, then ingestion may be considered. Moreover, the advantages and disadvantages of each administration route can help guide and personalize the way the medicine is delivered.

CBD-to-THC Ratios

Dosing cannabis is different from dosing for pharmaceuticals. Since cannabis contains more than one active ingredient, the dosing requires attention to ratios of CBD to THC and the timing of administration. Most cannabis experts advocate for having at least some amount of CBD when recommending THC. As the CBD:THC ratio increases, the THC-related effects decrease. Many patients prefer higher CBD:THC ratios during the day when lower psychoactivity is desirable,

Table 16.1 Administration routes, onset of action, duration of activity, advantages and disadvantages of whole flower or full extract cannabis oil

Route	Onset	Duration	Advantages	Disadvantages
Inhalation Smoke, vaporize or vape *Smoking* burns plant material. *Vaporizing* heats the flower. *Vaping* heats a liquid extract of cannabis.	1–5 minutes	1–6 hours	Ideal delivery for nausea, vomiting, or conditions with swallowing difficulties Greater ability to assess response and adjust dosing due to rapid onset of action	Potential cardiopulmonary irritation and worsening of respiratory conditions such as asthma and COPD from smoking or vaping as compared to vaporizing Higher abuse potential due to fast onset and greater absorption leading to greater activation of reward centers in the brain.
Topical: Cannabis or oil-based extracts added to lotions, balms, or patches	Variable	Variable	Option for pain, spasms, inflammation, and itching No psychoactive effects; unless high potencies used over large surface areas	Limited ability to deliver to deeper levels within the body
Liquid extracts: Oromucosal	10–45 minutes	2–8 hours	Convenient, discreet (minimal odor), and easy to dose correctly	Alcohol tinctures may irritate the mouth Inappropriate for people with a history of alcohol abuse
Ingestion	30–120 minutes	4–10 hours	Longer duration of activity: after absorption; it is directlytransported to liver, which metabolizes THC to 11-OH THC which is a more stable form	Difficult to achieve the correct dosage due to variation in absorption and activity Product may not have a homogenous distribution of cannabinoids

but they prefer a lower CBD:THC ratio in the evening or on the weekends[68] to allow for greater relaxation and soothing effects while promoting the opportunity for sleep.

1:1 CBD:THC. The equal balance of CBD and THC has been primarily studied in patients with multiple sclerosis or chronic pain, with favorable effects. At this ratio, the medicinal THC effects are noted but the adverse effects are much less. However, doses above therapeutic levels cause impairment.

2:1 to 5:1 CBD:THC. This range produces a lower risk of psychoactivity. The effects of CBD will increase, such as increased alertness and clear thinking.

6:1 to 30:1 CBD:THC. The CBD effects predominate but are enhanced slightly by the low levels of THC. This range is especially ideal for patients who are known to be sensitive to THC.

Cannabis–Medication Interaction

As with any medication, it is important to understand drug–drug interactions. The medications known to have potential interactions with cannabis include warfarin, statins at higher doses, erythromycin, azole antifungals, and stimulants. Cannabinoids are cleared via the liver through various isoforms of the cytochrome P450 pathways.[69] Although most interactions only occur in patients using high doses of cannabis, practitioners of cannabis medicine highlight the need to personalize the prescription.

Conclusion and Next Steps

Cannabis as a medicine has a long history and a recent resurgence in interest. Although the science of cannabis has given us a deeper appreciation of its medicinal properties, the research has been limited. By combining available clinical studies wgrowing clinical experience, dosing and formulations are becoming better understood, but many conditions have not been well studied. In sleep medicine, only a few studies have been done. Many more are needed, but the cannabis marketplace has moved forward without clinical backing. At the same time, most healthcare providers do not feel comfortable speaking to their patients about cannabis.

Herein lies the opportunity—and the next step. Discussions about the science of cannabis will help inform medical professionals and identify the science that is needed. Currently, cannabis cannot be *prescribed* for a patient; it can be *recommended.* The mindset for recommending cannabis is different from that used for current pharmaceuticals. Cannabis recommendations needs to be individualized. Clinicians can highlight how cannabis works and the role of CBD, THC, and terpenes. Most importantly, they can emphasize the need to start low and go slow. Above and beyond this, patients can be encouraged to seek safer products and have ongoing discussions with their medical teams regarding their cannabis use. These steps will support the call to action for standardized testing and greater research. The public is asking to learn about cannabis. This creates a unique opportunity for the medical profession to join them.

REFERENCES

1. Gallup. www.news.gallup.com/poll/243908/two-three-americans-support-legalizing-marijuana.aspx
2. BusinessWire. www.businesswire.com/news/home/20200116005248/en/Global-Cannabis-Sales-Grow-48-15-Billion
3. Rubin R. Medical marijuana is legal in most states, but physicians have little evidence to guide them. *JAMA.* 2017;317(16):1611–1613.
4. Pollio A. The name of cannabis: A short guide for nonbotanists. *Cannabis Cannabinoid Res.* 2016;1(1):234–238.
5. Musto DF. The Marihuana Tax Act of 1937. *Arch Gen Psychiatry.* 1972;26(2):101–108.
6. Forbes. www.forbes.com/sites/debraborchardt/2015/04/08/pfizer-eli-lilly-were-the-original-medical-marijuana-sellers/#1091902d3026
7. US Drug Enforcement Agency. www.dea.gov/drug-scheduling
8. Bostwick JM. Blurred boundaries: The therapeutics and politics of medical marijuana. *Mayo Clin Proc.* 2012;87(2):172–186. doi:10.1016/j.mayocp.2011.10.003.
9. US House of Representatives. https://uscode.house.gov/statutes/pl/115/334.pdf
10. National Academies of Sciences, Engineering, and Medicine; Health and Medicine Division; Board on Population Health and Public Health Practice; Committee on the Health Effects of Marijuana: An Evidence Review and Research Agenda. *The health effects of cannabis and cannabinoids: The current state of evidence and recommendations for research.* Washington, DC: National Academies Press 2017 Jan 12. 15.
11. Taschwer M, Schmid MG. Determination of the relative percentage distribution of THCA and D(9)-THC in herbal cannabis seized in Austria: Impact of different storage temperatures on stability. *Foren Sci Int.* 2015;254:167–171.
12. Reardon S. Marijuana gears up for production high in US labs. *Nature.* 2015;519(7543):269–270.
13. Schwabe A, Hansen C, Hyslop R, McGlaughlin M. Research grade marijuana supplied by the National Institute on Drug Abuse is genetically divergent from commercially available cannabis. 2019. 10.1101/592725
14. Russo EB. The case for the entourage effect and conventional breeding of clinical cannabis: No strain, no gain. *Front Plant Sci.* 2019;9:1969.

15. US Food and Drug Administration. www.fda.gov/news-events/public-health-focus/fda-regulation-cannabis-and-cannabis-derived-products-including-cannabidiol-cbd

16. Fasinu PS, Phillips S, ElSohly M, et al. Current status and prospects for cannabidiol preparations as new therapeutic agents. *Pharmacotherapy,* 2016;36(7):781–796.

17. Iffland K, Grotenhermen F. An update on safety and side effects of cannabidiol: A review of clinical data and relevant animal studies. *Cannabis Cannabinoid Res.* 2017;2(1):139–154.

18. Devinsky O, Marsh E, Friedman D, et al. Cannabidiol in patients with treatment-resistant epilepsy: An open-label interventional trial. *Lancet Neurol.* 2016;15(3):270–278.

19. World Health Organization. www.who.int/medicines/access/controlled-substances/CannabidiolCriticalReview.pdf

20. Huestis MA. *Pharmacokinetics and metabolism of the plant cannabinoids, δ 9-tetrahydrocannibinol, cannabidiol and cannabinol. Cannabinoids.* Berlin: Springer Berlin Heidelberg; 2005: 657–669.

21. Minoli G, Marazzi-Uberti E, Casadio S. Terpene compounds as drugs. 14. Terpenyl carbamates as central nervous system depressants. *J Med Chem.* 1972;15(9):998.

22. Russo E, Guy GW. A tale of two cannabinoids: The therapeutic rationale for combining tetrahydrocannabinol and cannabidiol. *Med Hypoth.* 2006;66(2):234–246.

23. Skaper SD, Di Marzo V. Endocannabinoids in nervous system health and disease: The big picture in a nutshell. *Philos Trans R Soc Lond B Biol Sci.* 2012;367(1607):3193–3200.

24. De Laurentiis A, Araujo HA, Rettori V. Role of the endocannabinoid system in the neuroendocrine responses to inflammation. *Curr Pharm Des.* 2014;20(29):4697–4706.

25. Turcotte C, Blanchet MR, Laviolette M, Flamand N. The CB_2 receptor and its role as a regulator of inflammation. *Cell Mol Life Sci.* 2016;73(23):4449–4470. doi:10.1007/s00018-016-2300-4.

26. Murillo-Rodriguez E, Blanco-Centurion C, Sanchez C, Piomelli D, Shiromani PJ. Anandamide enhances extracellular levels of adenosine and induces sleep: An in vivo microdialysis study. *Sleep.* 2003;26(8):943–947. doi:10.1093/sleep/26.8.943.

27. Vaughn LK, Denning G, Stuhr KL, deWit H, Hill MN, Hillard CJ. Endocannabinoid signaling: Has it got rhythm? *Br J Pharmacol.* 2010;160(3):530–543.

28. Hanlon EC, Tasali E, Leproult R, et al. Circadian rhythm of circulating levels of the endocannabinoid 2-arachidonoylglycerol. *J Clin Endocrinol Metab.* 2015;100(1):220–226.

29. Acuna-Goycolea C, Obrietan K, van den Pol AN. Cannabinoids excite circadian clock neurons. *J Neurosci.* 2010;30(30):10061–10066.

30. Saito VM, Wotjak CT, Moreira FA. Pharmacological exploitation of the endocannabinoid system: New perspectives for the treatment of depression and anxiety disorders? *Braz J Psychiatry.* 2010;32(Suppl 1):S7–S14.

31. Cousens K, DiMascio A. Delta 9 THC as a hypnotic. An experimental study of three dose levels. *Psychopharmacologia.* 1973;33(4):355–364.

32. Pivik RT, Zarcone V, Dement WC, Hollister LE. Delta-9-tetrahydrocannabinol and synhex1: Effects on human sleep patterns. *Clin Pharmacol Ther.* 1972;13(3):426–435.

33. Feinberg I, Jones R, Walker JM, Cavness C, March J. Effects of high dosage delta-9-tetrahydrocannabinol on sleep patterns in man. *Clin Pharmacol Ther.* 1975;17(4):458–466.

34. Barratt ES, Beaver W, White R. The effect of marijuana on human sleep patterns. *Biol Psychiatry.* 1974;8(1):47–54.

35. Feinberg I, Jones R, Walker J, Cavnes C, Floyd T. Effects of marijuana extract and tetrahydrocannabinol on electroencephalographic sleep patterns. *Clin Pharmacol Ther.* 1976;19(6):782–794.

36. MD Edge. www.mdedge.com/chestphysician/article/167690/sleep-medicine/impact-marijuana-sleep-not-well-understood

37. Babson K, Sottile J, Morabito D. Cannabis, cannabinoids, and sleep: A review of the literature. *Curr Psychiatry Rep.* 2017;19:23.

38. Copersino ML, Boyd SJ, Tashkin DP, et al. Cannabis withdrawal among non-treatment-seeking adult cannabis users. *Am J Addict.* 2006;15(1):8–14.

39. Bolla K, Lesage SR, Gamaldo CE, et al. Polysomnogram changes in marijuana users reporting sleep disturbances during prior abstinence. *Sleep Med.* 2010;11(9):822–829.

40. Dzodzomenyo S, Stolfi A, Splaingard D, Earley E, Onadeko O, Splaingard M. Urine toxicology screen in multiple sleep latency test: The correlation of positive tetrahydrocannabinol, drug negative patients, and narcolepsy. *J Clin Sleep Med.* 2015;11(2):93–99.

41. Tringale R, Jensen C. Cannabis and insomnia. *Depression.* 2011;4(12):60–68.

42. Vigil J, Stith S, Diviant J, et al. Effectiveness of raw, natural medical cannabis flower for treating insomnia under naturalistic conditions. *Medicines.* 2018;5:75.

43. Prasad B, Radulovacki MG, Carley DW. Proof of concept trial of dronabinol in obstructive sleep apnea. *Front Psychiatry.* 2013;4:1.

44. Carley DW, Prasad B, Reid KJ, et al. Pharmacotherapy of apnea by cannabimimetic enhancement, the PACE Clinical Trial: Effects of dronabinol in obstructive sleep apnea. *Sleep.* 2018;41:1–13.

45. Ramar K, Rosen IM, Kirsch DB, et al.; American Academy of Sleep Medicine Board of Directors. Medical cannabis and the treatment of obstructive sleep apnea: An American Academy of Sleep Medicine position statement. *J Clin Sleep Med.* 2018;14(4):679–681.

46. Megelin T. Letter to the Editor: Cannabis for restless legs syndrome: A report of six patients. *Sleep Med.* 2017;36:182–183.

47. Chagas MH, Eckeli AL, Zuardi AW, et al. Cannabidiol can improve complex sleep-related behaviours associated with rapid eye movement sleep behavior disorder in Parkinson's disease patients: A case series. *J Clin Pharm Ther.* 2014;39:564–566.

48. Fraigne J, Torontali Z, Snow M. REM sleep at its core: Circuits, neurotransmitters, and pathophysiology. *Front Neurol.* 2015;6:123.

49. Fraser GA. The use of a synthetic cannabinoid in the management of treatment-resistant nightmares in posttraumatic stress disorder (PTSD). *CNS Neurosci Ther.* 2009 Winter;15(1):84–88.

50. Cameron C, Watson D, Robinson J. Use of a synthetic cannabinoid in a correctional population for post traumatic stress disorder-related insomnia and nightmares, chronic pain, harm reduction and other indications: A retrospective evaluation. *J Clin Psychopharmacol.* 2014;34:559–564.

51. Lynch ME, Ware MA. Cannabinoids for the treatment of chronic non-cancer pain: An updated systematic review of randomized controlled trials. *J Neuro Immune Pharmacol.* 2015;10(2):293–301.

52. Russo EB, Guy GW, Robson PJ. Cannabis, pain, and sleep: Lessons from therapeutic clinical trials of Sativex, a cannabis-based medicine. *Chem Biodivers.* 2007;4(8):1729–1743.

53. Penn Medicine. www.pennmedicine.org/news/news-releases/2017/november/penn-study-shows-nearly-70-percent-of-cannabidiol-extracts-sold-online-are-mislabeled

54. Bonn-Miller, MO, Loflin M, Thomas BF, Marcu JP, Hyke T, Vandrey R. Labeling accuracy of cannabidiol extracts sold online. *JAMA.* 2017;318(17):1708–1709.

55. Cousijn J, Núñez AE, Filbey FM. Time to acknowledge the mixed effects of cannabis on health: A summary and critical review of the NASEM 2017 report on the health effects of cannabis and cannabinoids. *Addiction.* 2018;113(5):958–966.

56. Tan WC, Lo C, Jong A, Xing L. Marijuana and chronic obstructive lung disease—a population based study. *CMAJ.* 2009;180(8):814–820.

57. Tashkin DP, Coulson AH, Clark VA, et al. Respiratory symptoms and lung function in habitual heavy smokers of marijuana alone, smokers of marijuana and tobacco, smokers of tobacco alone, and nonsmokers. *Am Rev Respir Dis.* 1987;135(1):209–216.

58. Aldington S, Williams M, Nowitz M, et al. Effects of cannabis on pulmonary structure, function, and symptoms. *Thorax.* 2007;62(12):1058–1063.

59. Taskin DP, Calvarese BM, Simmons MS, Shapiro B. Respiratory status of seventy-four habitual marijuana smokers. *Chest.* 1980;78(5):699–706.

60. Hancox RJ, Poulton R, Ely M, et al. Effects of cannabis on lung function a population-based cohort study. *Eur Respir J.* 2010;35(1):42–47.

61. Taskin DP, Simmons MS, Sherrill D, Coulson AH. Heavy habitual marijuana smoking does note cause an accelerated decline in FEV1 with age. *Am J Respir Crit Care Med.* 1997;155(1):141–148.

62. Hoffmann D, Brunnermann KD, Gori GB, Wynder EL. On the carcinogenicity of marijuana smoke. In Runeckles VC, ed. *Recent advances in Phytochemistry.* New York: Springer US; 1975: 63–81. https://doi.org/10.1007/978-1-4684-0823-2_3

63. Baldwin GC, Tashkin DP, Buckley DM, Park AN, Dubinett S, Roth MD. Marijuana and cocaine impair alveolar macrophage function and cytokine production. *Am J Respir Crit Care Med.* 1997;156(6):1606–1613.

64. Kagen SL, Kurup VP, Sohnle PC, Fink JN. Marijuana smoking and fungal sensitization. *J Allergy Clin Immunol.* 1983;71(4):389–393.

65. Ungerleider JT, Andrysiak T, Tashkin DP, Gale RP. Contamination of marijuana cigarettes with pathogenic bacteria: Possible source of infection in cancer patients. *Cancer Treat Rep.* 1982;66(3):589–591.
66. Carter GT, Weydt P, Kyashna-Tocha M, Abrams DI. Medicinal cannabis: Rational guidelines for dosing. *Idrugs.* 2004 May;7(5):464–470.
67. Sañudo-Peña MC, et al. Activational role of cannabinoids on movement. *Eur J Pharmacol.* 2000;391(3):269–274.
68. Johnson JR, Burnell-Nugent M, Lossignol D, et al. Multicenter, double-blind, randomized, placebo-controlled, parallel-group study of the efficacy, safety, and tolerability of THC: CBD extract and THC extract in patients with intractable cancer-related pain. *J Pain Sympt Mgmt.* 2010;39(2):167–179.
69. Stout SM, Cimino NM. Exogenous cannabinoids as substrates, inhibitors, and inducers of human drug metabolizing enzymes: A systematic review. *Drug Metabol Rev.* 2014;46(1):86–95.

17

Sleep: A Traditional Chinese Medicine Perspective

ALEX HOLLAND

Traditional Chinese Medicine (TCM) developed through centuries of empirical observation. The language that evolved to convey these observations can appear, to those of us in the West, to be metaphorical in nature and thus can lose credibility when viewed beside our Western medical paradigm. But the language of TCM is far from metaphorical: it is deeply rooted in a far-reaching understanding of a worldview that extends beyond the significance of scientific data. For example, the Eastern concepts of *Yin* and *Yang* explain the balancing forces that permeate every facet of universal experience. There are no words in the English language that describe these two opposing, yet complementary, forces, and so even though the Chinese language appears to be cloaked in mystery, it is not. Once such terms and their implications are understood, TCM is revealed to represent a complete, viable, and integrated medical system.

TCM views human physiology from the perspective of energy, or vital force. A brief definition of some of the basic medical terms in the Chinese medical language will help to clarify the mechanisms relating to sleep and its disturbance.

In TCM, health is defined as the balanced integration of physical, mental, emotional, and spiritual states. Health is determined by the harmonious balance between the qualities and quantities of *Yin* and *Yang* in each of these human realms. *Yin* can essentially be equated to our tissues, our blood, and the moisture in our bodies; however, it plays a much more extensive role in its participation in balancing our health. *Yin* is also cooling and downward moving as it balances—similar to the one pole of a teeter-totter—the dynamic opposite, upward moving *Yang* pole. *Yang* maintains the qualities of activity, function, warming, and ascending movement. Although the constructs of *Yin* and *Yang* are relatively simple, the balance of their influence is the basis for health.

The Chinese Medical classics speak of the Three Treasures that form the foundation for all human activity and experiences. The Three Treasures, *Jing*, *Qi*, and *Shen*, are elements that significantly contribute to the qualities and balance of both *Yin* and *Yang*.

Of the Three Treasures, *Qi* can be viewed as the most dynamic, energetic, and vital force that, in Chinese culture, is said to permeate all things. In the body, *Qi* is the basis for all physiological processes and activities and is *Yang* in nature. *Qi* is the motivating factor that propels the blood, catalyzes all chemical reactions and physiological processes, and undergirds all thought and emotional experiences. *Qi* is foundational in determining how we maneuver and interact with the world.

Jing, often translated as "Essence," represents qualities that an individual inherits at conception from his or her parents. In large part, *Jing* corresponds to our DNA and expresses our constitutional predispositions, such as intelligence, vitality, and potential. *Jing* is said to be stored in the Kidneys and is *Yin* in nature. *Jing* supports all the activities of *Qi* and is a form of *Qi* itself. *Jing* is our reservoir for the primal source of *Yin* and *Yang* in the body and supports *Yin* qualities and *Yang* activity for all our body/mind systems.

Shen is often translated as "Mind" or "Spirit." *Shen* is a very rarified form of *Qi* and is *Yang* in nature. *Shen* is said to reside in the Heart and is said to express our consciousness. In TCM, when the tranquility of *Shen* is disturbed, insomnia and restless sleep often result. For sound sleep, it is important for *Shen* to be properly supported and nourished.

Jing, *Qi*, and *Shen* all work together to coordinate the basic physiological processes involved in all body/mind functions. In addition to the Three Treasures, another two essential substances are Blood and Body Fluids. These are both *Yin* qualities and are necessary for balancing all *Yang* activities. It would be analogous to needing lubrication in order for an engine to operate optimally. The activity and work of the engine expresses the *Yang*, and the lubrication is the *Yin*. Together they optimize the function of the engine.

A foundational objective of TCM is the maintenance of balance between the *Yin* and *Yang* of the body. As we have seen, *Yang* tends to rise and, in this process, can "pull up" the *Yin*. In opposition, *Yin* tends to sink and essentially pulls down or anchors the *Yang*. The give and take of these two contrasting forces together create the requirements for equilibrium in the body. If there is too much *Yang* and too little *Yin*, disharmonies will result. Conversely, if there is too much *Yin* and too little *Yang*, disharmonies will result. These disparities are common mechanisms that result in the variety of pathological sleep patterns.

Insomnia and hypersomnia are the result of the interplay of *Yin* and *Yang* between a number of organ systems, primarily the Heart, Liver, Spleen, and Kidneys. Working together, these systems are responsible for ensuring that the *Shen*, *Yin* and *Yang*, *Qi*, and Blood are appropriately maintained. When harmonized, the individual presents with a clear mind, emotional equanimity, and sound sleep.

Traditional Chinese Medicine Patterns

A *Pattern* is a configuration of signs and symptoms of an imbalance that leads to a specific diagnosis and resulting course of treatment. TCM diagnosis relies on the four traditional diagnostic methods: observation, listening/smelling, inquiring, and palpation. Pattern differentiation is based on the quantity and quality of the different components of the condition in relation to *Yin* and *Yang*, *Qi*, Blood, *Jing*, Body Fluids, and Essence. Pattern identification demonstrates the nature and location of the condition, prognosis, and treatment strategy, and indicates options for treatment.

TCM's view of the organ systems varies greatly from the Western perspective. Each organ system not only has a physiological function, but each also incorporates an emotional and a psycho-spiritual component. In the study of sleep disorders, there are essentially two organ systems that play a primary role in the quality of sleep: the *Heart* and the *Liver*. Other organ systems play a supporting role, but it is the Heart and Liver that greatly contribute to sleep disturbances.

In the body, *Liver Qi* tends to rise and is *Yang* in nature. If this *Yang* activity is not countered with appropriate *Yin* to stabilize it, resulting disorders develop: high blood pressure, headaches, dizziness, glaucoma, stroke, and emotional conditions such as anger, depression, and irritability. These conditions are located in the upper portions of the body, depicting the rising *Yang* nature of *Liver Qi*.

The Liver's psycho-spiritual component, called *Hun*, plays a prominent role in sleep. If the *Hun*, which is *Yang* in nature and tends to expand, is not rooted by enough of the *Yin* qualities such as Body Fluids or Blood, it will disturb the equanimity of the *Shen*. In this case, it is said that the *Hun* becomes untethered and wanders at night. This often results in symptoms of restless sleep with vivid dreams, a major contributing factor to insomnia.

Another organ system that is intimately linked with sleep is the *Heart*, where the *Shen* resides. When the *Shen* is fully supported and peaceful, individuals experience sound sleep. As with the *Hun*, the *Shen* needs to be properly anchored at night so that it does not become destabilized and wander.

The substances that support and anchor both the *Shen* and the *Hun* are Blood and Body Fluids, which contribute to the quality and quantity of *Yin* that reside in the Heart. Understanding the interconnectedness between Blood, Body Fluids, and *Yin* with *Shen* and *Hun* is crucial to understanding TCM differential diagnosis in the treatment of sleep disorders.

Insomnia specifically can also result from agitation or overstimulation from too much internal heat that will disturb the *Shen*. Additionally, stagnation, which is an excess accumulation of *Qi* and/or Blood, can agitate the *Shen*. All these factors are taken into consideration when determining the correct Pattern identification to appropriately treat insomnia.

When assessing a patient who presents specifically with insomnia, it is important to rule out transitory insomnia from true insomnia. Transitory insomnia may be due to numerous factors, including

- External noise
- Pain, breathing disorders, itching, and asthma
- Consumption of stimulants
- Eating late
- Emotional upset
- Disordered biorhythms of shift-workers
- Vigorous exercise before bedtime
- Sudden weather changes

Once any of these factors is eliminated, sleep will usually return to normal.

Acupuncture

Along with Chinese herbal medicine, acupuncture is one of the most commonly used TCM treatments for insomnia and hypersomnia. TCM adheres to the concept of a meridian system through which there is a distribution network for *Qi*. This distribution network is much like a giant web, linking different areas of the body together. This web of intricate and complex pathways makes up a comprehensive body map that supplies *Qi* to every part of the body. Within this web there are 12 primary meridian pathways upon which most of the acupuncture points are located. Through appropriate stimulation of the needles inserted at specific points along a meridian, the flow of *Qi* can either be increased or decreased. Because the meridians are connected to specific organ systems, acupuncture stimulation can have a direct effect on the function of specific organs or areas of the body and thus helps to reestablish the body's balance of *Yin* and *Yang*.

TCM Patterns for Insomnia

The etiological factors that cause insomnia are many and varied, as are the Patterns that depict the condition. The following sections describe the most common Patterns seen in clinical practice, along with their general signs and symptoms and sample herbal formulas.

LIVER QI STAGNATION, STAGNANT HEAT, LIVER FIRE

These three Patterns are a continuum that depicts a growing severity of insomnia. Typically, Liver Qi Stagnation occurs first, followed by the development of heat, and finally Liver Fire. These are all depicted by Figure 8 from Figure 17.1, where *Yin* is relatively normal but *Yang* increases with the severity of the condition.

Primary Clinical Features of Liver Qi Stagnation: Difficulty falling asleep, dream disturbed sleep, depression, moodiness, shoulder and neck tension, teeth grinding, temporal headache, hypochondriac discomfort, frequent sighing, dizziness, poor appetite, irregular menstruation, PMS, alternating diarrhea and constipation.

Treatment Principle: Course Liver, Regulate *Qi*, Nourish *Yin*, Eliminate Fire

Sample Herbal Prescriptions:
- *Xiao Yao San* is used when there is *Qi* stagnation without Heat.
- *Dan Zhi Xiao Yao San* is used when there is *Qi* stagnation with some Heat.
- *Long Dan Xie Gan Tang* is used when there is Liver Fire (extreme Heat).

HEART HEAT/FIRE

Heart Heat can result from a Deficiency of Yin (Figure 5) or an excess of Yang (Figure 7 or Figure 8).

Primary Clinical Features of Heart Heat/Fire: Frequent waking with nightmares, anxiety, restlessness, agitation, palpitations, thirst for cold water, mouth and tongue ulcers, concentrated urine, painful urination.

Treatment Principle: Clear Heart Heat/Fire, Calm the *Shen*

Sample Herbal Prescriptions:
- *Dao Chi San* is used when there is slight *Yin* Deficiency.
- *Huang Lian E Jiao Tang* is used when there is Heart Yin Deficiency following a fever condition.

STOMACH DYSFUNCTION

This Pattern describes food stagnation that results in insomnia due to obstruction of the stomach's natural function of descending *Qi* or resulting from stomach stagnation which generates Heat that rises to disturb the *Shen* (Figure 8).

Box 17.1 Diagnosis in Traditional Chinese Medicine

In Chinese diagnostics, imbalances are usually expressed in terms of *Excess* and *Deficiency*, two expressions that define the quantity and quality of the *Yin* and *Yang* in the body. Excess means pathological accumulation. Deficiency means a lack of a particular vital substance. Examples of pathologies include

Yin Excess

Presentation	System affected and result
• Obesity Body Fluids –	accumulation
• Phlegm Body Fluids –	increased viscosity of mucous
• Bruising Blood Stasis –	accumulation – clotting
• Thrombosis Blood Stasis –	accumulation – clotting

Yang Excess

Presentation	System affected and result
• Hyperactivity *Qi* –	too much energy available
• High Blood Pressure *Qi* –	too much energy rising
• Mania *Shen* –	too much energy infusing the mind/spirit
• Insomnia *Shen* –	too much energy infusing the mind/spirit

Yin Deficiency

Presentation	System affected and result
• Dryness Generalized *Yin* –	lack of moisture to lubricate
• Low Grade Fever Generalized *Yin* –	lack of moisture not cooling
• Insomnia Shen –	lack of *Yin* or Blood not anchoring *Shen*
• Busy Mind Shen –	lack of *Yin* or Blood not anchoring *Shen*

Yang Deficiency

Presentation	System affected and result
• Feeling Cold Generalized *Yang* –	"Fire" of *Yang* diminished
• Lack of Energy Generalized *Yang* –	lacking *Qi* for daily activity
• Physical Weakness Generalized *Yang* –	lacking *Qi* for daily activity

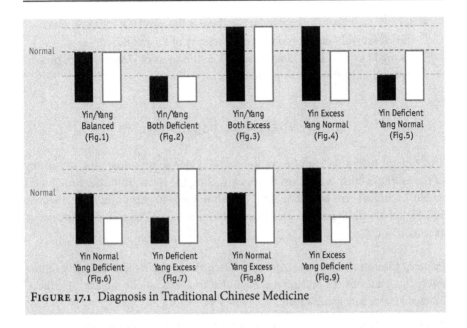

FIGURE 17.1 Diagnosis in Traditional Chinese Medicine

Primary Clinical Features of Stomach Dysfunction: Fullness and discomfort in the epigastric region, belching, acid reflux, abdominal distension and pain, gnawing hunger pains, bad breath, loose and foul-smelling stools or constipation.

Treatment Principle: Relieve Food Stagnation, Harmonize the Stomach, Calm the *Shen*

Sample Herbal Prescription:
- *Bao He Wan* is used to assist digestion and relieve bloating and gas.

PHLEGM HEAT HARASSING THE MIND

This Pattern results from the accumulation of Phlegm and resulting Heat in the Stomach that rises to unsettle the Mind, or *Shen*. Figure 8 represents this pathological presentation.

Primary Clinical Features of Phlegm Heat: Restless sleep, a sensation of heaviness, dizziness, nausea, a sensation of oppression in the chest, no appetite, palpitations, mental restlessness.

Treatment Principle: Clear Heat, Resolve Phlegm, Calm the *Shen*

Sample Herbal Prescription:

- *Shi Wei Wen Dan Tang* is used when there is Phlegm Heat in the Stomach and Heart with an accompanying Deficiency of *Qi* and Blood.
- *Huang Lian Wen Dan Tang* is used when the signs of Heat are more present and Phlegm is not so primary.

HEART AND SPLEEN BLOOD DEFICIENCY

This type of insomnia is more common and is due to an underlying deficiency of the Spleen, which is responsible for extracting the nutrient to make the Blood whole. In this case the lack of quality Blood is not able to anchor the *Shen*. Figure 5 and Figure 7 both depict the Deficiency of *Yin*, whereas Figure 8 depicts relative excess of *Yang*.

Primary Clinical Features of Heart and Spleen Blood Deficiency: Difficulty falling asleep, palpitations, poor appetite, inability to focus, slight anxiety, dizziness, blurred vision, pale complexion.

Treatment Principle: Tonify Spleen, Nourish Heart Blood, Calm the *Shen*

Sample Herbal Prescription:
- *Gui Pi Tang* is used to strengthen the Spleen's function of helping to create Heart Blood.

HEART AND KIDNEY *YIN* DEFICIENCY

At night, the *Yin* aspect of the body becomes more prominent and helps to anchor the *Shen*. When there is a Deficiency of *Yin* in both the Heart and Kidneys, the *Shen* is no longer able to be secured, giving rise to restlessness and frequent waking. Figure 5 and Figure 7 both depict the Deficiency of *Yin*, whereas Figure 8 depicts relative excess of *Yang*.

Primary Clinical Features of Heart and Kidney Yin Deficiency: Frequent waking, feeling warm with possible night sweats, agitation, palpitations, dry mouth and throat, dizziness, tinnitus, forgetfulness, lower back and knee aches.

Treatment Principle: Nourish Heart and Kidney *Yin*, Calm the *Shen*

Sample Herbal Prescription:
- *Tian Wang Bu Xin Dan* is used to nourish Heart and Kidney *Yin*.
- *Gui Zhi Jia Long Gu Mi Tang* is used following a significant shock that causes *Yin* deficiencies to occur in these two organ systems. This formula is used when "severed communication" between the Heart and Kidney energies results in insomnia with major emotional symptoms.

HEART AND GALL BLADDER *QI* DEFICIENCY

This Pattern is more of a constitutional condition, or it may result from a prolonged illness in which the *Shen* is unstable due to disruption by shock or fright. This Pattern is most appropriately represented by Figure 6.

Primary Clinical Features of Heart and Gall Bladder Qi Deficiency: Waking up early in the morning and being unable to fall back asleep, dreaming a lot, easily startled, timidity, lack of assertiveness, palpitations, tiredness, shortness of breath, depression.

Treatment Principle: Tonify Heart and Gall Bladder Qi, Calm the *Shen*

Sample Herbal Prescription:
- *An Shen Ding Zhi Wan* is used to tonify Heart Qi and also calm the spirit as well as open the senses.

LIVER *YIN* (BLOOD) DEFICIENCY

The *Hun* of the Liver is not anchored properly due to a deficiency of Liver Blood or *Yin* with the resulting functional aspect of Liver *Qi* agitating the *Shen*, resulting in difficulty sleeping. This Patten is most appropriately represented by Figure 5, Figure 7, or Figure 8, depending on the relative values of the balance of *Yin* and *Yang* in the body.

Primary Clinical Features of Liver Yin Deficiency: Frequent dreaming, talking in one's sleep, irritability, forgetfulness; in severe cases there will be sleep walking, dry throat or thirst, dry eyes, dizziness, palpitations, blurred vision.

Treatment Principle: Nourish Liver *Yin* (Blood), Root the *Hun*, calm the *Shen*

Sample Herbal Prescription:
- *Suan Zao Ren Tang* is used to nourish the *Yin* and is very effective for this type of insomnia.
- *Yin Mei Tang* is used specifically to nourish Liver *Yin* and root the *Hun* and is used when there are many unpleasant dreams.

TCM Patterns for Hypersomnia

TCM uses the same energetic and diagnostic principles to determine Patterns relating to hypersomnia that it does to diagnose insomnia. Hypersomnia is seen as a disorder in which there is not enough *Qi* to maintain wakefulness. *Qi* is either insufficient, or it is blocked and not able to rise to the head, which is the seat of alertness.

There are three primary Patterns that depict this condition. These Patterns are presented here along with their general signs and symptoms and sample herbal formulas.

SPLEEN *QI* DEFICIENCY

The Spleen orchestrates the absorption of nutrients, and when the Spleen becomes deficient, it can no longer extract the necessary nutrient *Qi* to maintain alertness. This is presented in Figure 6.

Primary Clinical Features of Spleen Qi Deficiency: Daytime drowsiness made worse with exertion, weakness of the limbs, sallow complexion, poor appetite, loose stools, abdominal distension.

Treatment Principle: Strengthen the Spleen and Tonify Qi

Sample Herbal Prescription:
- *Xiang Sha Liu Jun Zi Tang* is used to strengthen the Spleen and increase levels of *Qi*.

PHLEGM STAGNATION

This Pattern is seen most often in individuals who tend to be overweight and are subject to Phlegm accumulation. This Pattern tends to be more chronic and stubborn to treat. The Phlegm obstructs the *Yang* from rising to the head, causing sleepiness. This Pattern is best depicted with Figure 4 or Figure 9.

Primary Clinical Features of Phlegm Stagnation: Chronic sleepiness, tendency to obesity, poor concentration, heavy and tired limbs, a full feeling in the chest or epigastrium.

Treatment Principle: Transform Phlegm, Open Meridians to the Head

Sample Herbal Prescription:
- *Di Tan Tang* is used to help rid the body of excessive Phlegm Dampness and move *Qi* to the head.

KIDNEY *YANG* DEFICIENCY

This Pattern results from a decline of Kidney *Jing* and usually occurs in older individuals. The decline of *Jing* is synonymous with the decline of *Yang* (Figure 2, Figure 6, or Figure 9).

Primary Clinical Features of Kidney Yang Deficiency: Lethargy, apathy, lack of will-power, depression, chilliness, low back soreness and knee pain.

Treatment Principle: Tonify Kidney *Yang*, Stimulate the Rising of Q*i*

Sample Herbal Prescription:
- *Shi Bu Wan* is used to fortify the Kidney *Yang*, which will assist in raising Q*i* to the head.

TCM may be new to the West, but this in no way diminishes its time-tested mechanisms for the treatment of disease, including its proven efficacy in the treatment of insomnia and related sleep disorders.

Evidence for the Use of TCM

Conducting randomized controlled clinical trials using TCM is challenging given that the treatments are often individualized for each patient. As a result, there are limited data in the literature about the use of herbs or acupuncture for insomnia and even less for hypersomnia. However, the studies that have been performed overall suggest that both herbs and acupuncture can be effective for insomnia. In the United States, acupuncture is more often used than Chinese herbal medicine and has been shown to be effective in a systematic review of randomized control trials.[1-3] In a meta-analysis of 878 papers, the use of auricular acupuncture (AA) was shown to provide a statistical improvement in sleep.[4] A review including Chinese and English literature of randomized controlled studies indicate some effectiveness for treatment of insomnia.[3] Specific Chinese herbal formulas have also been shown to be an effective treatment for insomnia.[5,6]

These clinical findings support the proposition that acupuncture and Chinese herbal medicine can have a significant effect on the quality and duration of sleep. However, very little research has been conducted on the effects of acupuncture and Chinese herbal medicines in relation to the condition of hypersomnia, and more study is needed.

Conclusion

TCM may be relatively new to the West, but this in no way diminishes its time-tested mechanisms for the treatment of disease, including its proven efficacy in the treatment of insomnia and related sleep disorders.

REFERENCES

1. Huijuan Cao, Xingfang Pan, Hua Li, Jianping Liu. Acupuncture for treatment of insomnia: A systematic review of randomized controlled trials. *J Alt Compl Med.* 2009 Nov;15(11):1171–1186.
2. Kalavapalli R, Singareddy R. Role of acupuncture in the treatment of insomnia: A comprehensive review. *Compl Ther Clin Pract.* 2007 Aug;13(3):184–193.
3. Spence DW, Kayumov L, Chen A, Lowe A, Jain U, Katzman MA, Shen J, Perelman B, Shapiro CM. Acupuncture increases nocturnal melatonin secretion and reduces insomnia and anxiety: A preliminary report. *J Neuropsychiatry Clin Neurosci.* 2004 Winter;16(1):19–28. doi:10.1176/jnp.16.1.19. PMID: 14990755.
4. Hai Yong Chen, Yan Shi, Chi Sun Ng, Sai Man Chan, Ken Kin Lam Yung, Qing Ling Zhang. Auricular acupuncture treatment for insomnia: A systematic review. *J Alt Compl Med.* 2007 Aug;13(6):669–676.
5. Bo Yang, Aihua Zhang, Hui Sun, Wei Dong, Guangli, Yan Tingli, Xijun Wang. Metabolomic study of insomnia and intervention effects of suanzaoren decoction using ultra-performance liquid-chromatography/electrospray-ionization synapt high-definition mass spectrometry. *J Pharmaceut Biomed Analy.* 2012 Jan;58(25):13–124.
6. Yeung WF, Chung KF, Poon MM, et al. Chinese herbal medicine for insomnia: A systematic review of randomized controlled trials. *Sleep Med Rev.* 2012 Dec;16(6):497–507.

SUGGESTED READING

Holland A. *Voices of Qi: An introductory guide to Traditional Chinese Medicine.* Berkeley, CA: North Atlantic Books; 2000.

Kaptchuk TJ. *The web that has no weaver: Understanding Chinese medicine.* New York: Congdon & Weed; 1983.

Maciocia G. *The practice of Chinese medicine: The treatment of diseases with acupuncture and Chinese herbs.* New York: Churchill Livingstone; 1994.

Maclean W, Lyttleton J. *Clinical handbook of internal medicine: The treatment of disease with Traditional Chinese Medicine. Vol. 1: Lung, Kidney, Liver, Heart.* Sydney: University of Western Sydney; 1998.

18

Ayurveda and Sleep

VALENCIA PORTER

General Ayurvedic Principles

Ayurveda, in Sanskrit, means "the science of life," and it is a traditional medical system from India that developed more than 5,000 years ago. Ayurveda regards health as a balance of body, mind, and spirit. This balance can be achieved through a healthy lifestyle in accordance with nature and one's own mind–body constitution and includes the preventive practices of proper nutrition and exercise, nourishing relationships, good emotional health, and a regular daily routine.

According to Ayurveda, sleep is one of the primary pillars of health, with up to one-third or more of our lifetime spent in the sleep state.[1] The Ayurvedic saying that "sleep is the nurse of every living being" reflects its role in allowing the body and the mind to repair and rejuvenate.[2] During sleep the body achieves deep rest, metabolism slows, and the mind shifts its attention from the outside world to inner consciousness. One of the classical texts of Ayurveda, Vagbhata's *Ashtanga Hridayam*, states that lack of sleep is one of the causes of disease.[3] In addition, imbalanced sleep habits such as excessive sleep, untimely sleep, sleeping during the daytime (except during the hot summer), sleeping at sunrise or sunset, sleeping right after eating, and not sleeping the correct amount can reduce the life span and produce unhappiness.[4] Problems with sleep can manifest in different ways: difficulty falling asleep, waking in the middle of the night, difficulty falling back to sleep if awakened, and arising too early without being able to fall back asleep. While medications can help achieve the sleep state, this approach does not address underlying imbalances in the body which may have contributed to the sleep problem. Instead, Ayurveda takes a holistic approach aimed at producing physical and mental relaxation by bringing the mind and body back into harmony with nature and with one's own individual constitutional makeup.

Mind–Body Constitution

The Ayurvedic understanding of the body relates to the balance of five natural elements: space, air, fire, water, and earth. Three major constitutional types, called *doshas*, are described with physical, mental, and behavioral tendencies (*prakruti*) corresponding to the unique balance of the basic elements as described in Table 18.1.[4,5] This concept of unique psychophysiological body types is one of the most important ideas in Ayurveda, and recent gene studies have correlated genetic variances with these Ayurvedic phenotypes, which are known as *prakruti*.[6–8] *Vata*

Table 18.1 *Dosha* characteristics

Dosha	Vata	Pitta	Kapha
Principle	Movement/Change	Metabolism/ Transformation	Structure/Storage
Characteristics (Prakruti)	Light, thin build, variable appetite and digestion. Lively, spontaneous, unpredictable, communicative, creative, active mind	Medium, athletic build, strong appetite, excellent digestion. Goal-oriented, passionate, competitive, natural leaders	Solid, larger frame, good appetite, slower digestion. Even-keeled, methodical, reliable, slow to move, good stamina
Sleep-type	Light and interrupted; irregular sleep patterns	Sound, may need less than 8 hours; may awaken feeling overheated	Heavy, prolonged, may oversleep; wakes up slowly
Signs of imbalance (Vikruti)	Excessive movement, dryness, air • Nervous system disorders • Irritable bowel/ constipation • Anxiety • Insomnia • Chronic pain	Excessive physical or mental heat • Heartburn • Rashes • Hypertension • Inflammation • Anger • Irritability	Stagnation and accumulation • Weight gain • Fluid accumulation • Cysts and tumors • Congestion • Sluggishness • Withdrawal

controls movement including digestion, communication in the nervous system, breathing, and thoughts. *Pitta* oversees metabolism and digestion. *Kapha* controls structure and storage. These three basic principles of movement, metabolism, and structure are reflected throughout the body. A person may be dominant in one or two *doshas*, or they may be relatively equal among the three *doshas* (*tridoshic*). By knowing one's specific body type, diet, exercise, and daily routine can be optimized for a person's individual needs. Certain *dosha* types may be more prone to certain types of disorders.

With relation to sleep, *Vata* types tend to be more hyperaroused and are more prone to insomnia, restlessness, and anxiety. They may have difficulty falling asleep as well as having frequent waking during the night, and they sleep on average from 4 to 7 hours per night. Sleep talking, sleepwalking, and bruxism may occur more often in those with *vata dosha*. They may report a lot of dream activity but can have difficulty remembering them. By contrast, *pitta* types average 4–7 hours per night of sound sleep. Their dreams may be intense. They tend to have sleep disturbances affected by heat, including overeating of hot or stimulating foods, night sweats, and heated emotions such as anger, jealousy, and resentment. This may follow an argument or stressful situation or be part of a febrile illness. *Kapha* types tend to be heavy sleepers, requiring 8 or more hours of sleep. They may have difficulty waking up and can be slow to get moving in the morning. Their dreams tend to be calm and smooth. They can have issues with excessive sleep and daytime sleepiness. Insomnia may occur with congestion, and the root cause should be addressed.

Lifestyle and environment can cause imbalances in the *doshas* (*vikruti*) resulting in physical symptoms and disease. *Vata* tends to go out of balance more easily than *pitta* or *kapha* and is responsible for the early stages of many diseases. While sleep disturbances can have their root cause as an imbalance of one or more of the three *doshas*, because of the connection between sleep rhythms and unbalanced *vata dosha*, all doshic types must pay attention to *vata* balance when dealing with sleep issues. A 2015 cross-sectional study of 995 participants in a week-long yoga residential camp found that higher scores for *vata dosha* significantly predicted longer time to fall asleep and feeling less rested in the morning.[9] Causes of insomnia include stress, anxiety, excessive thinking, taking of drugs or stimulants, too much travel, overwork, and other *vata*-increasing factors. In general, treatments are designed to restore balance, but if imbalance is long-standing and toxicity accumulates, Ayurvedic cleansing therapies may be needed first, to reduce blockages that are preventing the body from returning to homeostasis. According to Ayurveda, treatment of the condition is of equal importance as eliminating the cause, rebuilding the body, and continuing support through rejuvenative practices.

Aligning Daily Routine with the Rhythms of Nature

Ayurveda recognizes natural rhythms that can impact our health including those that occur daily, monthly, and seasonally. Our internal experience is influenced by the larger rhythms of our environment. Many of the body's functions are governed by the circadian rhythm—hormone and enzyme production, neurological functions, temperature changes, electrolyte excretion, and sleep–wake cycle—affecting our energy levels and appetite.[1] Whereas in the past daily activities were largely dictated by the natural rhythm of the rising and setting of the sun, modern life has disconnected us from natural influences through artificial lighting, indoor temperature regulation, and the setting of our schedules by clock time. To reestablish balance, Ayurveda emphasizes living in harmony with natural rhythms versus going against the flow; resetting the biological clock to function in accord with the rhythms of nature is key.

Ayurveda recognizes that master cycles of the *doshas* circle around the time clock two times each (Figure 18.1) day. From 2:00 to 6:00 AM or PM, *vata* is dominant; from 6:00 to 10:00 AM or PM, *kapha* is dominant; and from 10:00 to 2:00 AM or PM, *pitta* is dominant. When the daily routine is aligned with these master cycles, our functioning is supported instead of in opposition to nature.

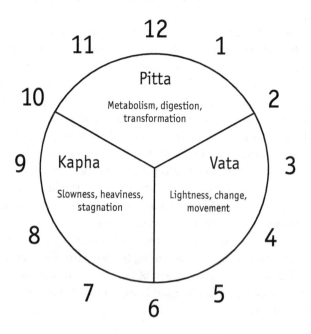

FIGURE 18.1 Dosha master cycles go around the time clock.

Daily Routine to Support Restful Sleep

- Rise with the sun around 6:00 AM, which is the junction point between *vata* and *kapha* periods. Waking up during the *vata* time period is associated with alertness, lightness, activity. The *kapha* time is heavy, dull, and sluggish, and waking up during *kapha* time can be difficult. For optimal energy and alertness, do not sleep past 7:00 AM. Establishing a regular rising time is the first step to regularity and balancing of *vata dosha*. Unless you are ill or have not slept well for several days, keep the same rising time each day, including weekends, because changing your patterns disrupts your rhythm. Waking up earlier also encourages an earlier bedtime.
- Meditation in the morning and in the afternoon/evening is encouraged.
- The best time for exercise is during the *kapha* period of morning from 6:00 to 10:00 AM. Exercise in the evening past 7:00 PM can aggravate insomnia by overstimulating the system too close to bedtime. At least 30 minutes of daily physical activity is recommended and should be appropriate for one's body type. *Vata* types should avoid excessive exercise, while *kapha* types respond well to vigorous exercise. Ayurvedic recommendations are to exercise to about 50% of one's capacity.
- Exposure to bright light or natural daylight is recommended during the day. Be fully awake and active during the day.
- Daytime napping is discouraged unless ill or convalescing. If one must nap, limit the time to less than 30 minutes so that deep sleep does not occur, which can increase the feeling of lethargy. Do not nap after 4:00 PM.
- The main meal should be eaten between 10:00 AM and 2:00 PM, when the influence of *pitta dosha* maximally supports digestion.
- Eat a light dinner, preferably before 7:00 PM. Heavy and late meals take a longer time and can be more difficult to digest which can result in increased metabolic activity and sleep disturbances.
- After dinner take a short walk for about 5–15 minutes to promote relaxation and aid digestion.
- In the evening, avoid engaging in exciting, intense, or overly focused physical or mental activities. Activities should be settled and relaxed, such as light reading, listening to calming music, light conversation, or other gentle activities. If one must attend to some focused activity or work at night, stop by 9:00 PM at the latest.
- Avoid watching TV or connecting to the internet in the evening. These both stimulate mental function and aggravate *vata*. In addition, the light from electronic screens (smartphones, tablets, computers, and TVs) has been shown to suppress melatonin, which can further exacerbate sleep issues.[10] Avoid use of electronic screens for 2–3 hours before bed. If one

must use them, blue-light blocking settings or glasses can help mitigate this effect.

- Prepare for bedtime at least 30 minutes before you intend to get into bed.
- If your mind is very active, journaling or another practice to download thoughts and concerns can help to reduce rumination at bedtime.
- Aim for a bedtime of 10:00 PM. The influence of *kapha dosha* before 10:00 PM supports sleep. Past 10:00 PM, the influence of *pitta* stimulates the mind, and it becomes difficult to fall asleep. The hours of sleep before midnight are more rejuvenating than sleep after sunrise, and sleep becomes lighter as the night progresses. If one is used to late hours, move the bedtime up by half an hour every week.

Balancing Through the Five Senses

Ayurveda recognizes that the state of one's being is the result of the genotype interacting with the environment and that, essentially, we are the metabolic end products of our sensory experiences. Inputs from each of our senses of sight, sound, smell, touch, and taste can support balance or contribute to imbalance. In the case of sleep disorders, overstimulation of some or all of the senses can aggravate *vata dosha* and lead to an agitated state of consciousness. Therefore, certain methods are recommended that can help promote balance through each of the senses throughout the day as well as at bedtime (Table 18.2).

Ayurvedic Oil Massage

The ancient Ayurvedic technique of self-*abhyangha* massage nourishes the body from head to toe, stimulates circulation and lymphatic drainage, softens the skin, and calms the mind. It is pacifying for *vata*. Although is recommended to perform this massage in the morning before bathing, for those with insomnia it can be helpful to perform the massage in the evening followed by a warm bath.[4] To do so, warm some food-grade oil such as sesame or almond oil (or coconut oil for *pitta dosha*) in a mug or with your hands and apply a small amount to the crown of your head, gently massaging the scalp. Using the flat part of your hands, make circular strokes over your head. Massage the face gently with oil: the forehead, temples, cheeks, around the mouth and noses, jaw, and ears. Apply oil and massage the neck and shoulders with circular motions. Then use long strokes to go along the long bones of the arms and circles around the elbow and wrist joints. Massage both hands including fingers and palms. Using broad strokes, massage the chest and the abdomen, moving up along the right side of the abdomen, then across,

Table 18.2 Balancing through the senses

Sense	Recommended balancing actions
Sight	• The bedroom should be visually pleasant and uncluttered. Looking out on nature or a picture of a natural scene is recommended. • Colors that are warm and soothing are best for restful sleep. • Avoid engaging mental activities in the bedroom such as reading, working, or watching television. • Avoid TV, particularly if violent or graphic. • Avoid use of electronic screens for 2–3 hours before bedtime. • Start dimming the lights as the sun goes down. When going to sleep, use blackout curtains or an eye mask to minimize light stimulation. • *Pitta* types are particularly sensitive to visual stimuli.
Sound	• Avoid sounds that are overly stimulating, dissonant, or otherwise unpleasant. • Pleasant, calming music or nature sounds are recommended. • Mantras "Ram Sham" or "Om Agasthi Shahina" can be repeated.
Smell	• Behaviors, emotions, and the autonomic nervous system are influenced by aromas, and certain aromas are useful for balancing *doshas*. For *vata* balancing, a mixture of warm, sweet and sour aromas can be calming and grounding such as lavender, sandalwood, chamomile, and vanilla. These can be used through aromatherapy diffusers, scented candles, or incense or rub a drop of essential oil on the temples or pulse points.
Touch	• Daily massage is helpful to rebalance *vata*. See text for instructions on how to do self-*abhyangha* massage, foot massage, and *marma* point therapy. • The bedroom should be well ventilated and about 68°F or cooler. If using an air conditioner or fan, be sure the air does not blow directly on the head as this exacerbates *vata*. • Taking a warm bath or shower before bed can help with mental and physical relaxation. This also initiates the cool-down response afterward, which helps to induce sleep.
Taste	• Each food has a particular influence on *vata*, *pitta*, and *kapha*. Eating foods that are known to reduce *vata* can bring more balance and alleviate insomnia. These include warm, cooked, heavier meals with nourishing foods that represent the sweet, sour, and salty tastes. Balanced sweet tastes include complex carbohydrates, healthy fats and oils, and quality sources of protein. Dairy, whole grains, and root vegetables are considered grounding foods. • Certain foods are agitating and should be avoided by people who have insomnia. These include stimulants such as caffeine and alcohol, carbonated beverages, cold food and drinks, dry foods, and rough foods. The tastes of spicy, bitter, and astringent should be minimized as they can aggravate *vata*. • Meals should be eaten regularly. • Lunch should be the main meal. • Avoid heavy food at dinner. A light dinner such as soup, pasta, rice, or lentils is recommended. • Warm milk or a cup of herbal tea can be taken after dinner. Chamomile, lavender, and valerian are relaxing choices.

and down along the left side of the abdomen, following the path of the large intestine. Massage the back in broad strokes as well as you can. Using a circular motion, massage both hips. Then take long strokes to go along the long bones of the legs, with circles around the knees and ankles. Massage both feet all the way to the toes, using the palm of your hand to massage the soles of your feet.

If there is not time enough to massage the entire body, it is recommended to massage the bottoms of the feet with oil.[4] The feet contain many vital points that relate to balancing the nervous system. After a few minutes, the oil can be wiped off with a cool damp cloth.

While massage can be relaxing, *marma points* are specific locations on the body that serve as gateways to the body's intelligence of mind, body, and spirit. Ayurveda describes 117 major *marma* points and three main *marma* sites: the head, heart, and base of the spine.[11] Toxins, stress, and negative emotions can accumulate at these sites, and, through manipulation of *marmas*, blockages can be removed and energy flow restored. Gentle touch of the *marma* points is a method of healing and is an important aid to help balance the *doshas*. Two major *marmas* that relate to sleep are located in the center of the forehead and on the lower abdomen just below the umbilicus, about three-quarters of the distance to the pubic bone.[1,11] Before bed, each of these areas can be gently massaged with a small amount of sesame oil (or coconut oil for *pitta* types) for about 1 minute using a very light, circular, clockwise motion.

Shirodhara massage is an Ayurvedic oil-dripping treatment that is often used to treat sleep problems. It consists of pouring a gentle stream of warm oil (sesame or herbal oil) over the forehead, rhythmically moving over the sixth chakra, and allowing the oil to flow over the scalp and through the hair. Recipients report states of relaxation and bliss. Prior studies, although limited, have demonstrated the effect of *Shirodhara* on improvement of subjective sleep quality.[12,13] A 2016 study examined sesame oil *Shirodhara* (SOS) against warm water *Shirodhara* (WWS) for 20 participants in a randomized, single-blinded, crossover study. In this study, each participant received seven 30-minute sessions within 2 weeks with either liquid, followed by a washout period of at least 2 months. Fifteen subjects completed the study, and it was found that SOS improved sleep quality over WWS as measured the Pittsburgh Sleep Quality Index (PSQI).[14]

Yoga for Restful Sleep

Yoga enhances coordination between the mind and body and can help to restore a healthy sleep pattern. Yoga and meditation help with stress and improve the general sense of well-being. With yoga, stress and tension that accumulates in the body can be released. In addition, the practice of self-awareness that is encouraged through yoga and meditation can also help one understand the cycle of natural rhythms through the day and one's relationship to those rhythms. Although studies are limited, a randomized controlled trial of 410 cancer survivors in 2013 found that a program of Gentle Hatha and Restorative yoga improved sleep quality and reduced medication use.[15] And a 2017 study of women with type 2 diabetes found that yoga was more effective than aerobic exercise in improving sleep quality.[16]

A gentle and mindful yoga practice in the evening before bed for 5–30 minutes can be beneficial. Helpful poses include the Child's Pose, Standing Forward Bend, Legs Up the Wall with Eyes Closed, Spinal Twist (seated or lying down), Reclining Butterfly (supported with pillows), and Corpse (Savasana).

Pranayama is the sister science of yogic breathing techniques that influences both the body and the mind. The technique of alternate nostril breathing (*Nadi Shodana*) quiets the mind and creates balance. To perform this technique, hold your right hand up, resting your pointer and middle fingers in between your eyebrows and place your thumb against your right nostril. Close your right nostril with your thumb, inhale through the left nostril. Close the left nostril with your ring finger, retain your breath for a brief moment. Release the thumb only, exhaling slowly through the right nostril. After exhaling completely, inhale through the right nostril keeping the ring finger on the left nostril. Close the right nostril with your thumb, pausing briefly, and then release the ring finger, exhaling through the left nostril. You have now completed one cycle. Repeat for 5–10 cycles. An alternate technique of relaxed belly breathing or diaphragmatic breathing can also be used. To do so, simply sit or lie comfortably and start to breathe in through your nose and out through your mouth. Allow your breathing to deepen, letting your belly be soft and relaxed during the breath. You may notice your belly move out during the inhale and back in during the exhale. Continue breathing slowly and deeply, allowing your mind and body to relax.

Meditation

A state of balance of the mind is important to achieving good sleep, and, in Ayurveda, a regular meditation practice is a core part of the daily routine. Meditation has been found to influence function of the brain, hypothalamo-pituitary adrenal axis, autonomic nervous system, and melatonin secretion, which all play a role in sleep.[17] A recent 2016 meta-analysis found that a form of meditation called *mindfulness meditation* significantly improved sleep parameters including total wake time and sleep quality.[18]

Various meditation techniques can be used to achieve a relaxation response, but the key is to have a regular daily practice. One simple practice is a breath awareness meditation. Sitting comfortably where you will not be disturbed, gently close your eyes. With a relaxed belly, allow your breath to flow in and out naturally. As you inhale, follow the flow of your breath in. As you exhale, follow the flow of your breath out. Do not force or try to control your breath. Just notice as it goes in and out. If your attention shifts to thoughts in your mind, sounds in your environment, or sensations in your body gently bring your attention back to your breath. Continue to meditate for 20–30 minutes. When done, sit for a moment with your eyes gently closed before resuming activity.

Yoga *nidra*, also known as yogic sleep, is a deeply restful state in between sleep and wakefulness. Yoga *nidra* quiets the mind, relieves stress, and promotes healing and relaxation. It is a very specific, guided meditation that typically is about 30 minutes long and brings awareness to each of the layers of the body, including the physical body, energetic body, emotional body, intellect, ego, and cosmic consciousness. Yoga *nidra* can be practiced on its own, at home, in a class, or as part of a traditional *asana* practice. A pilot study in 2014 of yoga *nidra* practice in women with sexual trauma found improvements in multiple parameters including improved quality of sleep.[19]

Ayurvedic Herbs

In Ayurveda, herbs are used as part of an overall strategy that includes creating balance at all levels of mind, body, and spirit. Like foods, each herb has a particular influence on *vata*, *pitta*, or *kapha*. Since sleep is affected by *vata*, many of the sleep-supportive herbs also support balancing *vata* (Table 18.3). Milk is often used with the herbs as a sedative and to enhance the tonic and nutritive effects of herbs.[20] Warm milk can be taken just before bedtime with herbs.

To make Cardamom-Nutmeg Milk, pour 1 cup of milk into a saucepan and bring it to a boil. Once it has boiled, remove it from the heat. Add two pinches of ground cardamom and two pinches of ground nutmeg. Sweeten to taste with sugar. Two to three threads of saffron can also be substituted for nutmeg. To increase digestibility of milk, two pinches of grated or finely chopped fresh ginger may be added before boiling; however do not use powdered dry ginger as it is too hot and stimulating to take prior to bed.

Ayurvedic Approach to Hypersomnia

Like the approach to insomnia, the Ayurvedic approach to addressing excessive sleep is to rebalance the body and mind. Establishment of a healthy daily routine

Table 18.3 Ayurvedic herbs for sleep

Herb	Properties	Use	Precautions
Jatamamsi root (*Nardostachys jatamansi*)	Similar to valerian in properties. Brain rejuvenative and sedative. Clears *pitta*, calms *vata*, reduces *kapha*. Cools and nourishes a "hot" and "exhausted" nervous system and aids digestion.	½ teaspoon of powder in a little honey. Or 250–500 mg three times per day. Often combined with gotu kola, brahmi, shankhapushpi.	Caution during pregnancy. High doses may cause nausea, colic, and urinary problems. Caution with sedative, antihypertensive, and antidepressive medications.
Ashwagandha root (*Withania somnifera*)	Rejuvenating adaptogenic herb. Dual action of energizing and calming. Useful in all conditions caused by stress and considered the best herb for nourishing *vata*. The name somnifera refers to its relaxing and sleep-promoting effects.	¼ to ½ teaspoon with warm water or 500 mg of an extract standardized to 2.5–5% with anolides, once or twice daily.	Precautions: High ama with congestion, excess *pitta*. Caution in pregnancy. Caution in individuals with hypoglycemia.
Brahmi leaf (*Bacopa monnieri*) or Gotu Kola Leaf (*Centella asiatica*)	There is some debate about which herb is the real Brahmi, however both have nervine activity and are useful for pacifying *vata*.	Bacopa dose: ¼ to ½ teaspoon with warm water or 200 mg standardized extract, once or twice daily. Gotu kola dose: ¼ to ½ teaspoon with warm water, once or twice daily or 50–250 mg of standardized extract, 2–3 times daily.	*Bacopa monnieri* is quite safe. Caution for gotu kola use in pregnancy. Large doses may cause headache or dizziness. Herb–drug interactions include: benzodiazepines, barbiturates, hypoglycemic agents, and cholesterol-lowering medication.

(continued)

Table 18.3 Continued

Herb	Properties	Use	Precautions
Jatiphala fruit/ seed (Nutmeg; *Myristica fragrans*)	Considered one of the best herbs for treating nervous disorders that can disrupt sleep. Also helps relax muscles and prevent pain associated with angina, fibromyalgia, and arthritis.	1/8 teaspoon powder in warm milk. May be combined with ashwagandha, brahmi, and jatamansi	Said to increase dullness of the mind in excess. Precautions in pregnancy and high *pitta*. Never use high doses (>6 g) as it may cause dizziness, heart palpitations, intoxication, and hallucinations.
Tagara root (Valerian; *Valeriana officinalis*)	Useful for cleansing accumulated *vata* from the nervous system. Often used in sleep formulas and teas in Western herbalism.	Take 1–2 hours before bedtime, or up to 3 times in the course of the day, with the last dose near bedtime. It may take a few weeks before effects are felt. Tea. Pour 1 cup boiling water over 1 teaspoonful (2–3 g) of dried root, steep 5–10 minutes. Or take with warm milk and ghee before bed. As extract take 250–600 mg per dose. May be used as part of a formula with ashwagandha, jatamamsi, nutmeg, and licorice. It can be added to a bath to help induce a deep sleep.	Caution in high *pitta*, depression and with central nervous system depressants including alcohol. Prolonged use should be avoided.

(*continued*)

Table 18.3 Continued

Herb	Properties	Use	Precautions
Shankhapushpi plant, juice (*Evolvulus alsinoides*)	Strengthens the nervous system and calms the mind. Considered by Charaka as the best of all the nervine herbs.	¼ to ½ teaspoon with warm water, once or twice daily.	Caution with sedative medications.

Sources: Frawley D, Lad V. *The yoga of herbs*, 2nd ed. Twin Lakes: Lotus Press; 2001; Pole S. *Ayurvedic medicine: The principles of traditional practice*. London: Churchill Livingstone; 2006.

in alignment with the rhythms of nature as outlined earlier is key. One should wake up no later than 7 AM and avoid napping during the day. Invigorating practices including *pranayama*, daily physical activity, and use of uplifting aromatherapy are recommended and can help to balance an underlying kapha aggravation.

Energizing breathing techniques such as Bellows Breath (*bhastrika*) increase oxygen flow and improve circulation. To perform this technique, sit comfortably with your spine upright and close your eyes. The breath is abdominal, using your diaphragm to move air while head and shoulders remain relaxed. Exhale fully, then begin to breathe deeply in and out through your nose. For the first 20 breaths take 2-second slow, forceful inhalations and 2-second slow, forceful exhalations. Perform the next 20 breaths faster with approximately 1-second each for inhalation and exhalation. Then, perform 20 rapid breaths, with approximately one-half second for inhalation and exhalation. After the 20 rapid breaths, take one more slow deep breath and then rest while observing the sensations in your body. Do not hyperventilate to the point where you are feeling lightheaded or dizzy. Another variation of the bellows breath is Skull Shining Breath (*Kapalabhati*), which involves forceful diaphragmatic exhalation followed by passive inhalation.

Stimulating aromas can be used, including cloves, camphor, cinnamon, eucalyptus, juniper, and marjoram. Mint and citrus aromas can also be uplifting. When performing daily massage, more vigorous strokes are used.

Foods should have qualities that bring balance to *kapha* and include lighter, warm, fresh foods such as steamed vegetables and vegetarian stir-fries. Heavy, dense foods should be avoided. In addition, foods with qualities of *tamas* (inertia or dullness) should be avoided. These include meat, poultry, fish, eggs, onions, garlic, alcohol, and other intoxicants including drugs. Fermented, overripe, overprocessed, stale, or leftover foods, as well as foods that are difficult to digest are considered tamasic. Overeating is also regarded as tamasic.

Conclusion

Sleep disturbances are widespread issues that are caused by and further aggravate various lifestyle-related factors that can impact health and disease. The use of prescription medications may not address the root cause of the sleep disturbance, and many patients are concerned about addiction, abuse, and the adverse effects of sleep medications. An Ayurvedic approach addressing the causative lifestyle factors and the unique individual should be considered when managing sleep problems.

REFERENCES

1. Chopra D. Restful sleep: *The complete mind/body program for overcoming insomnia.* New York: Harmony; 1996.
2. Agnivesha. *Charaka samhita.* In Sharma RK, Dash B, eds. Vol. 1. Varanasi: Chowkhamba Sanskrit Series Office; 2001.
3. Murthy KRS. *Vagbhata's Ashtanga Hridayam,* 5th ed. Varanasi: Krishnadas Academy; 2001.
4. Lad V. Ayurveda: *The science of self-healing.* Twin Lakes: Lotus Press; 2004.
5. Frawley D. *Ayurvedic healing: A comprehensive guide,* 2nd ed. Twin Lakes: Lotus Press; 2000.
6. Prasher B, Negi S, Aggarwal S, et al. Whole genome expression and biochemical correlates of extreme constitutional types defined in Ayurveda. *J Translational Med.* 2008;6:48. doi:10.1186/1479-5876-6-48.
7. Govindaraj P, Nizamuddin S, Sharath A, et al. Genome-wide analysis correlates Ayurveda Prakriti. *Sci Rep.* 2015;5:15786. doi:10.1038/srep15786.
8. Prasher B, Gibson G, Mukerji M. Genomic insights into ayurvedic and western approaches to personalized medicine. *J Genet.* 2016; 95(1):209–228.
9. Telles S, Pathak S, Kumar A, Mishra P, Balkrishna A. Ayurvedic doshas as predictors of sleep quality. *Med Sci Monit.* 2015; 21: 1421–1427.
10. West KE, Jablonski MR, Warfield B, Cecil KS, James M, et al. Blue light from light-emitting diodes elicits a dose-dependent suppression of melatonin in humans. *J Appl Physiol.* 2011;110:619–626.
11. Lad V, Durve A. *Marma points of Ayurveda: The energy pathways for healing body, mind, and consciousness with a comparison to Traditional Chinese Medicine.* Albuquerque: Ayurvedic Press; 2008.
12. Bharti, Makhija R, Kumar A, et al. Shirodhara: Pilot observations in anidra (insomnia). *J Ayurveda.* 2008;2:60–63.
13. Sahu A, Sharma A. A clinical study on anidra and its management with shirodhara and mansyadi kwatha. *J Ayurveda.* 2009;3:4–15.

14. Tokinobu A, Yorifuji T, Tsuda T, Doi H. Effects of Ayurvedic oil-dripping treatment with sesame oil vs. with warm water on sleep: A randomized single-blinded crossover pilot study. *J Alt Compl Med.* 2016; 22(1):52–58.

15. Mustian KM, Sprod LK, Janelsins M, et al. Multicenter, randomized controlled trial of yoga for sleep quality among cancer survivors. *J Clin Oncol.* 2013;31(26):3233–3241.

16. Ebrahimi M, Guilan-Nejad TN, Pordanjani AF. Effect of yoga and aerobics exercise on sleep quality in women with Type 2 diabetes: A randomized controlled trial. *Sleep Sci.* 2017;10(2):68–72.

17. Nagendra RP, Maruthai N, Kutty BM. Meditation and its regulatory role on sleep. Front Neurol. 2012;3:54. doi:10.3389/fneur.2012.00054.

18. Gong H, Ni CX, Liu YZ, Zhang Y, Su WJ, et al. Mindfulness meditation for insomnia: A meta-analysis of randomized controlled trials. *J Psychosom Res.* 2016;89:1–6.

19. Pence PG, Katz LS, Huffman C, Cojucar G. Delivering integrative restoration-yoga nidra meditation (iRest®) to women with sexual trauma at a veteran's medical center: A pilot study. *Int J Yoga Thera.* 2014;24:53–62.

20. Frawley D, Lad V. *The yoga of herbs*, 2nd ed. Twin Lakes: Lotus Press; 2001.

19

Manual Medicine and Sleep

MICHAEL KURISU

Introduction to Manual Medicine

As the name implies, in manual medicine the practitioner uses part(s) of his or her body (usually hands, but elbows, feet, and other body parts can be utilized) to influence or change specific imbalances in the patient. Emphasis is on the use of tactile sensation and perception as a centerpiece of healthcare for both diagnosis and treatment.

Manual medicine encompasses many different disciplines that share similar techniques and qualities. The main theme of these disciplines is that the body, or *soma*, is a therapeutic window into the patient. Manual medicine can effect changes in multiple tissues and can have a variety of pathophysiological effects. Techniques utilized by the manual medicine practitioner can change the resting tension in a muscle or tendon; change or "reset" a trigger point; alter the tension or torque within a ligament or fascial plane; change the alignment or asymmetry of bones or joints; help to alter structures that are impinging on nerves; release suppressed emotion which may be held in the myofascial tissues; improve lymphatic flow, visceral function, cerebral spinal fluid flow, and immune function; open up blocked energetic (*chi*) channels; and facilitate an integration of Spirit on the soma. As structural dysfunctions are released, a restoration of functional homeostasis ensues, and this is the goal of treatment.

Basic Diagnostic Parameters

The presence of objective findings of asymmetry, limited range of motion, and tissue texture changes are essential in formulating diagnosis and treatment. The term coined and used by the osteopathic profession is "somatic dysfunction," which is medically defined as "Impaired or altered *function* of related components of the somatic (body framework) system: skeletal, arthrodial, and myofascial structures and related vascular, lymphatic, and neural elements." Once a dysfunction is discovered, a treatment approach and manual techniques can be applied to physically correct the dysfunction.

Therapeutic Approaches

There is a vast array of different philosophies and practices of manual medicine. Going into detail about every practice is beyond the scope of this chapter, and the focus will be on the most common practice in the medical community and medical insurance industry.

OSTEOPATHIC MEDICINE

Osteopathy was founded in 1874 by A. T. Still, MD. He was a surgeon during the Civil War. Dr. Still withdrew from Western medicine when his family was struck by tragedy and two of his children passed away from meningitis. Frustrated that he could not offer anything besides drugs and archaic surgery, he sought to find a better form of healthcare.

A. T. Still came up with what has been termed the three tenets of osteopathic medicine:

1. The body is a unit; the person is a unit of body, mind, and spirit.
2. The body is capable of self-regulation, self-healing, and health maintenance.
3. Structure and function are reciprocally interrelated.
4. Rational treatment is based on an understanding of the basic principles of body unity, self-regulation, and the interrelationship of structure and function.

When using these tenets, the focus is on the health of each individual and not the disease process. Prevention and wellness thus became the center point of the philosophy of osteopathy.

Today doctors of osteopathy (DOs) are educated in fully accredited medical schools, are licensed to practice a full scope of medicine, and may select any established specialty. The education process is similar to allopathic (MD) schools. The main difference is philosophical, with osteopathic education focusing more on health and wellness, as opposed to the allopathic education, which focuses on treatment of disease. In addition to learning the science and clinical application of medicine, during their training, DOs spend several hundred hours learning the application of a variety of different manual medicine techniques. Many of the current techniques in all the fields of manual medicine can be traced back to the roots of osteopathy.

CHIROPRACTIC

Chiropractic was founded by Dr. Daniel David Palmer. He actually began working as a magnetic healer in Iowa and, through his readings, developed a theory that altered nerve flow was the cause of all disease and that misaligned spinal vertebrae had an effect on nerve flow. His postulation was that restoring these vertebrae to their proper alignment would restore health.

Today chiropractors have significant political clout and a large presence in the healthcare field. They have broad diagnostic skills and are also trained to recommend therapeutic and rehabilitative exercises, as well as to provide nutritional, dietary, and lifestyle counseling.

HEALING TOUCH

Healing touch is an internationally recognized modality. It is based on compassionate, noninvasive touch to restore harmony and balance energy that has been depleted due to stress, injury, illness, grief, or other medical conditions. It was developed by Janet Mentgen, RN, and is now used by thousands of nurses in many hospitals in the United States. There have been more than 100 publications on the benefits of healing touch.

MASSAGE

Massage has been around since the dawn of man; it is mentioned in records from ancient Chinese, Egyptian, and Biblical times. It was recommended by Hippocrates. There are now literally hundreds of different techniques of massage that are offered in a wide variety of settings. Like all forms of manual therapy, massage is mostly practitioner-dependent.

Treatment Techniques

There is great overlap within the different healing modalities of manual medicine. In general, all the different manual medicine treatment techniques can be divided into *direct* and *indirect* categories. Examples of direct techniques include but are not limited to high-velocity/low-amplitude, springing, post isometric relaxation (muscle energy), articulatory, inhibitory pressure, massage, rolfing, and trigger point therapy/injections. Indirect techniques involve manipulation at those points on the body where there is no physiological barrier. These techniques tend to be gentler, softer, and subtler and include but are not limited to balanced ligamentous tension, cranial-sacral, facilitated positional release, myofascial release, reiki, healing touch, strain/counterstain, and visceral techniques. Typical side effects of treatment include worsening pain and myalgia, fatigue, and nausea.

Contraindications for direct technique treatments	*Contraindications for indirect technique treatments*
• Acute trauma and hemarthrosis	• Acute trauma and hemarthrosis
• Congenital malformations	• Tissue instability (acute infection or
• Nearby vascular instability	inflammation)
(thrombosis, stenosis, or aneurysm)	
• Acute flare of rheumatic disease	
• Bone neoplasm	
• Connective tissue disease and	
hypermobility	

Key Points for Referrals

A referral to a provider who practices manual medicine is warranted if there is suspicion for an anatomical and musculoskeletal dysfunction for a specific disease process. In general, the laying on of hands can have a very relaxing effect on the body and should be recommended to any patient dealing with chronic pain and related stress or anxiety.

It is best to work with the patient's insurance company for better compliance. Osteopathic treatments and physical therapy tend to be covered by most insurance companies. Some insurance companies provide coverage for chiropractic care. Unfortunately, massage tends to be an out-of-pocket expense for the patient.

Manual Medicine and Sleep

Sleep loss and sleep disorders are among the most common yet frequently overlooked and readily treatable health problems. It is estimated that 50–70 million Americans chronically suffer from a disorder of sleep and wakefulness, hindering daily functioning and adversely affecting health and longevity.[1] A sleep disorder characterized by trouble initiating or maintaining sleep, *insomnia* is associated with impaired daytime function, injury due to accidents, and the development of depressive disorders. Persistent insomnia for less than 3 months is considered short-term, while chronic insomnia refers to 3 or more months of symptoms occurring at least three times per week.[2] Occasional, short-term insomnia affects 30–50% of the population.[3] The prevalence of chronic insomnia disorder in industrialized nations is estimated to be at least 10%.[4] In medically and psychiatrically ill populations, as well as in older age groups, the prevalence is significantly higher.

Insomnia has traditionally been treated with over-the-counter medications such as antihistamines and other prescription sleep aids. The desire to avoid adverse side effects and have less dependency on many sleep medications has led to an increased demand for nonpharmacologic treatments. There is a small but growing body of research that has demonstrated that manual medicine techniques can help decrease insomnia and have positive effects on other sleep disorders, which are often due to stress, pain, misalignment, or somatic dysfunction.

The goal of manual medicine is to evaluate somatic dysfunction and, through the application of a manual technique, promote proper alignment and therefore restore healing within the body of patients with these disorders. However, it should be noted that objectively evaluating somatic dysfunction in any individual and their physiologic changes after manual medicine has been applied is challenging to researchers and clinicians alike. The field of research in manual medicine continues to grow as we develop new technologies and methodologies for studying its effect.

Cutler and colleagues demonstrated that the compression of the fourth ventricle (CV4 technique) influenced the cranial rhythmic impulse and reduced muscle sympathetic nerve activity leading to reduced sleep latency in patients with insomnia.[5] This was the first study to demonstrate that cranial manipulation, specifically the CV4 technique of osteopathic manipulative treatment (OMT), can alter sleep latency and directly measure sympathetic tone in healthy humans. These findings also provide important insight into the possible physiologic effects of cranial manipulation.

A study involving retired professional football players from the National Football League and the Canadian Football League who had been medically diagnosed with postconcussion syndrome showed increases in nightly hours of sleep after manual medicine techniques were applied. Each participant received a 2-hour morning and afternoon session of specific manual medicine, including techniques of cranio-sacral therapy (CST), visceral manipulation (VM), and neural manipulation (NM) modalities.[6] Their hours of sleep averaged 2 hours on the first day of treatment and increased to 4 hours at the end of treatment and were continuing to increase, as noted at a 3-month evaluation. Ten sessions of specific CST/VM/NM techniques resulted in significant improvements in the number of hours slept per night as well as improved sleep quality in the postconcussion syndrome patients.

Since the majority of sleep disorders are multifaceted, sleep improvements are frequently reported in patients who incorporate a variety of lifestyle changes, including exercise, dietary changes, stress reduction, and limiting technology. In a university-based multisite study, adult patients received OMT and subsequently provided daily feedback on symptom severity and frequency for 7 days after the OMT session.[7] Compared to pre-OMT, patients reported statistically significant improvements in sleep quality and less sleep interference 7 days after receiving the OMT. Continued surveillance on practice outcomes may help identify priorities for osteopathic research and define evidence-based standards for OMT in the setting of sleep.

Patients who have a chronic sleep disturbance have proven levels of increased autonomic nervous system activity involving an increase in metabolism,[8] body temperature,[9] and heart rate.[10] Chronic insomniacs also display an increase in sympathetic output due to raised cortisol levels and recurrent activation of the hypothalamic-pituitary-adrenal (HPA) axis.[11] When compared to stress levels, a recent study revealed that breathing problems were more likely to be associated with insomnia, which the authors attributed to a below-normal drop in oxygen saturation.[12] Seated rib raising is an additional manual medicine "direct" technique that has been shown to regulate sympathetic and parasympathetic activity by normalizing the tone in the thoracolumbar region and promoting breathing. Targeting the somatic dysfunction and normalizing the sympathetic tone can potentially help regulate the nervous system dysfunction contributing to insomnia.

A 2010 review on manual medicine included studies that tested the effects of chiropractic therapy, spinal manipulative therapy, muscle relaxation techniques, cranial adjustments, and mind–body medical therapies for sleep disorders, notably insomnia.[13] Nine studies highlighted mind–body medical therapies for sleep disorders and pain in the cranio-mandibular and cervical spinal regions. There were no randomized clinical trials (RCTs) specific to chiropractic and insomnia although smaller scale studies utilizing osteopathic cranial manipulation for insomnia resulted in positive outcomes. An RCT using back massage performed by certified massage therapists in a Taiwanese cohort of postpartum women showed improvement in sleep quality as measured by the Pittsburgh Sleep Quality Index.[14] A small sample of postmenopausal women with climacteric symptoms such as hot flashes, insomnia, and mood disturbance reported positive changes in sleep and mood after therapeutic massage sessions.[15]

Manual medicine is a gentle, noninvasive and cost-effective treatment aimed at restoring normal movement, integrating all the body's systems, and promoting the body's natural ability to heal. Although a larger evidence base is needed to support the therapeutic outcomes, manual medicine remains a potentially promising treatment for psychiatric and chronic pain patients with comorbid insomnia, athletes battling sleeplessness, and the additional 30% of the American population burdened by sleep–wake disturbances. Further studies that employ psychometrically validated measurements, report sleep-related outcomes based on longer follow-up, and formally established larger clinical trials are needed in order to generate more robust conclusions.

REFERENCES

1. Colten, HR, Altevogt BM, eds.; Institute of Medicine (US) Committee on Sleep Medicine and Research. *Sleep disorders and sleep deprivation: An unmet public health problem.* Washington DC: National Academies Press (US); 2006: 3. Extent and health consequences of chronic sleep loss and sleep disorders. http://www.ncbi.nlm.nih.gov/books/NBK199161/.
2. Ellis JG, Perlis ML, Neale LF, Espie CA, Bastien CH. The natural history of insomnia: Focus on prevalence and incidence of acute insomnia. *J Psychiatr Res.* 2012;46(10):1278–1285.
3. Ohayon MM. Observation of the natural evolution of insomnia in the American general population cohort. *Sleep Med Clin.* 2009;4(1):87–92.
4. Sateia MJ, Buysse DJ, Krystal AD, Neubauer DN, Heald JL. Clinical practice guideline for the pharmacologic treatment of chronic insomnia in adults: An American Academy of Sleep Medicine Clinical Practice Guideline. *J Clin Sleep Med.* 2017 Feb;13(2):307–349.
5. Cutler MJ, Holland BS, Stupski BA, Gamber RG, Smith ML. Cranial manipulation can alter sleep latency and sympathetic nerve activity in humans: A pilot study. *J Alt Compl Med.* 2005;11(1):103–108.
6. Wetzler G, Roland M, Fryer-Dietz S, Dettmann-Ahern D. Craniosacral therapy and visceral manipulation: A new treatment intervention for concussion recovery. *Med Acupuncture.* 2017;29(4):239–248.
7. Degenhardt BF, Johnson JC, Gross SR, Hagan C, Lund G, Curry WJ. Preliminary findings on the use of osteopathic manipulative treatment: Outcomes during the formation of the practice-based research network, DO-Touch.NET. *J Am Osteopath Assoc.* 2014;114(3):154–170.
8. Bonnet MH, Arand DL. 24-Hour metabolic rate in insomniacs and matched normal sleepers. *Sleep.* 1995;18(8):581.
9. Lushington K, Dawson D, Lack L. Core body temperature is elevated during constant wakefulness in elderly poor sleepers. *Sleep.* 2000;23(10):504.

10. Freedman RR, Sattler HL. Physiological and psychological factors in sleep-onset insomnia. *J Abnorm Psychol.* 1982;91(9):380.

11. Vgontzas AN, Bixler EO, Lin HM, et al. Chronic insomnia is associated with nyctohemeral activation of the hypothalamic-pituitary-adrenal axis: Clinical implications. *J Clin Endocrinol Metab.* 2001; 86(94):3787.

12. Hynninen MJ, Pallesen S, Hardie J, et al. Insomnia symptoms, objectively measured sleep, and disease severity in chronic obstructive pulmonary disease outpatients. *Sleep Med.* 2013;14(33):1328.

13. Kingston J, Raggio C, Spencer K, Stalaker K, Tuchin PJ. A review of the literature on chiropractic and insomnia. *J Chiropract Med.* 2010;9(3):121–126.

14. Ko Y, Lee H. Randomized controlled trial of the effectiveness of using back massage to improve sleep quality among Taiwanese insomnia postpartum women. *Midwifery.* 2014;30(1):60–64.

15. Oliveira DS, Hachul H, Goto S, Bittencourt LRA. Effect of therapeutic massage on insomnia and climacteric symptoms in postmenopausal women. *Climacteric.* 2012:15:1, 21–29.

20

Energy Medicine and Sleep Disorders

ANN MARIE CHIASSON

Case Study

A 48-year-old male with insomnia presents to the office with a 2-month history of increasing difficulty sleeping. The patient states that he has delayed sleep onset and wakes once in the middle of the night to urinate. He cannot go back to sleep easily after using the bathroom; he finds he is ruminating about a difficult situation at work. He owns a business and is concerned about both financial aspects and personnel issues. Patient states he has mild anxiety, which mostly manifests as difficulty sleeping. He also notes his dreams are very busy and violent or disturbing at times. He is under the care of a family practitioner who has evaluated him for depression and anxiety. He does not meet the criteria for depression, and he does not want to use an anti-anxiety medication or a hypnotic for sleep because a previous trial interfered with his wakefulness during the day. He has decided to try energy treatments as a result of a suggestion from his wife.

The patient received a standard healing touch session with extra focus placed on his second chakra/lower *dan tien* area and his feet. The patient was also taught how to self-treat on the way to sleep by toe-tapping, an exercise that had him rotate his legs from the hips in and out to tap his toes together at the balls of the foot (the metatarsal phalanges joint.) In addition, he was taught a resting position in which he was to lay on his back and rest his hands on his hips, at the fold where the thigh meets the hip. A guided visualization CD for sleep was recommended. The following sleep recommendation was made: as he went to bed, he was to initially to lie on top of the covers, toe tap for 5 minutes, and then rest for at least 3 minutes in the sleep resting position and listen to as much of the guided visualization CD for sleep as needed until he began to fall asleep. If this did not let him fall into sleep, it was recommended he tap for 10 more minutes. As well, the same routine was recommended for any nighttime waking, to return to sleep. The patient returned for another treatment 3 weeks later. He reported that the toe-tapping had assisted him to begin to fall asleep, and, coupled with the CD, his sleep was about 50% improved. He received another treatment and left with the plan to continue this routine and return again in a month.

Energy Medicine: Scope and Definition

The field of *energy medicine* (EM) consists of modalities and techniques that work with the underlying energy field of the body to affect balance, health, and healing. In the broadest sense, the field of EM can be explained in the context of the organism: "in addition to a system of physical and chemical processes, the human being is made up of a complex system of energy."[1] These principles are ancient, although the term "energy medicine" was coined more recently to describe the scientific exploration of manipulating low levels of energy for healing: "Energy medicine is the application of extremely low-level signals to the body, including energy healer interventions and bio-electromagnetic device-based therapies, and is incomprehensible from the dominant biomedical paradigm of 'life as chemistry.'"[2]

The energy field, also called the *biofield*, is a system within (or underlying) the physical body; depending on the healing tradition, it is "a massless field, not necessarily electromagnetic, that surrounds and permeates living bodies and affects the body."[3] This biofield is considered the underlying organizing principle that is fundamental to all functioning of the physical body.[2]

> **Energy Medicine Reintegrates into Modern Medicine**
> Energy medicine may be a resurgence of "vitalism" or the belief that an underlying vital force exists in the body and is central to health. This concept predates Hippocrates, who espoused that the vital force was dependent on balance of the four humors. Mesmer also promoted this concept in the 1700s, calling it "magnetism." When medicine shifted to organ-based systems with the rise of the Paris Clinics in the early 1800s, the importance of the body's vital energy lost its place in modern medicine. The resurgence of EM can be interpreted as an integration of prior views of health and healing with modern-day medicine; this integration may end up augmenting our current views of health, healing, and illness.[4]

The body's biofield is a core tenet of many or most traditional healing paradigms developed prior to the advent of modern medicine.[4] This concept, that all life forms are regulated by a subtle field of energy, has been around for more than 4,000 years and has a name in most cultures; it is called *Qi* or *Chi* in Traditional Chinese Medicine (TCM), *ki* in the Japanese systems, *doshas* in Ayurvedic medicine, *mana* in the Hawaiian culture, and *pneuma* in ancient Greece, just to name a few.[5] While 94 cultures have been documented to have a concept that describes this underlying energy of the body, this enormous variation lacks a unified anatomy or set of characteristics. Thus, the scope of EM crosses boundaries with spiritual healing and hands-on energy healing, as well as with aspects of TCM, Ayurveda, mind–body medicine, and other traditional healing systems because each of these modalities works with the biofield (Box 20.1).[6] For the purpose of this chapter, we

Box 20.1 Healing modalities that affect the energy system of the body

Touch therapies: Classically considered energy healing therapies
   Healing touch, reiki, healing touch, zero balancing, orthobionomy, bio-touch, therapeutic touch, pranic therapy, Barbara Brennan healing, Rosalyn Bruyere healing, reconnective healing
Whole Medicine Systems
   Traditional Chinese Medicine (including acupuncture), Ayurveda, homeopathy
Manual therapies
   Qigong, yoga
Other Therapies
   Spiritual healing, shamanic healing, breathwork, mind-body therapies, sound healing

discuss EM with regard to those modalities that directly address the biofield or energy field and that are not also under the classification of another paradigm. These include but are not limited to therapeutic touch (TT), healing touch (HT), craniosacral therapy, reiki, joh rei, sound healing, zero balancing, Barbara Brennan's work, and Rosalyn Bruyere's healing.

The authenticity and measurement of the biofield is a central dilemma for the incorporation of EM practices into conventional medicine and has proved to be an impediment with respect to acceptance by conventional medical practitioners and researchers. This will likely continue until an agreed upon method is well-delineated to accurately measure the body's energy field.

MEASUREMENT OF THE BIOFIELD

While the science of the biofield has been best described as a "work in progress,"[7] conventional therapies certainly measure and/or manipulate electromagnetic fields (EMF) for healing, through the electrocardiogram (ECG), electroencephalogram (EEG), heart rate variability (HRV) monitors, laser therapies, cardiac pacemakers, and radiation therapy among many other electrical and electromagnetic technologies.[2] Furthermore, the interactivity of these fields is becoming recognized. The electrical pattern of the brain (measured by EEG) has been demonstrated to influence and be influenced by cardiac activity (measured by ECG); an ECG can develop synchronization with the EEG alpha waves of another subject at a distance of up to 5 feet.[8]

Currently, gas discharge visualization (GDV), which measures biophoton emissions; super conducting quantum interference devices (SQUID); and low-frequency pulsed EMF (PEMF) are being explored to measure the EMF of the body.[9] Biophoton emission has now been demonstrated in cell communication and function, both in human physiology and in energy healing.[2,10] Moreover, there is evidence that bioelectric activity has an effect on cell growth and signaling.[2] In addition, the GDV measurement technique has been demonstrated to measure the effect of a healer on the biofield of a subject's body; osteopathic treatment has affected the GDV in correlation with a decrease in stress and blood pressure.[11] The advent of devices that measure and/or affect the body's EMF is also evolving; these include nonthermal energy sources such as low-level lasers, vibration, sound, and direct electric current.[12] Research on human biofield detection has demonstrated that healers can sense the biofield and can do this with better accuracy with training.[13]

Energy Medicine Prevalence of Use

Despite the uncertainty of verification or distinct definition, EM modalities are being used in the United States. Data from the National Health Interview Survey (NHIS) from 2002 to 2012 reported that the prevalence of use of energy healing in the general population was 0.5%, although the definition of "energy healing" used was for reiki alone.[14] A more accurate recent estimate approximated that 3.8% of the general population use energy therapies, an estimate gathered from a larger definition that includes the most used forms of biofield therapies: HT, reiki, and TT.[15] The prevalence of use is much greater in persons suffering from chronic pain and chronic illness, with various studies reporting rates of greater than 20% in pain due to rheumatologic disorders.[16] Use appears to be higher in the United States than in Canada and Europe.[17]

Anatomy of the Energy Field

The anatomical composition of the energy field varies according to the belief system in each healing tradition. An overview of how these anatomical components interact can be described as layers within the body; different energy medicine techniques are targeted to and based on different layers of the biofield. A simple map of such layers is presented in Figure 20.1.[4] For example, the technique of zero balancing is targeted at the deepest layer; HT works at the chakra layer, TCM works both at the deepest layers of the *dan tiens* as well as with the meridians, and many indigenous and shamanic techniques target the matrix layer.

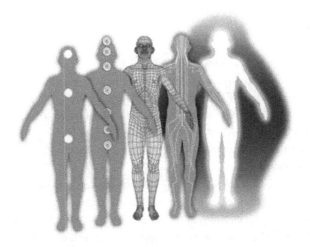

FIGURE 20.1 Summary of energy anatomy.

Energy Medicine and the Basis of Illness

Illness or disease first begins as an imbalance or blockage in the biofield. In the natural history of the disease, first the biofield field becomes unbalanced, next cellular or organ dysfunction develops, and, finally, clinical symptoms appear. Major cellular pathology typically appears weeks to years after a block in the natural flow of energy has occurred. As well, disruption of the biofield occurs concurrently with physical trauma. Pain, a symptom caused by blocked energy, can occur right away (i.e., trauma) or develop slowly, with poor energy flow over time. Infection is thought to occur from a weakness in the energy field that causes immunosuppression; this explains the transmission and expression variability of infectious agents from person to person. Anxiety is thought to be a result of an energy imbalance or an "ungrounded" energy field, with too much energy active higher in the body instead of centered on the lower *dan tien* or lower abdomen center.[4]

Factors that contribute to or cause energy blocks include external insults, genetic or hereditary causes, and physical or emotional trauma. Treatment is based on energy transfer and balancing in order to remove blocks and ultimately restore normal energy flow. Keeping the energy flowing and the energy field as clear as possible promotes health and healing.

HOW THE ENERGY BODY IS ALTERED

EM therapies rely on a variety of methods to shift or change the underlying energy field of the body. The most common technique involves the laying of the hands on or over the patient's body. However, different techniques employ vibration, light, sound, movement, magnets, or direct current.

The Healing Properties of Touch

The effect of touch, regardless of modality or tradition, is now coming to light as healing in its own right. The effect of touch is well-delineated in neonatal research; skin-to-skin contact between mother and infant stimulates oxytocin. Oxytocin has a host of positive and important effects including increased bonding, trust, and well-being. It is important to note that a lack of adequate endogenous oxytocin impairs social recognition and trust.[28]

Touch comes in many forms, ranging from massage to static hand placement energy healing techniques to non-contact touch that is close to the body. This inherent variety is one of the difficulties in researching touch and touch energy therapies. Despite this difficulty, touch has positive and healing effects on the body. Touch has been shown to decrease depression, shift EEG patterns, increase serotonin, decrease blood pressure, and decrease pain.[42]

In a clinical review of touch in critically ill patients, touch has been documented to stimulate vagal tone, increase HRV, modulate inflammation, and act on cytokines.[43] While the mechanism of action is unclear, the documented physiologic effects and benefits are becoming more evident. The affect or quality of touch has been demonstrated to be important, with early evidence of different receptors in skin that sense the effect; gentle and kind touch is more healing than rough touch.[42] As healers are commonly taught to use loving or compassionate touch, this also may be a factor in healing sessions.

Research on EM and Sleep

There is not an abundance of evidence from good-quality studies for the effect of biofield therapies on sleep. The inherent issues with the evidence for sleep stems primarily from three issues: almost all studies examined the effect of a biofield therapy on sleep as one of many factors of well-being assessed, most of the data collected was self-report, and there is no suitable "sham" touch control for comparison of biofield therapy effect. Reviews on biofield therapies are difficult to interpret due to the number of different types of small biofield studies; most reviews look at multiple types of therapies with practitioners of varying training and experience. Furthermore, since anxiety and pain can affect and/or cause sleep disorders, many studies correlated a decrease in anxiety and/or pain as a likely benefit for improved sleep. This review covers the data for sleep and certain studies on anxiety and pain assuming that the correlation between decreased anxiety and/or pain and better sleep is true.[15]

SLEEP IN CHRONIC PAIN PATIENTS

In a study in Brazil by Mart et al. in chronic pain patients, eight TT sessions were given to patients, and sleep, depression, and pain were assessed. Sleep was assessed by the Pittsburgh Sleep Quality Index. Patients who received the full course of TT demonstrated a significant improvement in sleep quality (p <0.05), as well as a decrease in pain and depression.[18] Another Brazilian study, by Weze et al., examined gentle touch therapy on 300 participants with chronic disease; the study consisted of four 1-hour treatments over a course of 6 weeks. This study found significant improvement in general health ratings including sleep disturbance reduction, stress reduction, pain reduction, and increased well-being (p <.0004). More specifically, sleep disturbance was improved by 3 points on a visual analog scale (VAS) (p <0.004) for those who slept too much, improved by 1 point on the VAS for those with slept well before the trial (p <0.017), and improved by 1 point for those who reported the worst sleep pre-intervention (p <0.004).[19]

Cranio-electrical stimulation (CES) uses small pulsed electrical impulses on the head to induce an effect similar to biofeedback; CES devices are now being widely marketed for insomnia and sleep. A small study done by Gilula on fibromyalgia patients using CES found a dramatic improvement in sleep from self-report questionnaires: poor sleep quality changed from 60% to 5% (p <.02).[20] However, a 2018 systematic review of CES for sleep alone in a variety of settings found most studies were of poor quality, and data for sleep and CES are inconclusive.[21]

SLEEP IN PALLIATIVE CARE PATIENTS

Senderovich et al. did a case control study from retrospective chart review on patients in a palliative care unit (PCU) to discern the benefit of TT. Patients who had one or more TT sessions were compared to a random selection of controls who had not chosen TT during their stay in the PCU. They found, through analyzing both qualitative and quantitative data, that TT patients had lower palliative performance scores (PPS) and significantly improved sleep. These findings suggest a strong benefit although are still based on the observations charted.[22]

SLEEP IN CANCER PATIENTS

A meta-analysis by Satija and Bhatnagar examined energy interventions in cancer patients. They concluded that energy therapies significantly induced the relaxation response and improved depression, anxiety, meaning, and spiritual well-being; however, this meta-analysis did not examine sleep alone.[23] One small study by

Biroco examined patients who had four reiki treatments while undergoing chemotherapy. This study concluded that self-report VAS anxiety scores were significantly improved (6.77 to 2.28, p <.000001). The study concluded that reiki improved sleep in cancer patients undergoing treatment.[24] A study by Marcus et al. of 145 self-report surveys from patients receiving biofield therapies at a chemo infusion center found that 86% of patients reported improved relaxation, 75% reported decreased anxiety, and 35% reported improved sleep.[25]

SLEEP IN ICU AND HOSPITALIZED PATIENTS

Biofield trials in the intensive care unit (ICU) have demonstrated positive data for sleep. One review by Richards et al. examined all useful complementary therapies for sleep in ICU patients. Their review of TT in critically ill ICU patients found that it significantly improved sleep and promoted relaxation that led to improved sleep. Limited qualitative data from this review found that TT either promoted sleep during the sessions or that patients slept longer after a TT session. They conclude that there is adequate evidence for biofield therapies for sleep in the ICU and advocate training ICU nurses in a biofield therapy.[26]

A trial done by Carniero et al. of a Brazilian biofield therapy (Brazilian spirits passe) significantly decreased anxiety and muscle tension in hospitalized patients; while sleep markers were not specifically explored, a reduction in muscle tension and anxiety could be inferred to assist with sleep in patient with difficulty sleeping.[27]

SLEEP IN THE NICU

Much work has been done with sleep and infants in the neonatal ICU (NICU). A handful of studies have been done on biofield therapies, but more research has been done on basic touch by parents or practitioners. While not therapies classified as biofield, kangaroo care, superior temporal sulcus (STS) touch, and massage all promote healing in ways similar to biofield therapies—from a transfer of energy, autonomic regulation, and the production of oxytocin from positive-quality touch.[28] One large review by Cleveland et al. examined 40 studies on STS, holding, or infant massage. This review concluded that both STS and infant massage helped consolidate sleep patterns in newborn infants.[29,30]

Harrison et al. examined 10 minutes of touch three times per week on pre-term NICU infants using 42 cases and 42 controls with normal care. They compared sleep and other measures between the two groups and found significantly decreased active non–REM sleep (p < 0.002) and a trend toward more quiet sleep.[31]

Yaksun touch, a Korean technique that massages the infant with one hand on the abdomen and keeps another hand stable on the back, has been examined in the NICU for its effect on sleep by two studies. A study by Bijari et al. examined Yaksun and gentle human touch (GTH) twice a day (15 minutes) on pre-term infants for 5 days versus a control group. Both the Yaksun and GHT groups had significantly improved sleep compared to the control group, while there was not a significant difference between the Yaksun and GHT groups in terms of the effect size.[32] This study points to the importance of quality of touch, not the specific touch technique. This model was also examined by authors Im and Kim on pre-term infants using a trial of twice a day for 15 minutes for 15 days. This study found that both GHT and Yaksun statistically improved sleep state scores compared to the control group, and both significantly decreased fussy state scores compared to the control group. Interestingly, the GHT infants slept during and after the sessions, while the Yaksun participants were active during the session but sleep more after the intervention.[33]

A large review by Erodgan and Atik on complementary therapies for sleep in the NICU found data for biofield therapies positive enough to recommend NICU nurses be trained in a biofluid or touch therapy; the authors stressed that touch is a low-tech intervention that can increase sleep and well-being in the NICU.[15]

SLEEP IN PRACTITIONERS LEARNING BIOFIELD THERAPIES

In a study by Tang et al., 26 practitioners learning HT were assessed for stress and sleep indicators by VAS before and after a 17.5-hour training course. The study found significant improvement in sleep, anxiety, and well-being from pre- to post-training.[34] Another study on nursing students by Kramer found that those taking courses focused on biofield or energy therapies reported decreased stress, improved concentration, and increased productivity through all self-report data. These students did not mention improved sleep.[35]

ANIMAL RESEARCH

Finally, a study by Buzetti et al. tested the effect of *Johrei* (a Japanese form of biofield healing) on sleep using a mouse model. This complex study design included testing true Johrei, sham Johrei, and no treatment at all on both sleep-interrupted and non-interrupted mice.[36] After the treatments, the researchers directly examined c-fos neurons in the brain; c-fos neuronal activity is known to be less active during sleep and more active during aroused states.[37] Their findings demonstrated that Johrei treatment was significantly associated with better sleep and lower c-fos activity in both mice with interrupted sleep and non-interrupted sleep. This study used a very interesting design as they were able to measure the actual effect of Johrei on the mouse brain tissue.[36]

SUMMARY OF THE DATA ON EM FOR PAIN, ANXIETY, AND STRESS

A few comprehensive systematic reviews have determined that energy therapies reduce pain and anxiety in certain populations. The strongest evidence to date was described in a 2010 systematic review of 66 biofield studies.[38] Results are summarized here:

> Pain measured by a visual analog scale: Evidence level 1
> Pain measured by comprehensive pain scales: Evidence level 4 (conflicting evidence)
> Pain in hospital patients: Evidence level 2
> Pain in postoperative patients: Evidence level 4 (conflicting evidence)
> Cancer pain: Evidence level 2 for acute pain
> Decreased anxiety in hospitalized patients: Evidence level 2
> Dose-response is present ($r = 0.321$, $p = 0.019$)

EM modalities show evidence for shifting autonomic nervous system function to improve health and reduce inflammation. Stress reduction has been demonstrated using TT following a natural disaster (Hurricane Hugo).[39] Wetzel demonstrated a significant increase in hemoglobin and hematocrit levels in healthy persons learning reiki, and Wardell et al. reported decreased blood pressure, increased IgA levels, changes in skin response, and a shift in cortisol following 30 minutes of reiki.[40] Experienced TT practitioners have been able to significantly alleviate anxiety, with the experience of the practitioner positively correlated with the amount of benefit.[41] EM may be a useful adjunct therapy for relaxation and stress management in persons with anxiety disorders.

SUMMARY ON THE EVIDENCE FOR EM AND SLEEP

For sleep, anxiety, and chronic pain, there appears to be enough evidence of effectiveness to support suggesting biofield therapies to those patients with a willingness to try them. The bulk of the evidence is for infants in the NICU, cancer patients, patients with chronic pain, and patients in the ICU. The evidence for the use of biofield therapies as a complementary therapy for sleep is evolving yet not strong enough to recommend them as solo first-line therapy. Nonetheless, since

---

Box 20.2 Energy therapies before sleep: Techniques to use for sleep hygiene

1. Toe-tapping: This is a qi gong technique that can stimulate sleep if done directly before going to sleep. The patient lies on their back, feet bare or with socks on, feet about 12 inches apart. The legs rotate, from the hips, in and out, allowing the metatarsal phalanges joints to tap together at a moderate pace, approximately once per second. The external rotation should go out as far as is comfortable, and the internal rotation stops with the balls of the feet tapping together. This can be done for 2–5+ minutes. Contraindications are pregnancy, recent hip surgery, or joint replacement. Using rhythmic music can help a rhythm to develop as faster tapping is easier.
2. Position before sleep: To achieve the correct energy circuit for sleep, the sleep position that promotes sleep best is to lie on one's back with both hands placed on the thighs right where the thigh meets the leg. If a position change is required for sleep, use this position for 3 minutes before changing position to allow one's self to drift off to sleep.
3. Gentle touch to the head at night: Placing hands on both sides of the head (the cranium) for 3+ minutes and then on both sides of the face (cheeks) for at least 2 minutes can promote energy balancing in the head to promote sleep.
4. Imagining healing energy: A technique from reiki that encourages patients to imagine they are surrounded by a blanket of healing energy as they crawl into bed for sleep.
5. Relaxing breath: Teach patients the 4–7–8 breath. Have them use 4–8 breaths on the way to sleep each night.
6. Guided imagery for sleep: Considered a mind–body technique instead of energy medicine, this is a powerful tool for patients to use with the other energy techniques for sleep. Suggest they buy a pre-recorded audio track to use nightly.

---

there are negligible harmful effects from biofield therapies and it is an easy intervention to use, it may be a good choice for those who have failed other therapies, have comorbid pain, or have a willingness or interest to try them.[15] Healthcare personnel can suggest to patients that they learn techniques from their practitioner so that they can self-administer just prior to sleep. A few of these are suggested in Box 20.2.

CONTRAINDICATIONS FOR ENERGY MEDICINE

Properly used, there are negligible adverse effects from EM modalities. The most common is an occasional increase in the symptom of pain in chronic pain patients following the first few treatments. Since pain is blocked energy, using an energy modality that adds energy to the human energy system can increase pain at or near the points of blockage. This pain typically diminishes within a few hours or a day and dissipates with subsequent treatments. Chronic pain patients need to go very slowly initially with energy modalities, spreading out sessions initially until they are comfortable with the effects of the sessions. If they do not experience pain after a session, then there is no need to lengthen the time between sessions. Skilled practitioners feel that a flair of symptoms represents the beginning of a release of blocked energy, and it typically diminishes and dissipates with subsequent treatments.

Due to the intimacy of healing sessions, patients who have had prior history of sexual abuse or trauma may require special care. Providing an extra layer of cover and having a companion in the room during the session can normally alleviate issues of trust or fear that patients may bring into the room with them. Advise patients to inform the EM practitioner of any issues before they begin to work with the practitioner.

> **Choosing an Energy Practitioner**
> When choosing a pracitioner for referral, I have a few considerations. I choose practitioners that do not "hex" or put down conventional medicine. I tend to choose practitioners that have more experience, at least 3 years, and preferably more than 10 years of expereince. Experience is not equal to expertise, yet I find healers who have been using these techniques longer are, as a group, better. I try to visit the healer myself prior to referring. I will often do this anonymously so I may have a "standard" session to see what my patients will experience.

Referral and Certification

When considering referral to an EM practitioner, it may be helpful to match the patients' belief system to modalities considered for referral. Patients who are seeking adjunctive therapies for pain or related symptoms with an openness or cultural alignment to EM may be appropriate for referral to EM (box 20.3). It can be a useful addition to their medical management, with few side effects. If a patient does not experience positive physical or mental effects within a series of 4–8 visits, discuss this with the patient; it may be more appropriate for them to use their resources on another adjunct complementary modality.

Most EM modalities have websites with certification guidelines and lists of certified practitioners. These include reiki, HT International, TT, polarity therapy, johrei, zero balancing, jin shin jytsu, Barbara Brennan Healing, and Rosalyn Bruyere's work. Since EM skills involve both expertise and sensitivity, counsel patients to consider choosing a practitioner with multiple years of experience.

> **Box 20.3 Energy medicine recommendations for patients with sleep disorders**
>
> Energy Healing has weak evidence data to support its use with pain, sleep, relaxation, and well-being.
>
> Include an energy modality in a multifaceted plan for a patient with sleep disorder if the patient has an open attitude to trying it.
>
> Counsel patients with a sleep disorder and chronic pain to "go slowly" with energy modalities to prevent a flare of symptoms. Encourage them to learn a self-healing energy modality to use at night while readying for sleep (see Box 20.2).
>
> Counsel patients that their sleep should be their guide. If they do not notice a difference in sleep or pain after 6–10 treatments, they may benefit from trying another modality.
>
> Energy modalities are safe, with negligible side effects.

Conclusion

EM is a collection of modalities that work with the body's biofield to promote health and healing. To date, there is minimal research specifically on EM in sleep disorders, although benefit has been shown in patients with chronic pain, cancer-related symptoms, hospitalized patients, and infants in the NICU. Referring patients with sleep issues, especially those with comorbid pain, may improve sleep and can be an important part of an integrative approach for sleep issues. Referral to an experienced practitioner is important, and patients should be educated to record symptoms to see if they have an improvement in quality of life and sleep. Patients who have an interest in EM modalities may be optimal patients to refer, yet belief is not required for benefit.

RESOURCES

This list does not incorporate all modalities, check individual modalities for more information.

- Healing touch: HealingTouchProgram.com
- Reiki schools: Reiki.org
- Barbara Brennan training: barbarabrennan.com
- Therapeutic Touch: http://therapeutic-touch.org

REFERENCES

1. Hurwitz W. Energy medicine In Micozzi MS, ed. *Fundamentals of complementary and alternative medicine*. New York: Churchill Livingstone; 2001: 238–256.

2. Rubik B, Muehsam D, Hammerschlag R, Jain S. Biofield science and healing: History, terminology, and concepts. *Glob Adv Health Med*. 2015 Nov;4(Suppl):8–14.

3. Rubik B, Pavek R, Greene E, Laurence D, Ward R, Al E. Manual healing methods. In Rubik B, et al., eds. *Alternative medicine: Expanding medical horizons: A report to the National Institutes of Health on alternative medical systems and practices in the United States* (NIH Publication). Washington, DC: US Government Printing Office; 1995: 113–157.

4. Chiasson A. *Energy healing: The essentials of self care*. Boulder, CO: Sounds True; 2013.

5. National Center for Complementary and Alternative Medicine (NCCAM). Energy medicine: An overview. *Backgrounder*. National Institute for Health; 2003.

6. Di Nucci EM. Energy healing: A complementary treatment for orthopaedic and other conditions. *Orthop Nurs*. 2005;24(4):259–269.

7. Jain S et al. Biofield science and healing: An emerging frontier in medicine. *Global Adv Health Med*. 2015;4(Suppl):42–51.

8. McCraty R. The energetic heart: Bioelectromagnetic communication within and between people. In Rosch PJ, Markov MS, eds. *Bioelectromagnetic medicine*. New York: Marcel Dekker; 2005:511–530.

9. Di Nucci EM. Energy healing: A complementary treatment for orthopaedic and other conditions. *Orthop Nurs*. 2005;24(4):259–269.

10. Ives J, van Wijk E, Bat N, et al. Ultraweak photon emission as a non-invasive health assessment: A systematic review. *PLoS One*. 2014;9(2):e87401.

11. Konstantin K, Shelkov O, Shevtsov A, et al. Stress reduction with osteopathy assessed with GDV electrophotonic imaging: Effects of osteopathy treatment. *J Alt Compl Med*. 2012;18(3):251–257. doi:10.1089/acm.2010.0853. Erratum in: J Altern Complement Med. 2012 Sep;18(9):887. PMID: 22420738.

12. Muehsam D, Chevalier G, Barsotti T, Gurfein B. An overview of biofield devices. *Glob Adv Health Med*. 2015 Nov;4(Suppl):72–78.

13. Schwartz GE. Biofield detection: Role of bioenergy awareness training and individual differences in absorption. *J Alt Compl Med*. 2004 Feb;10(1):167–169.

14. Clark TC, Black LI, Stussman BJ, Barnes PM, Nahin RL. Trends in the use of complementary health approaches among adults: United States, 2002–2012. *Natl Health Stat Report*. 2015 Feb 10;(79):1–16.

15. Erodgan Z, Atkin D. Complementary health approaches used in the intensive care unit. *Holist Nurs Pract*. 2017 Sept?Oct;31(5):323–343.

16. Hagen LE, Schneider R, Stephens D, Modrusan D, Feldman BM. Use of complementary and alternative medicine by pediatric rheumatology patients. *Arthritis Rheum*. 2003;49(1):3–6.

17. Harris LR, Roberts L. Treatments for irritable bowel syndrome: Patients' attitudes and acceptability. *BMC Compl Alt Med.* 2008;8:65.

18. Marta IE, Baldan SS, Berton AF, Pavam M, da Silva MJ. [The effectiveness of therapeutic touch on pain, depression and sleep in patients with chronic pain: Clinical trial.] *Enferm USP.* 2010 Dec;44(4):1100–1106.

19. Weze C, Leathard HL, Grange J, Tiplady P, Stevens G. Evaluation of healing by gentle touch. *Public Health.* 2005 Jan;119(1):3–10.

20. Gilula MF. Cranial electrotherapy stimulation and fibromyalgia. *Expert Rev Med Devices.* 2007 Jul;4(4):489–495.

21. Shekelle PG, Cook IA, Miake-Lye IM, Booth MS, Beroes JM, Mak S. Benefits and harms of cranial electrical stimulation for chronic painful conditions, depression, anxiety and insomnia: A systematic review. *Ann Intern Med.* 2018 Mar 20;168(6):414–421.

22. Senderovich H, Ip ML, Berall A, et al. Therapeutic touch in a geriatric palliative care unit: A retrospective review. *Complement Ther Clin Pract.* 2016 Aug;24:134–138.

23. Satija A, Bhatnagar S. Complementary therapies for symptom management in cancer patients. *Indian J Palliat Care.* 2017 Oct-Dec;23(4): 468–479.

24. Birocco N et al. The effects of Reiki therapy on pain and anxiety in patients attending a day oncology and infusion services unit. *Am J Hosp Palliat Care.* 2012 Jun;29(4):290–294.

25. Marcus DA, Blazek-O'Neill B, Kopar JL. Symptomatic improvement reported after receiving Reiki at a cancer care infusion center. 2013 Mar;30(2):216–217.

26. Richards K, Nagel C, Markei M, Elwell J, Barone C. Use of complementary and alternative therapies to promote sleep in critically ill patients. *Crit Care Nurs Clin North Am.* 2003 Sept;15(3):329–340.

27. Carniero EM, Moraes GV, Terra GA. Effectiveness of spiritist passe (spiritual healing) on the psychophysiological parameters in hospitalized patients. *Adv Mind Body Med.* 2016 Summer;30(3):4–10.

28. Ishak WW, Kahloon M, Fakhry H. Oxytocin role in enhancing well-being: A literature review, *J Affect Disord.* 2011;130:1–9.

29. Cleveland L, Hill CM, Pulse WS, DiCioccio HC, Field T, White-Traut R. Systematic review of skin-to-skin care for full-term, healthy newborns. *J Obster Gynecol Neonatal Nurs.* 2017 Nov-Dec;46(6):857–869.

30. van den Hoogen A, Teunis CJ, Shellhaas RA, Pillen S, Benders M, Dudink J. How to improve sleep in a neonatal intensive care unit: A systematic review. *Early Hum Dev.* 2017 Oct;113:78–86.

31. Harrison LL, Williams AK, Berbaum ML, Stem JT, Leeper J. Physiologic and behavioral effects of gentle human touch of preterm infants. *Res Nurs Health.* 2000;23:(6):435–446.

32. Bijari BB, Iranmanesh S, Eshghi F, Baneshi MR. Gentle human touch and Yakson: The effect on preterm's behavioral reactions. *ISRN Nurs.* 2012;2012:1–6.

33. Im H, Kim E. Effect of Yakson and gentle human touch versus usual care on urine stress hormones and behaviors in preterm infants: A quasi-experimental study. *Int J Nurs Stud.* 2009;46:450–458.

34. Tang R, Tegeler C, Larrimore D, Cowgill S, Kemper KJ. Improving the well-being of nursing leaders through healing touch training. *J Alt Compl Med.* 2010 Aug;16(8):837–841.

35. Kramer D. Energetic modalities as a self-care technique to reduce stress in nursing students. *J Holist Nurs.* 2017 Dec;36(4):366–373.

36. Buzzetti RA, Hinojosa-Kurtzberg M, Shea TJ, Ibuki Y, Sirakis G, Parthasarathy S. Effect of Johrei therapy on sleep in a murine model. *Explore.* 2013 Mar-Apr;9(2):100–105.

37. Qiu MH, Chen MC, Huang ZL, Lu J. Neuronal activity (c-fos) delineating interactions of the cerebral cortex and basal ganglia. *Front Neuroanat.* 2014 Mar 26;8:13.

38. Jain S, Mills PJ. Biofield therapies: Helpful or full of hype? A best evidence synthesis. *Int J Behav Med.* 2010 Mar;17(1):1–16.

39. Olson M, Sneed N, Bonadonna R, Ratliff J, Dias J. Therapeutic touch and post-Hurricane Hugo stress. *J Holist Nurs.* 1992;10(2):120–136.

40. Miles P, True G. Reiki: Review of biofield therapy, history, theory, practice, and research. *Altern Ther Health Med.* 2003;9(2)62–72.

41. Ferguson CK. *Subjective experience of therapeutic touch (SETTS): Psychometric examination of an instrument.* PhD. dissertation. Austin: University of Texas at Austin; 1986.

42. Field T. Touch for socioemotional and physical well-being: A review. *Developm Rev.* 2010 Dec;30(4):367–383.

43. Papathanassoglu ED, Mpouzika MD. Interpersonal touch: Physiological effects in critical care. *Biol Res Nurs* 2012 Oct;14(4):431–443.

21

Aromatherapy for Sleep

VALERIE CACHO AND MINDY GREEN

Introduction

Aromatherapy is defined as using the essential (volatile) oil extracted from an aromatic plant to improve health and well-being. Essential oils can be targeted for use in specific physical and emotional conditions such as burn wounds and anxiety; they can also be used as supportive agents to bring balance to overall health or aid in palliative care treatments. They are commonly used through inhalation or topical application. When inhaled, essential oils enter the body via the olfactory system and activate the limbic/emotional system, producing physiologic benefits to the mind and body.[1] Research on aromatherapy demonstrates improvement in depression, anxiety, stress, and fatigue as well as blood pressure, pulse, pain, and sleep.[2] Aromatherapy is often combined with other integrative modalities such as acupuncture, massage, and yoga, or it is used in a targeted approach to reduce stress and discomfort in fields such as palliative care. Lavender, which has numerous clinical studies to support its therapeutic use, is an essential oil with sleep-promoting properties. Additional soporific and calming oils with supporting research that will be further discussed include sweet marjoram, sandalwood, jasmine, bergamot, cedarwood, bay laurel, and frankincense. The essential oils of peppermint, sweet orange, and rosemary have stimulating and energizing properties which are useful for people who are excessively tired. This chapter examines the neurobiology and chemistry of aromatherapy and its clinical applications for insomnia and hypersomnia.

History of Aromatherapy

Though the term "aromatherapy" was not coined until the early twentieth century, the fat extraction from fragrant plants has been in use for more than 6,000 years according to historical records found in ancient Egypt and India. From ancient times to the present day, aromatic plants have been a part of the phyto-therapeutic protocol, as both herbs and essential oils. Egyptians used fragrant oils in religious ceremonies, such as mummification, and as medicine. Ayurveda, the traditional medical system of India, incorporates aromatherapy in its meditation practices for balancing the body and mind. In Ayurveda, specific essential oils are used in massage to treat the different "*doshas*" or constitutional types. There are biblical references to using fragrant resins or extracts in ceremonies, as when, per the book of Matthew, the Magi brought frankincense and myrrh as gifts for the Christ child. Lavender was used in medieval times as the remedy for seizures and migraines.[3] Distilled essential oils were not widely available until the 1700s for the noble class and the 1800s for the common consumer. In 1982, the French physician, Jean Valnet, published the book, *The Practice of Aromatherapy*, at a time when essential oil use was increasing in Britain and the United States.[4] Valnet became well-known for his medical application of aromatherapy for wound care on soldiers during World War II.

Science of Aromatherapy

Essential oils were popularized through the study of the chemical constituents after Gattefosse, a French chemist, experienced an extraordinary personal healing with lavender following a burn in his laboratory in 1910.[5] The burgeoning science during the early twentieth century led to the isolation and further study of essential oil components that are frequently seen in published research papers today. Occasionally a whole oil is studied, but, as is typical for an allopathic approach to therapeutics, scientists are searching for the "active compound" in any given plant.

Steam distillation is the main extraction process by which the volatile oils (found in leaves, flowers, seeds, peels, roots, rhizomes, bark, resins, or tree branches) are separated from the various plant parts. Other extraction processes include cold pressing of citrus oils (although in this case, the process may contribute to sun sensitization of the dermis). Hexane processing results in "absolutes," and carbon dioxide (CO_2) extraction creates CO_2 products, but these are less available in the marketplace; jasmine is the only one addressed here.

Through studies on individual constituents, researchers have discovered the pharmacokinetics of how essential oils interact with the human body. Several biochemical constituents of essential oils can produce hypnotic, sedative, or anti-anxiety effects, including acids and esters, coumarins, aldehydes, and monoterpenols. These compounds cross the blood–brain barrier to modulate neuronal function by inducing the secretion of serotonin and endorphins that impact the autonomic nervous system (ANS).[6] The inhalation of different fragrances creates measurable electroencephalographic (EEG) changes from sleepy to alert states (Figure 21.1).[7]

The scientific connection between scent and psyche has been conclusively linked by several authorities to the olfactory system and the limbic brain, including how aroma affects emotions and mental processes. Avery Gilbert, a scent scientist and former president of the Sense of Smell Institute, has published extensively on these findings.[8] Additionally, former Yale psychiatry professor Gary Schwartz believes that fragrance may provide valuable complementary treatment for a host of problems related to emotions.

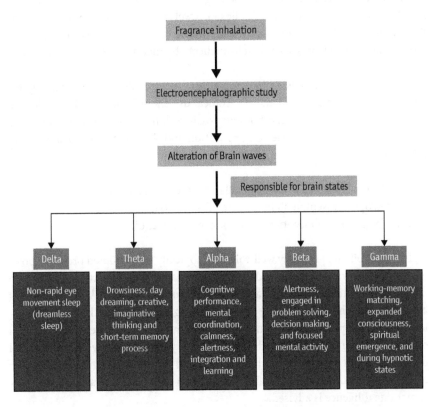

FIGURE 21.1 Fragrance inhalation and electroencephalographic changes.
From Sowndhararajan K, Kim S. Influence of fragrances on human psychophysiological activity: With special reference to human electroencephalographic response. Viernstein H, ed. *Scientia Pharmaceutica*. 2016;84(4):724–752.

Essential Oils 101

In aromatherapy practice the selection of an essential oil is individualized or custom formulated depending on the therapeutic effect(s) desired and the patient's preference of aroma. Commercial products are pre-blended for direct use on the skin, but undiluted oils must be added to a carrier oil, such as sunflower, apricot, coconut, almond, or other fatty oil. Perception of an essential oil as pleasant or unpleasant significantly impacts the user's experience, which can lead to therapeutic benefit without objective evidence to support its utility.[5] The safest and most common application is through direct inhalation from the vial or drops on a cotton gauze or through vaporization with a diffuser. Cutaneous absorption occurs through massage when the essential oil(s) is mixed with a carrier oil or lotion. Oral application is controversial, as not all oils are safe for ingestion and this delivery route should not be undertaken by the public. Currently, there are a few legitimate companies marketing essential oils as dietary supplements, mostly as capsules. One example is Silexan, a well-researched oral lavender essential oil capsule, which is discussed further in the lavender section of this chapter. One should not self-prescribe or self-medicate by ingesting homemade essential oil preparations.

The essential oils discussed here are generally nontoxic and nonirritating, especially when used as an inhalation. Topical use should not exceed 2% dilution. Individual reactions may vary, but any possible skin irritation is temporary and can be quelled by plain carrier oil application and the use of a lower dilution in future applications.

2% dilution (10 drops of essential oil in 1 ounce of carrier oil)
1% (5 drops of essential oil in 1 ounce of carrier oil)
0.5% (2–3 drops of essential oil in 1 ounce of carrier oil)

Essential oils are generally well-tolerated topically when diluted properly, however some safety concerns include contact dermatitis from direct exposure to an undiluted oil, photosensitivity reaction with sun or ultraviolet (UV) light (tanning bed) exposure, the unwitting use of synthetic fragrance oils, and the potential toxicity to a developing baby with use during pregnancy or breastfeeding. Essential oils also should not be used by children under 2 years of age. Given that essential oil quality is not monitored by the US Food and Drug Administration (FDA) or other organizations, the quality and composition of the oils are variable, and consumer due diligence is advised.

It is imperative that the product guarantee botanical sourcing and not be synthetically produced or contain artificial fragrance. Labels should be searched for the scientific (Latin) name of the plant, and, when in doubt, the manufacturer should be contacted. Essential oils should be stored away from heat and light and have a reasonable shelf life of about 2 years for citrus oils and 5 years for others. For accidental or excessive use that results in skin irritation, simple application of an unscented vegetable oil such as olive, almond, or sunflower to the affected area can be used as treatment. Further information is provided by the International Fragrance Association guidelines (http://www.ifraorg.org/en-us/standards), which are followed by most large cosmetics companies.

Aromatherapy for Sleep Promotion

Using aromatherapy to induce sleep is an attractive therapy given the low side-effect profile of essential oils when compared to hypnotic pharmaceutical agents. The mechanisms by which the oils produce their hypnotic, sedative, or anti-anxiety effects have not been completely elucidated because they affect multiple biochemical and psychological systems.[6] There are a limited number of appropriately designed clinical trials using aromatherapy for sleep, and most studies have small sample sizes of around 10–60 subjects. Studies on the use of essential oils for relaxation, stress reduction, and parasympathetic nervous system (PNS) support are included in this section.

LAVENDER (*LAVANDULA ANGUSTIFOLIA, LAVANDUA* SPP.)

Lavender is an aromatic evergreen shrub native to the Mediterranean and used widely in perfumes, cosmetics, and household cleaning solutions for its floral fragrance. It is the most popular essential oil associated with sleep given its anxiolytic and sedative effects. The active constituents of lavender that produce sedation, linalool and linalyl acetate, are involved with serotonergic transmission.[9] In a small study of geriatric patients dependent on benzodiazepines, substitution of the benzodiazepine with a lavender essential oil resulted in the restoration of sleep after withdrawal of the benzodiazepine.[3] Decreases in sympathetic nervous system (SNS) drive as measured by the lowering of blood pressure, heart rate, and skin temperature have been observed in healthy volunteers after inhalation of lavender essential oil.[10] Additionally, lavender increases non–rapid eye movement (NREM) sleep and decreases nighttime awakenings.[11] An oral lavender oil capsule studied in Germany, Silexen, has been found to be comparable to the benzodiazepine lorazepam in a 6-week controlled clinical trial for patients with general anxiety disorder. Silexen is a safe, non–habit forming alternative to lorazepam and was also shown to alleviate anxiety related to disturbed sleep.[12] As compared to benzodiazepines, no withdrawal symptoms are associated with abrupt discontinuation of Silexen.[13] In the United States, Silexan (also sold as Lasea) is marketed as the dietary supplement Calm Aid by Nature's Way.

Inhalation of lavender essential oil has been shown to be beneficial in the healthy population and in people with insomnia. In a randomized controlled study (RCT) of 18 healthy Japanese students, exposure to lavender essential oil at bedtime for 5 days resulted in an improvement in subjective levels of sleepiness upon awakening.[14] For healthy adults and nursing home residents with insomnia, various RCTs on the inhalation of lavender prior to bedtime have shown clinical improvement in the Pittsburgh Sleep Quality Index (PSQI), a questionnaire measuring sleep quality and disturbance.[10,15,16] Improvements in sleep quality, stress, and anxiety levels were observed in acutely hospitalized patients in intensive care units in Turkey and South Korea after inhalation of lavender.[17,18]

SWEET MARJORAM (*ORIGANUM MAJORANA;* AKA *MAJORANA HORTENSIS*)

Similar to lavender, sweet marjoram is native to the Mediterranean and is best known as a culinary herb. Historically it has been used for respiratory and musculoskeletal conditions. Sweet marjoram contains linalyl acetate, linalool, terpinen-4-ol, and other monoterpenes which are proposed to support sleep, but study data are inconclusive. In a study of 50 female night shift nurses, sweet marjoram inhalation resulted in improvements in daytime dysfunction, sleep quality, and sleep disturbance when compared to controls.[19]

SANDALWOOD (*SANTALUM ALBUM, S. SPICATUM*)

As sandalwood (*Santalum album*) is considered an endangered plant in India, so essential oils from cultivated Australian (*S. spicatum*) plants are recommended. The main constituent of sandalwood attributed to sedation is santalol. A Viennese study of 36 healthy adults measured various physiological parameters of ANS activity along with self-ratings of arousal after inhaling sandalwood (*S. album*, Santalaceae) essential oil or alpha-santalol via a nebulizer for 20 minutes. In the alpha-santalol cohort, both attentiveness and relaxation scores were higher, offering a treatment for situations in which one would need to be simultaneously alert and calm.[20]

JASMINE (*JASMINE OFFICINALE* AND *J. GRANDIFLORUM*)

Jasmine is a fragrant white-flowered shrub native to west Asia and India and is known for its strong floral aroma. It is extracted with hexane as an *absolute*, not distilled as an essential oil, because heat destroys the fragrance. Historical uses include the treatment of liver dysfunction, headaches, pain, and insomnia.

Inhaled jasmine essential oil is associated with increased sleep efficiency, improved cognitive processing speed, and decreased levels of anxiety in healthy college students.[21]

BERGAMOT (*CITRUS BERGAMIA*)

Bergamot is an inedible citrus fruit native to southern Italy and Greece and is a hybrid between lemon and bitter orange. It is extracted through cold expression, not distillation. Bergamot's peel is the source of the essential oil which is used medicinally for its antiseptic, antibacterial, analgesic, and anti-anxiety effects.[22] Limonene, the main constituent of bergamot, has been shown to induce the release of serotonin, a neurotransmitter involved in mood stabilization.[23] Anxiety, physiological stress, and a heightened SNS response are major contributors to sleep disturbances, and studies suggest that bergamot may be beneficial in reducing the stress response. In a small study performed on healthy female university students inhaling bergamot essential oil for 15 minutes, lower levels of cortisol were measured from their saliva. PNS activity, as measured by high-frequency heart rate variability, was significantly increased in the bergamot-exposed group, suggesting a modulating effect of bergamot on the ANS toward a resting state. Moreover, positive effects on mood, anxiety, and fatigue were observed in the bergamot group.[24] After 10 minutes of inhaling diffused bergamot essential oil, highly stressed elementary teachers in Taiwan had statistically significant reductions blood pressure and heart rate. They also exhibited increased PNS activity, thus supporting the claim of bergamot's ability to alleviate stress.[25]

Any topical use of bergamot should only be from a "bergapten-free" product. This is the photosensitizing agent that is problematic with UV light exposure. This should be noted on the product label, or the manufacturer can be contacted for further information.

CEDARWOOD (*CEDRUS ATLANTICA, C. DEODARA*)

Cedrus atlantica is found native in Algeria in the Atlas Mountains and is characterized as a sweet and woody fragrance. Cedarwood should not be confused with several species of *Juniperus*, often labeled with the common name of "cedar." Cedarwood is used medicinally in skin care and for arthritis, congestion, and cough. Research shows that cedrol, a sesquiterpene alcohol found in cedarwood and several other conifer oils (*Cupressus* spp., *Juniperus* spp.) can promote relaxation in stressful events.[26] The autonomic effects of inhaled cedrol were examined in healthy adults by measuring blood pressure, heart rate, and respiratory rate. Researchers found a significant increase in PNS and a decrease in SNS activity with exposure to cedrol, exemplifying its relaxation effect.[27]

BAY LAUREL (*LAURUS NOBILIS*)

Native to the eastern Mediterranean region and popularized by the Romans, bay laurel is described as spicy and strong in scent. It has been used to treat conditions of the digestive system, bronchitis, and flu. Bay laurel is also used as a fragrant herb for cooking. A piperonyl also known as heliotropin is extracted from several plants of the Lauraceae family and has been shown to promote sleep both objectively and subjectively in healthy adults and those with insomnia. Polysomnogram data performed on 12 university students exposed to heliotropin for 30 minutes after lights-off showed a decrease in sleep latency and an increase in total sleep time, sleep efficiency, and total amount of REM sleep as compared to controls. Adults with insomnia who inhaled heliotropin prior to bedtime reported feeling refreshed in the morning.[28]

FRANKINCENSE (*BOSWELLIA* SPP.)

The etymology of the word "frankincense" is French, meaning "pure incense"; it is also known by its ancient name, *olibanum*. The essential oil is created from the oleogum resin of trees in the *Boswellia* genus found in west Africa and the Middle East. The biological activities of *Boswellia* essential oils include acetylcholine esterase inhibition, and it is known as an antioxidant, antimicrobial, anticancer, and antibiofilm agent.[29]

A small study was performed in a cancer center in the United Kingdom to determine the utility of aromatherapy on cancer patients with sleep problems. Patients were provided with aroma sticks (small personal inhalers) of Frankincense (*Boswellia carterii*) used in a blend with mandarin (*Citrus reticulata*) and lavender essential oils (*Lavandula angustifolia*). By self-report before and after two nights of using the aroma stick, 64% of patients noted improvement in sleep.[30]

OIL BLENDS

A combination of intentionally formulated blends of essential oils can also be designed to promote relaxation and sleep quality, as shown by the following research studies.

In a small study in Japan, adults with dementia living in care facilities received inhaled aromatherapy with the following oils: true lavender (*Lavandula angustifolia*); true lavender blended with sweet orange (*Citrus sinensis*); or a blend of Japanese cypress (*Chamaecyparis obtusa*), Virginian cedarwood (*Juniperus virginiana*), cypress (*Cupressus sempervirens*), and pine (*Pinus* spp.) oil. Longer sleep time and decreased early morning awakenings were found during the 20 days of nightly exposure to the oils.[31]

Poor sleep and fatigue are commonly observed in patients with end-stage renal disease on hemodialysis. A randomized clinical study of 62 hemodialysis patients examined the effects of a 1:1 lavender and sweet orange essential oil blend using the PSQI and Piper fatigue scales. Nightly inhalation of these oils for 1 month prior to bedtime resulted in improved sleep quality and decreased levels of fatigue.[32]

An RCT of the essential oil blend of lemon, eucalyptus, tea tree, and peppermint in a ratio of 4:2:2:1 was performed to evaluate its effects on stress and sleep quality. Participants in the aromatherapy group were exposed to this blend day and night through a pendant and aromatherapy stone, respectively, for 4 weeks. Compared to controls, those in the aromatherapy group had lower levels of perceived stress and depression and improved sleep quality.[33]

A nursing invention study was performed on 56 patients in an intensive care unit in Korea. Patients received aromatherapy before and after percutaneous intervention for coronary artery disease. A blend of lavender (*L. officinalis*), roman chamomile (*Chamaemelum nobile*), and neroli (*Citrus aurantium*) in a 6:2:0.5 ratio was given to each patient. Patients reported lower anxiety and improved sleep quality compared to those only receiving conventional nursing care.[34]

Historically and anecdotally, other essential oils used by aromatherapists to promote relaxation and induce sleep include geranium (*Pelargonium graveolens*), Roman chamomile (*Chamaemelum nobile, Anthemis nobilis*), German chamomile (*Matricaria recutita, M. chamomilla*), clary sage (*Salvia sclaria*), orange (*Citrus sinensis*), vetiver (*Vetiveria zizanioides*), and ylang ylang (*Cananga odorata*).

Aromatherapy as a Stimulant

There is a dearth of research supporting the use of aromatherapy as a stimulant, as compared to its use for relaxation and sleep. The handful of evidence supporting essential oils that boost energy and increase arousal and alertness is discussed here.

PEPPERMINT (*MENTHA PIPERITA*)

Peppermint is a popular herb found throughout American and Europe. Peppermint is a stimulating scent and has been demonstrated to increase alertness and attention.[35] Researchers discovered that subjects exposed to peppermint oil showed less pupil dilation, an objective measure of daytime sleepiness also known as the *pupillary unrest index*, suggesting that peppermint oil reduces sleepiness.[36]

Twenty-one healthy adults underwent a polysomnogram with intermittent exposure to peppermint oil or water that they inhaled from vials. An increased amount of NREM sleep and total sleep time was observed in those exposed to peppermint oil. As compared to water, peppermint oil was found to improve mood and reduce sleepiness.[37]

SWEET ORANGE (*CITRUS SINENSIS*)

Sweet orange is an evergreen tree native to China, and its fruit is ingested commonly as food or beverage. Sweet orange oil is non-photosensitizing, and, in one study, the essential oil was given to healthy male graduate students before taking an anxiety-provoking word color test. The intervention group had lower levels of anxiety and reported feeling more energetic.[38]

ROSEMARY (*ROSMARINUS OFFICINALIS*)

Rosemary is an aromatic shrub of the mint family cultivated throughout the world and used to enrich the flavor of meats, foods, and spirits. It is considered an antioxidant in addition to its antispasmodic, analgesic, antiseptic, and tonic effects. Rosemary essential oil has been used medicinally for digestive, respiratory, nervous, and circulatory conditions. Inhaling rosemary aroma has been associated with increased alertness via EEG changes showing decreased frontal alpha and beta power in addition to its known effects of stimulating the SNS.[39,40]

Historically and anecdotally, the following essential oils have been used to stimulate energy and uplift the mood: spearmint, eucalyptus, pine, fir, spruce, tea tree, ginger, cinnamon, clary sage.

Conclusion

Essential oils are an effective adjunct to a variety of integrative therapies for healthy adults or those who suffer from a sleep disturbance, anxiety, or stress. The simplest way to understand how the sense of smell can help reduce stress is to observe what happens during the inhalation of an aroma that is perceived as pleasing: we take a deeper breath. The act of inhaling deeply can reduce heart rate, calm the nervous system, and contribute to a host of relaxing physiological events. Smelling a pleasant fragrance is soothing to the nervous systems for a variety of reasons that the recipient need not even be aware of. Aromatherapy is an easy, inexpensive, and relaxing therapy that contributes to a calmer demeanor and a better night's sleep or provides a stimulating effect to improve daytime energy. Tables 21.1 and 21.2

Table 21.1 Aromatherapy formulas for supporting sleep and relaxation

Peaceful Dreams	Nighty Night	Somnifera	Floral Slumber	Pillow Deep
Lavender 6 drops	Bergamot 4 drops	Sandalwood 5 drops	Rose 4 drops	Lavender 4 drops
Neroli 2 drops	Lavender 3 drops	Cedarwood 3 drops	Lavender 4 drops	Frankincense 4 drops
Frankincense 2 drops	Sweet marjoram 3 drops	Bay laurel 2 drops	Ylang Ylang 2 drops	Sweet Marjoram 2 drops

Table 21.2 Aromatherapy formulas for supporting stimulation and to boost mood

Get up and go	Accelerate	Hearten	Rise and Shine	Spice Me Up
Rosemary 6 drops	Rosemary 4 drops	Pine 5 drops	Fir 4 drops	Spruce 4 drops
Orange 2 drops	Eucalyptus 3 drops	Spearmint 3 drops	Orange 3 drops	Ginger 3 drops
Peppermint 2 drops	Ginger 3 drops	Clary Sage 2 drops	Rosemary 3 drops	Cinnamon 3 drops

provide suggested formulations for at-home treatments for those with difficulty initiating or maintaining sleep, or who are excessively sleepy.

REFERENCES

1. Hwang E, Shin S. The effects of aromatherapy on sleep improvement: A systematic literature review and meta-analysis. *J Alt Compl Med.* 2015;21(2):61–68.
2. Won SJ, Chae YR. The effects of aromatherapy massage on pain, sleep, and stride length in the elderly knee osteoarthritis. *J Korean Biol Nurs Sci.* 2011;13:142–148.
3. Koulivand P, Ghadiri M, Gorji A. Lavender and the nervous system. *Evidence-Based Compl Alt Med.* 2013: Article ID 681304.
4. PDQ Integrative, Alternative, and Complementary Therapies Editorial Board. Aromatherapy and essential oils (PDQ®): Health professional version. 2017 Dec 13. PDQ Cancer Information Summaries [Internet]. Bethesda (MD): National Cancer Institute (US); 2002. https://www.ncbi.nlm.nih.gov/books/NBK65874/
5. Thomas D. Aromatherapy: Mythical, magical, or medicinal? *Holistic Nurs Pract.* 2002;17(1):8–16.
6. Lillehei A, Halcon L. A systemic review of the effect of inhaled essential oils on sleep. *J Alt Compl Med.* 2014;20(6):441–451.
7. Sowndhararajan K, Kim S. Influence of fragrances on human psychophysiological activity: With special reference to human electroencephalographic response. Viernstein H, ed. *Scientia Pharmaceutica.* 2016;84(4):724–752.

8. Gilbert AN. *What the nose knows: The science of scent in everyday life.* New York: Crown Publishers; 2008.

9. Pergentino de Sousa D, Hocayen P, Andrade L, Andreatini R. A systemic review of the anxiolytic-like effects of essential oils in animal models. *Molecules.* 2015;20:18620–18660. doi:10.3390/molecules201018620.

10. Sayorwan W, Siripornpanich V, Pirapunyaporn, Hongratanaworakit T, Kotchabhakdi N, Ruangrungshi N. The effects of lavender oil inhalation on emotional states, autonomic nervous system, and brain electrical activity. *J Med Assoc Thai.* 2012 April;95(4):598–606.

11. Chien L, Cheng S, Liu C. The effect of lavender aromatherapy on autonomic nervous system in midlife women with insomnia. *Evidence-Based Compl Alt Med.* 2011;2012: Article ID 740813.

12. Woelk H, Schläfke S. A multi-center, double-blind, randomized study of the Lavender oil preparation Silexan in comparison to Lorazepam for generalized anxiety disorder. *Phytomedicine.* 2010 Feb. 17:94–99.

13. Gastpar M, Müller WE, Volz HP, Möller HJ, Schläfke S, Dienel A, Kasper S. Silexan does not cause withdrawal symptoms even when abruptly discontinued. *Int J Psychiatry Clin Pract.* 2017;21(3):177–180.

14. Hirokawa K, Nishimoto T, Taniguchi T. Effects of lavender aroma on sleep quality in healthy Japanese students. *Percept Motor Skills.* 2012;114(1):111–122.

15. Lewith G, Godfrey A, Prescott P. A single-blinded, randomized pilot study evaluating the aroma of *Lavandula augustifolia* as a treatment for mild insomnia. *J Alt Compl Med.* 2005; Aug 1(4):631–637.

16. Faydali S, Cetinkaya F. The effect of aromatherapy on sleep quality of elderly people residing in a nursing home. *Holistic Nurs Pract.* 2018;Jan/Feb;32(1):8–16.

17. Karadag E, Samancioglu S, Ozden D, Bakir E. Effects of aromatherapy on sleep quality and anxiety of patients. *Nurs Crit Care.* 2017;22(2):105–112.

18. Cho E, Lee M, Hur M. The effects of aromatherapy on intensive care unit patients' stress and sleep quality: A nonrandomised controlled trial. *Evidenced-Based Compl Alt Med.* 2017: Article ID 2856592.

19. Chang Y, Lin C-L, Chang L-Y. The effects of aromatherapy massage on sleep quality of nurses on monthly rotating night shifts. *Evidence-Based Compl Alt Med.* 2017: Article ID 3861273.

20. Heuberger E, Hongratanaworakit T, Buchbauer G. East Indian sandalwood and alpha-santalol odor increase physiological and self-rated arousal in humans. *Planta Med.* 2006;72:792–800.

21. Raudenbush R, Koon J, Smith J, Zoladz P. Effects of odorant administration on objective and subjective measures of sleep quality, post-sleep mood and alertness, and cognitive performance. *N Am J Psychol.* 2003;5(2):181–192.

22. Navarra M, Mannucci C, Delbo M, Calapai G. *Citrus bergamia* essential oil: From basic research to clinical application. *Front Pharmacol.* 2015 Mar;6: Article 36.

23. Yun J. Limonene inhibits methamphetamine-induced locomotor activity *via* regulation of 5-HT neuronal function and dopamine release. *Phytomedicine.* 2014 May;21(6):883–887.

24. Watanabe E, Kuchta K, Kimura M, Rauwald HW, Kamei T, Imanishi J. Effects of bergamot (*Citrus bergamia* (Risso) Wright & Arn.) essential oil aromatherapy on mood states, parasympathetic nervous system activity, and salivary cortisol levels in 41 healthy females. *Forsch Komplementmed.* 2015;22:43–49.

25. Chang K, Shen C. Aromatherapy benefits autonomic nervous system regulation for elementary school faculty in Taiwan. *Evidence-Based Compl Alt Med.* 2011: Article ID 946537.

26. Komori T, Tamura Y, Mitsui M, Matsui J, Uei D, Aoki S. A preliminary study to investigate relaxation and sleep-inducing effects of cedrol. *Open Access J Sci Tech.* 2016;4: Article ID 101228.

27. Dayawansa S, Umeno K, Takakura H, et al. Autonomic responses during inhalation of natural fragrance of Cedrol in humans. *Auton Neurosci.* 2003 Oct 31;108(1–2):79–86.

28. Yamagishi R, Yokomaku A, Omoto F, et al. Sleep-improving effects of the aromatic compound heliotropin. *Sleep Biol Rhythms.* 2010 Oct;8:254–260.

29. Hussain H, Al-Harrasi A, Al-Rawahi A, Hussain J. Chemistry and biology of essential oils of genus *Boswellia*. *Evidence-Based Compl Alt Med.* 2014;2014:792517.

30. Dyer J, Cleary L, McNeill S, Rahsdale-Lowe M, Osland C. The use of aromasticks to help with sleep problems: A patient experience survey. *Compl Ther Clin Pract.* 2010;22:51–58.

31. Takeda A, Watanuki W, Koyama S. Effects of inhalation aromatherapy on symptoms of sleep disturbance in the elderly with dementia. *Evidence-Based Compl Alt Med.* 2017;2017: Article ID 1902807.

32. Muz G, Tasci S. Effect of aromatherapy via inhalation on the sleep quality and fatigue level in people undergoing hemodialysis. *Appl Nurs Res.* 2017 Oct;27:26–35.

33. Lee M, Lim S, Song J, Kim M, Hur M. The effects of aromatherapy essential oil inhalation on stress, sleep quality and immunity in healthy adults: Randomized controlled trial. *Eur J Integrat Med.* 2017;12:70–86.

34. Cho M-Y, Min ES, Hur M-H, Lee MS. Effects of aromatherapy on the anxiety, vital signs, and sleep quality of percutaneous coronary intervention patients in intensive care units. *Evidence-Based Compl Alt Med.* 2013; Article ID 381381. http://doi.org/10.1155/2013/381381

35. Barker S, Grayhem P, Koon J, Perkins J, Whalen A, Raudenbush B. Improved performance on clerical tasks associated with administration of peppermint odor. *Percept Motor Skills.* 2003;97:1007–1010.

36. Norrish M, Dwyer KL. Preliminary investigation of the effect of peppermint oil on an objective measure of daytime sleepiness. *Int J Psychophysiol.* 2005 Mar;55(3):291–298.

37. Goel N, Lao R. Sleep changes vary by odor perception in young adults. *Biol Psychol.* 2006 Mar;71(3):341–349.

38. Goes TC, Antunes FD, Alves PB, et al. Effect of sweet orange aroma on experimental anxiety in humans. *J Alt Compl Med.* 2012;18:798–804.

39. Diego MA, Jones NA, Field T, et al. Aromatherapy positively affects mood, EEG patterns of alertness and math computations. *Int J Neurosci.* 1998;96:217–224.
40. Sayorwan W, Ruangrungsi N, Piriyapunyporn T, Hongratanaworakit T, Kotchabhakdi N, Siripornpanich V. Effects of inhaled rosemary oil on subjective feelings and activities of the nervous system. *Scientia Pharmaceutica.* 2013;81(2):531–542.

22

Functional Medicine and Sleep

JOSÉ COLÓN

The field of functional medicine is relatively recent, but it has become increasingly popular as patients seek complementary approaches to conventional medicine. While various definitions of functional medicine exist, the Cleveland Clinic uses the following: "Functional Medicine is a personalized, systems-oriented model that empowers patients and practitioners to achieve the highest expression of health by working in collaboration to address the underlying causes of disease." Important points in that definition are both the patient-oriented approach and the goal of determining underlying causes of disease.

The systems-biology model of functional medicine consists of seven core physiological processes, defined as Assimilation and Elimination, Detoxification, Defense, Cellular Communications, Cellular Transport, Energy, and Structure. This model differs from the conventional organ systems approach in which individual organs are viewed as having different disease processes. Through the lens of functional medicine, the function of each core process and their interconnections are assessed to determine their role in creating health or contributing to a progressive state of chronic disease.

The appropriate treatment of sleep disorders involves taking a detailed history, conducting a physical exam, and obtaining any necessary diagnostic studies such as polysomnography. Through that process a diagnosis may be revealed; for example, a polysomnogram may identify sleep apnea, or a multiple sleep latency test (MSLT) may be consistent with narcolepsy. At other times, studies may be unrevealing, resulting in a blanket diagnosis of insomnia or somatization. In conventional medicine, an evaluation may end when a diagnosis is reached, at which point a treatment plan is initiated. In functional medicine, however, this is often a point of entry. Accurate diagnosis in sleep medicine is critically important as many sleep disorders may present with a complaint of nonrestorative sleep, but each requires different treatment modalities.

The Functional Medicine Approach to Sleep Disorders

A functional medicine approach seeks to find the underlying upstream causes and any triggering factors that have led to the diagnosis. Dr. Patrick Hanaway, former director of the Institute for Functional Medicine (IFM), states, "Functional medicine is like a root cause analysis." This root cause approach can be applied to many medical disorders, including sleep disorders. Interestingly, Dr. Hanaway's statement mirrors that of Kryger's *Principles and Practice of Sleep Medicine*, "Insomnia may best be viewed as a symptom rather than a disease process. Often, it accompanies another cause or disorder." The functional medicine approach to diagnosis demands not only that a determination is made of what disease a patient is suffering from, but also that the underlying physiological dysfunctions and underlying causes are identified.[1] Underlying both integrative medicine and functional medicine is the belief that good medicine is based in good science (Figure 22.1).

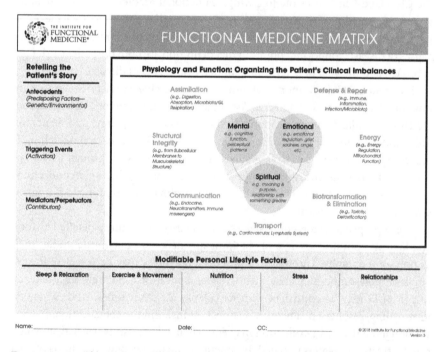

FIGURE 22.1 The Functional Medicine Matrix from the Institute for Functional Medicine.

Functional medicine recognizes that illness does not occur in isolation. Similarly, sleep disorders do not occur in a vacuum because clinical imbalances that lead to illnesses may subsequently affect sleep, and sleep disruption and circadian dysregulation affect chronic disease. The Functional Medicine Matrix helps clinicians examine the body systems, symptoms, and risk factors associated with a specific condition. The matrix provides a template for the clinician to organize the patient's clinical imbalances in the following biological systems, called *nodes*: defense and repair, energy, biotransformation and elimination, transport, communication, structural integrity, and assimilation.

The left section of the matrix is useful in retelling the patient's story by tracking antecedents, triggering events, and mediators/perpetuators. The bottom of the matrix details lifestyle factors like sleep and relaxation, exercise and movement, nutrition and hydration, stress and resilience, and relationships and networks. As a whole, the Functional Medicine Matrix assists the clinician in organizing and prioritizing each patient's health issues, including sleep disorders, as elicited by a thorough personal, family, social, and medical history. The matrix is a tool for organizing what seem to be disparate issues into a complete story to help the clinician gain a comprehensive perspective of the patient and subsequently facilitate discussion of complex health issues, including chronic disease and sleep disorders.

In conventional medicine it is common to have several diagnoses, each with a distinct treatment plan. If the underlying root causes are not identified, a medication may ameliorate the symptoms, but the disease process may still progress. Medications have the potential to cause side effects, which can lead to new diagnoses that are perceived as separate illnesses. One of the key principles of functional medicine is that no illness typically happens in isolation, but rather presents over time in association with an emerging picture of clinical concern.

Viewing the patient's presenting signs and symptoms through the lens of the patient's timeline and seven core physiological processes of the functional medicine approach offers a vivid illustration of this. It is important to identify the "ATMs"—that is, the Antecedents, Triggering Events, and Mediators/Perpetuators of disease—as well as to identify modifiable personal lifestyle factors that influence health; without addressing these, disease progression is likely to occur. Upon determining the imbalances, two simple questions can be asked: (1) Does the patient need to eliminate something (toxin, allergen, infection, poor diet, stress)?[2] Does the patient have an unmet individual need that is required for optimal function?

To address sleep disorders using a functional medicine approach, it is important to review and leverage the scientific literature identifying the causes of sleep disturbances. It is equally important to understand the deleterious effects that disruptions in sleep and sleep disorders create on the rest of the body when viewed through a systems biology approach. In this chapter we explore and provide examples of the bidirectional nature of system imbalances and sleep.

Assimilation

The process of assimilation is a key component of quality sleep, with influences observed down to the molecular level. Assimilation includes digestion, absorption, the microbiota, and respiration. Food provides both macronutrients and micronutrients that must be broken down in the process of digestion, and the absorption of these nutrients can impact sleep-related hormone production and conversion. For example, 3% of dietary tryptophan is used to synthesize serotonin,[3] 95% of which is found within the gastrointestinal tract,[2] while melatonin is a hormone produced downstream in the tryptophan/serotonin pathway.[4]

There are more bacterial cells in the intestinal tract than there are human cells in the human body, and these bacteria form the gastrointestinal microbiome.[5] Impairments in assimilation of nutrients for us or our microbiome can alter the gut–brain paradigm and affect sleep.

Reviewing food logs and medication lists can be helpful in assessing assimilation. Medications are commonly noted to have "side effects," however biochemistry-based science commonly reveals these to be direct effects on assimilation. For example, some cardiovascular medications can negatively affect assimilation in ways that impact sleep. Digoxin reduces tubular magnesium reabsorption, and both loop and thiazide-like diuretics increase magnesiuresis[6]; low magnesium levels have been associated with poorer sleep quality. Beta-blockers have been shown to decrease melatonin release via specific inhibition of adrenergic beta 1-receptors.[7] Studies show that insomnia is associated with an increased risk of developing cardiovascular disease,[8] but medications used to treat this may in turn detrimentally affect sleep.

In viewing assimilation through the functional medicine lens, there are several approaches that can be taken to identify or treat imbalances that may affect sleep. Running micronutrient analyses may identify deficiencies that can contribute to insomnia or fatigue, and identifying such a deficiency may assist in targeting certain foods or guide the selection of appropriate supplementation for replenishment. In a patient who requires cardiac medications that affect the assimilation of magnesium or melatonin, supplementation for adequate support may be appropriate. In a patient with restless legs syndrome (RLS), commercially available small intestinal bowel overgrowth (SIBO) testing may be appropriate as SIBO has been associated with RLS. Methods of repairing dysbiosis, treating SIBO, and other clinical approaches to treating gastrointestinal imbalances can be conducted through functional medicine's classical "4R" approach: the Remove, Replace, Reinoculate, and Repair protocol.[5,9] More recent approaches include a "5R" approach that includes Rebalance, which uses the practice of relaxation techniques to rectify stress–life–work imbalances that can adversely affect gut integrity.

Biotransformation and Elimination

When assessing sleep and sleep disorders through the systems of biotransformation and elimination, the burden of toxic exposures must be considered. Toxic exposures and an elevated body burden may affect sleep, and likewise sleep has implications for detoxification as well.

Sleep has an important role in optimal detoxification. The brain has a unique waste management system, known as the *glymphatic system*, which is active during sleep. The glymphatic system pumps cerebral spinal fluid through the brain's tissues, flushing the metabolic waste from the brain into the bloodstream and the liver for elimination.[10]

Sleep is also very important for optimal liver health, which is crucial for the elimination of toxic substances. Short sleep duration and poor sleep quality have been significantly associated with an increased risk of nonalcoholic fatty liver disease in middle-aged adults,[11] and obstructive sleep apnea (OSA) is associated with liver injury due to hypoxia.[12] Liver disease has also been demonstrated to impair sleep quality. Patients with cirrhosis often have sleep–wake abnormalities, and the quality of their sleep has been observed to be significantly worse than that of healthy subjects.[13]

Toxic exposures can affect sleep as well. Loge-transformed bisphenol A (BPA) levels may be associated with fewer hours of sleep among US adults.[14] Arsenic, heavy metals, phthalate, pesticides, polyaromatic hydrocarbons, and polyfluoroalkyl compounds have been associated with sleep disturbances, and their elimination has been suggested to improve sleep health.[15]

In viewing biotransformation and elimination through the functional medicine lens, there are several approaches that can be taken to identify or treat imbalances that may affect sleep. The Toxin Exposure Questionnaire (TEQ-20) is used to identify possible sources of exposure from the community and home including occupations, hobbies, medications, and dental work. In a toxic exposure history, the timeline is critical to identifying when the sleep disturbance presented and how it has fluctuated over time. Tests for toxins and for measures of oxidative stress are commercially available. Once a toxin or an imbalance in the detoxification system is identified, measures for lowering the toxic burden can be implemented through diet, lifestyle, and other strategies. There is no one single "detoxification protocol" for better sleep per se; however, identification of *xenobiotics* (substances that are foreign to the body or to an ecological system) that are contributing to impaired sleep may help determine the appropriate detoxification methods. In functional medicine, when a detoxification protocol is prescribed, adequate sleep and identification of sleep disorders should be included as part of the protocol.

Defense and Repair

The processes of defense and repair involve the interactions among our immune system, inflammation, infections, and, once again, our microbiota. These systems have bidirectional findings on sleep health.

Sleep and the circadian system exert a strong regulatory influence on immune functions. Research following a systems approach of neuroimmunology indicates that sleep enhances immune defense, confirming the popular wisdom that "sleep helps healing."[16] Furthermore, sleep loss impairs immune function, and sleep is altered during infection, which may impact survival.[17]

Sleep affects the immune system, but infections also can affect sleep. For example, Lyme disease causes profound sleep disruption and fatigue,[18] babesiosis is associated with insomnia,[19] and up to 70% of HIV patients experience sleep disturbances.[20]

Similarly, inflammatory disorders and autoimmune disorders have been associated with poor-quality sleep. Disrupted sleep is associated with an increased risk of developing autoimmune disorders such as rheumatoid arthritis,[21] multiple sclerosis,[22] and celiac disease.[23] Symptoms of insomnia can predate the diagnosis of autoimmune conditions; one study noted that chronic insomnia requiring hypnotics may be associated with a 70% increased risk for future autoimmune disease.[24] Furthermore, inflammatory immune-mediated conditions may be the cause of sleep disorders. Narcolepsy has been directly associated with previous strains of flu vaccine and the influenza infection as well.[25,26]

In functional medicine, a standard approach to understanding a patient's complex problems is to take a chronologic history, which can unveil how antecedents, triggers, and mediators affect their current health. The same is true for sleep health when evaluating factors involved in defense and repair. Testing to look for previous or current infections may be considered. In lifestyle prescriptions, adequate sleep may be prescribed as a means of improving the immune system and decreasing inflammation. Viewed through the lens of the timeline, complaints of sleep difficulties may be found to result from inflammatory conditions, and implementing strategies for prevention and treatment of chronic disease using exercise, diet, and nutraceuticals can be part of an effective lifestyle prescription.

Cellular Communications

Our bodies are factories of chemical reactions that are stimulated by the messages of cellular communications around the clock during both wake and sleep.[5] Alterations in sleep–wake cycles can lead to disruption in neurotransmitters, immune messengers, hormones, and the endocrine system. Conversely, system imbalances that alter neuroendocrine communication can disrupt sleep.

Melatonin is produced by the pineal gland during the dark phase of the light–dark cycle, and it regulates the sleep–wake cycle and the circadian clock. Cortisol is produced by the adrenal glands in response to stress and is also known for its diurnal variation linked to the sleep–wake cycle. In healthy individuals, melatonin and cortisol have opposite patterns of production. While melatonin rises at night and peaks during the early hours of the morning, cortisol is at its lowest levels throughout the night. Disruption of the normal circadian cortisol cycle, as occurs during excessive stress, may lead to high nocturnal cortisol levels. Symptoms of elevated cortisol levels include irritability/anxiety, fatigue/low energy, night sweats, muscular tremors, poor sleep/sleep disturbance, hot flashes, insomnia, and trouble falling or staying asleep.[9] Disrupted sleeping patterns may in turn lead to increased exposure to light at night, which may suppress production of nocturnal melatonin, leading to low levels in the blood as circulating melatonin is rapidly and efficiently hydroxylated and conjugated with sulfate in the liver to form its primary metabolite, 6-sulfatoxymelatonin (MT6s).[27] These metabolites are excreted into urine and saliva.

There are many safe and effective supplements and botanicals that can improve both the quantity and quality of sleep. Complementing these with a functional medicine approach may allow for personalized treatment. This approach to sleep may include obtaining diurnal measurements of melatonin and cortisol profiles through commercially available testing. Although many patients empirically try melatonin for sleep, it may be of no benefit if a deficiency does not exist. If testing demonstrates disruption in the cortisol circadian rhythm, the use of botanicals as adaptogens for hormonal disturbances may be effective. For example, phosphatidylserine supplementation has been shown to attenuate the serum cortisol response under conditions of stress,[28] and rhodiola exerts an antifatigue effect and decreases cortisol response.[29]

Neurotransmitter function also affects sleep and wake states. Neurotransmitters and surrogate measures of neurotransmitters can be measured through noninvasive salivary and urinary measures, which are commercially available, and these can be coupled with melatonin, cortisol, and hormonal measurements as well. This practical approach to testing does not require obtaining cerebrospinal fluid (CSF) and bypasses the need for venipuncture, which can affect catecholamines and cortisol levels. Low levels of histamine neurotransmitters have been found to be an identifiable cause of sleepiness,[30] while pathologically high levels of dopamine have been associated with anxiety and mood disorders.[31] Both disorders are known to be associated with poor sleep, and, interestingly, low levels of dopamine have also been associated with poorer sleep quality.[32] Abnormal gamma-aminobutyric acid (GABA) activity has been implicated as a potential contributor to daytime sleepiness.[33] Low serotonin can be a biomarker for depression,[34] which may exacerbate sleep symptoms, and serotonin is also required for the production of melatonin.

Upon identification of imbalances in neurotransmitters, adaptogens and lifestyle measures can be implemented to achieve balance. For example, a patient with fatigue or brain fog who is found to have high GABA may benefit from dehydroepiandrosterone (DHEA) supplementation,[35] or a patient with low serotonin may require further evaluation and treatment of gut dysfunction.[36]

We can further illustrate a functional medicine approach by examining hormonal disturbances in women. During perimenopause, estrogen levels fluctuate, causing hot flashes that can affect both sleep and circadian patterns.[37] The functional medicine approach is to examine what the causes and treatments of hot flashes have in common, which is epinephrine. While estrogen may be the rheostat, the on/off switch is epinephrine, and hot flashes are an aberration of the temperature control mechanism.[9] The thermal control center is norepinephrine sensitive. Estrogen downregulates norepinephrine receptors in the hypothalamus, while decreases in estrogen upregulate norepinephrine receptors, leading to sensitivity to hot flashes.[38] Identification of adrenal imbalance can help direct personalized treatment, such as using rhodiola to create balance if high norepinephrine levels are identified.[39] There are also comprehensive kits commercially available that can measure neurotransmitters, hormones, and adrenal function together through noninvasive saliva and urine measures.

Transport

Processes of transport include the cardiovascular and lymphatic systems, and we have previously discussed how the glymphatic system is activated during sleep. Sleep also affects the cardiovascular system in a similar method.

Sleep deprivation increases sympathetic nervous system activity and may serve as a common pathophysiologic pathway for both hypertension and diabetes.[40] Untreated sleep apnea is associated with adverse cardiogenic effects, such as atrial fibrillation, and treatment with positive airway pressure may help induce conversion of atrial fibrillation to normal sinus rhythm in OSA.[41] Improving sleep in cardiac patients can improve cardiac outcomes, and in patients with insomnia and stable heart failure, cognitive-behavioral therapy for insomnia has been found to be effective therapy.[42] When addressing patients with cardiovascular disease, it is important to identify and treat sleep disorders such as sleep apnea, as it may be a perpetuator, or potentially even a trigger, of their disease.

Energy

Energy regulation, oxidative-reduction imbalances, and mitochondrial function are the core of many sleep complaints. The mitochondria generate energy by oxidative metabolism in the form of adenosine triphosphate (ATP), producing energy for muscle contractions, nerve impulses, and all energy-consuming processes in the body, including the synthesis of complex molecules.[43,44] Many patients who present with sleep complaints do so because they are fatigued. These patients may benefit from workups that evaluate for mitochondrial stress. For example, there is evidence that mitochondrial dysfunction is present in some chronic fatigue syndrome (CFS) patients. In these patients, an "ATP profile" test is a tool that can differentiate between patients who have depleted energy levels due to stress and psychological factors from those who have insufficient energy due to dysfunction of cellular respiration. Individual factors indicate which remedial actions, in the form of dietary supplements, drugs, and detoxification, are most likely to be of benefit.[45]

Sleep is affected by disruptions of mitochondrial function, which is what occurs with exposure to electromagnetic frequency (EMF). Mitochondria help maintain the proper flow of calcium within various components of the cell, and EMF activation of voltage-gated calcium channels (VGCCs) increases the production of cellular free radicals.[46] Sleep disturbance and insomnia are commonly reported neuropsychiatric symptoms following EMF exposure.[47]

In functional medicine, the goal is to find the roots of the underlying conditions. In patients presenting with sleep disturbances, a detailed history of exposures affecting energy balance and an assessment of markers of oxidative stress are important tools in the process. Simple measures such as reducing foods that lead to oxidative stress and identifying and supplementing of nutritional deficiencies for proper mitochondrial electron chain transport can lead to significant improvements. The IFM's Mito Food Plan is a therapeutic food plan derived to help support mitochondrial and brain function. It has a targeted macronutrient and micronutrient composition that may support better sleep.

Structural Integrity

"Structural integrity" is a broad term that refers to all forms of structure in the body, from subcellular membrane function to musculoskeletal structure. Structural integrity can influence sleep, and sleep disorders can affect structural integrity.

Sleep disorders secondary to structural integrity issues can be seen in obesity, neuromuscular disease, and chronic pain. Obesity contributes to collapse of the upper airway in OSA and may also cause obesity hypoventilation syndrome.[48] Structural problems due to neuromuscular disease may lead to loss of muscle tone and result in various forms of sleep-disordered breathing, and[49] chronic spine pain has been shown to impair overall sleep quality.[50]

Eczema can affect the structural integrity of skin and is one of the most common skin conditions of childhood. For children with severe eczema, constant itching and scratching can have many consequences, including sleep disturbances.[51] Insomnia in some infants with comorbid atopy shows that cow's milk allergy has been found to be a cause of insomnia in infants.[52] A functional medicine approach to sleep may include prescribing an elimination diet if eczema or allergies are affecting sleep.

Sleep disorders such as OSA also may affect structural integrity. Snoring originates in the upper airway and results in vibrations of the pharyngeal wall and associated structures. These vibratory stimuli can cause damage to endothelial cells in the arterial wall.[53] Furthermore, OSA is a disorder of sympathetic activation with impaired vascular response to hypoxia and oxidative stress. The intermittent hypoxia and impaired endothelial vascular control in OSA are likely to compromise perfusion and delay healing in patients with chronic wounds.[54] It is appropriate in functional medicine to assess for signs and symptoms of sleep apnea in a patient with complex medical problems.

The Mental, Emotional, and Spiritual Overlap

The Functional Medicine Matrix Model acknowledges that optimal health includes balancing mental, emotional, and spiritual aspects that may affect the seven physiological systems and sleep as well. Mental aspects include cognitive function and perceptual patterns, while emotional aspects address regulation and reactions to grief, sadness, or anger. Spirituality embodies having a sense of meaning and purpose, as well as having a relationship with something greater. All of these aspects affect our systems and sleep as well.

Antecedents, Triggers, and Mediators (ATMs)

Antecedents include predisposing factors such as genetic or environmental factors. The impact of the microbiome on sleep has been previously described, and early predisposing factors to alterations in the microbiome include vaginal versus cesarean delivery and formula versus breastfeeding. Antibiotic exposures and exposures to foods in early childhood can affect the microbiome as well. Adverse childhood experiences (ACEs) are other types of antecedents that have been shown to be associated with multiple sleep disturbances. In particular, family conflict at 7–15 years of age is associated with the development of insomnia, and childhood sexual abuse in women has been shown to lead to sleep disturbances years later.[55]

Triggering events are known as *activators of conditions*. Divorce has been associated with poor-quality sleep.[56] Postpartum depression can adversely impact sleep, and insomnia during pregnancy may be a marker for postpartum recurrence of depression among women with a previous history of depression.[57]

With regard to sleep issues, *mediators* are what keep physiologically driving the sleep disorder forward in a perpetuating cycle. Interestingly, functional medicine's approach to ATMs directly mirrors that of the "3P" model of insomnia describing predisposing, precipitating, and perpetuating factors relevant to the development and maintenance of insomnia.[58]

Modifiable Personal Lifestyle Factors

The Functional Medicine Matrix Model acknowledges that modifiable lifestyle factors and personal behaviors are foundational to optimal health; hence they are positioned at the base of the Matrix. Part of the process of a functional medicine evaluation includes identifying negative factors that are contributing to a patient's system imbalances as well as identifying positive factors that the patient is already practicing. In partnership with the patient, lifestyle can be part of the treatment plan of reversing chronic disease. The Functional Medicine Prescription and Lifestyle Plan routinely includes personalized lifestyle measures oriented toward achieving better health. Dr. Dean Ornish received the Linus Pauling Award from the IFM for his work on lifestyle as treatment for cardiovascular disease and cancer, and its effect on gene expression. Fellow Linus Pauling winner Dr. Terry Wahls, a VA functional medicine physician, has likewise shown that lifestyle can help treat chronic disease through her work with multiple sclerosis. Both physician-champions of wellness implemented aspects of relaxation or sleep, and they are the first modifiable personal lifestyle factors addressed at the bottom of the Functional Medicine Matrix.

Exercise and movement are the second modifiable personal lifestyle factors that are addressed on the Matrix, and regular exercise has been demonstrated to improve sleep. Population data show that people sleep significantly better and feel more alert during the day if they get at least 150 minutes of exercise a week.[59] Low levels of physical activity have been associated with moderate-severe OSA, whereas exercise in individuals with OSA is associated with lower levels of depression, fatigue, blood pressure, and C-reactive protein (CRP) levels.[60]

Nutrition is the next modifiable risk factor addressed on the Matrix. A common functional medicine prescription is to move away from a standard American diet (SAD) and prescribe a modified-Mediterranean Diet. For a patient with narcolepsy, a low glycemic diet or nutritional ketosis may be beneficial. Medicinal foods should also be considered as they can target gut health, as in a patient with dysbiosis and RLS. An anti-inflammatory diet may be recommended for a patient with insomnia due to generalized pain or rheumatologic disease.

The next modifiable personal lifestyle factor is stress. The myriad stressors of daily life can impact sleep quality and duration. Central nervous system hyperarousal can lead to insomnia, and a therapeutic approach to insomnia should be multidimensional, with the goal of reducing both emotional and physiologic hyperarousal and its underlying factors throughout the 24-hour sleep–wake period.[61] While sleep hygiene is commonly given as instructions by healthcare providers, mindfulness meditation has been shown to be more effective for treatment of insomnia than sleep hygiene alone.[62]

The final modifiable personal lifestyle factor is that of relationships. While healthy relationships can be beneficial to one's health, dysfunctional relationships can be detrimental. The association between sleep and relationships is likely to be bidirectional and reciprocal: the quality of close relationships influences sleep and sleep disturbances, and sleep disorders influence the quality of those close relationships.[63] In men, better sleep efficiency predicts less negative partner interaction the following day. In women, less negative partner interaction during the day predicts greater actigraphy-based sleep efficiency that night.[64] Intimacy and sexual relations can be important in healthy relationships; sexual activity is beneficial for sleep.[65] Also, sexual intercourse typically occurs in bed, which is associated with sleep.

GO TO IT: Retelling the Patient Story and the Therapeutic Encounter

This chapter is by no means a comprehensive list of all the causes of insomnia or sleepiness, but rather it provides examples of how lifestyle and clinical imbalances affect sleep health. How does one apply a root cause analysis to a patient's sleep complaint? In applying the functional medicine operating system, one uses the "GO TO IT" heuristic for patient management, which trains physicians to Gather, Organize, Tell, Order, Initiate, and Track. The model includes the *Gathering* of the patient's medical history and influential lifestyle factors on the functional medicine timeline with care given to identify ATMs, followed by *Organizing* the relevant details and clinical imbalances within the Matrix Model. The patient is engaged in the therapeutic encounter by the physician taking the time to *Tell* the patient's story back to them for both accuracy and additional input. Next, the practitioner identifies the clinical priorities and considers the patient's goals to create a therapeutic plan and sequence for care; this is identified as the *Order* step in the heuristic. The process guides the *Initiate* step that indicates what further assessments are required and informs the care plan. *Track*, the final aspect of the functional medicine heuristic, includes following the patient's progress and adjusting case management for ongoing modifications to care.

Once the information and history have been gathered and organized into the Matrix, perhaps one of the most influential features of the functional medicine approach includes providing a timeline to the patient. The timeline is a clinical tool for organizing the patient's history and identifying antecedents and triggers of current symptoms. This may allow a patient to realize that his or her sleep complaint came around a time of a certain medication or diagnosis and that the symptoms preceded a life event or are due to lifestyle factors. This may motivate the patient to make changes if perpetuating factors are identified. Importantly, the telling of the patient story may be therapeutic; for many, feeling understood is often the root of hope.

Once the pivotal retelling of the story has been accomplished, the partnership in rapport and care is established, and patient and practitioner can organize their priorities. Patient goals and modifiable risk factors are determined with an eye to identifying imbalances in the matrix. Initiating care is the next step, which allows for further assessments or adjuvant care as needed. Results are tracked as therapy is initiated. An example of tracking data may include following biomarkers or the Multiple Symptoms Questionnaire (MSQ) in functional medicine. This can also be done in sleep medicine with the Epworth Sleepiness Scale, the RLS Rating Scale, or through the use of sleep logs. Tracking assessments allow the patient and provider to determine the effectiveness of the therapeutic approach and identify clinical outcomes at each visit.

Root-Cause Medicine

As discussed in the opening, it is not uncommon in conventional medicine to have several different diagnoses, with individual treatments for each, such as type 2 diabetes, hyperlipidemia, gout, hypertension, nonalcoholic fatty liver disease, Alzheimer's, obesity, sleep apnea and hypersomnia, or insomnia with sleep apnea. In functional medicine these disorders are not viewed as separate, but rather as symptoms of an underlying root cause. To give an oversimplified example, the 10 diagnoses just provided may be a result of the standard American diet (SAD). Such a diet is highly glycemic and leads to insulin resistance, which may cause stress on the mitochondria and impair energy production, leading to fatigue. The standard American diet commonly lacks vegetables and fruits, resulting in insufficient phytonutrients for sleep and mitochondrial support. The insulin resistance stimulates HMGCoA reductase to produce cholesterol, and elevated cholesterol levels often result in the prescription of a statin, further stressing the mitochondria and commonly associated with fatigue. The high consumption of sugar can lead to both nonalcoholic fatty liver disease, which may compromise the ability to detoxify, and increased uric acid formation, which can lead to gout. Excess sugar consumption also disrupts endothelial cells, leading to hypertension which may lead to prescriptions for cardiovascular drugs that contribute to insomnia. Insulin resistance is commonly associated with obesity, which is associated with sleep apnea. Insulin resistance also leads to what is being coined as "type 3 diabetes" or Alzheimer's, which is commonly predated by insomnia and circadian rhythm disturbances.

In conventional medicine, "The eyes see only what the mind knows."[66] This may explain why highly skilled clinicians may view the 10 different diagnosis, including sleep disorders, as separate, unrelated entities and overlook a common underlying root cause. In the interest of brevity, the example just given was oversimplified because there is typically not just one cause, but rather a combination of associated root causes. In both integrative medicine and functional medicine, the patient is viewed as a whole person, not as a person with multiple distinct and different diseases. While testing or protocols may play a role, fundamentally, functional medicine is centered on root-cause medicine, viewing the patient's state of health over time and considering the multiple factors that may have impacted or influenced the expression of symptoms and disease. It focuses on patterns and connections, which in turn allows the identification of causes of clinical imbalances, and it encourages a medical and lifestyle plan to restore balance. This approach can be applied to sleep disorders and general health as well.

REFERENCES

1. Pizzorno JE. Clinical decision making: A functional medicine perspective. *Global Adv Health Med.* 2012;1(4):8–13. doi:10.7453/gahmj.2012.1.4.002.
2. Sanger GJ. 5-Hydroxytryptamine and the gastrointestinal tract: Where next. *Trends Pharmacol Sci.* 2008;29:465–471.
3. van Praag HM, Lemus C. Monoamine precursors in the treatment of psychiatric disorders. In Wurtman RJ, Wurtman JJ, eds. *Nutrition and the brain.* New York: Raven Press; 1986: 89–139.
4. Marz RB. *Medical nutrition from Marz.* 2nd ed. Portland, OR: Omni-Press; 1999: 200–205.
5. Bland JS. *The disease delusion: Conquering the causes of chronic illness for a healthier, longer and happier life.* New York: HarperCollins; 2014.
6. Crippa G, Sverzellati E, Giorgi-Pierfranceschi M, Carrara GC. Magnesium and cardiovascular drugs: Interactions and therapeutic role. *Ann Ital Med Int.* 1999;14:40–45.
7. Stoschitzky K, et al. Influence of beta-blockers on melatonin release. *Eur J Clin Pharmacol.* 1999 Apr;55(2):111–115.
8. Spiegelhalder K, Scholtes C, Riemann D. The association between insomnia and cardiovascular diseases. *Nat Sci Sleep.* 2010;2:71–78.

9. Institute for Functional Medicine et al., eds. *Textbook of functional medicine.* Federal Way, WA: Institute for Functional Medicine; 2010.

10. Louveau A, Smirnov I, Keyes TJ, et al. Structural and functional features of central nervous system lymphatics. *Nature.* 2015;523(7560):337–341.

11. Kim C-W, Yun KE, Jung H-S, et al. Sleep duration and quality in relation to non-alcoholic fatty liver disease in middle-aged workers and their spouses. *J Hepatol.* 2013;59(2):351–357.

12. Veasey S. Good soldier falls: The liver in sleep apnea. *J Appl Physiol.* 2007;102(2):513–514.

13. Montagnese S, Middleton B, Skene DJ, Morgan MY. Sleep-wake patterns in patients with cirrhosis: All you need to know on a single sheet. A simple sleep question-naire for clinical use. *J Hepatol.* 2009;51(4):690–695.

14. Beydoun HA, Beydoun MA, Jeng HA, Zonderman AB, Eid SM. Bisphenol-A and sleep adequacy among adults in the National Health and Nutrition Examination Surveys. *Sleep.* 2016;39(2):467–476.

15. Shiue I. Urinary arsenic, pesticides, heavy metals, phthalates, polyaromatic hydrocarbons, and polyfluoroalkyl compounds are associated with sleep troubles in adults: USA NHANES, 2005–2006. *Environm Sci Pollut Res Int.* 2017;24(3):3108–3116.

16. Besedovsky L, Lange T, Born J. Sleep and immune function. *Pflugers Archiv.* 2012;463(1):121–137. doi:10.1007/s00424-011-1044-0.

17. Imeri L, Opp MR. How (and why) the immune system makes us sleep. *Nat Rev Neurosci.* 2009;10(3):199–210.

18. Greenberg HE, Ney G, Scharf SM, Ravdin L, Hilton E. Sleep quality in Lyme dis-ease. *Sleep.* 1995 Dec;18(10):912–6.

19. Eskow ES, Krause PJ, Spielman A, Freeman K, Aslanzadeh J. Southern extension of the range of human babesiosis in the Eastern United States. *J Clin Microbiol.* 1999;37(6):2051–2052.

20. Taibi DM. Sleep disturbances in persons living with HIV. *J Assoc Nurs AIDS Care.* 2013;24(1 Suppl):S72–S85.

21. Hsiao YH, Chen YT, Tseng CM, et al. Sleep disorders and increased risk of autoim-mune diseases in individuals without sleep apnea. *Sleep.* 2015;38(4):581–586.

22. Veauthier C. Sleep disorders in multiple sclerosis. Review. *Curr Neurol Neurosci Rep.* 2015 May;15(5):21.

23. Zingone F, Siniscalchi M, Capone P, et al. The quality of sleep in patients with coe-liac disease. *Aliment Pharmacol Ther.* 2010 Oct;32(8):1031–1036.

24. Kok VC, Horng J-T, Hung G-D, et al. Risk of autoimmune disease in adults with chronic insomnia requiring sleep-inducing pills: A population-based longitudinal study. *J Gen Intern Med.* 2016;31(9):1019–1026.

25. Duffy J, Weintraub E, Vellozzi C, et al. Narcolepsy and influenza A(H1N1) pan-demic 2009 vaccination in the United States. *Neurology.* 2014;83(20):1823–1830.

26. Han F, Lin L, Mignot E, et al. Narcolepsy onset is seasonal and increased following the 2009 H1N1 pandemic in China. *Ann Neurol.* 2011;70(3):410–417.

27. Waller KL, Mortensen EL, Avlund K, et al. Melatonin and cortisol profiles in late midlife and their association with age-related changes in cognition. *Nat Sci Sleep.* 2016;8:47–53.

28. Starks MA, Starks SL, Kingsley M, et al. The effects of phosphatidylserine on endocrine response to moderate intensity exercise. *J Int Soc Sports Nutr.* 2008 Jul 28;5:11.

29. Olsson EM, von Schéele B, Panossian AG. A randomised, double-blind, placebo-controlled, parallel-group study of the standardised extract shr-5 of the roots of Rhodiola rosea in the treatment of subjects with stress-related fatigue. *Planta Med.* 2009 Feb;75(2):105–12.

30. Scammell TE, Mochizuki T. Is low histamine a fundamental cause of sleepiness in narcolepsy and idiopathic hypersomnia? *Sleep.* 2009;32(2):133–134.

31. Bonomaully M, Khong T, Fotriadou M, Tully J. Anxiety and depression related to elevated dopamine in a patient with multiple mediastinal paragangliomas. *Gen Hosp Psychiatry.* 2014 Jul-Aug;36(4):449.e7–e8.

32. Seay JS, McIntosh R, Fekete EM, et al. Self-reported sleep disturbance is associated with lower CD4 count and 24-h urinary dopamine levels in ethnic minority women living with HIV. *Psychoneuroendocrinology.* 2013;38:2647–2653.

33. Rye DB, Bliwise DL, Parker K, et al. Modulation of vigilance in the primary hypersomnias by endogenous enhancement of GABAA receptors. *Sci Transl Med.* 2012;4(161):161ra151.

34. Nichkova MI, Huisman H, Wynveen PM, et al. Evaluation of a novel ELISA for serotonin: Urinary serotonin as a potential biomarker for depression. *Analys Bioanal Chem.* 2012;402:1593–1600.

35. Genud R, Merenlender A, Gispan-Herman I, et al. DHEA lessens depressive-like behavior via GABA-ergic modulation of the mesolimbic system. *Neuropsychopharmacology.* 2009;34:577–584

36. Evrensel A, Ceylan ME. The gut-brain axis: The missing link in depression. *Clin Psychopharmacol Neurosci.* 2015;13(3):239–244.

37. Prior JC. Perimenopause: The complex endocrinology of the menopausal transition. *Endocr Rev.*1998;19(4):397–428.

38. Freedman RR. Menopausal hot flashes: Mechanisms, endocrinology, treatment. *J Steroid Biochem Molec Biol.* 2014;142:115–120.

39. Verpeut JL, Walters AL, Bello NT. Rhodiola is an adaptogen that can reduce norepinephrine levels. *Citrus aurantium* and *Rhodiola rosea* in combination reduce visceral white adipose tissue and increase hypothalamic norepinephrine in a rat model of diet-induced obesity. *Nutr Res (New York, NY).* 2013;33(6):10.1016.

40. Nagai M, Hoshide S, Kario K. Sleep duration as a risk factor for cardiovascular disease: A review of the recent literature. *Curr Cardiol Rev.* 2010;6(1):54–61.

41. Walia HK, Chung MK, Ibrahim S, Mehra R. Positive airway pressure-induced conversion of atrial fibrillation to normal sinus rhythm in severe obstructive sleep apnea. *J Clin Sleep Med.* 2016;12(9):1301–1303.

42. Redeker NS, Jeon S, Andrews L, Cline J, Jacoby D, Mohsenin V. Feasibility and efficacy of a self-management intervention for insomnia in stable heart failure. *J Clin Sleep Med* 2015;11(10):1109–1119.

43. Alberts B, Johnson A, Lewis J, Raff M, Roberts K, Walter P. *Molecular biology of the cell*. New York: Garland Science; 2002.

44. Voet D, Voet JG, Pratt CW. *Fundamentals of biochemistry*. New York: Wiley; 2006.

45. Myhill S, Booth NE, McLaren-Howard J. Chronic fatigue syndrome and mitochondrial dysfunction. *Int J Clin Exp Med*. 2009;2(1):1–16.

46. Pall ML. Electromagnetic fields act *via* activation of voltage-gated calcium channels to produce beneficial or adverse effects. *J Cell Molec Med*. 2013;17(8):958–965.

47. Pall ML. Microwave frequency electromagnetic fields (EMFs) produce widespread neuropsychiatric effects including depression. *J Chem Neuroanat*. 2016 Sep;75(Pt B):43–51.

48. Romero-Corral A, Caples SM, Lopez-Jimenez F, Somers VK. Interactions between obesity and obstructive sleep apnea: Implications for treatment. *Chest*. 2010;137(3):711–719.

49. Aboussouan LS. Sleep-disordered breathing in neuromuscular disease. *Am J Respir Crit Care Med*. 2015 May 1;191(9):979–989.

50. Marty M, Rozenberg S, Duplan B, et al. Quality of sleep in patients with chronic low back pain: A case-control study. *Eur Spine J*. 2008;17(6):839–844.

51. Santiago S. Food allergies and eczema. *Pediatr Ann*. 2015 Jul;44(7):265–267.

52. Kahn A, Mozin MJ, Casimir G, Montauk L, Blum D. Insomnia and cow's milk allergy in infants. *Pediatrics*. 1985 Dec;76(6):880–884.

53. Puig F, Rico F, Almendros I, Montserrat JM, Navajas D, Farre R. Vibration enhances interleukin-8 release in a cell model of snoring-induced airway inflammation, *Sleep*. 2005 Oct;28(10):1312–1316.

54. Patt BT, Jarjoura D, Lambert L, et al. Prevalence of obstructive sleep apnea in patients with chronic wounds. *J Clin Sleep Med*. 2010;6(6):541–544.

55. Kajeepeta S, Gelaye B, Jackson CL, Williams MA. Adverse childhood experiences are associated with adult sleep disorders: A systematic review. *Sleep Med*. 2015;16(3):320–330.

56. Newton TL, Burns VE, Miller JJ, Fernandez-Botran GR. Subjective sleep quality in women with divorce histories: The role of intimate partner victimization. *J Interpers Violence*. 2016 May;31(8):1430–1452.

57. Dørheim SK, Bjorvatn B, Eberhard-Gran M. Can insomnia in pregnancy predict postpartum depression? A longitudinal, population-based study. Mazza M, ed. *PLoS ONE*. 2014;9(4):e94674.

58. Spielman AJ, et al. A behavioral perspective on insomnia treatment. *Psychiatric Clin N Am*. 1987;10:541–553.

59. Loprinzi PD, Cardinal BJ. Association between objectively measured physical activity and sleep, NHANES 2005–2006. *Mental Health and Physical Activity*. 2011; 4(2):65–69.

60. Simpson L, McArdle N, Eastwood PR, et al. Physical inactivity is associated with moderate-severe obstructive sleep apnea. *J Clin Sleep Med.* 2015;11(10):1091–1099.

61. Basta M, Chrousos GP, Vela-Bueno A, Vgontzas AN. Chronic insomnia and stress system. *Sleep Med Clin.* 2007;2(2):279–291.

62. Black DS, O'Reilly GA, Olmstead R, Breen EC, Irwin MR. Mindfulness meditation and improvement in sleep quality and daytime impairment among older adults with sleep disturbances: A randomized clinical trial. *JAMA Intern Med.* 2015;175(4):494–501.

63. Troxel WM, Robles TF, Hall M, Buysse DJ. Marital quality and the marital bed: Examining the covariation between relationship quality and sleep. *Sleep Med Rev.* 2007 Oct;11(5):389–404. doi:10.1016/j.smrv.2007.05.002. PMID: 17854738; PMCID: PMC2644899.

64. Hasler BP, Troxel WM. Couples' nighttime sleep efficiency and concordance: Evidence for bidirectional associations with daytime relationship functioning. *Psychosom Med.* 2010 Oct;72(8):794–801. doi:10.1097/PSY.0b013e3181ecd08a

65. Kruger D, Hughes S. Tendencies to fall asleep after sex are associated with greater partner desires for bonding and affection. *J Soc Evolut Cult Psychol.* 2011;5(4):239–247.

66. Jairath UC, Spodick DH. The eyes see only what the mind knows. *J Emerg Med.* 2000;19(3):275–276. doi: 10.1016/s0736-4679(00)00237-7. PMID: 11033275.

23

Hypnosis and Guided Imagery

JACLYN L. LEWIS-CROSWELL

Hypnosis

Hypnosis and how it works has been pondered for hundreds of years. Jack Watkins, a pioneer in the study and practice of hypnosis, once said, "Seventy years of amazement, and we still don't know what it is." James Braid coined the term "hypnosis" in the nineteenth century; at the time he considered hypnosis to be a form of sleep. Today, it is considered to be a different state from sleep although hypnotized patients may drift into sleep spontaneously.[1] Only in the past 70–80 years has hypnosis been more scientifically investigated, and only in the past two decades have we had the tools of electroencephalography (EEG) and functional magnetic resonance imaging (fMRI) imaging to study the effects of hypnosis on the brain.[1]

Hypnosis is commonly defined as a state of attention, with receptive concentration containing three features: dissociation, absorption, and suggestibility. Some describe hypnosis as an "altered state of consciousness," while others refer to it as a state of relaxation with focused attention.[2] According to the Society of Psychological Hypnosis, "hypnosis is a procedure involving cognitive processes (like imagination) in which a subject is guided by a hypnotist to respond to suggestions for changes in sensations, perceptions, thoughts, feelings, and behaviors." People can be trained to guide themselves through a hypnotic procedure, coined "self-hypnosis." Hypnosis or hypnotherapy is a trance-like state of mind that can create a state of deep relaxation. This state of consciousness is characterized by focused attention and reduced peripheral awareness, with an enhanced capacity for response to suggestion. As a result, the mind can concentrate intensely on a specific thought, memory, feeling, or sensation without distractions, resulting in increased suggestibility that can be used to change certain thoughts or behaviors.[3] This shift in consciousness enables subjects to tap into their natural abilities, allowing them to make changes more quickly.[1,4,5]

A session of hypnosis between a provider and patient will typically involve the following steps:

1. Establish rapport and a trusting, working relationship with the patient. Hypnosis is a cooperative experience and not something the practitioner "does to" the patient; therefore the relationship is critically important. The patient is educated about hypnosis and informed about what to expect.[6]

2. Once informed consent is received, the practitioner leads the patient into a hypnotic trance with the use of a *hypnotic elicitation*, which is a procedure designed to induce hypnosis. A hypnotic elicitation can vary greatly between practitioners but may include a relaxation elicitation, such as progressive muscle relaxation, guided imagery, body scan, hand levitation, or eye roll.

3. After the elicitation, a deepening technique is completed to assist with further relaxation effect. As an example, the patient is told to imagine going down an elevator and to feel more relaxed with each level the elevator descends. Worry, stress, and anxiety get off the elevator on each floor that the door opens. By the time the elevator reaches the first floor, the patient is completely relaxed and worry free.[6]

4. The practitioner then utilizes post hypnotic suggestions that are directed toward changing some kind of thought, behavior, perception, emotion, sensation, or physiologic process, imagery, and relationship. [6] The suggestions are based on a previously agreed approach to treatment that has been created utilizing the patient's view of their symptoms. The hypnotic suggestions may focus on an immediate response that occurs during the session, or they may occur as a posthypnotic effect, that will occur after and outside of the session.[6]

An example of a hypnotic suggestion to deepen sleep may include something like, "Now you will experience a heaviness, and as your body feels heavy you will go into deep sleep. With each exhalation you will fall deeper and deeper asleep." An example of a posthypnotic suggestion for a patient experiencing a nocturnal eating disorder is, "When you get out of your bed, you will notice your feet hit the floor, and that sensation will be alerting to you, and you will find you are then in control of your decisions. And one day, I don't know when, your innermost unconscious mind knows that you will sleep deeply all the way through the night. From that night on, you will sleep through each night with this problem no longer bothering you, no longer disturbing you, and you can sleep soundly and easily." Kohler and Kurz describe a similar protocol for sleep walkers in their book, *Hypnosis in the Management of Sleep Disorders*.[1]

There are many different ways of providing hypnotic suggestions. Some are directive, others are implied or passive, and some suggestions are confusional while others use symbolism or metaphors. [1,6] A posthypnotic suggestion may include external reminders. For a patient presenting with insomnia, the suggestion could be, "When you brush your teeth prior to going to bed, the brushing will instill relaxation in your body and once you finish brushing your teeth you will feel sleepy enough to get into bed and fall asleep immediately once your head hits the pillow." [7]

5. Finally, the practitioner will re-alert the patient. The importance of ensuring that the patient or participant is fully re-alerted cannot be emphasized enough. Some research has been done regarding the importance of the re-alerting the patient for safety and comfort.[8,9] The alerting process can be direct or indirect. An example of a direct re-alerting method is, "I will count from 1 to 5 and when I say 5 you will be alert, refreshed and at ease. 1: begin feeling your chest expand with your breath., 2: begin to notice the sounds inside and outside the room, and feel the chair supporting your body, and feel your feet touching the ground., 3: begin to rouse from this relaxing state., 4: blink your eyes open., And 5: open your eyes, feeling alert, refreshed and at ease, sound in mind and sound in body."

An indirect re-alerting example is, "Once your inner mind knows you can manage this problem, you will open your eyes feeling alert, refreshed, and confident in your ability to handle (the problem presented)." (The original authors of these examples are unknown but many in the field of hypnosis use something similar to these examples to re-alert their participants.) Regardless if a direct or indirect re-alerting is used, it is important that the patient is fully alert in mind and body before terminating the session. On many occasions, a patient feels disoriented or confused due to not being re-alerted completely. Research indicates that an assessment of the patient's alertness should be conducted before and after a hypnotic intervention. The hypnotherapist can direct the patient to look around the room and ask the patient questions to determine how aware she is of her surroundings and how connected the patient feels to her body.[8,9]

THE DEVELOPMENT OF HYPNOTHERAPY

Although it wasn't called hypnosis, the phenomenon of hypnosis has been documented since the sixteenth century. The first official documentation of hypnosis goes back to the time of Franz Mesmer and his dissertation titled, "On the Influence of the Planets." Mesmer believed that there was a "peculiar animal gravitation,", and history suggests that Mesmer was using magnetic science. Mesmer thought the magnets were healing his patients and was surprised when later his patients responded equally well to other nonmagnetized objects, such as tea cups, bread, wood, animals, or other people. We now know that Mesmer's patients reacted to his touch through hypnotic elicitation and suggestion. Many books or texts on hypnosis indicate that hypnosis is considered a natural phenomenon that can occur automatically in most people. [2,10-12]

There are many misconceptions about hypnosis due to several factors, including its start through Mesmer's less than reputable history, demonstrations by stage hypnotists, and hypnotists who put signs out indicating that they can cure an ailment or help someone stop smoking in one session. It is unfortunate that many people base their assumptions about hypnosis on stage hypnosis or the use of hypnosis in comedy acts. Stage hypnotists screen volunteers and select individuals who are cooperative, with possible exhibitionist tendencies, and who are extremely responsive to hypnosis. Stage hypnosis creates myths and fears that, discourage people from seeking legitimate medical hypnotherapy for treatment that can provide relief and even healing.

Another myth about hypnosis is that people lose consciousness or have amnesia. The truth is that a small percentage of subjects who go into very deep levels of trance may have some spontaneous amnesia regarding the experience of hypnosis, but the majority of people remember everything from a hypnotic session. Most of what is accomplished during hypnosis can be done in a medium-depth trance, after which subjects generally have full recall. Another frequent concern that patients cite is a fear of losing control or "going crazy." The patient is not under the control of the hypnotherapist and always has control over his or her own behaviors. Hypnosis is not something done to the patient; rather, it is a collaborative activity, and the patient learns to use it as a skill to overcome a symptom they wish to alleviate. The hypnotherapist acts as the facilitator who serves to guide the patient. [4-6]

Many patients fear they are not hypnotizable, but research indicates that most people respond to hypnosis. There are some patients who lack the ability to use visualization or have difficulty relinquishing reality-bound thinking in the hypnotic context, and others may have difficulty forming rapport and trust with the hypnotherapist. These patients are less able to utilize hypnosis or benefit from its use. [13] However, even people who initially are low on a hypnotizability scale can learn to use hypnosis with good instruction, willingness, and practice. In fact, natural experiences of self-hypnosis occur all the time and include daydreaming, driving for several miles to a destination without any memory of the event, and losing a sense of time while playing an instrument or creating art. [1,5-7]

"Hypnosis is best considered a therapeutic modality rather than a therapy in its own right. It should be offered within the context of a complete psychological and medical treatment plan and offers the advantage to facilitate sensations, perceptions, thoughts, feelings, or behaviors." [7] Hypnosis has also been described as "the art of securing a patient's attention and then effectively communicating ideas that enhance motivation and change perceptions."[6] Hypnotherapy sessions are individualized, and the most effective suggestion for each client will differ. Hypnosis is also most effective when it is combined with other (non-hypnotic) interventions. It is not uniformly appropriate or effective for all medical or psychological problems or all people. It is best when used eclectically by a provider trained to treat the specific presenting problem. Professionals use hypnosis as one treatment modality, and it is important not to self-identify as "hypnotists" but instead as physicians, psychologists, social workers, marriage and family therapists, etc., who use hypnosis as one type of treatment intervention in addition to other clinically relevant treatment tools.[6] As the historic stigma of hypnosis is discredited and people come to understand that hypnosis is a scientific, evidence-based treatment, then more patients and providers will accept the use of hypnosis for the treatment of medical conditions.

USING HYPNOSIS TO TREAT SLEEP DISORDERS

Hypnosis can be effective in treatment of rapid eye movement (REM) parasomnia, including nightmare disorder, and non–REM (NREM) parasomnia, including sleep walking, nocturnal sleep-related eating disorder, night terrors, and parasomnia overlap disorder. It can also be used for insomnia as well as pain, which can be a cause of secondary insomnia.

Hypnosis has been found to be an effective treatment for nightmares. In a small case series of 10 patients with nightmares who were treated with hypnosis, 71% of respondents had improvement or were symptom-free at 18 months, and 67% at 5-year follow-up maintained improvement of their symptoms.[14] Another study with three subjects showed that brief hypnotic therapy of 1–5 sessions was beneficial for repetitive nightmares. [1] Transformation of the nightmare can occur while the patient is reliving or replaying it under hypnosis. Case reports describe two combat veterans with posttraumatic stress disorder (PTSD) and nightmares whose nightmares resolved with dream substitution and rehearsal during hypnotic trance.[15] A study from as far back as 1959 discussed the use of hypnosis for patients whose nightmares are secondary to trauma—not to alter the actual memory of the traumatic event, but to add elements that enable the patient to cope with the frightening content of the nightmare.[16] Another hypnotic technique is to have the patient imagine that the nightmare is playing on a movie or television screen while controlling it with a remote control. In some interventions the patient learns to stop the movie prior to the "bad part," or the patient may learn to "change the ending" of the nightmare to a more pleasant scene. Hypnosis intervention is individualized and specialized for each patient's needs, and therefore a scripted or recorded session of hypnosis is not necessarily generalizable to the population at large because it may miss the specific issue that needs to be addressed for a given individual.[1]

Hypnosis has been found to be an effective treatment for NREM parasomnias such as sleep walking and night terrors.[17] In one study, subjects with sleep walking and nocturnal sleep eating disorder were treated with posthypnotic suggestions that were repeated over 3 weeks. Every subject in the active treatment group improved on all parameters by the end of the 3 weeks and remained symptom free at 1 year follow-up; the most improvement occurred for patients early in the treatment phase. The results suggest that patients who are free of psychiatric illness tend to respond well to hypnotic suggestions for treatment of sleep walking. [17] Another study looked at 12 men in the military who were facing discharge secondary to sleep walking. Six of the them engaged in hypnosis, and four reported total alleviation of the sleep walking.[18]

Hauri, Silber, and Boeve published a frequently cited 5-year follow-up study regarding the treatment of parasomnias with hypnosis. This study looked at sleep walking, night terrors, nightmares, epic dreaming, and sleep eating. Patients were asked to listen to a recorded hypnotic intervention daily for at least 2 weeks. Of the 18 patients who completed all three follow-ups, 5 (28%) had no spells or were much improved throughout the study, 4 (22%) had no spells or were much improved initially but showed but little or no improvement at later follow-ups, 3 (17%) had no improvement initially but improved on later follow-ups, and 6 (33%) had little or no improvement on any of the three follow-ups.[14]

It has been suggested that part of the efficacy of hypnosis for parasomnias is related to the relaxation effect induced by hypnosis and leads, to improved sleep. In a review of hypnosis for the treatment of parasomnias, the authors noted that relaxation induced by hypnosis was a significant contributing factor to therapeutic efficacy in three patients with NREM parasomnias, and they concluded that hypnosis is a relatively simple, noninvasive, inexpensive, and effective means of treating nightmares, sleep walking, and sleep terror disorders.[19] Another published case study is of a patient treated with hypnosis for parasomnia overlap disorder. The patient had sleep walking, sleep talking, and dream enhancement and was treated with three sessions of hypnosis, which were recorded and repeated at home. The patient's symptoms improved initially and continued throughout the duration of treatment. [20]

Hypnosis has been used for insomnia, and in one study by Cordi, et al., participants who listened to hypnotic suggestions to "sleep deeper" had an increase in slow wave sleep of 81%. Time awake was reduced by 67%, and other sleep stages were unaffected by the hypnotic suggestions. They also found that subjects who had low hypnotic ability on previous testing spent less time in slow wave sleep after being given the posthypnotic suggestion to "sleep deeper."[21] This finding suggests that assessing a patient's hypnotic suggestibility prior to engaging in hypnosis is important in identifying those who can benefit from this intervention to increase slow wave sleep or improve sleep quality.

Hypnotherapy can be useful for the patient with insomnia because it can be a key to turning off anxiety patterns and creating healthy lifestyle patterns; however, the published literature is sparse. [22] Chronic insomnia is frequently associated with depression, pain, anxiety, and lifestyle change. An article by Patterson suggests that insomnia with these associated disorders is most likely to improve with the use of hypnosis and other techniques such as progressive relaxation and ego-strengthening (using posthypnotic suggestions to improve self-efficacy).[23] Although this article found hypnosis to be effective as an intervention for insomnia in highly hypnotizable individuals, cognitive-behavioral therapy for insomnia (CBT-I) continues to be first-line treatment for insomnia, and is discussed in detail in another chapter. Hypnosis is a good option to help the patient with deepening sleep or increasing slow wave sleep once the behavioral intervention of CBT-I is completed.[24]

Hypnosis can be an effective primary intervention for insomnia, and several researchers have published research supporting this. In a retrospective review of 84 children and adolescents with insomnia, 75 patients were offered hypnosis for treatment and returned for follow-up after the first hypnosis session: 90% of the patients reported a decrease in time to sleep onset, and, of the patients who reported difficulty with wake after sleep onset (WASO), 52% reported resolution of WASO and 38% reported improvement.[25] While CBT-I is recognized as first-line therapy for insomnia, hypnosis may provide an alternative for those patients in whom CBT-I is not successful, or who have residual sleep issues after completing treatment. For example, if a patient is still not sleeping optimally after CBT-I, he can be taught to use self-hypnosis prior to bedtime. Self-hypnosis can elicit the relaxation response, leading to better, deeper sleep.

Hypnosis can also be used to treat factors contributing to insomnia such as chronic pain, which can be very disruptive to sleep because pain can lead to alpha intrusion or arousals that decrease slow wave sleep and increase lighter stages of sleep. Hypnosis has been found in many research studies to be an effective tool to assist with pain reduction, that can lead to improved sleep.[23,26] In one study, patients who were taught to use self-hypnosis for pain control were able to change their coping strategies from passive to active, resulting in reduced pain perception and improvement of their global impression of treatment effectiveness. Patients who felt they had greater pain control also had lower disability and decreased belief that hurt signifies harm.[27] A large body of research supports the efficacy of hypnosis for pain control, which may in turn improve sleep disrupted by pain.

Guided Imagery

Guided imagery, similar to clinical hypnosis in many ways, is also a therapeutic technique that has been used for sleep. While the term "guided imagery" may suggest an experience focused simply on visualization, guided imagery is actually a narrated multisensory experience, incorporating other senses such as sounds and scents. Guided imagery is often regarded as a treatment for relaxation and stress reduction, but it has been used for many other health complaints, including arthritis and pain, depression, and asthma. It is also often utilized during hypnosis as part of the deepening technique or post hypnotic suggestion.

Guided imagery has been used in sports psychology, in which the athlete imagines winning a game or performing perfectly, with often successful results. In a similar manner, people can worry themselves unwell, because the same mechanism is in place when visualizing poor outcomes. The good news, according to Dr. Rossman from the Academy for Guided Imagery, is that the person who is a good worrier is usually a good candidate for using visualization to improve performance or elicit relaxation. Brain scans completed during guided imagery/visualization have demonstrated activation of the cerebral cortex and centers of the primitive brain; when imagery is imagined, the visual cortex is active, and when sounds are imagined, the auditory cortex is active.[22]

A formal guided imagery session with a practitioner typically includes an assessment of which symptoms the patient might want to explore, the imagery process, and an evaluation of the patient after the imagery process. The imagery process may begin with relaxation and include various guided imagery techniques such as healing imagery, interactive imagery dialogue, and evocative imagery. While formal guided imagery sessions are done with a practitioner, guided imagery can be done utilizing audio recordings, a method that reduces cost and inconvenience. Many published studies have examined the efficacy of guided imagery through the use of audio recordings.

While guided imagery can be utilized with minimal downside by most people, there are patients in whom guided imagery should be used with caution, including patients with a history of trauma, suicide, or unstable medical problems. Practitioners of guided imagery, like those who practice hypnosis, should have an appropriate level of training.

The literature for guided imagery has grown significantly, and the majority of studies have been published in the past decade.[28] A growing body of evidence suggests that guided imagery is effective for numerous conditions. Giacobbi, et al. conducted a scoping review of guided imagery and analyzed 320 randomized controlled trials that used guided imagery as an intervention for various complaints, including insomnia. The review found that the majority of studies showed positive outcomes related to physical, psychological, and functional changes.[29] A subgroup analysis of studies from four selected journals demonstrated an improvement in 10 of 13 studies (76.9%), suggesting that guided imagery results in improved outcomes. Since the conditions treated varied widely, a meta-analysis was not conducted, and quantitative data were not obtained in that review.

Guided imagery has been used for sleep issues, often in conjunction with progressive muscle relaxation. The published data are limited but does suggest that guided imagery may be effective. In one study, patients with cancer used guided imagery during their treatment and were assessed after treatment.[30] Sleep was one of the metrics analyzed, and it was found that the use of guided imagery resulted in a significant improvement in sleep quality. In another study, the use of relaxation and guided imagery for pain, fatigue, and sleep disturbance found a trend toward improvement in fatigue and sleep, but pain remained problematic for the majority of the patients at the end of treatment.[31]

Imagery rehearsal therapy can be considered a form of guided imagery that has been used to treat nightmares related to PTSD and subsequent sleep disruption.[32] This therapy treats nightmares by creating and rehearsing an altered dream script, and a meta-analysis of 13 studies found that imagery rehearsal had large effects on nightmare frequency, sleep quality, and PTSD symptoms from initial to post-treatment assessments. Results were sustained for 6–12 months of follow-up. Imagery rehearsal therapy can also be used during hypnosis, as previously described.

Although the data are somewhat limited for guided imagery and insomnia, guided imagery has been found to be effective for multiple conditions including stress and anxiety, which are frequently contributing factors to insomnia. Given its low cost and ease of use, a trial of guided imagery as an adjunctive measure to CBT-I may be beneficial in appropriately selected patients. Relaxation strategies including guided imagery and progressive muscle relaxation can be included in insomnia treatment classes, and insomnia patients can be encouraged to practice these relaxation techniques daily to induce the parasympathetic nervous system to prepare the body for sleep.

Hypnosis Versus Guided Imagery

While guided imagery and hypnosis are not identical, the distinction between the two is not well delineated. Both have similarities in that they may use suggestion, imagery, and the mind to address a clinical condition. Hypnosis utilizes a more formalized procedure with the elicitation of trance and the creation of post hypnotic suggestion, but imagery is frequently used as a part of the hypnosis process. Patients may respond to either form of therapy, although those who are more hypnotizable may find guided imagery and hypnosis more beneficial than those who are not.

The findings of one study suggest that the imagery that patients experience during hypnosis may be in part related to their degree of hypnotizability.[33] Imagery and perception share cortical patterns when activated, but in this study it was discovered that high- and low-hypnotizable subjects may experience visual and tactile imagery tasks differently. Both sets of subjects had similar visual imagery ability, but low-hypnotizable subjects required more effort to obtain this imagery. High-hypnotizable patients also obtained better imagery when tactile instructions were given as compared with low-hypnotizable subjects, who again required more effort. This study found that low-hypnotizable subjects' main imagery modality was that of visualization while high-hypnotizables may have utilized visual and tactile imageries.

Overall, the literature suggests that both clinical hypnosis and guided imagery can be effective in the treatment various sleep conditions. While neither would be a replacement for CBT-I, the first-line treatment for insomnia, they can be used during or after a course of CBT-I. They can also be used for other sleep disorders such as nightmares and NREM parasomnias, and they can help with conditions that interfere with sleep, such as pain. Practitioners of guided imagery and clinical hypnosis should have proper training in either technique. Numerous audio recordings of guided imagery are available for purchase as apps and CDs, but careful vetting of the practitioner is recommended to ensure that the therapeutic techniques are appropriately performed. Audio recordings also exist for hypnosis, but the lack of an individualized post hypnotic suggestion may render them less effective for a given patient's needs.

In summary, clinical hypnosis and guided imagery are low-cost, low-risk interventions that may yield significant benefits, and, although further study is needed, they may be used to effectively address a variety of sleep issues and issues related to sleep.

Resources

HYPNOSIS SOCIETIES

American Society of Clinical Hypnosis (ASCH)
National Pediatric Hypnosis Training Institute (NPHTI)
Society for Clinical and Experimental Hypnosis (SCEH)
Milton H. Erickson Foundation. [6]

GUIDED IMAGERY SOCIETIES

Academy for Guided Imagery (AGI)

REFERENCES

1. Kohler WC, Kurz PJ. *Hypnosis in the management of sleep disorders.* New York: Routledge; 2017.
2. Hammond DC. *Hypnotic induction & suggestion.* Bloomingdale, IL: American Society of Clinical Hypnosis; 1998.
3. Aurora RN, Zak RS, Auerbach SH, et al. Best practice guide for the treatment of nightmare disorder in adults. *J Clin Sleep Med.* 2010;6(4):389–401.
4. American Psychological Association Division 30 (APA division 30). 2017 Jul 5. http://www.apadivisions.org/division-30/index.aspx
5. American Society of Clinical Hypnosis. 2017 Jul 5. http://www.asch.net/
6. Hammond C. *The handbook of hypnotic suggestions and metaphors.* Bloomingdale, IL: American Society of Clinical Hypnosis; 1990.
7. Becker P. Hypnosis in the management of sleep disorders. *Sleep Med Clin.* 2015;10:85–92.
8. Howard HA. Promoting safety in hypnosis: A clinical instrument for the assessment of alertness. *Am J Clin Hypnosis.* 2017;59(4):344–362.
9. Kluft RP. The importance of dehypnosis or re-alerting in safeguarding patients and workshop participants. *Focus.* 2006;48(1): 6–7.
10. Gordon J. *Handbook of clinical and experimental hypnosis.* New York: Macmillan; 1967.
11. Temes R. *Medical hypnosis: An introduction and clinical guide.* New York: Churchill Livingstone; 1999.
12. Yapok M. *Trancework,* 3rd ed. New York: Routledge Taylor & Francis Group; 2003.
13. Gfeller J, Lynn SJ. Enhancing hypnotic susceptibility: Interpersonal and rapport factors. *J Pers Soc Psychol.* 1987 Mar. doi:10.1037//0022-3514.52.3.
14. Hauri PJ, Silber MH, Boeve BF. The treatment of parasomnias with hypnosis: A 5-year Follow-Up Study. *J Clin Sleep Med.* 2007;3(4):369–373.
15. Eichelman B. Hypnotic change in combat dreams of two veterans with post-traumatic stress disorder. 1985 Feb. doi:10.1176/ajp.142.1.112.
16. Erikson MH. Further clinical techniques of hypnosis: Utilization techniques. *Am J Clin Hypnosis.* 1959;2:3–21.
17. Hurwitz TD, Mahowald MW, Schenck CH, Schluter JL, Bundlie SR. A retrospective outcome study and review of hypnosis as treatment of adults with sleepwalking and sleep terror. *J Nerv Ment Dis.* 1991;179(4):228–233.
18. Reid WH. Treatment of somnambulism in military trainees. *Am J Psychother.* 1975;29(1):101–106.
19. Kennedy G. A review of hypnosis in the treatment of parasomnias: Nightmare, sleepwalking, and sleep terror disorders. *Austral J Clin Exp Hypnosis.* 2002;30(2):99–155.
20. Kohler WC, Kurz PJ, Kohler EA. A case of successful use of hypnosis in the treatment of parasomnia overlap disorder behavioral sleep medicine. *Behav Sleep Med.* 2015; 13:349–358.

21. Cordi MJ, Schlarb AA, Rasch B. Deepening sleep by hypnotic suggestion. *Sleep.* 2014;37(6):1143–1152.
22. Ross H, Lac KB. Mind-body therapies for better sleep. *Advances.* Winter 2007/ 2008;22(3–4):28–31.
23. Patterson D. Hypnosis: An alternate approach to insomnia. *Can Fam Physician.* 1982.28:768–770.
24. Qaseem A, Kansagara D, Forciea MA, Cooke M, Denberg TD. Management of chronic insomnia disorder in adults: A clinical practice guideline from the American College of Physicians. *Ann Intern Med.* 2016;165(2):125–133.
25. Anbar R, Slothower D, Molly P. Hypnosis for treatment of insomnia in school-age children: A retrospective chart review. *BMC Pediatr.* 2006 Aug 16. http://www.biomedcentral.com/I471-2431/6/23
26. Morone NE, Greco CM. Mind-body interventions for chronic pain in older adults: A structured review. *Pain Med.* 2007;8(4):359–375.
27. Vanhaudenhuyse A, Gillet A, Malaise N, et al. Psychological interventions influence patients' attitudes and beliefs about their chronic pain. *J Tradit Compl Med.* 2017 May 11;8(2):296–302. doi:10.1016/j.jtcme.2016.09.001.
28. Rossman M. Guided imagery and interactive guided imagery. In Rakel D, ed. *Integrative medicine*, 4th ed. Philadelphia: Elsevier; 2018: 930–936.
29. Giacobbi PR Jr, Stewart J, Chaffee K, Jaeschke AM, Stabler M, Kelley GA. A scoping review of health outcomes examined in randomized controlled trials using guided imagery. *Prog Prev Med.* 2017 Dec;2(7):e0010.
30. Shu-Fen Chen, Hsiu-Ho Wang, Hsing-Yu Yang, Ue-Lin Chung. Effect of relaxation with guided imagery on the physical and psychological symptoms of breast cancer patients undergoing chemotherapy. *Iranian Red Crescent Med J.* 2015 Nov;17(11):e31277.
31. Nooner AK, Dwyer K, DeShea L, Yeo TP. Using relaxation and guided imagery to address pain, fatigue, and sleep disturbances: A pilot study. *Clin J Oncol Nurs.* 2016;20(5):547–552.
32. Casement MD, Swanson LM. A meta-analysis of imagery rehearsal for post-trauma nightmares: Effects on nightmare frequency, sleep quality, and post-traumatic stress. *Clin Psychol Rev.* 2012 Aug;32(6):566–574.
33. Carli G, Cavalloro F, Santarcangelo E. Hypnotizability and imagery modality preference: Do highs and lows live in the same world? *Contemp Hypnosis.* 2007;24(2):64–75. www.interscience.wiley.com. doi:10.1002/ch.331.

24

Pharmaceutical Sleep Medications and Medications That Affect Sleep

MICHAEL BESHIR AND KAYLA COOK

Introduction

Sleep disturbance is one of the most prevalent complaints that impacts individuals of all races and ages throughout the world. It is estimated that approximately 10–15% of the adult population suffer from insomnia disorder alone.[1] Much of this is often attributable to factors such as poor sleep hygiene, psychological stress, respiratory issues, pain, and the widespread use of psychoactive substances like caffeine and nicotine. While some causes of insomnia are easily identifiable and widely accepted as significant culprits, diagnosing the disorder remains a challenge to many providers. In fact, as recently as 2014, the *International Classification of Sleep Disorders* (ICSD) reclassified the disorder because the previous classification failed to better identify the cause and improve diagnosis.[2,3] Previously, insomnia was divided into three categories: primary insomnia, secondary insomnia, and comorbid insomnia. Currently it is designated as either *short-term insomnia* (lasting less than 3months and caused by an identifiable trigger) or *chronic insomnia* (persisting for more than 3 months and often without an identifiable trigger). In this chapter, we discuss medications used in the treatment of insomnia as well as medications used for other purposes that contribute to either insomnia or hypersomnia.

Medications Used in the Treatment of Insomnia

In this section, we explore the pharmacological options available for use in treating patients with insomnia, their risks and downsides, as well as important age considerations. As age increases, so does the prevalence of insomnia. According to the American Academy of Sleep Medicine (AASM), insomnia is defined as the subjective perception of difficulty with sleep initiation, duration, consolidation, or quality that occurs despite adequate opportunity for sleep, which results in some form of daytime impairment.[4] Persistent insomnia is the presence of symptoms at least three times per week and present for a duration of 3 months or longer.[5] While cognitive-behavioral therapy and nonpharmacological management have been proved effective first-line treatments, pharmacotherapy remains the most widely used treatment option for patients with insomnia.[6,7]

Pharmacotherapy for treatment of insomnia should only be utilized on an as-needed basis and for the shortest duration of therapy as possible.[8] When used for longer periods some medications such as benzodiazepines may lose effectiveness due to tolerance, or dependence may develop.[9] Additionally, the safety and efficacy of long-term pharmacotherapy for insomnia has not been studied.

Evaluating duration of action is especially important when selecting which sedative-hypnotic agent is most appropriate for treatment of insomnia. It is helpful to consider whether a patient is having difficulty initiating sleep or maintaining sleep throughout the night. If insomnia is primarily due to trouble initiating sleep upon going to bed, a faster acting medication with a shorter half-life may be the most beneficial.[10,11] In cases where there is difficulty maintaining sleep, such as frequent awakenings or problems returning to sleep after awakening, a medication with a longer time to peak effect and longer half-life would be more suitable. Age is another important factor when choosing therapy, and the American Geriatrics Society (AGS) Beers Criteria includes many medications for use in treatment of insomnia that should be avoided in older adults.[12]

BENZODIAZEPINES

Benzodiazepines, a class of sedative-hypnotic medications, are important in the setting of short-term insomnia. Benzodiazepines can be divided into three major categories depending on half-life. Short-acting benzodiazepines have a half-life of less than 12 hours. Intermediate-acting benzodiazepines have a half-life of 12–24 hours, and long-acting benzodiazepines may have half-lives of more than 24 hours. The half-life of a long-acting benzodiazepine may be due to the production of active metabolites that may contribute to the sedating effects of the medication being seen long after drug has been eliminated.[13]

Benzodiazepines act as sedatives by potentiating the action of inhibitory neurons within the central nervous system (CNS). Gamma-aminobutyric acid (GABA) is the fundamental sedating neurotransmitter released in the CNS. The benzodiazepine acts by binding to a subunit of the $GABA_A$ receptor, the BZ receptor, of postsynaptic GABA neurons.[14,15] While the class of benzodiazepines is broad and many drugs exist, only five have been approved by the US Food and Drug Administration (FDA) for use in treatment of insomnia: temazepam (Restoril), triazolam (Halcion), flurazepam (Dalmane), quazepam (Doral), and estazolam.

In the setting of insomnia, benzodiazepines take effect quickly. Results in sleep improvement are seen after as little as one dose, though tolerance to benzodiazepines develops quickly, and symptoms of rebound insomnia when withdrawing therapy may be seen after as little as 10 days of therapy.[16,17] Benzodiazepines should be prescribed with caution especially in the older adult population. The AGS Beers' Criteria includes benzodiazepines as high-risk medications and potentially inappropriate to use in the elderly. Benzodiazepines have been linked to increased risk of falls leading to fractures, prolonged sedation, respiratory depression, and death in elderly patients.[12] If use of benzodiazepines is unavoidable, dose reduction is recommended as well as use of agents with shorter half-lives (e.g., temazepam) over longer acting benzodiazepines. Half-life can as much as double when used in the elderly population, and close monitoring for daytime sedation is required.[18] In the inpatient setting, use of benzodiazepines increases risk of delirium significantly.[18,19] All benzodiazepines may result in common side effects, including drowsiness, dizziness, and lethargy.[18]

Triazolam

Triazolam is a short-acting benzodiazepine FDA approved for short-term use in insomnia, preferably for 14 days or less.[17] Triazolam has an onset of only 15–30 minutes, with a half-life of 1.5–5.5 hours.[20] With its rapid onset, triazolam is ideal for use in those with sleep onset insomnia; it can be taken immediately before bed and should be taken on an empty stomach. However, in patients who are a high fall risk, the fast onset may increase risk for falls and fractures. No dosage adjustment is required in the setting of renal or hepatic dysfunction. Triazolam does not produce an active metabolite, which decreases risk of accumulation upon repeated dosing. In patients with a low body weight, a decreased dose may be recommended. In addition to the class-wide side effects, the most commonly reported side effects of triazolam include ataxia, headache, and nausea.[20–22]

Temazepam

Temazepam is an intermediate-acting benzodiazepine with a half-life of 3.5–18.4 hours, with peak effects seen in as little as 1 hour.[23] Due to the longer half-life, temazepam dosage adjustments are required when used in elderly and debilitated patients to reduce risk of side effects due to dose accumulation.[24] Temazepam, unlike triazolam, can cause a daytime "hangover effect" likely due to its extended half-life. Dose reductions are not required in renal or hepatic dysfunctions, although these patients should be closely monitored for daytime sedation. With long-term use of temazepam, withdrawal or rebound symptoms can be seen if dose is abruptly decreased or discontinued, and the dose should be reduced slowly to prevent symptoms of withdrawal.[23-25]

Estazolam

Estazolam is an intermediate-acting benzodiazepine with a half-life ranging from 10 to 24 hours, which may contribute to next-day sedation. Peak action occurs on average 2 hours after dose is taken, but onset is as early as 30 minutes. For this reason, estazolam should be taken right before bed, preferably on an empty stomach. Estazolam produces inactive metabolites that do not influence the drug's duration of action. In addition to the common class side effects, estazolam may cause "hangover effect" and abnormality in thinking. No dosage adjustments for renal or hepatic function are required, although empiric dose reduction is recommended for the elderly and debilitated populations. Estazolam is substrate of CYP3A4, and use of estazolam with other drugs metabolized by CYP3A4 should be evaluated for interaction and either therapy or dose adjustments should be considered. Smoking increases clearance of estazolam, likely due to CYP3A4 induction.[26]

Flurazepam

Flurazepam is a long-acting benzodiazepine useful in both sleep onset and sleep maintenance insomnia. Flurazepam is rapidly absorbed, with peak effects seen in 30–60 minutes and with a half-life of only 2.3 hours for the parent compound. However, metabolism of the drug produces an active metabolite (N-desalkylflurazepam) that may continue circulating for as long as 90 hours after a single dose. In older adults (>61), this is lengthened further, with the metabolite present for up to 160 hours. Though no renal or hepatic dose adjustments are required, next-day sedation and drowsiness may be increased in these populations and patients should be closely monitored. When discontinuing chronic treatment, doses should be reduced slowly to avoid symptoms of withdrawal and rebound insomnia.[27]

Quazepam

Quazepam is also a long-acting benzodiazepine. Like flurazepam, quazepam produces active metabolites which dramatically extend the half-life of the drug.

Time to peak effect observed is approximately 2 hours, and half-life of the parent compound is 39 hours. Half-life of active metabolite N-desalkyl-2-oxoquazepam is 73 hours. Notably, when compared to younger adults, the half-life of quazepam doubles in the elderly population, and empiric dose reduction in geriatric patients is recommended due to the increased risk of confusion and next-day sedation. Withdrawal symptoms and rebound insomnia may occur if long-term treatment is discontinued abruptly.[28]

DRUG INTERACTIONS

Drug interactions should be evaluated when prescribing benzodiazepines for use in insomnia. Due to benzodiazepine metabolism through the liver, other medications that are also metabolized by CYP enzymes may compete with benzodiazepines, leading to increased half-life and prolonged effects. Major inhibitor interactions include macrolide antibiotics, HIV protease-1 inhibitors, amiodarone, diltiazem, and grapefruit juice. Alternatively, drugs that induce enzymes of the liver may lead to an increased clearance of benzodiazepines and reduced effects. Major inducers to consider when prescribing include anticonvulsants like carbamazepine, phenytoin, and fosphenytoin, as well as rifampin and the herbal supplement St. John's Wort.[15,29] Concomitant use with opioids is not advised, and the FDA has issued a black box warning due to increased risk of impaired cognition, respiratory depression, coma, and death.[30,31] Alcohol may also contribute to the risk of oversedation as well as respiratory depression when used with benzodiazepines and should be avoided.

Z-DRUGS AND OTHER HYPNOTICS

Z-drugs are another common class of hypnotics that also exerts action via the BZ receptor. Their structural dissimilarity prevents them from being classified as benzodiazepine and leads to the advantage of exhibiting their effects more selectively within the $GABA_A$ receptor.[32] Z-drugs are more selective for the BZ receptor, which allows the agent to exert hypnotic activity without the additional anxiolytic and anticonvulsant effects of the benzodiazepines. This specificity may reduce the occurrence of therapy limiting side effects such as daytime sedation, fatigue, and cognitive impairment associated with benzodiazepines.[33] There have been less instances of withdrawal side effects when discontinuing treatment with Z-drugs, and, when compared to benzodiazepines, abuse is less frequent. For these reasons, the Z-drugs are considered a safer option when selecting pharmacotherapy for insomnia.[6,8,11,33]

However, parasomnias, or activities completed during sleep that patients cannot recall the next day, have been observed with use of Z-drugs.[33] As with benzodiazepines, Z-drugs are included on the AGS Beers Criteria as high-risk medications to be avoided in the elderly due to increased instances of side effects such as delirium, falls, motor vehicle accidents, and increased hospitalizations.[12] There are three FDA-approved hypnotics for treatment of insomnia, classified as Z-drugs: zaleplon (Sonata), zolpidem (Ambien, Ambien CR, Intermezzo), and eszopiclone (Lunesta).

Zaleplon

Zaleplon has a fast onset, and peak effects are observed about 1 hour after ingestion; it has an extremely short half-life of less than 1 hour. The fast-acting kinetics makes zaleplon an effective choice for patients who have difficulty initiating sleep. The fast onset of action allows zaleplon to be taken immediately before bed. High-fat meals should be avoided before taking zaleplon as absorption and effects may be delayed by as much as 2 hours. Incidences of daytime fatigue and prolonged sedation is decreased owing to the short half-life. However, zaleplon may not be an effective treatment option for patients who require therapy for sleep maintenance, and efficacy has not been studied for long-term use. Renal dosing is not required, but in the setting of hepatic dysfunction or advanced age empiric dose reduction is recommended for use of zaleplon.[34,35]

Zolpidem

Zolpidem was the first Z-drug approved for use in insomnia by the FDA. Zolpidem is commercially available in multiple dosage forms including immediate-release (IR), extended-release (CR), and orally disintegrating (ODT) tablets, as well as an oral metered dose spray. Different options in dosage formulations can be an advantage when treating special populations such as patients who may have difficulty swallowing.[36]

Zolpidem immediate-release has a short half-life of 2.5 hours with a peak onset at 1.6 hours. This makes zolpidem immediate-release an effective option for treatment of sleep initiation, but its effects may not last long enough to impact sleep maintenance. The zolpidem extended-release formulation has a similar half-life to zolpidem IR, but the drug is designed to be released over a longer period. This makes zolpidem extended-release a potentially more effective option for use in sleep maintenance insomnia. Zolpidem extended-release may also be effective for long-term use. Zolpidem sublingual tablets (Intermezzo) have the benefit of a very short half-life of 3 hours and may be uniquely beneficial for patients with sleep disturbances causing awakening in the middle of the night.[36]

All formulations of zolpidem should be taken on an empty stomach. Eating a meal prior to taking zolpidem can delay onset of effects up to 2 hours. In the setting of hepatic dysfunction and cirrhosis, clearance of zolpidem is decreased, leading to prolonged effects. Empiric dose reductions for hepatic dysfunction are recommended. Interestingly, females have decreased clearance of zolpidem when compared to males, and dose reduction is also recommended when initiating therapy to prevent next-day sedation and cognitive side effects. The most common side effects reported are headache, drowsiness, and dizziness. Cardiac side effects such as tachycardia, hypertension, and chest pressure have also been reported. Zolpidem is a major substrate of the hepatic enzyme CYP34A, and a minor substrate for CYP1A2, CYP2C19, and CYP2C9. Due to the high potential for drug–drug interactions, the patient's current medication regimen should be closely examined before initiating therapy with zolpidem for treatment of insomnia.[12,37–39]

Eszopiclone

Eszopiclone has the longest action of the Z-drugs. With a half-life in adults of 6 hours and an extended half-life of up to 9 hours in elderly patients, eszopiclone can be used effectively for both sleep initiation and sleep maintenance. Due to the longer half-life, next-day fatigue may be more common when using eszopiclone compared to other Z-drugs. Patients may also report a metallic taste in the mouth when using eszopiclone. Eszopiclone clearance decreases in the setting of hepatic dysfunction and in those older than 65, thus making dose reduction appropriate in these populations as well as in debilitated patients. Similar to zolpidem, eszopiclone should be taken on an empty stomach because eating prior to dose may delay onset of action. Eszopiclone is a major substrate of CYP3A2, so reviewing closely for potential drug–drug interactions is important when deciding to initiate therapy.[12,40]

SEDATING ANTIDEPRESSANTS

Tertiary Amine TCAs (Sedating TCAs): Doxepin, Amitriptyline, Trimipramine

Tertiary amine tricyclic antidepressants (TCAs) possess sedating properties largely from their ability to block histamine receptors and, to a lesser degree, their α_1 adrenergic receptor antagonism [3 Amitriptyline has been shown to decrease sleep onset latency (SOL), and in numerous studies patients reported increased drowsiness.[41,42] Similarly, doxepin decreased SOL but is also associated with decreased wake after sleep onset (WASO), increased total sleep time (TST), and better sleep efficiency. In fact, low dose doxepin in 3mg and 6mg doses are so effective as a sedative that it is the only antidepressant to have received FDA indication for this purpose.

Mixed Serotonergic Antidepressants: Trazodone, Nefazodone

Trazodone and nefazodone are classified as mixed serotonergic (or mixed 5-HT) antidepressants for their dual actions as 5-HT2 antagonists/5-HT reuptake inhibitors and their ability to enhance 5-HT_{1A} neurotransmission. Due to their poor receptor selectivity and their prominent antihistaminergic properties, their use as antidepressants is limited by the resulting somnolence. Behind TCAs and monoamine oxidase inhibitors (MAOIs), trazodone is considered the most sedating of all other antidepressants and is now primarily used for this purpose.[43] At low doses, trazodone is often coadministered with selective serotonin reuptake inhibitors (SSRIs) or serotonin-norepinephrine reuptake inhibitors (SNRIs) to counteract their disruptive effects on sleep. It has been shown to decrease SOL, decrease WASO, increase rapid eye movement (REM) latency, increase slow wave sleep (SWS), and improve TST.[44]

Serotonin and α2-Adrenergic Receptor Antagonists: Mirtazapine

Mirtazapine enhances central serotonergic and noradrenergic activity blocking central presynaptic α_2 autoreceptors. It also antagonizes 5-HT_2 and 5-HT_3 receptors, resulting in lower anxiety and gastrointestinal side effects, respectively. Like trazodone, mirtazapine also blocks histamine receptors and causes excessive sedation when used at the higher antidepressant dose. At doses of less than 30 mg it produces predominantly antihistaminergic effects and can serve as an excellent sleep aid.[45] Its favorable effects on sleep parameters include significant reductions in SOL, large increases in TST and sleep efficiency, with minimal changes to REM sleep variables.[44]

SUVOREXANT AND LEMBOREXANT

Suvorexant (Belsomra) and Lemborexant (Dayvigo) are an orexin receptor antagonists. Orexin is a peptide involved with the body's endogenous sleep–wake cycle. Orexin receptors work in the body to promote wakefulness. For this reason, these medications work by downregulating orexin receptor function to promote sleep. They are safe for use in the elderly and does not cause dependence or withdrawal symptoms. The most common side effect seen ~~suvorexant~~ is somnolence, which resolves when use is discontinued. Use of these medications in severe hepatic disease has not been studied and therefore is not recommended. Suvorexant and Lemborexant are safe for use in patients with moderate hepatic dysfunction, though dose adjustments may be required when used in combinations with CYP3A4 inhibitors as well as with drugs with CNS depressing properties. Several important moderate to severe drug–drug interactions to watch for when initiating therapy with Suvorexant or Lemborexant include macrolide antibiotics, HIV-1 protease inhibitors, ketoconazole, itraconazole, diltiazem, and grapefruit juice. No dosage adjustments are required for renal dysfunction or increased age.[12,41,42,45]

MELATONIN RECEPTOR AGONISTS

Melatonin receptor agonists are another treatment option for insomnia. Melatonin is a hormone produced endogenously by the pineal gland of the brain. Stimulation of melatonin receptor (MT_1) induces drowsiness, while (MT_2) primarily functions by synchronizing the circadian rhythm and sleep–wake cycle by indicating to the body that it is dark outside. Many patient-specific and environmental factors can alter the release of endogenous melatonin, making this an attractive molecular target for treating insomnia.[43]

As age increases secretion of melatonin decreases, which may contribute to decreased sleep quality in the elderly.[43] Use of bright lights and devices that produce light, such as smartphones, at night may also cause melatonin production to decrease. While good sleep hygiene includes a cool, dark room that may help to counteract insomnia due to slowing of melatonin release, additional intervention may still be necessary.[44,46] The only current prescription option approved by the FDA for insomnia is ramelteon, which is a melatonin receptor agonist that binds to both melatonin receptors MT_1 and MT_2, thus promoting the feeling of drowsiness and sedation.[47] Ramelteon has a short half-life of 1–3 hours, making it a viable option for patients with sleep induction disturbances. Additionally, it has an active metabolite (M-II) that can extend its half-life by 2–6 hours, making it potentially useful for sleep maintenance.

Ramelteon does not interact with benzodiazepine receptors and consequently does not promote CNS depression, physical dependence, or withdrawal symptoms when therapy is discontinued. Side effects when taking ramelteon include headache, somnolence, and nasopharyngitis. It is a major substrate of CYP1A2, so drug interactions with mexiletine, ciprofloxacin, and fluvoxamine are important to consider. Empiric dose reductions in patients with mild-moderate hepatic dysfunction are recommended, and use should be avoided in severe cases. Dosage reductions are not required when using ramelteon in the elderly.[47,48]

OVER-THE-COUNTER MEDICATIONS

Melatonin

In addition to the previously discussed prescription options, over-the-counter (OTC) medications are another important option to consider when treating insomnia. In the United States and Canada, exogenous melatonin is a commonly available FDA-designated "dietary supplement" available in all doses without a prescription.[49] In some other countries, melatonin use has been restricted to prescription use only. Melatonin is commercially available in a range of doses from 0.3 to 10 mg[50,51] and is sold most commonly as oral tablets although transmucosal controlled-release tablets, sublingual melatonin sprays, and transdermal patches are alternative forms of administration. Use of higher doses may increase risk of side effects such as headaches and next-day grogginess.

Use of melatonin may be beneficial for both short- and long-term insomnia, including disorders due to sleep–wake disorders and jet lag. When used for jet lag or circadian disorders, the timing of melatonin administration is critical. Typical dosing of melatonin for use in insomnia is 0.3–5 mg nightly for 4 weeks. Melatonin has a half-life of roughly 50 minutes, so a second dose could be considered for patients experiencing nighttime awakening.[52] For elderly patients, a lower dose of 1–2 mg immediate-release tablets nightly before bedtime is recommended; controlled-release should be avoided due to risk of prolonged sedation.[51,52] Given the fairly short half-life of melatonin, controlled-release formulations may potentially be more effective for patients with sleep maintenance insomnia. A sublingual formulation may be helpful for sleep onset insomnia or for dosing after a nighttime awakening.

Though melatonin itself has not been shown to cause dependence, chronic use of high-dose melatonin may impact endogenous nocturnal production of melatonin.[53-55] It has been suggested that treatment with melatonin may be particularly useful in the elderly suffering from early morning awakening, but further studies are still needed.

Melatonin may also have an important role in treatment of REM sleep behavior disorder (RBD), a sometimes violent parasomnia in which patients may act out their dreams.[56] Actions may include flailing of arms, kicking, hitting, or other potentially injurious behaviors. Clonazepam is the current first-line treatment, but melatonin may be a viable option as well.[56] In a placebo-controlled trial, melatonin significantly reduced the frequency of potentially harmful behaviors when compared with baseline.[57] With fewer drug interactions and a more favorable side-effect profile, melatonin appears to be a promising treatment option, especially in the elderly population and in patients at high risk for polypharmacy.[56]

Histamine Receptor (H₁) Antagonists

First-generation antihistamines diphenhydramine and doxylamine are widely used in OTC allergy products but are also available for use in treatment of occasional insomnia. Through competition for histamine receptor (H₁) sites, diphenhydramine and doxylamine promote sedation. Diphenhydramine has a half-life of about 9 hours in adults that is extended to 13.5 hours when used in the elderly. Similarly, doxylamine has a half-life of 10–12 hours. Diphenhydramine and doxylamine peak effect is within 2 hours of administration, and they should be taken 30 minutes before bedtime. The longer half-life may contribute to side effects of daytime sedation and drowsiness after using antihistamines for sedation.[58-60]

Histamine receptor (H₁) antagonists cause potent anticholinergic side effects. Anticholinergic side effects include confusion, blurry vision, dry mouth and skin, urinary retention, and hyperthermia. These side effects are particularly important to consider in the elderly. The Beers Criteria includes both diphenhydramine and doxylamine as medications to avoid in adults older than 65 due to increased risk of anticholinergic side effects and toxicity. Other medications that may also cause anticholinergic toxicity can increase side effects when using histamine receptor antagonists and should be avoided. Additionally, use of alcohol and medications that increase CNS depression should be avoided in combination with histamine receptor antagonists as they may contribute to further CNS depression.[58-60]

Valerian Root

Valerian root (*Valeriana officinalis*) is a herbal therapy possessing sedative properties that may be useful in insomnia. Though the exact mechanism of action is unknown, it is thought to have an effect on GABA receptors. Side effects when taking valerian may include dizziness or drowsiness and potentially abdominal pain if ingested in large quantities. No significant/severe drug interactions have been identified with use of valerian for treatment of insomnia.[61]

Drug-Induced Sleep Disturbance

In the first part of this chapter, we looked at drugs used in the treatment of insomnia and discussed specifics pertaining to their use. In this section, we look at drugs used for other purposes that can lead to some form of sleep disturbance. This includes either drug-induced insomnia or drug-induced hypersomnia. We will attempt to explain the mechanisms by which these drugs result in sleep changes and also discuss the impact that stimulants and restless leg syndrome (RLS) can have on sleep quality.

DRUG-INDUCED INSOMNIA

Although the overall incidence of drug-induced insomnia is unknown, its prevalence for certain drugs is reported to be as high as 55%.[62] Nonetheless, due to its subjective nature and the inherent patient-to-patient variability in symptoms and drug regimens, drug-induced insomnia is often underdiagnosed. Although more robust diagnostic tools, such as polysomnography, daytime multiple sleep latency testing (MSLT), and actigraphy can be employed, their cost is often prohibitive, leading the AASM to recommend against their routine use.[63] For our purposes, however, we will use polysomnographic parameters to objectively discuss the impact that different drugs have on sleep quality. Table 24.1 displays the sleep parameters and various sleep components to which they correspond.

INSOMNIA AS AN ADVERSE EFFECT

It is well-established that insomnia can be secondary to drug use; however, the precise mechanism by which this occurs is less clear for some drug classes. Some adverse effects have strong associations with the offending drugs, such as gastrointestinal irritation caused by nonsteroidal anti-inflammatory drugs (NSAIDs) or hypersensitivity reactions seen with penicillin. Insomnia, however, with its complicated multifactorial etiology, is more difficult to attribute to a drug when

Table 24.1 Polysomnographic parameters of sleep

Polysomnographic parameter	Sleep component
Sleep onset latency (SOL)	Sleep initiation
Total sleep time (TST)	Sleep duration
Wakefulness after sleep onset (WASO)	Sleep consolidation
Sleep efficiency Slow wave sleep (SWS) time REM latency (time to REM sleep) Total REM time	Sleep quality

it occurs as a side effect. Physicians often attribute the insomnia to poor sleep hygiene or an underlying condition.

PSYCHOTROPIC DRUGS

The two major classes of psychotropic drugs implicated in sleep disturbance are antidepressants and antipsychotics. Although their effects on sleep are considered secondary to their intended purpose, those effects can be desirable depending on the patient's underlying disease state and comorbidities. Within these classes of - drugs are several generations of agents that are generally comparable in efficacy but exhibit a vast array of different side effects. These effects are often a consequence of a drug's specific mechanism of action and the set of neurotransmitters it employs but can also be related to its pharmacokinetic and pharmacodynamics profiles.

Antidepressants

With increasing rates of depression among the adult population, the role of antidepressant drugs continues to rise. In a 2011 National Health and Nutrition Examination survey by the Department of Health and Human Services (DHHS), it was estimated that 11% of Americans over the age of 12 were taking antidepressants.[64] While their efficacy in depression and anxiety is undeniable, they add yet another layer of challenges to the already complicated relationship between insomnia and depression. Patients suffering from depression often complain of difficulty falling asleep, frequent awakenings, early morning awakening, and non-refreshing sleep.[65] Conversely, insomnia can cause daytime fatigue, distress, impairment of daytime functioning, and reduced quality of life, which are all risk factors for depression. The challenge with antidepressants is that their impact on this bidirectional relationship between insomnia and depression is largely variable and not easy to ascertain. They predictably alleviate depressive symptoms but can either improve or exacerbate insomnia depending on the balance between their sedating and activating properties. Most literature on antidepressants will make some reference to this point, and some will even classify the drugs based on this property.

Effects of Antidepressants on Sleep
Due to their varying mechanisms and receptor selectivity, some antidepressants can be activating while others tend to be sedating. Activating antidepressants often exacerbate insomnia by increasing 5-HT2 receptor activity and potentiating

noradrenergic and dopaminergic neurotransmission. Examples of activating agents include SSRIs, SNRIs, norepinephrine and dopamine reuptake inhibitors (NDRI), MAOIs, and activating/secondary amine TCAs. On the other hand, sedating antidepressants generally have strong antihistaminergic action and can cause hypersomnia. These include sedating/tertiary amine TCAs, trazodone, and mirtazapine.[66]

SSRIs: Fluoxetine, Paroxetine, Sertraline, Citalopram, Escitalopram, Fluvoxamine. By their serotonergic mechanism of action, SSRIs are generally thought of as the more activating class of antidepressants. They can sometimes lead to restlessness and sleep disturbance.[67] Many patients report attenuation of symptoms over time, but some can persist and negatively impact quality of life. Of the SSRIs, the effects of fluoxetine on sleep are the most extensively studied and appear to reflect those of other agents within this class.[64,65,67,68] A study of 119 participants found no statistically significant difference between fluoxetine, paroxetine, and sertraline in their activating and/or sedating properties.[69] Pooled subjective data from the other fluoxetine studies indicated that it was more likely to cause insomnia when compared to placebo, but, interestingly, rates of somnolence reporting were also high.[65,68,70] This also coincides with rates of sleep disturbance reported for other drugs within this class. According to data from the FDA, the incidence of treatment-emergent insomnia with administration of an SSRI was nearly 17% as compared to 9% for patients receiving placebo.[65,71] Similarly, the average incidence of treatment-emergent somnolence was 16% for SSRIs versus 8% for placebo. Fluvoxamine for the treatment of obsessive compulsive disorder (OCD) was associated with both the highest rate of treatment-emergent insomnia at 31.3% and treatment-emergent somnolence at 26.9%. The drug with the lowest incidence of insomnia was citalopram for the treatment of major depressive disorder (MDD), which occurred in less than 2% of patients. For hypersomnia, escitalopram for MDD was the least offending drug, occurring in approximately 6% of patients.

Objective parameters of the impact of SSRIs on sleep are obtained through polysomnographic testing (Table 24.2), which show decreased REM, increased wakefulness after sleep onset, and reduced sleep efficiency.

SNRIs: Desvenlafaxine, Venlafaxine, and Duloxetine. Polysomnographic studies of SNRI effects on sleep are limited, but they are consistent with the subjective complaints of insomnia. WASO is increased, REM onset latency is significantly increased, and total REM time is decreased (Table 24.2). Periodic limb movements that are involuntary in nature, repetitive, and affect the lower extremities can occur in patients receiving venlafaxine and persist for several days after discontinuation. These are also confirmed by increased polysomnographic activity and are likely a contributing factor to sleep disturbance. Like the SSRIs, the average rates of treatment-emergent insomnia and treatment-emergent hypersomnia were significantly higher in patients receiving SNRIs than in those receiving placebo. Of the patients on SNRIs, 13% reported treatment-emergent insomnia and 10%

Table 24.2 **Effects of various drugs on sleep parameters**

Drug class	Sleep parameter						
	SOL	WASO	SWS	REM Latency	Total REM	TST	Sleep efficiency
SSRIs		↑		↑	↓		↓
SNRIs		↑			↓		
Trazodone, nefazodone	↓	↓	↑	↑		↑	
Mirtazapine	↓		=			↑	
Bupropion				↓	↑		
Tertiary amine TCAs	↓	↓		↑	↓	↑	↑
Secondary amine TCAs	↑	↑					↓
MAOIs	↑				↓		
Typical antipsychotics	↓	↓	=	↑		↑	↑
Atypical antipsychotics	↓	↓	↑		↑	↑	↑

MAOI, monoamine oxidase inhibitors; REM, rapid eye movement; SNRI, serotonin-norepinephrine reuptake inhibitors; SOL, sleep onset latency; SSRI, selective serotonin reuptake inhibitors; SWS, slow wave sleep; TCA, tricyclic antidepressant; TST, total sleep time; WASO, wakefulness after sleep onset.

reported treatment-emergent hypersomnia, as compared to those receiving placebo whose corresponding rates were 7% and 5%, respectively. Venlafaxine for treatment of generalized anxiety disorder was associated with both the highest rates of treatment-insomnia and treatment emergent somnolence, each occurring at a rate of 24%. Conversely, levomilnacipran for treatment of MDD was associated with the lowest rates of both, each occurring at a rate of less than 2%. When used for MDD maintenance, duloxetine also had a less than 2% incidence of treatment-emergent somnolence.[71]

In addition to subjective reports of insomnia and daytime somnolence, parasomnias are also a complaint with SNRI use. Polysomnographic testing of venlafaxine shows increased WASO, increased REM onset latency, and a decrease in total REM time. There also appeared some activity in the lower extremity electrodes that could explain the occasional complaints of involuntary leg movements.

Norepinephrine and Dopamine Reuptake Inhibitor (NDRI)—Bupropion. Bupropion is the sole agent in this class and is considered one of the more activating antidepressants. Reports of insomnia depend on several factors but can be as high as 20% in patients with depression or seasonal affective disorder. Despite this, bupropion is one of the few antidepressants that shows favorable REM effects. It shortens REM latency and increases total REM sleep time.

Secondary Amine TCAs (Activating TCAs). Because of their affinity for various unintended targets such as the cholinergic, histaminergic, and α-adrenergic receptors, TCAs lead to many adverse effects that limit their use in depression. Reports of arrhythmias, sedation, weight gain, orthostatic hypotension, and anticholinergic effects are well-documented and appear to be dose-dependent. Interestingly, the propensity to cause these effects shows a stronger correlation with an identifiable structural feature that is not common to all TCAs: the presence of a tertiary amine in their chemistry. It is for this reason that TCAs are often subclassified by their chemical structure as either secondary amines or tertiary amines. Tertiary amine TCAs are more sedating, more likely to induce hypersomnia, and will be discussed in greater detail later in the hypersomnia section of this chapter. Secondary amine TCAs, which include drugs such as desipramine and nortriptyline, are more activating and more likely to cause insomnia. Studies looking at the effects of desipramine on sleep found that it was associated with increases in SOL, increases in WASO, reduced TST, and less sleep efficiency.[66,72] Similarly, nortriptyline's effects on sleep parameters showed a trend consistent with insomnia: increased SOL, increased REM latency, and overall REM suppression.[73]

Monoamine Oxidase Inhibitors (MAOIs). By inhibiting monoamine oxidase (MAO), the enzyme responsible for the degradation of 5-HT, norepinephrine, and dopamine, MAOIs result in increased levels of these neurotransmitter in a nonselective manner. Adverse effects and drug interactions are very common with this drug class and can lead to serious and potentially fatal consequences. Insomnia complaints are frequently reported, especially with tranylcypromine, which has a structure similar to amphetamines.[65] MAOIs are associated with increased SOL, less sleep efficiency, and increased WASO.[74,75] REM suppression is also common with continued use but often rebounds after discontinuation of drug.

Stimulants

Stimulant drugs include methylphenidate and amphetamine salts and are primarily used to treat attention deficit-hyperactivity disorder (ADHD) and are also used to treat central disorders of hypersomnolence (CDH). Additional stimulant medications specific to the treatment of CDH include modafinil, armodafinil, pitolisant and solriamfetol. They medications are discussed in in detail in chapter 30. The precise mechanisms of methylphenidate and amphetamine salts are not well understood, but they act on the dopaminergic and noradrenergic systems to promote the release of catecholamines from their storage sites.[76] In relation to sleep, experts disagree on whether stimulants improve or impair sleep parameters.[77] Some investigators claim that properly treating ADHD with stimulants can improve sleep as baseline rates of insomnia in untreated ADHD can to be as high as 20%.[78,79] In a meta-analysis of methylphenidate's adverse effects, three studies found that patients receiving the drug were at least twice as likely to complain of insomnia as their counterparts who received placebo.[80] Another meta-analysis of seven studies looking at sleep effects of both methylphenidate and amphetamines found that they increase SOL, decrease TST, and decrease sleep efficiency. It is important to note, however, that these undesired effects became less severe over time in patients who remained on stimulants, suggesting that they may be temporary as the body adjusts to the medication. Additionally, SOL results were more favorable for once-daily extended-release formulations than for three times daily immediate-release stimulants since the latter remain in the system for longer. Thus, insomnia could be more linked stimulant levels in the blood and may be improved by optimizing frequency of administration.

Drug-Induced Hypersomnia

According to the third edition of the ICSD, "hypersomnia due to a medication or substance" is one of eight disorders under the broad category of "Central Disorders of Hypersomnolence".[81] An important distinction is made that these disorders are characterized by excessive daytime sleepiness that is not attributable to nocturnal interruptions in sleep or abnormalities of circadian rhythm. In the *Diagnostic and Statistical Manual of Mental Disorders* (DSM-V), hypersomnia is defined as a prolonged nocturnal episode or daily sleep amounts exceeding 9 hours.[2,82] For our purposes, hypersomnia will refer to the excessive daytime sleepiness that occurs as a direct consequence of drug therapy. Our focus will be on drugs with non-sleep primary indications that cause hypersomnia through their sedating properties. Hypersomnolence resulting from drug-induced insomnia or disruption of sleep architecture will not be discussed. Refer to the earlier section "Antidepressants" for a discussion of these drugs effects on hypersomnolence.

ANTIPSYCHOTICS

Antipsychotics are subdivided into first-generation (typical) and second-generation (atypical) agents. Chlorpromazine, fluphenazine, haloperidol, pimozide, and thioridazine are some of the more common first-generation drugs. Second-generation agents include aripiprazole, clozapine, lurasidone, olanzapine, paliperidone, risperidone, ziprasidone, and quetiapine. Although they cause less extrapyramidal side effects and are better tolerated overall, atypical antipsychotics are more associated with sedation. This is because, in addition to blocking histamine receptors as do the first-generation drugs, they also strongly antagonize 5-HT$_2$ receptors.[65] Sleep architecture studies show that both generations of antipsychotics increase

TST, improve sleep efficiency, decrease SOL, and decrease WASO. SWS appeared unchanged by first-generation antipsychotics but was increased by the second-generation agents.[80]

Restless Leg Syndrome

RLS is a sleep-related movement disorder characterized by an urge to move the lower legs, which is sometimes described as a "creeping" sensation. It is worse at night and is typically relieved by movement. These nocturnal symptoms often interfere with sleep and can lead to excessive daytime somnolence secondary to insomnia. Although the pathophysiology is not well understood, a number of associations have been made to reduced CNS iron stores and interference with the dopaminergic system. The reduced CNS iron theory is substantiated by consistently low CSF ferritin in RLS cases when compared to placebo and occurs even when systemic iron studies are normal. The relationship between dopamine and RLS is complex, but they appear to have a positive correlation. This is evidenced by the improvement of RLS symptoms when patients receive dopamine-potentiating drugs.[83]

RLS is often exacerbated, or potentially precipitated, by several types of drugs. Those include antihistamines (particularly the sedating agents), dopamine antagonists (antipsychotics), and antidepressants (mirtazapine, TCAs, and some SSRIs). Antidepressant-induced RLS is most associated with mirtazapine, where rates of new or worsening RLS were as high as 28%.[65] Further supporting the dopaminergic etiology is that the antidepressant bupropion, which blocks reuptake of dopamine, may reduce RLS.[84] Treatment options for RLS include pramipexole, ropinirole, rotigotine transdermal patch, gabapentin, and pregabalin.[85]

Conclusion

While some drugs play an important role in the treatment of sleep disorders, others can drastically disrupt sleep architecture and lead to sleep disturbances. Benzodiazepines offer multiple reliable options for the treatment of insomnia but have many safety concerns and high abuse potential. Z-drugs and the orexin receptor antagonist suvorexant are generally safer than benzodiazepines but can also lead to intolerable side effects and drug interactions. Melatonin receptor agonists are promising treatment options but require further research.

Psychotropic drugs, on the other hand, are the most common cause of drug-induced sleep disturbance. Unfortunately, the exact mechanism is not clearly defined and diagnostic tools are limited. Both drug-induced insomnia and hypersomnolence are common with these drugs since some possess activating properties while others are more sedating. Familiarity with these drug properties is therefore vitally important for a thorough evaluation and accurate diagnosis.

REFERENCES

1. Schweitzer PK, Randazzo AC. Drugs that disturb sleep and wakefulness. In Kryger MH, Roth T, Dement WC, eds. *Principles and practice of sleep medicine.* 6th ed. Philadelphia: Elsevier; 2017: 542–560.

2. American Psychiatric Association. Sleep-wake disorders. http://www.dsm5.org/proposedrevision/Pages/Sleep-WakeDisorders.aspx

3. Everitt H, Baldwin DS, Stuart B, Lipinska G, Mayers A, Malizia AL, Manson CCF, Wilson S. Antidepressants for insomnia in adults. *Cochrane Database Syst Rev.* 2018;5:CD010753.

4. American Academy of Sleep Medicine. *International classification of sleep disorders,* 2nd ed. Westchester, IL: American Academy of Sleep Medicine; 2005.

5. Roth T. Insomnia: Definition, prevalence, etiology, and consequences. *J Clin Sleep Med.* 2007;3(5 Suppl):S7–S10.

6. Sateia MJ, Buysse DJ, Krystal AD. Clinical practice guideline for the pharmacologic treatment of chronic insomnia in adults: An American Academy of Sleep Medicine clinical practice guideline. *J Clin Sleep Med.* 2017 Feb;13(2):307–349.

7. Katz DA, McHorney CA. Clinical correlates of insomnia in patients with chronic illness. *Arch Intern Med* 1998;158:1099.

8. Schutte-Rodin S, Broch L, Buysse D, Dorsey C, Sateia M. Clinical guideline for the evaluation and management of chronic insomnia in adults. *J Clin Sleep Med.* 2008;4(5):487–504.

9. Vinkers CH, Olivier B. Mechanisms underlying tolerance after long-term benzodiazepine use: A future for subtype-selective GABA(A) receptor modulators? *Adv Pharmacol Sci.* 2012:416864. doi:10.1155/2012/416864.

10. Pagel JF, Parnes BL. Medications for the treatment of sleep disorders: An overview. *Prim Care Companion, J Clin Psychiatry.* 2001;3(3):118–125.

11. Saddichha S. Diagnosis and treatment of chronic insomnia. *Ann Indian Acad Neurol.* 2010;13(2):94–102. doi:10.4103/0972-23277.64628.

12. American Geriatrics Society, Beers Criteria Update Expert Panel. American Geriatrics Society 2019 Updated AGS Beers Criteria for potentially inappropriate medication use in older adults. *J Am Geriatr Soc.* 2019:1–21. doi:10.1111/jgs.15767.

13. Griffin CE, Kaye AM, Bueno FR, Kaye AD. Benzodiazepine pharmacology and central nervous system-media effects. *Ochsner J.* 2013;13(2):214–223.

14. Ali NJ, Olsen RW. Chronic benzodiazepine treatment of cells expressing recombinant GABA(A) receptors uncouples allosteric binding: Studies on possible mechanisms. *J Neurochem.* 2001;79:1100.

15. Greenblatt DJ, Shader RI, Divoll M, Harmatz JS. Benzodiazepines: A summary of pharmacokinetic properties. *Br J Clin Pharmacol.* 1981;11(Suppl 1):11S.

16. Brett J, Murnion B. Management of benzodiazepine misuse and dependence. *Aust Prescr.* 2015;38(5):152–155. doi:10.18773/austprescr.2015.055.

17. Asnis GM, Thomas M, Henderson MA. Pharmacotherapy treatment options for insomnia: A primer for clinicians. *Int J Mol Sci.* 2015 Dec;17(1):50.

18. Praharaj SK, Gupta R, Gaur N. Clinical practice guideline on management of sleep disorders in the elderly. *Indian J Psychiatry.* 2018;60(Suppl 3):S383–S396.

19. National Clinical Guideline Centre (UK). Delirium: Diagnosis, prevention and management. *NICE Clin Guidelines.* 2010 Jul;103:8. https://www.ncbi.nlm.nih.gov/books/NBK65564/

20. Upjohn Co. *Halcion (triazolam) prescribing information.* New York: Pharmacia & Upjohn Co.; 2018.

21. Pakes GE, Brogden RN, Heel RC. Triazolam: A review of its pharmacological properties and therapeutic efficacy in patients with insomnia. *Drugs.* 1981;22(2):81–110.

22. Greenblatt DJ, Harmatz JS, Shapiro L. Sensitivity to triazolam in the elderly. *N Engl J Med.* 1991;324(24):1691–1698.

23. Mallinckrodt Inc. *Restoril (temazepam) prescribing information.* Hazelwood, MO: Mallinckrodt Inc.; 2018 Dec.

24. Divoll M, Greenblatt DJ, Harmatz JS. Effect of age and gender on disposition of temazepam. *J Pharm Sci.* 1981;70(10):1104–1107.

25. Nelson J, Chouinard G. Guidelines for the clinical use of benzodiazepines: Pharmacokinetics, dependency, rebound, and withdrawal. Canadian Society for Clinical Pharmacology. *Can J Clin Pharmacol.* 1999;6(2):69–83.

26. Actavis Pharma. *Estazolam prescribing information.* Parsippany, NJ: Actavis Pharma, Inc.; 2018 Dec.

27. Mylan Pharmaceuticals. *Flurazepam hydrochloride prescribing information.* Morgantown, WV: Mylan Pharmaceuticals Inc.; 2016 Sep.

28. Galt Pharmaceuticals. *Doral (quazepam) prescribing information.* Atlanta, GA: Galt Pharmaceuticals, LLC. 2018 Dec.

29. Dresser GK, Spence JD, Bailey DG. Pharmacokinetic-pharmacodynamic consequences and clinical relevance of cytochrome P450 3A4 inhibition. *Clin Pharmacokinet.* 2000;38:41.

30. Park TW, Saitz R, Ganoczy D, et al. Benzodiazepine prescribing patterns and deaths from drug overdose among US veterans receiving opioid analgesics: Case-cohort study. *BMJ.* 2015;350:h2698.

31. Jones CM, Paulozzi LJ, Mack KA, Centers for Disease Control and Prevention (CDC). Alcohol involvement in opioid pain reliever and benzodiazepine drug abuse-related emergency department visits and drug-related deaths—United States, 2010. *MMWR Morb Mortal Wkly Rep.* 2014;63:881.

32. Gunja N. The clinical and forensic toxicology of Z-drugs. *J Med Toxicol.* 2013;9(2):155–162. doi:10.1007/s13181-013-0292-0.

33. Brandt J, Leong C. Benzodiazepines and Z-drugs: An updated review of major adverse outcomes reported on in epidemiologic research. *Drugs R D.* 2017;17(4):493–507.
34. Pfizer Inc. *Sonata (zaleplon) prescribing information.* New York: Pfizer Inc.; 2019 Jan.
35. Pharmacy Quality Alliance. Use of high-risk medications in the elderly (HRM). 2015. http://pqaalliance.org/images/uploads/files/HRM2015.pdf
36. Zolpidem. Lexi-Drugs. Lexicomp. Wolters Kluwer Health, Inc. Riverwoods, IL. http://online.lexi.com
37. Langtry HD, Benfield P. Zolpidem: A review of its pharmacodynamic and pharmacokinetic properties and therapeutic potential. *Drugs.* 1990;40(2):291–313.
38. Salva P, Costa J, Clinical pharmacokinetics and pharmacodynamics of zolpidem. Therapeutic implications. *Clin Pharmacokinet.* 1995;29(3):142–53.
39. Taylor JR, Vazquez CM, Campbell KM, Pharmacologic management of chronic insomnia. *South Med J.* 2006;99(12):1373–1377.
40. Suovion. *Lunesta (eszopiclone) prescribing information.* Marlborough, MA: Sunovion Pharmaceuticals Inc.; 2018 Dec.
41. Merck. *Belsomra (suvorexant) prescribing information.* Whitehouse Station, NJ: Merck, Sharpe & Dohme; 2018 Jul.
42. Kishi T, Matsunaga S, Iwata N. Suvorexant for primary insomnia: A systematic review and meta-analysis of randomized placebo-controlled trials. *PLoS One.* 2015;28:e0136910.
43. Lynch HJ, Jimerson DC, Ozaki Y, et al. Entrainment of rhythmic melatonin secretion in man to a 12-hour phase shift in the light/dark cycle. *Life Sci.* 1978;23:1557.
44. Chang AM, Aeschbach D, Duffy JF, Czeisler CA. Evening use of light-emitting eReaders negatively affects sleep, circadian timing, and next-morning alertness. *Proc Natl Acad Sci U S A.* 2015;112:1232.
45. Ardeljan AD, Hurezeanu R. Lemborexant. StatPearls. Treasure Island (FL): StatPearls Publishing; 2021 Jan.
46. Stepanski EJ, Wyatt JK. Use of sleep hygiene in the treatment of insomnia. *Sleep Med Rev.* 2003;7:215.
47. Nguyen NN, Uy SS, Song JC, Ramelteon: A novel melatonin receptor agonist for the treatment of insomnia. *Formulary.* 2005;40:146–155.
48. Hatta K, Kishi Y, Wada K. Ramelteon for delirium in hospitalized patients. *JAMA.* 2015;314(10):1071–1072.
49. Laudon M, Frydman-Marom A. Therapeutic effects of melatonin receptor agonists on sleep and comorbid disorders. *Int J Mol Sci.* 2014 Sep 9;15(9):15924–15950. doi:10.3390/ijms150915924.
50. Schroeck JL, Ford J, Conway EL, et al. Review of safety and efficacy of sleep medicines in older adults. *Clin Ther.* 2016;38(11):2340–2372.
51. Melatonin (Natural Products Database), Lexicomp Online. Hudson, Ohio: Wolters Kluwer Clinical Drug Information, Inc. 2019 Jun 14.

52. Tordjman S, Chokron S, Delorme R, et al. Melatonin: Pharmacology, functions and therapeutic benefits. *Curr Neuropharmacol.* 2017;15(3):434–443.

53. Witt-Enderby PA, Bennett J, Jarzynka MJ, et al. Melatonin receptors and their regulation: biochemical and structural mechanisms. *Life Sci.* 2003;72:2183.

54. Brzezinski A, Vangel MG, Wurtman RJ, et al. Effects of exogenous melatonin on sleep: A meta-analysis. *Sleep Med Rev.* 2005;9:41.

55. Buscemi N, Vandermeer B, Hooton N, et al. The efficacy and safety of exogenous melatonin for primary sleep disorders. A meta-analysis. *J Gen Intern Med.* 2005;20:1151.

56. McGrane IR, Leung J, Louis E, et al. Melatonin therapy for REM sleep behavior disorder: A critical review of evidence. *Sleep Med.* 2015;16(1):19–26. doi:10.1016/j.sleep.2014.09.011.

57. Kunz D, Mahlberg R. A two-part, double-blind, placebo-controlled trial of exogenous melatonin in REM sleep behaviour disorder. *J Sleep Res.* 2010;19(4):591–596. doi:10.1111/j.1365-2869.2010.00848.x. Epub 2010/06/22.

58. Church MK, Maurer M, Simons FE, et al. Risk of first-generation H(1)-antihistamines: A GA(2)LEN position paper. *Allergy.* 2010;65(4):459–466.

59. Pharmaceuticals Associates. *Diphenhydramine hydrochloride prescribing information.* Greenville, SC: Pharmaceuticals Associates Inc.; 2008 Sep.

60. Chattem. *Unisom (doxylamine) prescribing information.* Chattanooga, TN: Chattem; 2013.

61. Andreatini R, Sartori VA, Seabra ML, Leite JR. Effect of valepotriates (valerian extract) in generalized anxiety disorder: A randomized placebo-controlled pilot study. *Phytother Res.* 2002;16:650.

62. Auger RR, Burgess HJ, Emens JS, et al. Clinical practice guideline for the treatment of intrinsic circadian rhythm sleep-wake disorders. An update for 2015. *J Clin Sleep Med.* 2015;11(10):1199–1236.

63. Gebara MA, Kasckow J, Smagula SF, et al. The role of late life depressive symptoms on the trajectories of insomnia symptoms during antidepressant treatment. *J Psychiatr Res.* 2018;96:162–166.

64. Pratt LA, Brody DJ, Gu Q. Antidepressant use in persons aged 12 and over: United States, 2005–2008. Hyattsville (MD): U.S. Department of Health and Human Services; Centers for Disease Control and Prevention. 2011. http://www.cdc.gov/nchs/data/databriefs/db76.pdf

65. Doghramji K, Jangro WC. Adverse effects of psychotropic medications on sleep. *Psychiatr Clin North Am.* 2016;39(3):487–502.

66. Kupfer DJ, Perel JM, Pollock BG, et al. Fluvoxamine versus desipramine: comparative polysomnographic effects. *Biol Psychiatry.* 1991;29:23–40.

67. American Psychiatric Association. *Practice guideline for the treatment of patients with major depressive disorder.* 3rd ed. Arlington, VA: American Psychiatric Association; 2010.

68. Tisdale JE, Miller DA, Forsyth L. *Sleep disorders: Drug-induced diseases, prevention, detection, and management.* Bethesda, MD: ASHP; 2010.

69. Fava M, Hoog SL, Judge RA, Kopp JB, Nisson ME, Gonzales JS. Acute efficacy of fluoxetine versus sertraline and paroxetine in major depressive disorder including effects of baseline insomnia. *J Clin Psychopharmacol.* 2002;22(2):137–147.

70. Beasley CM Jr, Sayler ME, Weiss AM, et al. Fluoxetine: Activating and sedating effects at multiple fixed doses. *J Clin Psychopharmacol.* 1992;12(5):328–333.

71. Wichniak A, Wierzbicka A, Walęcka M, Jernajczyk W. Effects of antidepressants on sleep. *Curr Psychiatry Rep.* 2017;19(9):63. doi:10.1007/s11920-017-0816-4.

72. Shipley JE, Kupfer DJ, Griffin SJ, et al. Comparison of effects of desipramine and amitriptyline on EEG sleep of depressed patients. *Psychopharmacology.* 1985;85:14–22.

73. Reynolds CF III, Buysse DJ, Brunner DP, et al. Maintenance nortriptyline effects on electroencephalographic sleep in elderly patients with recurrent major depression: Double-blind, placebo- and plasma-level-controlled evaluation. *Biol Psychiatry.* 1997;42:560–567.

74. Wyatt RJ, Fram DH, Kupfer DJ, et al. Total prolonged drug-induced REM sleep suppression in anxious-depressed patients. *Arch Gen Psychiatry.* 1971;24(2):145–155.

75. Kupfer DJ, Bowers MB Jr. REM sleep and central monoamine oxidase inhibition. *Psychopharmacologia.* 1972;27(3):183–190.

76. Kidwell KM, Van dyk TR, Lundahl A, Nelson TD. Stimulant medications and sleep for youth with ADHD: A meta-analysis. *Pediatrics.* 2015;136(6):1144–1153.

77. Preuss U, Ralston SJ, Baldursson G, et al. Study design, baseline patient characteristics and intervention in a cross-cultural framework: Results from the ADORE study. *Eur Child Adolesc Psychiatry.* 2006;15:(Suppl 1):i4–i14.

78. Harpin VA. Medication options when treating children and adolescents with ADHD: Interpreting the NICE guidance 2006. *Arch Dis Child Educ Pract Ed.* 2008;93(2):58–65.

79. Storebø OJ, Pedersen N, Ramstad E, et al. Methylphenidate for attention deficit hyperactivity disorder (ADHD) in children and adolescents: Assessment of adverse events in non-randomised studies. *Cochrane Database Syst Rev.* 2018;5:CD012069.

80. Sharpley AL, Vassallo CM, Cowen PJ. Olanzapine increases slow-wave sleep: Evidence for blockade of central 5-HT(2C) receptors in vivo. *Biol Psychiatry.* 2000;47(5):468–470.

81. Sateia MJ. International classification of sleep disorders-third edition: Highlights and modifications. *Chest.* 2014;146(5):1387–1394.

82. Thorpy MJ. Classification of sleep disorders. *Neurotherapeutics.* 2012;9(4):687–701. doi:10.1007/s13311-012-0145-6.

83. Connor JR, Boyer PJ, Menzies SL, et al. Neuropathological examination suggests impaired brain iron acquisition in restless legs syndrome. *Neurology.* 2003;61:304.

84. Kim SW, Shin IS, Kim JM, et al. Bupropion may improve restless legs syndrome: A report of three cases. *Clin Neuropharmacol.* 2005;28(6):298–301.

85. Aurora RN, Kristo DA, Bista SR, et al. The treatment of restless legs syndrome and periodic limb movement disorder in adults: An update for 2012: Practice parameters with an evidence-based systematic review and meta-analyses: An American Academy of Sleep Medicine Clinical Practice Guideline. *Sleep.* 2012;35(8):1039–1062.

25

Insomnia and Integrative Therapies

ROBERT MAURER AND PARAM DEDHIA

Insomnia Therapy

OVERVIEW

Despite our robust biochemistry and physiology evolved to promote sleep, insomnia is common. Sleep is vulnerable to many factors that can limit the ability to fall asleep at the desired time. This is also true of the many potential challenges to maintain sleep without an excessive number of awakenings. Understanding these factors provides key insights into the treatment of insomnia and is essential to deliver a personalized and therefore effective treatment approach for insomnia.[1,2]

Of all the topics in sleep health, insomnia is one of the most common sleep complaints. It is also one of the most common sleep challenges for which adults seek medical advice. In recent decades, the focus on treatment has ultimately relied on pharmaceuticals. There are many limits that this approach creates. The intention of this chapter is to highlight the management of insomnia with a focus on cognitive-behavioral therapy for insomnia (CBT-I), mindfulness-based therapy for insomnia (MBTI), and other nonpharmacologic therapies.[3-5]

DEFINING INSOMNIA

To appropriately evaluate and target different therapies, it is important to start with the established definition of insomnia. For the purposes of this chapter, we use the paradigms established by both the American Association of Sleep Medicine (AASM; *International Classification of Sleep Disorders* [ICSD-3])[6] and the American Psychiatric Association (APA; *Diagnostic and Statistical Manual of Mental Disorders* [DSM-5]).[7] Insomnia is defined by three cardinal features:

1. A persistent difficulty with sleep initiation, duration, consolidation, or quality
2. Occurs despite adequate opportunity and circumstance for sleep
3. Results in some form of daytime impairment

From a clinical perspective, this is associated with a range of daytime symptoms. To reiterate, without the report of daytime impairment, the challenge with sleep initiation and sleep maintenance would not be diagnosed as insomnia. The classic complaint is fatigue, malaise, or daytime sleepiness. Patients may speak of their reduced motivation, initiative, or energy throughout the day. At other times, the symptoms are less obvious and not initially recognized by the patient or caregiver. Disrupted or disordered sleep can result in poor attention and concentration and possibly memory impairment. As medical reviews do not always go beyond the physical symptoms, it is important to appreciate the symptoms of hyperactivity, impulsivity, and aggression as potential signs of sleep disruption, especially in children. Patients may highlight mood disturbances and irritability within the time course of insomnia. Sometimes insomnia has a more public presentation, with impaired performance in social, family, occupation, or academic settings. At times, it shows itself through errors or accidents. For both the clinician and patient, a symptom review allows for a greater understanding of the patient's current life experiences as well as an opportunity to prioritize treatment. Individuals are not classified as having insomnia if they are, by choice, not allowing sufficient opportunity for sleep. Finally, the diagnosis of insomnia needs to be part of a comprehensive sleep review to determine that another sleep disorder, medical condition, mental health concern, or medication is not contributing to the insomnia. Evidence suggests that insomnia, left untreated, may adversely affect the outcome of both the sleep disturbance and comorbid conditions related to sleep.

TIME COURSE AND CATEGORIES OF INSOMNIA

The time course of signs and symptoms is important to appreciate when individualizing the definition of insomnia. Typically, insomnia is not noted on every night of sleep. Most people erroneously believe that sleeplessness needs to be an every night occurrence for insomnia to exist. More commonly, one or more nights of poor sleep are then followed by a more restful night of sleep with improved quantity and/or quality.

Two classic categories are *acute insomnia* and *chronic insomnia*. The key difference between acute and chronic insomnia is that chronic sleep insomnia is a sleep disturbance and its associated with daytime dysfunction that has existed for 3 months or longer and occurs at least 3 nights per week. Acute insomnia may evolve into chronic insomnia. Given the natural history of acute insomnia, most individuals will seek help only after repeated challenges to obtaining restorative sleep and after attempting to unsuccessfully address their insomnia by themselves. Therefore chronic rather than acute insomnia is the presentation most commonly seen in the medical office setting.

Acute Insomnia

Acute insomnia, also referred to as *adjustment insomnia* or short-term insomnia, usually lasts a few days or weeks and occurs in response to an identifiable stressor. By definition symptoms are present for less than 3 months. Stressors can be physical, psychological, psychosocial, or interpersonal. Symptoms usually resolve when the stressor is eliminated or when the individual adapts to the stressor. Occasionally, sleep problems persist and lead to chronic insomnia. This may occur due to the development of unhelpful sleep habits during the acute insomnia period.

When acute sleep disturbance is left untreated, the patient is at risk of evolving into chronic insomnia. This results in sleep-specific symptoms such as difficulty falling and staying asleep. Again, by definition, insomnia is associated with significant waking distress or impairment. Although the initial sleep disturbance that disrupted healthy sleep may have eased or been removed, it is common that unhelpful and often unintended thoughts and behaviors may perpetuate a state of mental and physical hyperarousal. With the increased effort to sleep, there is often increased cognitive and emotional distress related to sleep and associated with fears related to the ability to sleep, rigid expectations about sleep, and increased attention to solving difficulties with sleep. All of these create a vicious cycle of insomnia fueled by hyperarousal.

Chronic Insomnia

Chronic insomnia may also be diagnosed in individuals who report a pattern of repeated occurrence of sleep difficulties for weeks at a time over several years, even though an individual episode may not last a full 3 months. Some individuals recall an initial stressful event that triggered insomnia, but others report nearly lifelong symptoms without an identifiable trigger. Night-to-night variability and a waxing and waning course related to psychosocial stressors and psychiatric or medical comorbidities are common.

Key History Details on Sleep Patterns

ESTIMATION OF SLEEP DURATION

Given the negative bias of the brain, people with insomnia often overestimate the amount of time it takes them to fall asleep and underestimate their total sleep time when compared with objective data from in-laboratory polysomnography. Although it is not essential to have a formal overnight sleep study to diagnosis insomnia unrelated to a comorbid sleep disorder, the information can be helpful when available. Because limited biomarkers correlate with sleep disorders, it is important to partner with patients to understand their perception of their sleep in order to guide the evaluation, diagnosis, and treatment of insomnia.[8]

TIMING OF SLEEP

Those with restorative sleep are often able to get to sleep within about 10–20 minutes of going to bed with the intention to sleep. Moreover, they typical experience less than 30 minutes awake during the night. Early morning awakening is defined as termination of sleep at least 30 minutes prior to the desired wake-up time.

AWAKENINGS

Night time arousals normally occur and can be misinterpreted as poor sleep. It may be helpful to normalize the patient's distress. This is not to say that an underlying sleep disorder is not present, but the opportunity exists to educate and partner with the patient to differentiate normal awakenings from underlying etiologies disrupting and disordering sleep.

Treatment

Although insomnia is widespread, it is often treatable. As with all disorders, insomnia can be best treated following a thorough history and evaluation that allows for a greater range of optimal options for treatment. Although signs and symptoms are important in making the diagnosis, using these as targets for therapy is not sufficient to appropriately treat the problem. It is necessary to highlight systems and identify etiologies to develop personalized and optimized therapy. It is commonly shown that sleep quality is only as strong as its weakest link. Those with insomnia often have one or more contributors to inadequate sleep. Contributing factors include psychiatric illness, underlying sleep disorders, medical illnesses, medications, poor sleep hygiene, and stress. It is important to determine whether the insomnia is associated with another condition, medication, or substance since these may also need to be a focus of treatment.

Prior to therapy, it is important to prioritize treatment goals with the patient. Classic opportunities include

- Improve sleep quality and/or time
- Decrease time of sleep onset (sleep onset latency [SOL] <30 minutes)
- Limit the time awake after sleep onset (wakefulness after sleep onset [WASO] <30 minutes)
- Reduce number of awakenings
- Increase total sleep time (total sleep time [TST] >6 hours)
- Improve sleep efficiency (>85% of bed time is sleep time)
- Decrease sleep-related psychological distress
- Eliminate daytime impairments in order to promote energy, attention, memory, and cognitive function; reduce fatigue; and improve somatic symptoms

In recent years, there has been a frequent and increasing reliance on pharmacological treatments, and, although these can be helpful when appropriately selected, they are typically most effective as short-term treatments. Furthermore, many patients still experience sleep disturbance despite taking these drugs. Chronic use of hypnotics may lead to dependence on and tolerance of the drugs. Many patients are so overwhelmed when presenting for insomnia in the clinical setting that these limitations do not seem like significant concerns at the time of starting therapy, but most hypnotics pose a risk due to their potential side-effect profile. Therefore careful patient selection and thorough education while initiating a prescription is essential, and a similar process is needed when renewing these medications. The treatment of insomnia presents an opportunity to move beyond pills and speak to skill sets.

COGNITIVE-BEHAVIOR THERAPY FOR INSOMNIA

CBT-I is the leading nonpharmacological treatment for insomnia, and it has substantial evidence to support treatment effectiveness. CBT-I is now a first-line treatment for the disorder. It has been endorsed by the American Academy of Sleep Medicine[9] and the American College of Physicians.[10,11] Its techniques address dysfunctional behaviors and thoughts that interfere with healthy sleep. It usually requires from 4 to 10 visits.

CBT-I Studies

CBT-I studies have shown results either equivalent[12,13] or superior to medication.[14,15] *Combination therapies* provide medication and CBT-I for the duration of CBT and then taper the medication during the course of treatment, but it has been reported that the use of medication prior to initiating CBT is less effective.[16] The medication creates the risk of dependency, and, in the elderly, there is a serious risk of falls. The decision regarding medication use should consider patient motivation and the risks associated with untreated insomnia, which includes substance abuse, depression, and medical comorbidities. CBT-I alone achieves excellent results in the 64–70% range.[17–19]

Research on effectiveness is summarized in two meta-analytic publications. The review by Morin et al.[19] summarized 37 CBT-I outcome studies conducted between 1998 and 2004. All were peer-reviewed, randomized controlled studies, and had one or more of the same outcome measures: SOL, number of awakenings during the night (NA), WASO, TST, or sleep efficiency (ratio of total sleep time to time in bed, expressed as a percentage). Sleep diaries were used to assess results. All interventions were with individuals rather than groups. The studies averaged a 64% improvement. SOL was reduced from 61 to 28 minutes following active treatment compared to a change from 74 to 70 minutes for the control. The control groups were patients on waiting lists who kept diaries but had no formal invention. The second meta-analysis was conducted by Trauer.[15] Twenty studies involving 1,162 patients were included. Individual and group interventions were included. Control groups included sleep hygiene instructions, patient education, or placebo pills. Five of the studies used polysomnography and reported results similar to sleep diaries. Outcomes were measured at the conclusion of treatment, at early follow-up (4 weeks to less than 6 months), and again at 6–12 months. The results for SOL, NA, WASO, and TST were all statistically significant. Average improvement across all measures of sleep outcome was 70% improvement from baseline. A qualification on both of these meta-analyses is that all studies excluded patients with comorbid conditions such as depression or anxiety.

Sleep Hygiene

Sleep hygiene is often the first strategy offered to patients, but it is the least effective.[2,20,21] It should be introduced as a technique that will make CBT-I more effective. Patients often look at the list of sleep hygiene suggestions, assume it is CBT-I, and believe they have already tried this approach and it hasn't worked. The most important sleep hygiene instructions are to ask the patient to wake up at the same time every day and avoid alcohol and naps. One practical strategy is to review the entire sleep hygiene list with the patient, ask them which of the recommendations they are already doing, which ones they have questions about, and which ones they are willing to try. Many sleep hygiene lists were developed before the advent of ubiquitous electronic devices like computers and smartphones that emit light that suppresses melatonin and delays the night time cue to go to sleep that comes with darkness. Clearly this is an important element to be discussed. CBT-I uses the term "buffer zone" to describe the hour or more before bedtime when relaxing activities are recommended. It is important to remind the patient that it may take weeks for CBT-I to be effective.

Sleep Diary

Using the sleep diary method, the patient is asked to keep a record of sleep for 2 weeks. This can be especially helpful to reduce recall errors. Each morning the patient charts when they went to bed, their estimate of when they fell asleep (sleep latency), how many times they awoke and how long they were awake, when they woke up (WASO), and when they got out of bed. The purpose of the diary is to assess *sleep efficiency*: ratio of total sleep time to time in bed, expressed as a percentage For example, the patient reports she went to bed at 10:00 PM, estimates that she fell asleep around midnight, awoke once for about 30 minutes, and was out of bed at 6:00 AM with their family. She was in bed 8 hours and slept approximately 5.5 hours, resulting in a sleep efficiency of 69% (sleep efficiency of 85% and greater is ideal). The diary can reveal poor sleep habits and help identify circadian rhythm disorders. Moreover, it may provide the patient with self-awareness and insight while they are completing the sleep log.

Food Diary

A food diary is often helpful. While there are limited and incomplete studies researching the impact of eating habits on insomnia, clinically, we have treated many patients who eat sparingly during the day and then consume a large meal at night. They report daytime fatigue and difficulty falling asleep or staying asleep. The body is receiving most of its fuel supply—food—at exactly the wrong time of day. When the patient is advised to eat three meals during the day, with breakfast and lunch intake larger than dinner, insomnia is frequently resolved.

CBT-I Strategies

There are three key CBT-I strategies:

1. Stimulus control
2. Sleep restriction
3. Cognitive restructuring

Stimulus control is based on the theory of *operant conditioning*. Insomnia frequently starts with a life crisis that makes sleep difficult. Although the crisis has resolved, the patient now enters the bed worried about whether they will be able to sleep. The worry is now perpetuating the insomnia. The stimulus control strategy uses the following specific instructions designed to break the association between bed and worry:

1. You have come to associate the bed with sleep struggles. These instructions will help you to view the bed as an opportunity for restful, effortless sleep.
2. When you get in bed, if you are unable to sleep, get out of bed and engage in a restful and pleasant activity until you feel sleepy.
3. Feeling "sleepy" is when you can barely keep your eyes open. Being "tired" is when you do not feel rested and alert.
4. Examples of pleasant activities include reading magazines, knitting, watching light entertainment on TV such as comedies, and using relaxation and/or meditation techniques. Avoid electronic devices such as computers and phones.
5. When sleepy, return to bed. If you find yourself unable to sleep, leave the bedroom again and engage in a relaxing, pleasant activity until you are sleepy.
6. Continue this practice for as many nights as necessary to achieve quality sleep. It can often take 1–2 weeks.

Sleep restriction is usually very effective. The principle is to increase the drive to sleep and reduce nighttime awakenings by reducing the time in bed. The sleep diary is essential in calculating the time when the patient is advised to get into bed. Returning to our previous example, if the patient is achieving an estimated 5.5 hours of sleep in spite of spending 8 hours in bed, she is encouraged to go to bed at 12:30 AM if 6:00 AM is the preferred wake time: 5.5 hours is the most that is ever restricted. If the patient is reluctant, there is an alternative: she can start delaying bedtime by 15 minutes a week. Each week, sleep is delayed an additional 15 minutes with the goal of reaching a 12:30 AM bedtime. Once an 85% efficiency of sleep time per amount of bedtime is achieved, 15 additional minutes are added back to the overall sleep time each week if necessary. So, the same patient would go to bed at 10:15 PM and proceed weekly toward the 12:30 AM goal. Once healthy sleep is restored, the process can be reversed: the patient goes to bed 15 minutes earlier while maintaining consolidated sleep (sleep efficiency of 85% or better). As with stimulus control, it is important to negotiate what activities the patient will engage in for the hours before bedtime. Some patients report improved sleep within days, but others require 4–6 weeks for complete success.

Both stimulus control and sleep restriction can result in increased fatigue in the short run. The patient should be cautioned to avoid driving or other activities if the fatigue is a challenge. Safety naps, usually 20–30 minutes maximum, are encouraged if the fatigue is a barrier to adherence.

Cognitive restructuring is sometimes necessary to achieve results with CBT-I. Commonly, many with chronic insomnia worry that their inadequate sleep will significantly limit and impair their daytime lives. This creates a pattern that worsens insomnia. In CBT-I, the counselor elicits the unhelpful beliefs that are contributing to the insomnia. Questionnaires such as the Dysfunctional Beliefs and Attitudes about Sleep (DBAS) elicit beliefs such as "After a poor night's sleep, I know it will interfere with my activities the next day" and "I have little ability to manage the negative consequences of disturbed sleep." Some patients attribute all of their problems in life to insomnia. As a part of cognitive restructuring, the counselor helps the patient to recognize the negative consequences of these perspectives. For some patients, journaling about their worries early in the evening can lead to less rumination at bedtime.

Relaxation Training

Relaxation training is considered an adjunct to other methods and is rarely used alone. Its techniques include progressive muscle relaxation (PMR), controlled breathing, and meditation. PMR involves tensing and relaxing 16 different muscle groups (more details are provided in the section on nonpharmacological approaches). Controlled breathing allows for an awareness of inhalation, pause, and exhalation. Meditation seeks to curate awareness and often provides both physical and psychological well-being through relaxation.

Online CBT-I

Online CBT-I has been effective in improving Insomnia Sleep Index scores, sleep efficiency, TST, SOL, and time awake after sleep onset.[22] Whereas traditional practice focuses on face-to-face CBT-I, the opportunity to offer CBT-I online allows for greater availability and provides, for those hesitant to commit to the structured program, a chance to explore how CBT-I works. For those generations raised with a digital interface, online CBT-I may be used with greater frequency. Data demonstrate that comparable efficacy can be found when comparing online and face-to-face CBT-I, with patient preference being important.

Negative Predictors of CBT-I

In recent years, four key predictors of reduced success of CBT-I have been noted. First and perhaps most obvious is poor adherence.[23] CBT-I requires significantly more motivation than medication treatment. It is ideal for patients who are averse to taking medication or for whom medication has not worked. CBT-I can lead to increased daytime fatigue which may increase risks for accidents or falls. Daytime "safety naps" are permitted. In some studies of CBT-I, the dropout rate was as high as 34%, although the studies were done with group CBT and/or patients on chronic hypnotic medications.[24,25] Second, patients with a TST of less than 6 hours are less likely to benefit from CBT-I.[26] Of the many implications that may result, short sleep time is a risk factor for cardiovascular disease.[27] Vgontzas et al. have proposed that varying insomnia phenotypes might respond differently to insomnia treatment. Those experiencing insomnia with short sleep duration might respond better to biological interventions such medications.[28,29] As one can imagine, this is debatable. Those with insomnia and a more normal sleep duration might have a more positive response to behavioral interventions targeting cognitive-emotional arousal, altering unhealthy sleep-related behaviors and beliefs, and changing sleep misperceptions. Third, patients with childhood-onset insomnia are more difficult to treat than are those with adult-onset insomnia.[20] It is speculated that certain conditions early in life limit the development of coping skills, the ability to self-soothe, and resiliency. These are needed to manage life stressors effectively without suffering significantly from their emotional impacts. It also could be the case that the poorer treatment response occurs because these individuals have suffered from insomnia for a much longer period of time than other patient populations. Fourth, current psychiatric comorbidity is strongly predictive of negative treatment outcome with CBT-I.[30] This may simply be a result of the cognitive dissonance and resultant behaviors that promote hyperarousal and difficulty in gaining insight from CBT-I. The presence of a psychiatric disorder must therefore be one of the leading considerations in the choice of treatment modalities being proposed to patients with insomnia. CBT-I techniques are used with posttraumatic stress disorder (PTSD), bipolar, and suicidal patients only if they are being treated by a counselor at the same time and with the counselor's recommendation.[13,15]

MINDFULNESS-BASED THERAPY FOR INSOMNIA

MBTI combines the principles and practices of mindfulness meditation with some of the behavioral strategies used in CBT-I as an integrative approach to treatment. MBTI is focused on helping people who are distressed about their sleep problems while suffering from insomnia. The intention is to have them see their sleep challenges in a different way and provide some tools to help them sleep better.

Mindfulness meditation cultivates a practice of being in the present moment without holding judgment. This allows for clarity, self-compassion, and reducing one's suffering. The practice of mindfulness is rooted in the observation of impermanence— the awareness that change is the nature of all things. Therefore, thoughts are not necessarily absolute facts; they are simply mental constructs that are ever-changing rather than solely fixed. One of the keys of MBTI to promote better sleep is *meta-cognitive processing*, which includes

- being aware of thoughts in the mind at the present moment while not holding judgment about them,
- appreciating that these thoughts are essentially mental events that come and go, and
- letting go of the attachment to these thoughts and desires.

The core of MBTI is an eight-session group intervention with each session 2.5 hours in duration. Each session has three primary activities: (1) formal meditations, (2) period of discussion, and (3) insomnia-related activities and CBT-I instruction. Each week presents a theme involving the principles of mindfulness integrated with behavioral sleep medicine along with the practice of mindfulness meditation. A meditation retreat is an elective that the patient may choose to deepen their experience and treatment.

Between sessions, participants are given a home meditation practice of 30 minutes for 6 days per week to further the teaching and experience of the group session. Guided meditations may be given to promote home practice. Individuals are asked to complete a daily diary to record their meditation and sleep patterns.

Research studies have provided empirical support for the efficacy of MBTI. It has been shown to reduce pre-sleep arousals to promote sleep onset, WASO, and the ability to return to sleep during the night. Favorable response rates have been noted at the end of the MBTI program, with a rate of response of 60% and a 33% remission rate post-treatment. Furthermore, after 6 months, there was a response rate of 79%, and a 50% remission rate. MBTI is rooted in mindfulness-based stress reduction (MBSR), which is the standard mindfulness-based therapy. MBSR has been shown to produce significant improvements in the Insomnia Severity Index (ISI), Pittsburgh Sleep Quality Index (PSQI), and diary-measured TST, SOL, and sleep efficiency.[31] Moreover, MBTI was superior when compared to MBSR in decreasing insomnia from baseline to 6-month follow-up.[32-36]

Nonpharmacological Practices to Promote Sleep

Whether directly related to thoughts, behaviors, and stressors or having these manifest as a result of other sleep disorders or conditions, there are many causes of insomnia and factors that may perpetuate insomnia. CBT-I and MBTI provide a comprehensive review and approach, and it is important to highlight the modalities within these systems. When possible, it is best to personalize and individualize therapy. Hence, it may be helpful to consider other modalities that could be used in tandem with CBT-I or MBTI—or as standalone opportunities—to further reduce the burden of insomnia. In practical application, CBT-I and MBTI are often combined with other therapies toward improving the initiation and maintenance of sleep as well as the ability to return back to sleep during the night. Therapies and approaches are inherently limited; one size cannot fit all. Although the modalities discussed here are supported by research, the limited medical literature posts results with a range of results—positive, negative, and mixed in different patient populations and with different comorbidities. It is important to understand these different techniques so that their selection can be aligned with patients who may be open to these approaches and who are clinically appropriate.

PROGRESSIVE MUSCLE RELAXATION

PMR dates back to the 1930s as an anxiety-reduction technique. Through a learned script or audio guidance, PMR teaches a person to create muscular and therefore mental relaxation through a two-step process: (1) tensing particular muscle groups, such as the neck and shoulders or a series of muscle groups from head-to-toe or toe-to-head, and (2) releasing the tension on the muscles while creating awareness of the experience and relaxation. This can lower overall tension and stress levels, promote relaxation when feeling anxious, and reduce physical ailments. By tensing and releasing, patients become aware of relaxation within the body and are able to be more aware when tension is starting or building within the body. PMR may be helpful for conditions that cannot be fully improved through medications, such as dementia.[37] Moreover, even in conditions responsive to pharmacotherapy, there are benefits to using a therapy without risk of drug effects[38] or as a supplement to pharmacological treatment.

While a useful adjunct to CBT-I, the research suggests that this strategy is only moderately effective[12,39] as a stand-alone strategy. PMR techniques are thought to either counteract physiological arousal or diminish cognitive activation, such as rumination or worry. One study of the effects of PMR on the sleep quality of cancer patients found that sleep onset and TST were significantly improved.[40]

YOGA

Yoga, which literally means "union," was developed up to 5,000 years ago on the Indian subcontinent as a comprehensive system for well-being on all levels: physical, mental, emotional, and spiritual. Yoga is often equated with hatha yoga—the physical techniques grounded in postures and breathing techniques. Types of hatha yoga include ashtanga, vinyasa, iyengar, satyananda, and power yoga. As sleep is thought to be a rebalancing of the sympathetic and parasympathetic systems toward rest and restoration, breathing promotes vagal tone and relaxation through parasympathetic relaxation. In a National Institutes of health (NIH) survey[41] of persons 18 years and older, 59.3% noted that yoga improved their sleep, yet the survey did not identify type of yoga or frequency of use. In this survey, users of yoga were more likely to report wellness outcomes as compared to those using natural products and spinal manipulation.

In another study focused on a gerontology population, 69 nursing home residents were randomly allocated to three groups: yoga (physical postures, relaxation techniques, voluntarily regulated breathing, and lectures on yoga philosophy), ayurveda (a herbal preparation), and wait-list control (no intervention).[41] After 6 months the yoga group showed a significant decrease in the time taken to fall asleep (approximate group average decrease of 10 minutes) and an increase in the total number of hours slept (approximate group average increase of 60 minutes) and feeling of being rested in the morning based on a rating scale. The statistical finds all noted significance ($P < 0.05$). The comparison groups showed no significant change.

Yoga nidra, a meditation and self-hypnosis technique that does not require intense mental effort or concentration, has been shown to increase parasympathetic dominance and thus relaxation. This has been reported to improve sleep parameters. Clinical studies are in process to determine its benefits and efficacy.[42]

Tai Chi

Tai chi, with principles tracing back to the fourteenth century, emerged initially within China during the middle of the nineteenth century. Tai chi is a form of inner martial art that is practiced as a dynamic form of moving meditation. While gently exercising the whole body, it brings calmness and peace of mind by emphasizing the principles of relaxation. Its teachers encourage the cultivation of inner strength and harmony of both body and mind.

In a study of older adults 59–86, sleep quality was reviewed in persons randomly assigned to 25 weeks of tai chi.[43] This research used PSQI for assessment. The PSQI is a self-reported questionnaire that assesses sleep quality over a 1-month interval. The component scores consist of subjective sleep quality, sleep latency, sleep duration, habitual ciency, sleep disturbances, use of sleeping medication, and daytime dysfunction. Scores range from 0 to 21, with 5 and greater identifying sleep disturbance. Among adults with moderate sleep complaints, subjects in the tai chi condition were more likely to achieve a treatment response as defined by a PSQI score of less than 5, compared to those given health education. Subjects in the tai chi condition with poor sleep quality also showed significant improvements in PSQI global score as well as in the sleep parameters of rated sleep quality, habitual sleep efficiency, sleep duration, and sleep disturbance. All finds demonstrated clinical significance (at least $P < 0.05$).

In determining which modalities to consider, it is important to individualize therapy. In a study of 123 older adults with chronic and primary insomnia, CBT-I was compared to tai chi.[44] CBT-I performed better than tai chi in remission of clinical insomnia, as ascertained by a clinician, and also showed greater and more sustained improvement in sleep quality, sleep parameters, fatigue, and depressive symptoms than tai chi. These results noted significance with P-values of less than 0.01. One of the limitations of this study is that it did not state patient preference or consider this factor in its analysis. However, in another randomized, partially blinded study of breast cancer survivors with insomnia, tai chi was found to be non-inferior to CBTI. Both produced clinically meaningful improvements in insomnia. Therefore, tai chi may be considered for the treatment of insomnia, particularly in patients who may not be willing to do CBTI.[45]

A key benefit of yoga and tai chi is that they espouse a set of principles and methods that can be made accessible to people of different ages and ability. As in any field, some aspects of yoga and tai chi are too subtle to be learned from books or lectures and must be acquired through direct experience. These modalities place a time-honored emphasis on the student–teacher relationship to deepen learning and understanding through personal experience.

BIOFEEDBACK

Biofeedback is a technique for developing greater awareness of and voluntary control over the physiological processes affected by stress. With the use of sensors to monitor autonomic nervous system and/or body function, a patient is trained to gain voluntary control of their stress levels. These may include heart rate, blood pressure, and muscle tension, all of which increase under stress. The intention is to recognize the stress as well as relieve it through relaxation. Depending on the type of technique used, patients can hear, see, and measure their stress levels and learn to relax. The therapist acts as a coach, teaching patients how to relax and thereby further reduce stress and anxiety. The most commonly used forms of treatment are electromyelography (EMG) biofeedback, respiratory biofeedback, thermal biofeedback, and neurofeedback. A systematic review of studies on biofeedback's effectiveness found no consistent improvement in total sleep time, sleep efficiency, or subjective reports of sleep quality. Some studies found improvement in sleep onset efficiency and the frequency of awakenings after sleep onset.[46]

ELECTRICAL STIMULATION

Of the many forms of electrical stimulation used for medical applications, cranial electrical stimulation (CES) has gained most attention in recent years. This modality delivers low levels of alternating electrical current to the head[47] and has been shown to have positive effects in the treatment of sleep disturbances. Moreover, it has been used in various patient populations to promote improvement of depressive symptoms, perceived stress, and other disorders that impact sleep.[48] It is believed that CES stimulates the vagus nerve, causing a parasympathetic response and relaxation. Additionally, it may also increase the blood and cerebrospinal fluid levels of specific neurotransmitters to promote relaxation. CES is FDA approved for the treatment of insomnia, yet the research on its effectiveness is limited and the results are mixed.[49]

HEART RATE VARIABILITY

A healthy heart is not a metronome. It demonstrates beat-to-beat fluctuations, with heart rate modulated by the combined effects of the sympathetic and parasympathetic nervous systems. Therefore, measurement of changes in heart rate over time (heart rate variability [HRV]) provides information about autonomic functioning. HRV has been used to identify people at high risk for stress related conditions, understand the autonomic components of different disorders, and evaluate the effect of different interventions.[50] HRV measures the variation between heartbeats within a specific timeframe. HRV is governed by the autonomic nervous system. The parasympathetic branch has more immediate effects on only a few beats and leads to a heart rate that is less than the intrinsic level, thus giving more room for variability between successive heartbeats. The sympathetic branch creates an impact on several consecutive beats and creates an accumulative effect that increases the heart rate from the intrinsic level, thus giving less time and opportunity for variability between heartbeats. Hence, sleep is promoted by more parasympathetic and less sympathetic regulation, which would be revealed by a lower heart rate and higher HRV. Physical and mental states can affect the autonomic system and impact HRV. With this in mind, different programs have been designed to promote greater HRV, such as biofeedback tools and exercise programs.

HRV has been shown in a recent study to improve sleep. In this case-controlled study with 24 subjects and 24 controls, patients with major depression and PSQI scores higher than 6 were recruited. The HRV group received a weekly 60-minute protocol for 6 weeks, and the control group of matched age and sex received medical care only. In the HRV group, symptoms of depression and anxiety, sleep quality, and pre-sleep arousal were significantly improved over the control group. Further studies will be needed to determine the length of time this intervention requires and if ongoing training is needed.[51,52]

NIGHTTIME BATHING

Physiological mechanisms that cool the body may promote sleep. In a small study, six female volunteers aged 22–24 bathed in warm water (95°F above room temperature) for 90 minutes.[53] After the warm bath, they reported significant increases in sleepiness at bedtime, slow wave sleep, and stage 4 sleep. REM sleep was reduced, particularly in the first REM sleep period. In comparison, those in a cool bath demonstrated no significant changes in any parameter. In another study, a range of age groups (30 young (ages 17–22) and 30 older adults (65–83)) were given a trial of nighttime bathing. During the first half of the sleep night, fewer body movements and less restless sleep were reported after bathing by both young and elderly subjects.[54] Overall, the results suggest that a bath before sleep enhances the quality of sleep, particularly in the elderly. Overall, a practical benefit from showering or bathing is that it can be part of a soothing routine. With such a pleasurable cue prior to bedtime, the physical relaxation can also become a mental and emotional easing as well. When showering and bathing, the patient can incorporate the senses through the use of as dim lighting, soothing scents, and relaxing music or welcomed silence. Some learning theories promote using the five senses to allow for parallel inputs to create new or strengthening pathways toward a conditioned soothing that can proceed bedtime.

EXERCISE

The benefits of exercise on sleep have been noted through different pathways, including the adenosine triphosphate (ATP)-adenosine theory,[55] the thermogenic model,[56] and the relaxation response following exercise.[57] Administering adenosine or its agonists to experimental subjects promotes sleepiness. Adenosine has been shown to promote both homeostatic drive to sleep as well as promote non–REM sleep, including slow wave sleep. The duration of wakefulness and the amount of brain activity and physical activity throughout the day has been shown to increase adenosine levels. The molecule adenosine is in progressively higher concentration in the brain during waking periods, especially with extended periods of wakefulness. This helps explain why we experience greater fatigue and deeper sleep after long days and when we are physically exhausted. In addition to the adenosine concept to promote sleep, exercise-mediated hyperthermia has led to increases in slow wave sleep. Some have noted that the cooling effect after exercise-induced hyperthermia may promote sleep; thus, the timing of exercise before bed is controversial, with recommendation ranging from 3 to 5 hours prior to bedtime to allow for this sleep promoting cooling to occur. Last, physical relaxation from reduced mental and physical tension in body has been noted to help sleep. This has been linked to reducing hyperarousal and lowering inflammation levels within the body through relaxation.

Research on the effects of exercise on sleep is limited but consistently finds that moderate-intensity movement such as walking, if done regularly, can improve sleep onset and quality of sleep.[58,59]

A meta-analysis of 23 studies was undertaken to determine if vigorous exercise before bed had a negative effect on sleep. The studies reviewed here do not support the hypothesis that evening exercise negatively affects sleep, but rather the opposite. However, SOL, TST, and sleep efficiency might be impaired after vigorous exercise ending 1 hour or less before bedtime.[60]

NUTRITION

Many people seek to eat foods that may promote sleep, but no one food has been proved to combat insomnia. Because of the interest in using melatonin to promote sleep and balance the circadian cycle, there is equal interest in tryptophan-rich foods, given that this amino acid is converted into 5-HTP and then serotonin before becoming melatonin. Although turkey is often thought of as a tryptophan-rich food, the US Department of Agriculture National Nutrient Database notes the following foods to be higher in melatonin: mozzarella cheese, roasted soybeans, pumpkins seeds, parmesan cheese, oat bran, cheddar cheese, and tofu. Studies have suggested that tryptophan-rich foods are helpful,[61] but these have been correlational studies, rather than prospective studies looking at causality. Hence, it is difficult to discern if a higher intake of tryptophan-rich foods translates into bioactive melatonin for the body or improves sleep.

With greater appreciation of the circadian rhythm, factors beyond light exposure have been shown to influence sleep timing. At this time, it may be more helpful to appreciate that meal frequency, timing of meals, and the quantity of food are more often noted to be important factors in sleep rather than focusing on foods that induce sleep. As noted in the section regarding CBT-I, eating large meals before bed often disrupts sleep quantity and quality, and maintaining scheduled meals, such as breakfast, may be helpful to stabilize and strengthen the circadian system.

In regards to sodium intake, there are concerns about sodium's negative health impacts, especially with the globalization of the Western diet. A high-sodium diet may increase the possibility of reduced sleep maintenance and increased sleep fragmentation.[62] Furthermore high-sodium diets may worsen circadian rhythm–related sleep disruptions.[63] A model in *Drosophila* shows that these sleep changes occur through a dopaminergic-dependent system.

A recent review of the medical literature looked to evaluate the extent to which macronutrients and specific foods may promote optimal sleep.[64] Researchers reviewed high-carbohydrate and high-fat diets and their impact on sleep quality. They highlighted evidence to suggest that dietary patterns favoring high carbohydrate intake are associated with reduced SOL but less slow wave sleep and increased REM sleep. They noted that high fat intakes promoted higher slow wave sleep but lower sleep efficiency, reduced REM, and increased arousals. The studies were not robust enough to offer firm conclusions, and this issue must be studied using randomized controlled trials. The review also commented on studies looking at specific foods such as milk products, fish, fruits, and vegetables that show sleep-promoting effects. However, definitive recommendations could not be drawn since the studies were too diverse, short, and small. Nevertheless, they offered the comforting note that their findings are in line with other dietary recommendations for health in the general population: increasing fruit and vegetable intake, choosing whole grains that are high in fiber, and favoring vegetable oils that are low in saturated fat.

Conclusion

In promoting sleep, better health is promoted. In addressing the disruptors of sleep, we address thoughts and behaviors that may move us away from sleep and health. The treatment of insomnia offers an opportunity to address the most common challenge in those not achieving restorative sleep. With a thorough understanding of the diagnostic criteria of insomnia, we can discern and personalize opportunities. Of the many approaches and recommendations for treating insomnia and encouraging a healthy lifestyle related to sleep, there is significant value in learning about CBT-I, MBTI, and nonpharmacological approaches to help our patients get to sleep, stay asleep, and live robust daytime lives.

REFERENCES

1. Chesson A Jr, Hartse K, Anderson WM, et al. Practice parameters for the evaluation of chronic insomnia. An American Academy of Sleep Medicine report. Standards of Practice Committee of the American Academy of Sleep Medicine. *Sleep.* 2000;23:237.

2. Schutte-Rodin S, Broch L, Buysse D, et al. Clinical guideline for the evaluation and management of chronic insomnia in adults. *J Clin Sleep Med* 2008;4:487.

3. National Institutes of Health. National Institutes of Health State of the Science Conference statement on Manifestations and Management of Chronic Insomnia in Adults, June 13-15, 2005. *Sleep.* 2005 Sep;28(9):1049–1057.

4. Ong J, Sholtes D. A mindfulness-based approach to the treatment of insomnia. *J Clin Psychol.* 2010;66(11):1175–1184.

5. Ford ES, Wheaton AG, Cunningham TJ, et al. Trends in outpatient visits for insomnia, sleep apnea, and prescriptions for sleep medications among US adults: Findings from the National Ambulatory Medical Care survey 1999–2010. *Sleep* 2014;37:1283.

6. American Academy of Sleep Medicine. *International classification of sleep disorders.* 3rd ed. Darien, IL: American Academy of Sleep Medicine; 2014.

7. American Psychiatric Association. *Diagnostic and statistical manual of mental disorders.* 5th ed. Arlington, VA: Author; 2013.

8. Lineberger MD, Carney CE, Edinger JD, et al. Defining insomnia: Quantitative criteria for insomnia severity and frequency. *Sleep.* 2006;29(4):479–485.

9. Edinger JD, Arnedt JT, Bertisch SM, et al. Behavioral and psychological treatments for chronic insomnia disorder in adults: an American Academy of Sleep Medicine clinical practice guideline. *J Clin Sleep Med.* 2021 Feb 1;17(2):255–262

10. Qaseem A, Kansagara D, Forcisa MA, et al. Management of chronic insomnia disorder in adults: A clinical practice guideline from the American College of Physicians. *Ann Intern Med.* 2106;165:125.

11. Brasure M, Fuchs E, MacDonald R, et al. Psychological and behavioral interventions for managing insomnia disorder: An evidence report for a clinical practice guideline by the American College of Physicians. *Ann Intern Med.* 2016;165:113.

12. Morin CM, Colecchi C, Stone J, et al. Behavioral and pharmacological therapies for late-life insomnia: A randomized-controlled trial. *JAMA.* 1999;281:991.

13. Morin CM, Vallieres A, Guay B, et al. Cognitive behavior therapy, singly and combined with medication, for persistent insomnia: A randomized controlled trial. *JAMA.* 2009;301:2005.

14. Beaulieu-Bonneau S, Ivers H, Guay B, Morin CM. Long term maintenance of therapeutic gains associated with cognitive-behavioral therapy for insomnia delivered alone or combined with Zolpidem. *Sleep.* 2017;40(3):1–6.

15. Trauer M, Qian MY, et al. Chronic behavioral therapy for chronic insomnia. A systematic review and meta-analysis. *Ann Intern Med.* 2015:163(3):191–205.

16. Vallieres A, Morin CM, Guay, B. Sequential combination of drug and cognitive behavioral therapy for chronic insomnia: An exploratory study. *Behav Res Ther.* 2005;43:1611.

17. Morin CM, Culbert JP, Schwartz SM. Nonpharmacological interventions for insomnia: A meta-analysis of treatment efficacy. *Am J Psychiatry*.1994;151:1172–1180.

18. Morin CM. Cognitive-behavioral approaches to the treatment of insomnia. *J Clin Psychiatry.* 2004;65(Suppl 16):33–40.

19. Morin CM, Bootzin RR, Buysee DJ, et al. Psychological and behavioral treatment of insomnia: Update of the recent evidence (1998–2004), *Sleep.*2006;29:1398–1414.

20. Edinger JD, Wohlgemuth WK, Radtke RA, Marsh GR, Quillian RE. Cognitive behavioral therapy for treatment of chronic primary insomnia: A randomized controlled trial. *JAMA.* 2001;285(14):1856–1864.

21. Guilleminault C, Clerk A, Black JJ, et al. Nondrug treatment trials in psychophysiologic insomnia. *Arch Intern Med.* 1995;155:838.

22. Seyffert M, Lagisetty P, Landgraf J, et al. Internet-delivered cognitive behavioral therapy to treat insomnia: A systematic review and meta-analysis. *PLoS One.* 2016;11(2):e0149139.

23. Dong L, Soehner AM, Bélanger L, Morin CM, Harvey AG. Treatment agreement, adherence, and outcome in cognitive behavioral treatments for insomnia. *J Consult Clin Psychol.* 2018 Mar;86(3):294–299.

24. Ong JC, Kuo TF, Manber R. Who is at risk for dropout from group cognitive behavior therapy for insomnia? *J Psychom Res.* 2008;64:419–425.

25. Morgan K, Thompson J, Dixon S, Tomeny M, Mathers N. Predicting longer-term outcomes following psychological treatment for hypnotic-dependent chronic insomnia. *J Psychom Res.* 2003;54(1):21–29.

26. Bathgate CJ, Edinger JD, Krystal AD. Insomnia patients with objective short sleep duration have a blunted response to cognitive behavioral therapy for insomnia. *Sleep.* 2017;40(1):zsw012.

27. Bertisch SM, Pollock BD, Mittleman MA, et al. Insomnia with objective short sleep duration and risk of incident cardiovascular disease and all-cause mortality: Sleep Heart Health Study. *Sleep.* 2018;41(6):zsy047.

28. Vgontzas AN, Fernandez-Mendoza J. Insomnia with short sleep duration: Nosological, diagnostic, and treatment implications. *Sleep Med Clin.* 2013 Sep 1;8(3):309–322.

29. Vgontzas AN, Fernandez-Mendoza J, Liao D, Bixler EO Insomnia with objective short sleep duration: The most biologically severe phenotype of the disorder. *Sleep Med Rev.* 2013 Aug;17(4):241–254.

30. van de Laar M, Pevernagie D, van Mierlo P, Overeem S. Psychiatric comorbidity and aspects of cognitive coping negatively predict outcome in cognitive behavioral treatment of psychophysiological insomnia. *Behav Sleep Med.* 2015;13(2):140–156.

31. Gross CR, Kreitzer MJ, Reilly-Spong M, et al. Mindfulness-based stress reduction versus pharmacotherapy for chronic primary insomnia: A randomized controlled clinical trial. *Explore (NY).* 2011 Mar-Apr;7(2):76–87.

32. Ong JC, Manber R, Segal Z, Xia Y, Shapiro S, Wyatt JK. A randomized controlled trial of mindfulness meditation for chronic insomnia. *Sleep.* 2014 Sep 1;37(9):1553–1563.

33. Kreitzer MJ, Reilly-Spong M, Wall M, Winbush NY, Patterson R, Mahowald M, Cramer-Bornemann M. Mindfulness-based stress reduction versus pharmaco-therapy for chronic primary insomnia: A randomized controlled clinical trial. *Explore (NY)*. 2011 Mar-Apr;7(2):76–87.

34. Martires J, Zeidler M. The value of mindfulness meditation in the treatment of insomnia. *Curr Opin Pulm Med*. 2015 Nov;21(6):547–552.

35. Zhang JX, Liu XH, Xie XH, Zhao D, Shan MS, Zhang XL, Kong XM, Cui H Mindfulness-based stress reduction for chronic insomnia in adults older than 75 years: A randomized, controlled, single-blind clinical trial. *Explore (NY)*. 2015 May-Jun;11(3):180–185.

36. Gong H, Ni CX, Liu YZ, Zhang Y, Su WJ, Lian YJ, Peng W, Jiang CL. Mindfulness meditation for insomnia: A meta-analysis of randomized controlled trials. *J Psychosom Res*. 2016 Oct;89:1–6. Epub 2016 Jul 26.

37. Ikemata S, Momose Y. Effects of a progressive muscle relaxation intervention on dementia symptoms, activities of daily living, and immune function in group home residents with dementia in Japan. *Jpn J Nurs Sci*. 2017;14(2):135–145. doi:10.1111/jjns.12147.

38. Canter A, Kondo CY, Knott JR. A comparison of EMG feedback and progressive muscle relaxation training in anxiety neurosis. *Br J Psychiatry*. 1975 Nov;127:470–477.

39. Chesson AL, Anderson WM, Littner M, et al. Practice parameters for the nonpharmacologic treatment of chronic insomnia. *Sleep*. 1999;22:1128–1133.

40. Wang F, Feng F, Vitello M, et al. The effects of meditative movement on sleep quality. A systematic review. *Sleep Med Rev*. 2016;36:43–52.

41. Stussman BJ, Black LI, Barnes PM, Clarke TC, Nahin RL. *Wellness-related use of common complementary health approaches among adults: United States, 2012*. National health statistics reports no. 85. Hyattsville, MD: National Center for Health Statistics; 2015.

42. Markil N, Whitehurst M, Jacobs PL, Zoeller RF. Yoga Nidra relaxation increases heart rate variability and is unaffected by a prior bout of Hatha yoga. *J Alt Compl Med*. 2012 Oct;18(10):953–958.

43. Irwin MR, Olmstead R, Motivala SJ. Improving sleep quality in older adults with moderate sleep complaints: A randomized controlled trial of Tai Chi Chih. *Sleep*. 2008;31(7):1001–1008.

44. Irwin MR, Olmstead R, Carrillo C, et al. Cognitive behavioral therapy vs. Tai Chi for late life insomnia and inflammatory risk: A randomized controlled comparative efficacy trial. *Sleep*. 2014;37(9):1543–1552.

45. Irwin MR, Olmstead R, Carrillo C, Sadeghi N, Breen EC, Witarama T, Yokomizo M, Lavretsky H, Carroll JE, Motivala SJ, Bootzin R, Nicassio P. Cognitive behavioral therapy vs. Tai Chi for late life insomnia and inflammatory risk: a randomized controlled comparative efficacy trial. *Sleep*. 2014 Sep 1;37(9):1543–1552.

46. Melo DLM, Carvalho LBC, Prado LBF, et al Biofeedback therapies for chronic insomnia: A systematic review. *Appl Psychophysiol Biofeedback*. 2019 Dec;44(4):259–269.

47. Kirsch D. *The science behind cranial electrotherapy stimulation*. Edmonton: Medical Scope Publishing Corporation; 2002.

48. Tyers S, Smith R. Treatment of fibromyalgia with cranial electrotherapy stimulation. *Original Internist*. 2001;8(3):15–17.

49. Shekelle PG, Cook IA, Miake-Lye IM, et al. Benefits and harms of cranial electrical stimulation for chronic pain conditions, anxiety and insomnia. *Ann Intern Med*. 2018;168(6):414–421.

50. Stein PK, Pu Y. Heart rate variability, sleep and sleep disorders. *Sleep Med Rev*. 2012 Feb;16(1):47–66. doi:10.1016/j.smrv.2011.02.005. Epub 2011 Jun 11.

51. Bonnet MH, Arand DL. Heart rate variability: Sleep stage, time of night, and arousal influences. *Electroencephalogr Clin Neurophysiol*. 1997 May;102(5):390–396.

52. Lin IM, Fan SY, Yen CF, et al. Heart rate variability biofeedback increased autonomic activation and improved symptoms of depression and insomnia among patients with major depression disorder. *Clin Psychopharmacol Neurosci*. 2019 May 31;17(2):222–232.

53. Horne JA, Reid AJ. Night-time sleep EEG changes following body heating in a warm bath. *Electroencephalogr Clin Neurophysiol*. 1985 Feb;60(2):154–157.

54. Kanda K, Tochihara Y, Ohnaka T. Bathing before sleep in the young and in the elderly. *Eur J Appl Physiol Occup Physiol*. 1999 Jul;80(2):71–75.

55. Bjorness TE, Greene RW. Adenosine and sleep. *Curr Neuropharmacol*. 2009 Sep;7(3):238.

56. Gilbert SS, van den Heuvel CJ, Ferguson SA, Dawson D. Thermoregulation as a sleep signaling system. *Sleep Med Rev*. 2004 Apr;8(2):81–93.

57. Horne JA, Moore VJ. Sleep EEG effects of exercise with and without additional body cooling. *Electroencephalogr Clin Neurophysiol*. 1985 Jan;60(1):33–38.

58. Passo GS, Poyares D, et al. Effects of moderate aerobic exercise on chronic primary insomnia. *Sleep Med*. 2011;12(10):1018–1027.

59. Yang PY, Ho KH, Chen HC, Chien MY. Exercise training improves sleep quality in middle-aged and older adults with sleep problems: A systematic review. *J Physiother*. 2012;58(3):157–163.

60. Stutz J, Eiholzer R, Spengler CM. Effects of evening exercise on sleep in healthy participants: A systematic review and meta-analysis. *Sports Med*. 2019 Feb;49(2):269–287. doi:10.1007/s40279-018-1015-0.

61. Peuhkuri K, Sihvola N, Korpela R. Diet promotes sleep duration and quality. *Nutr Res*. 2012 May;32(5):309–319.

62. Grandner MA, Jackson N, Gerstner JR, Knutson KL. Sleep symptoms associated with intake of specific dietary nutrients. *J Sleep Res*. 2014;23(1):22–34.

63. Xie J, Wang D, Ling S, Yang G, Yang Y, Chen W. High-salt diet causes sleep fragmentation in young Drosophila through circadian rhythm and dopaminergic systems. *Front Neurosci*. 2019;13:1271.

64. St-Onge MP, Mikic A, Pietrolungo CE. Effects of diet on sleep quality. *Adv Nutr*. 2016 Sep 15;7(5):938–949.

26

Hypnotic Medication Use

KADDY REVOLORIO AND JENNIFER L. MARTIN

The use of sleeping medications (hypnotics) is prevalent in the United States, with an estimated 4% of adults 20 years of age and older indicating that they have used sleep medications in the past month.[1] One in six adults who are diagnosed with a sleep disorder and one in eight adults who report difficulty with sleep report using sleep medications.[1] Approximately 65% of all hypnotic prescriptions in the United States are to individuals who take 30 doses or more per month and have been taking hypnotics for an average of 5 years or longer.[2] Additionally, about half of hypnotic medication sales go to individuals who are 60 years of age and older.[2] Long-term use of hypnotics has been shown to have a number of potential effects, including memory impairment, risks of tolerance and dependence, altered sleep physiology, and, in older adults, long-term use has been shown to increase the risk of falls, motor vehicle accidents, and mortality.[2,3] Additionally, older adults and individuals with a remote or recent substance abuse history have been identified to be at a higher risk for hypnotic drug dependence, particularly with benzodiazepines.[4,5]

Treatments for Insomnia Disorder: Recommendations and Patient Preferences

The American College of Physicians published clinical guidelines for the treatment of insomnia in 2016.[6] They identified cognitive-behavioral therapy for insomnia (CBT-I) as the first line of treatment and pharmacological treatments as a second line of treatment. However, studies have found that individuals with insomnia most often report sleep difficulties in primary care settings where most hypnotic prescriptions originate, and the setting where individuals seek care can influence the type of services received.[7] Primary care providers are more likely to provide pharmacological treatments instead of behavioral treatments for insomnia,[8] likely due to factors such as insufficient knowledge about behavioral treatments and insufficient time to deliver such interventions.

While information on patient preferences for pharmacological versus behavioral treatments is limited, there is some evidence that patients prefer nonpharmacological approaches. In particular, women and younger individuals tend to prefer behavioral treatments over pharmacological treatments of psychiatric disorders.[9] In a study examining the acceptability of pharmacological treatments versus nonpharmacological treatments of insomnia among women veterans, nonpharmacological treatments of insomnia were rated as very acceptable significantly more often than were pharmacological treatments for insomnia.[10] This may indicate a potential mismatch between patient preference for treatment and treatments they are given.

Identifying Patients Who Should Discontinue Use of Hypnotics

Despite extensive evidence regarding nonpharmacological treatments for insomnia and evidence to support hypnotic discontinuation interventions, identifying which patients to target for hypnotic discontinuation remains unclear. Conceptually, there are some patients who seek to discontinue use on their own, and there are other patients who need to discontinue use for health-related reasons. Many patients are likely to discontinue use on their own, and we did not identify any studies related to what leads patients to discontinue use without the support of their healthcare providers. In general, most newer generation hypnotic medications can be safely discontinued by patients; however, some medications should be discontinued under medical supervision (e.g., long-acting benzodiazepines). There is also relatively little research on differences in hypnotic discontinuation success rates between individuals who seek hypnotic discontinuation on their own versus individuals who need to get off hypnotics, for example, due to health risks leading to a provider recommendation for discontinuation. The studies just discussed included only individuals interested in hypnotic discontinuation.[3,11–13] Understanding if there is a difference between these two distinct populations can facilitate understanding of how best to increase motivation to discontinue hypnotics prior to engaging the patient in a combined tapering plan plus behavioral insomnia treatment.

The first step is to identify patients who may need to discontinue hypnotics due to contraindications such as being at higher risk for falls and cognitive impairment, which are common clinical concerns in geriatric populations. Another subset of patients who should be identified are those who need to discontinue hypnotics because they meet criteria of the *Diagnostic and Statistical Manual of Mental Disorders* (DSM-5) for Sedative, Hypnotic, or Anxiolytic Use Disorder.[14] Individuals who meet criteria may often take these medications in larger amounts over a longer period than intended, have a persistent desire to cut down or unsuccessful attempts at reducing use, spend a large amount of time acquiring these medications, crave these medications, experience impairment in various areas of functioning and continue using, and experience tolerance to these medications and withdrawal symptoms.[14] Sedative, Hypnotic, or Anxiolytic Use Disorder is highest in adults aged 18–29 and occurs at a 0.5% rate; it is lowest in individuals older than 65, at a .04% rate in prevalence.[14] Clinically, we are less likely to see individuals who meet criteria for this disorder than we are to encounter individuals who need to discontinue hypnotic use due to a contraindication to continue taking these medications. However, one area that should be addressed with individuals in both these populations who may not necessarily have a strong desire to discontinue hypnotic use is their motivation to discontinue and any ambivalence that they may be experiencing regarding discontinuing hypnotics. Typically, hypnotic medication discontinuation is carried out on an outpatient basis; however, some individuals who meet criteria for dependence may require closer monitoring and/or inpatient treatment.

Interventions to Support Discontinuing Use of Hypnotic Medications

Discontinuing the use of hypnotic medications after long-term use can be challenging, and this is especially difficult with benzodiazepines.[11,13] Individuals withdrawing from hypnotics can experience withdrawal symptoms, anticipatory anxiety, and a fear of rebound insomnia.[11,15] Often, these physiological and psychological symptoms can lead to hypnotic-dependent insomnia.[16] If done carefully, individuals can successfully discontinue hypnotic medications. To date, there have been several studies examining the effectiveness of hypnotic discontinuation with the use of a withdrawal schedule and behavioral treatments.[3,11–13]

In order for individuals to safely withdraw from hypnotics, they are typically placed on a graduated tapering schedule where they decrease their dosage weekly. Individuals can complete this on their own with regular follow-up meetings with their medical providers. Some hypnotic tapering protocols also include behavioral components addressing sleep difficulties as well as cognitions related to discontinuing hypnotic use. The remainder of this chapter provides a brief description of the various interventions used with individuals who are discontinuing hypnotic use.

HYPNOTIC MEDICATION TAPERING

A hypnotic taper intervention typically includes an initial meeting with a healthcare provider for a consultation where the focus is on coming up with an individualized withdrawal schedule. Part of this consultation also includes information on withdrawal procedures. To date there are no national clinical guidelines for tapering; however, some healthcare systems (e.g., Veteran's Healthcare Administration Pharmacy Benefits Management and National Center for Posttraumatic Stress Disorder [PTSD]; Kaiser Permanente Healthcare)[17-19] have developed their own resources to support patients and providers. These supportive tools generally suggest educating patients about the potential risks of chronic use of benzodiazepines and other hypnotics, then developing an individualized tapering schedule. For example, Kaiser Permanente Healthcare has provided guidelines for gradual tapering and for rapid discontinuation.[18] Their guidelines for gradual discontinuation include decreasing the patient's dose by 10% every week or every 2–4 weeks. The guidelines for rapid discontinuation include decreasing the patient's dose by 25% every week. The VA's National Center for PTSD has suggested benzodiazepine taper guidelines.[17] Their guidelines include switching patients to longer acting benzodiazepines first then reducing the dose by 50% during the first 2–4 weeks and maintaining patients on that does for 1–2 months, and then reducing the dose by 25% every 2 weeks until the medication has been discontinued. Similarly, the University of Montreal has developed its own guidelines for sedative-hypnotic tapering.[19] Their schedule includes taking a half-dose 2 days per week during the first 2 weeks, taking a half-dose for 5 days each week during weeks 3 and 4, taking a half-dose daily during weeks 5 and 6. Patients then reduce to a quarter of the initial dose on 2 days per week during weeks 7 and 8, take a quarter-dose 3 days per week during week 9 and 10, and take a quarter-dose 5 days per week during weeks 11 and 12. Then they take a quarter-dose daily during weeks 13 and 14, and introduce no medication 4 times a week during weeks 15 and 16; finally, they take no medication during weeks 17 and 18. In research, some hypnotic taper studies have used an initial schedule which includes broad anchor points for reducing the initial dosage by 25% by week 2, 50% by week 4, and 100% by weeks 8–10.[16] The taper may also need to be adjusted based on withdrawal symptoms and psychological factors including anticipatory anxiety and difficulty coping.[11] Some individuals may also have difficulty in completing the final cessation step and should be reminded that the small quantity of the medication that they are taking is probably producing little benefit to their sleep.[16] Subsequently, these worries should be addressed as they may contribute to residual sleep disturbances after the hypnotic taper intervention.[20]

Table 26.1 shows the tapering plan one might use for an older patient with a history of falls and concern for mild cognitive impairment.

Table 26.1 Tapering schedule for an older patient taking 10mg zolpidem nightly.

	Monday	Tuesday	Wednesday	Thursday	Friday	Saturday	Sunday
Week 0	10mg	10mg	10mg	10mg	10mg	10mg	10mg

Assess sleep quality (based on caregiver and patient report).

	Monday	Tuesday	Wednesday	Thursday	Friday	Saturday	Sunday
Week 1	7.5mg	7.5 mg	7.5mg	7.5mg	7.5 mg	7.5mg	7.5 mg
Week 2	7.5mg	7.5 mg	7.5mg	7.5 mg	7.5mg	7.5 mg	7.5mg

Re-assess sleep quality (based on caregiver report and/or diary). If sleep quality has returned to baseline, reduce dose by 25%, if not, continue with current dose for an additional week.

	Monday	Tuesday	Wednesday	Thursday	Friday	Saturday	Sunday
Week 3	5mg	5mg	5mg	5mg	5mg	5mg	5mg
Week 4	5mg	5mg	5mg	5mg	5mg	5mg	5mg

Re-assess sleep quality (based on caregiver report and/or diary). If sleep quality has returned to baseline, reduce dose by 25%, if not, continue with current dose for an additional week.

	Monday	Tuesday	Wednesday	Thursday	Friday	Saturday	Sunday
Week 5	2.5mg	2.5mg	2.5mg	2.5mg	2.5mg	2.5mg	2.5mg
Week 6	2.5mg	2.5mg	2.5mg	2.5mg	2.5mg	2.5mg	2.5mg

Re-assess sleep quality (based on caregiver report and/or diary). If sleep quality has returned to baseline, eliminate medication, if not, continue with current dose for an additional week.

	Monday	Tuesday	Wednesday	Thursday	Friday	Saturday	Sunday
Week 7	Discontinue medication 0mg	0mg	0mg	0mg	0mg	0mg	0mg
Week 8	0mg	0mg	0mg	0mg	0mg	0mg	0mg

Re-assess sleep quality (based on caregiver report and/or diary). If sleep quality is not satisfactory, begin or continue with non-pharmacological treatments.

If the patient is still reporting poor sleep quality at the end of the taper, the provider can emphasize the importance of regularizing sleep by having a regular bedtime and rise time. The provider can also provide some information regarding healthy sleep hygiene practices and help normalize that patients will have some difficulty with sleep on occasion. However, the patient with access to behavioral treatments who is still reporting poor sleep quality after the completion of the hypnotic taper should be referred to complete a behavioral treatment for insomnia program at this point.

Morin and colleagues[11] conducted a study examining differences between supervised tapering and CBT for discontinuing benzodiazepine use in older adults with insomnia and found that after the supervised tapering intervention, 48% of individuals were benzodiazepine free. Similarly, Baillargeon and colleagues[13] conducted a study comparing a combined CBT and hypnotic tapering intervention with a hypnotic tapering intervention and found that after the tapering (alone) intervention, 38% of individuals were no longer using hypnotics. This study also found that 3 months after completing the tapering-only intervention, 34% were not using hypnotics, and that 12 months after the intervention, 24% were not using hypnotics. Belleville and colleagues[12] conducted a study examining differences in outcome between a hypnotic taper intervention and a combined hypnotic taper intervention with a self-help CBT component and found that after the hypnotic taper intervention, 64% of individuals were not taking hypnotics, and 6 months after the intervention 54% were not taking hypnotics. Supervised hypnotic taper interventions have been shown to have some limitations in reducing long-term hypnotic use. In the following sections, combined cognitive behavioral and supervised hypnotic taper interventions will be discussed to discover if there are added benefits to hypnotic tapering outcomes.

Hypnotic Medication Tapering plus Cognitive-Behavioral Therapy

Cognitive behavioral interventions in combination with hypnotic taper interventions have been widely used for benzodiazepine discontinuation.[21–23] Cognitive behavioral interventions that are combined with taper interventions typically include psychoeducation, relaxation exercises, and cognitive restructuring of thoughts related to withdrawal symptoms and relapse.[22,23] These interventions vary in length from the previously mentioned studies, and the tapering schedules that are followed range from 4 to 16 to weeks in length.[21,23] The length of the cognitive behavioral interventions also varies in the two studies discussed in this section: one group intervention is 5 weeks in length, and the other group is 20 weeks in length.[21,23] Oude Voshaar and colleagues[23] found that group CBT did not significantly increase benzodiazepine discontinuation when compared to a taper-only intervention. This study also found that 58% of individuals in the CBT group and taper intervention were able to discontinue use, and 62% of individuals in the taper-only intervention were able to discontinue benzodiazepine use.[23] O'Connor and colleagues[21] found that in a group CBT and taper intervention, 83% of individuals were not using benzodiazepines at 3-month follow-up in comparison to 39% of individuals in the taper-only intervention. Additionally, a meta-analysis of current approaches for benzodiazepine discontinuation found that the addition of psychological interventions was slightly more effective than taper-only interventions, and this effect was also seen at follow-up.[24] However, generalizing the results of these studies has its limitation due to their use of these interventions only with benzodiazepines, and we are interested in the effectiveness of these interventions broadly applied to all hypnotic medication use.

Hypnotic Medication Tapering plus CBT for Insomnia

To address insomnia symptoms in individuals who are discontinuing hypnotic use, CBT-I is commonly used. Treating the underlying insomnia can help decrease anticipatory anxiety and fear of rebound insomnia that individuals discontinuing hypnotics often experience.[11,15] CBT-I in combination with hypnotic taper interventions has been found to be successful in helping individuals discontinue hypnotic medications.[11–13]

CBT-I typically includes education about sleep, sleep hygiene strategies, sleep restriction therapy, stimulus control, and cognitive restructuring, and it can include relaxation strategies.[25] Cognitive restructuring used within CBT-I can also help disrupt beliefs about sleep and hypnotic use that can contribute to the continuation of hypnotic drug use and perpetuate insomnia, as depicted in Figure 26.1.

When implementing CBT-I, some clinical considerations should be made. The following example illustrates clinical considerations to be made when a patient is receiving CBT-I and completing a hypnotic taper concurrently. The patient is on a high hypnotic medication dose (e.g., 20 mg Ambien), and they begin encountering difficulty during the taper and report not being able to fall asleep if the medication falls below a certain point (e.g., 10 mg Ambien). Assuming that the patient cannot fall asleep at a half dose, a CBT-I provider may want to consider identifying and addressing any thoughts and fear around rebound insomnia. If the patient has thoughts about rebound insomnia and reports that this is keeping them from falling asleep, the CBT-I provider can move forward and engage in cognitive restructuring by first identifying the patient's thought (e.g., "My insomnia is going to come back if I don't take my medication"), challenging their thought by asking the patient to provide evidence for and against this thought, and finally by having the patient come up with a more balanced thought about their medication

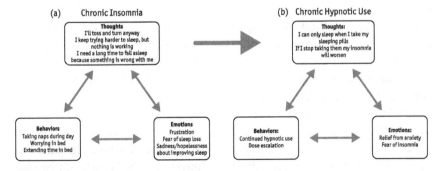

FIGURE 26.1 Cognitive-behavioral model of insomnia (A) and chronic hypnotic medication use (B).

discontinuation. If the patient continues to experience fear around going below a specific dose, and it is getting in the way of them falling asleep, the CBT-I provider can consider teaching relaxation strategies (e.g., diaphragmatic breathing, progressive muscle relaxation) for the patient to engage in before bedtime or when the patient is awake in the middle of the night. This example provides some clinical considerations to make and by no means includes an exhaustive list of the clinical considerations that CBT-I providers could make. In some instances, it may be necessary to slow the tapering schedule to address these cognitive issues.

CBT-I has also been shown to be effective for hypnotic-abusing individuals with chronic insomnia, and individuals who were discontinuing hypnotics have more improvement in sleep efficiency after CBT-I do than individuals who never used hypnotics.[25] A few studies have examined the effectiveness of a combined CBT-I and hypnotic taper intervention.[11–13] Morin and colleagues[11] provided weekly group CBT-I for 10 weeks to individuals who were concurrently briefly meeting weekly with their physicians for a supervised medication taper for 10 weeks. This study found that 85% of individuals in a combined CBT-I and supervised hypnotic tapering intervention were no longer taking benzodiazepines after the intervention.[11] Baillargeon and colleagues[13] combined CBT-I and supervised hypnotic taper intervention concurrently administered over the course of 8 weeks and found that 77% of individuals were no longer using hypnotics, 67% were no longer using at 3-month follow-up, and 70% were no longer using 12 months after the intervention.[13] Belleville and colleagues used a combined CBT-I and hypnotic taper intervention by providing self-help materials covering components of CBT-I for the first 5 weeks that individuals were enrolled in an 8-week hypnotic taper schedule. These individuals met twice with their physician, once to set their taper schedule and once in the middle of treatment to monitor withdrawal symptoms, and they received weekly phone calls from a therapist to check in about their withdrawal schedule and adherence to the CBT-I interventions.[12] After the intervention, 72% of individuals were no longer taking hypnotics, and, 6 months after the intervention, 47% were no longer taking hypnotics.[12] This study found that the combined CBT-I and hypnotic taper intervention did not significantly differ from a hypnotic taper-only intervention, and the combined intervention did not have an added effect in maintaining abstinence. Their results may have been due to the self-help nature of the CBT intervention provided, in comparison to the therapist-administered interventions that were used in the studies by Morin and colleagues[11] and Baillargeon and colleagues.[13]

Providing both interventions at the same time will allow individuals who may be experiencing fear of rebound to address those fears while completing a behavioral treatment for insomnia. However, providing two treatments at the same time may be overwhelming to some individuals. Introducing the behavioral treatment prior to beginning the hypnotic taper may be beneficial to some people who are ambivalent about discontinuing hypnotics to show them that they are able to have improvements in sleep through behavioral changes and that behavioral therapy can address their worries and fears related to discontinuing hypnotics. Belleville and colleagues implemented the behavioral intervention at the beginning of the taper intervention, and it ended prior to the taper intervention.[12] The study by Oude Voshaar and colleagues[23] provided the behavioral intervention halfway through the taper intervention, and it ended 2 weeks after the taper intervention concluded. Interestingly, these two studies did not find an added benefit of using a combined CBT and hypnotic taper intervention because they did not find a difference between the combined intervention and a hypnotic taper-only intervention. The collective findings of these studies may suggest that added benefits are seen when behavioral interventions and hypnotic taper interventions are similar in length and are implemented concurrently.

The studies that concurrently implement CBT-I and hypnotic taper have the best outcomes, and part of this may be due to individuals learning that they are able to improve sleep while decreasing the amount of hypnotics that they previously relied on for sleep. However, implementing both treatments concurrently is not always feasible. Completing a supervised hypnotic taper without any behavioral interventions may be more readily accessible. Including a behavioral treatment typically requires an additional professional trained in CBT-I. A study by Morgan and colleagues[20] found that they were able to implement CBT-I in a primary care setting by training primary care counselors. This study found that implementing this treatment in primary care was not only cost effective but also helped reduce sleep latency, improved sleep efficiency, and reduced the frequency of hypnotic medication use.[20] Training primary care providers in this treatment can be helpful in making a combined taper and CBT-I intervention more accessible to individuals needing both treatments. Due to hypnotic taper interventions being effective for some people, an additional behavioral treatment may not always be indicated. Studies that implement taper intervention and behavioral intervention concurrently have been more successful than those that provide both treatments at different times. For some individuals, a self-guided hypnotic tapering schedule is enough to discontinue medications, and, for others, concurrently receiving a supportive intervention and hypnotic tapering is more effective. Belleville and Morin examined differences between individuals who completed a hypnotic discontinuation intervention and were not taking medications at the 6-month follow-up and compared them to individuals who completed this intervention but continued to use hypnotics.[26] This study found that individuals who were successful in discontinuing hypnotic medications had a decrease in insomnia and anxiety symptoms and had positive perceived health and higher self-efficacy.[26] These findings may suggest that the characteristics that made these individuals more successful in remaining free of hypnotic medications are areas that can be addressed in behavioral treatments.

Provider Beliefs and Attitudes About Hypnotic Medications

Another area of importance to highlight are the beliefs and attitudes of providers regarding prescribing hypnotics and limiting hypnotic medication use, especially within primary care, where hypnotic medications are widely prescribed.[8] Siriwardena and colleagues[27] found that providers had negative attitudes toward hypnotic medications and positive attitudes about reducing prescriptions for hypnotics for sleep problems. However, these same practitioners often continued prescribing hypnotic medications due to feeling pressure to prescribe from patients and having insufficient resources available to reduce prescribing hypnotic medications.[27] Similarly, Davy and colleagues[28] found that practitioners were ambivalent about prescribing hypnotic medications yet often prescribed them to avoid confrontation with patients or to express empathy.[28] CBT-I referrals were rarely offered, and many providers were unaware of the utility of CBT-I.[28] Although prescribers may not see prescribing hypnotic medications as favorable, they continue to prescribe these medications in the absence of alternatives.

To limit hypnotic medication prescribing, practitioners must collaborate with patients, build trusting relationships, and discuss the risks and benefits of these medications openly. Moreover, there seems to be a lack of knowledge of and resources for alternatives such as CBT-I. The accessibility of behavioral treatments such as CBT-I can potentially have an impact on provider beliefs and would give patients treatment options.

Future Directions for Treatment Research

Due to the wide range of hypnotic discontinuation rates in hypnotic taper-only interventions and in combined interventions, looking at supplemental interventions may be helpful. In both approaches, there seems to be an increase in hypnotic use at follow-up. *Motivational interviewing* (MI) can be used to supplement hypnotic taper interventions. MI has been widely used in the area of addiction.[29] Although not all individuals who complete a hypnotic taper suffer from addiction, MI can be used with those individuals who are ambivalent about a behavioral change. These findings may point to the use of MI for retention in treatments, which may be most useful when longer hypnotic tapering protocols are used. Using MI can help address some of the ambivalence seen in individuals who need to discontinue hypnotic medications, and helping these individuals realize that they have a choice can empower them and move them in the direction of change. For example, Zahradnik and colleagues[30] conducted a study using two sessions of a brief MI intervention for problematic prescription drug use in patients who were not seeking treatment. At the 3-month follow-up, 52% of participants had reduced their daily dosage in comparison to 30% of individuals in the control group. Additionally, 18% of individuals who received the MI condition discontinued use of their prescription drugs in comparison to 9% of individuals in the control group.[30] This study's findings are promising because they suggest that a brief MI intervention can help individuals who are not seeking treatment to reduce their use of problematic prescriptions. These findings can also suggest that for individuals who may not want to discontinue hypnotic medication use, Motivational Interviewing may be a starting point for treatment.

Conclusion

Hypnotic taper interventions as well as hypnotic taper interventions combined with CBT-I are generally useful in helping patients discontinue use. Interventions that include CBT-I seem to have greater long-term benefits as patients experience long-lasting improvements in sleep. Making these interventions more accessible can help many long-term users discontinue hypnotic medications and may prevent the adverse consequences of hypnotic medication use in those who wish to or need to discontinue use. Additional research to incorporate motivational enhancement strategies and better understand the optimal timing and structure of hypnotic medication tapering and CBT-I is needed.

Acknowledgments

This material is the result of work supported with resources from and use of facilities at the VA Greater Los Angeles Healthcare System, Geriatric Research, Education and Clinical Center and the Department of Psychology.

REFERENCES

1. Chong Y, Fryar CD, Gu Q. *Prescription sleep aid use among adults: United States, 2005–2010.* NCHS Date Brief; 2013.
2. Kripke DF. Chronic hypnotic use: Deadly risks, doubtful benefit. *Sleep Med Rev.* 2000;4(1):5–20.
3. Lichstein KL, Nau SD, Wilson NM, et al. Psychological treatment of hypnotic-dependent insomnia in a primarily older adult sample. *Behav Res Ther.* 2013;51(12):787–796.
4. Morgan K, Dallosso H, Ebrahim S, Arie T, Fentem PH. Prevalence, frequency and duration of hypnotic drug use among the elderly living at home. *Br Med J.* 1988;296:601–602.

5. Longo LP, Johnson B. Addiction: Part I. Benzodiazepines: Side effects, abuse, risk and alternatives. *Am Fam Physician.* 2000;61(7):2121–2128.

6. Qaseem A, Kansagara D, Forciea MA, Cooke M, Denberg T; American College of Physicians. Management of chronic insomnia disorder in adults: A clinical practice guideline from the American College of Physicians. *Ann Intern Med.* 2016;165(1):125–133.

7. Jenkins MM, Colvonen PJ, Norman SB, Afari N, Allard CB, Drummond SP. Prevalence and mental health correlates of insomnia in first-encounter veterans with and without military sexual trauma. *Sleep.* 2015;38(10):1547–1554.

8. Simon GE, VonKorff M. Prevalence, burden, and treatment of insomnia in primary care. *Am J Psychiatry.* 1997;154(10):1417–1423.

9. McHugh RK, Whitton SW, Peckham AD, Welge JA, Otto MW. Patient preference for psychological vs pharmacologic treatment of psychiatric disorders: A meta-analytic review. *J Clin Psychiatry.* 2013;74(6):595–602.

10. Culver NC, Song Y, Kate McGowan S, et al. Acceptability of medication and nonmedication treatment for insomnia among female veterans: Effects of age, insomnia severity, and psychiatric symptoms. *Clin Ther.* 2016;38(11):2373–2385.

11. Morin CM, Bastien C, Guay B, Radouco-Thomas M, Leblanc J, Vallieres A. Randomized clinical trial of supervised tapering and cognitive behavior therapy to facilitate benzodiazepine discontinuation in older adults with chronic insomnia. *Am J Psychiatry.* 2004;161(2):332–342.

12. Belleville G, Guay C, Guay B, Morin CM. Hypnotic taper with or without self-help treatment of insomnia: A randomized clinical trial. *J Consult Clin Psychol.* 2007;75(2):325–335.

13. Baillargeon L, Landreville P, Verreault R, Beauchemin JP, Gregoire JP, Morin CM. Discontinuation of benzodiazepines among older insomnia adults treated with cognitive-behavioural therapy combined with gradual tapering: A randomized trial. *Can Med Assoc J.* 2003;169(10):1015–1020.

14. American Psychiatric Association. *Diagnostic and statistical manual of mental disorders.* 5 ed. Washington DC: American Psychiatric Association; 2013.

15. Salzman C. The APA Task Force report on benzodiazepine dependence, toxicity, and abuse. *Am J Psychiatry.* 1991;148(2):151–152.

16. Belanger L, Belleville G, Morin C. Management of hypnotic discontinuation in chronic insomnia. *Sleep Med Clin.* 2009;4(4):583–592.

17. Veterans Administration. Pain management. 2013. https://www.va.gov/PAINMANAGEMENT/docs/OSI_6_Toolkit_Taper_Benzodiazepines_Clinicians.pdf

18. Sparks A. Benzodiazepine and Z-drug safety guideline. Kaiser Permanente. 2014. https://wa.kaiserpermanente.org/static/pdf/public/guidelines/benzo-zdrug.pdf

19. Tannenbaum C. Canadian Institutes of Health Research. 2014. http://www.criugm.qc.ca/fichier/pdf/BENZOeng.pdf

20. Morgan K, Dixon S, Mathers N, Thompson J, Tomeny M. Psychological treatment for insomnia in the management of long-term hypnotic drug use: A pragmatic randomised controlled trial. *Br J Gen Pract.* 2003;53(497):923–928.

21. O'Connor K, Marchand A, Brousseau L, et al. Cognitive-behavioural, pharmacological and psychosocial predictors of outcome during tapered discontinuation of benzodiazepine. *Clin Psychol Psychother.* 2008;15(1):1–14.

22. Voshaar RC, Gorgels WJ, Mol AJ, et al. Predictors of long-term benzodiazepine abstinence in participants of a randomized controlled benzodiazepine withdrawal program. *Can J Psychiatry.* 2006;51(7):445–452.

23. Voshaar RC, Gorgels WJ, Mol AJ, et al. Tapering off long-term benzodiazepine use with or without group cognitive-behavioural therapy: Three-condition, randomised controlled trial. *Br J psychiatry.* 2003;182:498–504.

24. Parr JM, Kavanagh DJ, Cahill L, Mitchell G, Young RMD. Effectiveness of current treatment approaches for benzodiazepine discontinuation: A meta-analysis. *Addiction.* 2009;104(1):13–24.

25. Zavesicka L, Brunovsky M, Matousek M, Sos P. Discontinuation of hypnotics during cognitive behavioural therapy for insomnia. *BMC Psychiatry.* 2008;8:80.

26. Belleville G, Morin CM. Hypnotic discontinuation in chronic insomnia: Impact of psychological distress, readiness to change, and self-efficacy. *Health Psychol.* 2008;27(2):239–248.

27. Siriwardena AN, Apekey T, Tilling M, Dyas JV, Middleton H, Orner R. General practitioners' preferences for managing insomnia and opportunities for reducing hypnotic prescribing. *J Eval Clin Pract.* 2010;16(4):731–737.

28. Davy Z, Middlemass J, Siriwardena AN. Patients' and clinicians' experiences and perception of the primary care management of insomnia: Qualitative study. Health Expectations, 18, 1371–1383. *Health Expectations.* 2013;18(5):1371–1383.

29. Miller WR, Rollnick S. *Motivational interviewing: Helping people change*, 3rd ed. New York: Guilford; 2013.

30. Zahradnik A, Otto C, Crackau B, et al. Randomized controlled trial of a brief intervention for problematic prescription drug use in non-treatment-seeking patients. *Addiction.* 2009;104(1):109–117.

27

Integrative Sleep Medicine and Chronic Pain Management

ASHWIN MEHTA

Introduction

This chapter describes the interrelated nature of sleep disorders and chronic pain, which are intrinsically linked by inflammation. Addressing this link is a pivotal step toward improving quality of life. The prevalence of opioid abuse in the United States has reached endemic proportions, and health systems nationwide are increasingly interested in nonpharmacologic, integrative approaches to addressing chronic pain. The importance of a multidisciplinary approach to pain management is underscored, and promising integrative modalities toward addressing sleep quality in patients with chronic pain are presented.

The field of sleep medicine draws from neurology, pulmonology, otolaryngology, dentistry, and psychiatry, among others. The multidisciplinary nature of sleep diagnostics makes perfect sense because often patients present with comorbid, associated conditions such as chronic pain, fatigue, teeth grinding, and depression. Thus, isolated attempts to address a singular aspect of this self-perpetuating cycle may provide transient relief for one condition while contributing to a deterioration of the others. As evidenced by recent research, this constellation of interrelated conditions often gives rise to a progressively worsening and self-perpetuating cycle if not curtailed by proactive treatment strategies.

Given the significant link between pain and poor sleep quality, it is essential for clinicians to screen patients who present primarily with chronic pain for sleep concerns, and conversely, to screen those who complain of suboptimal sleep quality for any discomfort that is further contributing to sleep disturbance. Effective treatment of a patient who is experiencing concomitant pain and poor sleep quality requires a provider to identify this complex of symptoms, delve deep into clinical inquiry to establish the root causes, and devise a comprehensive plan that breaks the cycle at multiple stages. Evidence suggests that addressing this debilitating symptom cluster with a nuanced, integrative approach has the best chance of improving outcomes. Treatment recommendations that include nutritional interventions coupled with exercise prescriptions, sound sleep hygiene, and mindfulness are most effective to ameliorate this knot of suffering.[1]

The relationship between pain, poor sleep quality, and depression has been evaluated in numerous pain populations including those with fibromyalgia, neuropathy, and cancer. According to data compiled in a report by the National Sleep Foundation, 66% of those who have chronic pain also report poor sleep quality. Up to 30% of patients with depression are not satisfied with their sleep quality. Furthermore, the medications most commonly used to treat depression, including selective serotonin reuptake inhibitors (SSRIs), are notorious for suppressing rapid eye movement (REM) sleep, often considered the most restorative stage of sleep.[2] Chronic pain causes sleep disturbance as alpha waves intrude into the deeper stages of sleep including stage 3 and REM. Conversely, sleep deprivation lowers pain thresholds and slows the healing process. Adequate duration and quality of sleep is important to reverse the oxidative stress that we incur during our waking lives. This oxidative damage is thought to be a primary contributor to the daytime fatigue suffered by those with suboptimal sleep. Core body temperature drops during deep sleep, and the science regarding heightened immune system functions during stage 3 and REM sleep is also emerging.[3] Sleep deprivation significantly alters metabolism and impairs the primary adipokines that regulate satiety, often giving rise to late-night snacking and eventual obesity. Any prolonged disruption in sleep architecture can impair these processes and exacerbate both chronic pain and depression.[4]

The physiologic effects of prolonged sleep loss on immune function are evidenced by studies that show diminished natural killer cell activity in sleep-deprived individuals. Research has shown decreased production of antibodies required for immunity in sleep-deprived participants who received the influenza vaccination. Significant changes in circulating levels of cytokines including increased tumor necrosis factor (TNF-alpha) and interleukin (IL-6) have been observed in the context of sleep deprivation. Increased inflammatory markers such as C-reactive protein are also prevalent in the setting of chronic sleep loss. Therefore, the link between pain and inflammation builds a strong case for simultaneously treating sleep disorders as part of a comprehensive chronic pain management plan.[5]

Understanding the Relationship Between
Sleep and Pain

Patients with chronic pain often present with a constellation of associated conditions, including poor sleep quality. The prevalence of sleep deprivation in patients with chronic neck and back pain was found to be 42.22% in a retrospective evaluation of 1,016 patients.[6] Chronic pain and sleep disturbances have a bidirectional and reciprocal relationship. In a cohort of 250 veterans, it was established that changes in pain significantly predict changes in sleep and vice versa.[7] The degree to which pain intensity correlates with sleep loss has also been demonstrated. In one particular study, each incremental increase on a 10-point visual analogue pain scale was associated with a 10% increase in likelihood of reporting sleep disturbance.[8]

REM sleep is a period during which almost all muscles in the body are atonic. The near complete loss of muscle tone leads to a significant drop in core body temperature, and it is thought that the body resolves oxidative damage as well as inflammation during this crucial sleep stage.[9] Disrupted sleep architecture that inhibits cycling into REM sleep can therefore cause the accumulation of inflammatory mediators and worsen pain. Substance P is another important neurotransmitter implicated in the transmission of pain signals from the periphery to the central nervous system. Prolonged, high concentrations of this pro-nociceptive agent are a central aspect of pain syndromes such as fibromyalgia and are thought to be the reason for low pain thresholds in patients with this condition. Substance P is resorbed during the deeper stages of sleep, and insufficient sleep duration or inadequate sleep quality can exacerbate chronic pain by sustained increase of this mediator.[10]

Improving sleep quality is therefore an essential aspect of treating chronic pain and mood disorders. One of the most common associations in the arena of pain management is the interrelated nature of insomnia and depression.[11] Apart from the experience of disabling pain, these individuals become increasingly frustrated over time due to their perceived loss of control over one of life's most simple and basic physiologic functions—sleep. This loss of control further exacerbates depression through a learned helplessness that dissolves away confidence and belief in their ability to make a positive change in physical health. Ultimately, in its most pronounced form, pain and depression go hand in hand with insomnia that is perpetuated by anxiety about sleep itself.[12] For this reason, screening for sleep disorders such as insomnia, obstructive sleep apnea (OSA), narcolepsy, and restless legs syndrome (RLS) is an important initial step in treating the patient with depression and chronic pain.

Sleep Disorders Associated with Pain

A Case Vignette

Stef is a 61-year-old obese woman with a history of hypertension and rheumatoid arthritis who has undergone several courses of steroids as well as various disease-modifying antirheumatic drugs (DMARDs), which had to be changed because of toxicities. Presently, she reports poor sleep quality, snoring, almost daily fatigue, physical deconditioning, pain in her hands and feet, difficulty focusing on tasks that require sustained attention, lapses in short-term memory, and negative moods. She has gained more than 17 pounds since the onset of her treatment, is largely sedentary (body mass index [BMI] of 38), and has a tendency to eat unhealthy, late-night snacks even after a full dinner. She admits to poor sleep hygiene, including television at bedtime and high caffeine intake (2–3 large cups of coffee daily) accompanied by a diet high in refined sugars and processed foods.

INSOMNIA, PAIN, AND INTEGRATIVE TREATMENTS

About 15% of Americans suffer from chronic insomnia, making insomnia the most common sleep disorder in the US population. Insomnia is defined as a subjective difficulty falling or maintaining sleep which is associated with daytime functional impairment, described as fatigue, daytime sleepiness, and memory or concentration difficulties among other complaints. Multiple studies, including a large cohort from the Atherosclerosis Risk in Communities (ARIC) Study, have found that self-reported complaints of insomnia are associated with an increased risk of coronary heart disease, myocardial infarction, or death.[13] This is thought to be due to the significant inflammatory burden that sleep loss inflicts on the body. In addition, individuals with sleep apnea frequently complain of insomnia, highlighting the need for providers to screen aggressively given the possibility of multiple sleep disorders that have a tendency to cluster in any given patient. This is particularly important in the depressed patient because insomnia often presents in conjunction with psychiatric diseases, mainly depression, generalized anxiety, and post-traumatic stress disorder.[14]

Pain patients often experience disrupted sleep and insomnia due to their chronic pain. Furthermore, sleep state misperception is commonly experienced by individuals who are taking medications to treat chronic pain. In recent research, Chan and colleagues described broad variations in sleep perception, defined as the subjective notion of how well (and how long) one has slept, among patients with insomnia who are also taking opioid medication for fibromyalgia.[15] Insomnia is very common in individuals who are grappling with chronic pain and depression.

The presence of insomnia can also impact the experience of pain itself. The association between chronic low back pain and insomnia was elucidated by the Norwegian HUNT study. In a sample of 30,669 rural participants, individuals with insomnia were found to have twice the odds of reporting chronic low back pain. This same study sought to establish C-reactive protein as a mediator of this relationship, albeit unsuccessfully.[16]

The treatment of insomnia that is coupled with depression or chronic pain requires a more comprehensive, integrative approach due to the interrelated nature of these conditions.[17] Multiple modalities of therapy are often required for successful treatment., including cognitive-behavioral therapy for insomnia (CBT-I), exercise, and mindfulness, among others.

Cognitive Behavioral Therapy for Insomnia

Some of the most pertinent literature regarding the application of cognitive behavioral treatments for insomnia (CBT-I), comes from studies done on patients with fibromyalgia. The research done by McCrae and colleagues evaluating Sleep and Pain Interventions in Fibromyalgia (SPIN) reveals that, in patients with chronic pain, CBT-I improves insomnia symptoms as measured by self-report. Additionally, CBT-I also gave rise to long-term pain reduction that persisted at 6 months, relative to control.[18]

Exercise for Insomnia

It is important to prescribe an exercise plan in conjunction with medical management and CBT-I.[19] Regular exercise increases sleep drive and is also thought to elevate mood. There are significant anti-inflammatory benefits of exercise that can play a complementary role in pain management. Exercise prescriptions must be comprised of three important components including duration, frequency, and intensity. It is essential for the provider to screen for obstacles that a given patient may have to effectively carrying out an exercise plan.[20] Patients with a history of trauma, surgery, significant physical deconditioning, gait imbalances, or a history of falls may do well in a physical therapy program prior to the initiation of an exercise plan. To begin with, an exercise prescription that sets a target of 30 minutes of aerobic exercise, moderate intensity, for 5 days each week is a suitable starting point for most patients and meets the American Heart Association's recommendation for minimal physical activity to effectively prevent cardiovascular disease.[21] Interestingly, those forms of exercise that draw from ancient healing traditions and also have a mindfulness component, such as yoga, tai chi, and baduanjin qigong, show promise to alleviate both musculoskeletal pain and improve sleep quality.[22]

Mindfulness for Insomnia

All patients who demonstrate the cluster of symptoms that include pain, insomnia, and depression should receive a mindfulness recommendation.[23] Mindfulness has been shown to be effective in mitigating pain, elevating mood, and priming the body and brain for improved sleep quality. For this reason, mindfulness is an effective tool that can be applied prior to bedtime, as part of an individualized routine to encourage good quality sleep.[24] Mindfulness is not one modality, but in fact a family of methods that serve to bring one's awareness and attention into the present moment.

Guided imagery, creative visualization, breathing exercises, traditional forms of meditation, devotional practices such as prayer, biofeedback, and even journal-writing provide the same general benefits to individuals over time. To date, there are no validated tools to help the clinician decide which modalities may be of maximal benefit to a patient given certain personality traits and characteristics. Clinical observation suggests that type A personalities with result-driven mindsets who prefer real-time measures of success may try biofeedback as an initial step toward a regular mindfulness practice.[25] Individuals with artistic tendencies may gravitate more toward creative visualization and guided imagery programs. Mathematical and analytical people may enjoy a fixed-gaze meditation or other similar concentration exercises, in conjunction with breath work. People with roots in organized religion may already have a devotional or prayer practice, and these should be encouraged as an adjunct to any pain management plan.

These are broad generalizations and are only meant to serve as a starting point. Suffice it to say that there is often a period of trial and error when coaching a patient to incorporate mindfulness as part of a bedtime ritual. Therefore, it is important for the provider to set reasonable expectations when first starting a client with a daily mindfulness routine. Often, it is useful to convey appropriate goals such as 15–20 minutes of mindfulness in the mornings or nightly, and twice daily for more advanced practitioners.[26] Potential challenges to implementing such a practice should also be addressed preemptively. For example, spousal nighttime television watching would be a significant distraction, and, for this reason, it is helpful to enlist the assistance and cooperation of the bed partner when initiating steps to promote wellness using an integrative approach.[27]

Nutritional Recommendations for Insomnia

Certain herbs and supplements may also be of value when treating insomnia in patients with chronic pain, but these are only useful after important dietary changes have been implemented by the patient. An anti-inflammatory diet rich in fresh fruits, vegetables, beans, legumes, nuts, seeds, whole grains, cold-water fish, whole soy foods, mushrooms, herbs, and spices is best.[28] Caffeine consumption must be documented in any patient with sleep disturbances. It is important to keep in mind that regular caffeine use may be an indication that the patient is making efforts to reduce the daytime symptoms of sleep loss such as fatigue, somnolence, difficulty focusing on tasks that require sustained attention, and reduced memory functions. The common practice of masking daytime symptoms of poor-quality sleep with stimulants such as caffeine is another reason sleep disorders pose a diagnostic challenge. Reduction of caffeine intake is a difficult habit to break because a morning cup of tea or coffee is such a common ritual to begin the day. For this reason, substituting one cup of organic green tea for coffee is a helpful first step, reducing caffeine intake by roughly half.

Patients with insomnia who present along with hypertension, depression, or constipation should be evaluated for a magnesium deficiency. Achieving a magnesium level of at least 2.0 mg/dL is an important aspect of alleviating the poor sleep quality that accompanies depression.[29] Sublingual melatonin is indicated when there is a component of jet lag or history of circadian rhythm disorder contributing to the insomnia.[30] Promising research has evaluated the efficacy of chamomile to improve sleep quality, and the tea is particularly useful if there are accompanying symptoms of nocturnal reflux. Passionflower tea can be beneficial to address insomnia; lemon balm and lavender aromatherapies have demonstrated anxiolytic properties as well.[31] Valerian and hops have been shown to improve sleep quality in some studies and are thought to act via the glutamic acid decarboxylase and gamma-aminobutyric acid (GABA) inhibitory pathways. In summary, the first-line treatments for insomnia including medication and CBT are insufficient to address poor sleep quality in patients with chronic pain and depression. Therefore, the ideal management of this cluster of conditions must also include an exercise prescription, a mindfulness recommendation, nutritional guidance, and a focus on proper sleep hygiene.

OBSTRUCTIVE SLEEP APNEA

OSA is a common condition, and the prevalence can be as high as 36% in some populations, such as in the obese.[32] Occurring in 5–15% of the general population, OSA is characterized by repetitive occlusions of the airway during sleep. These episodes result in oxyhemoglobin desaturation, inspiratory effort against an obstructed airway, and arousal from sleep.[33]

The link between OSA and pain syndromes has only recently been elucidated. The rampant increase in the use of opioid medication likely contributes to sleep disturbances. Among patients using narcotic medications to address chronic pain syndromes, the prevalence of sleep-disordered breathing is disproportionately high compared to the general population.[34] Research indicates that OSA is present in 35–57% of patients managed in long-term pain clinics, and one concerning demographic finding was that the mean age was 31.8 ± 12.3 years and that 60% were women. This is a departure from the traditional thinking regarding risk factors for OSA using the STOP-BANG criteria where increasing age (A) and male gender (G) are included in the screening index. This would suggest that clinicians in a pain management practice ought to have higher clinical suspicion for sleep-disordered breathing and would do well to consider earlier polysomnography in the population of patients receiving opioids for chronic pain. In one observational study among non-obese, long-term opioid users, the apnea/hypopnea index was as high as 43.9 ± 1.2, which represents severe OSA.

Nocturnal hypoxia is also greater among patients using narcotics than would be predicted by severity of sleep-disordered breathing. The persistence of central apneas in spite of treatment with continuous positive airway pressure (CPAP) for patients with comorbid chronic pain and OSA further complicates treatment and may warrant bilevel positive airway pressure (BiPAP) or adaptive servo-ventilation (ASV).[35] This complex treatment algorithm warrants improved communication and coordination of care between pain management practitioners and sleep specialists, with the goal of minimizing doses of narcotic medications while improving overall sleep quality by treating a largely underdiagnosed entity such as OSA.

RESTLESS LEGS SYNDROME

RLS is a common sleep disorder characterized by an unpleasant sensation of the legs, associated with the urge to move them. The symptoms are prominent at rest, mainly during nighttime, and relieved with leg movement.[36] RLS could be idiopathic or secondary to iron deficiency anemia, uremia, pregnancy, neuropathy, radiculopathy, and myelopathy, among other causes. According to the Restless Legs Syndrome Foundation, up to 40% of people with RLS complain of symptoms that would also indicate depression. The link between RLS and depression has been established in patients with renal disease, particularly those who are on renal replacement treatment such as hemodialysis. RLS contributes to conditions prevalent within the population such as depression, anxiety, and insomnia.[37] Therefore, patients with poor-quality sleep, depression, and pain must be evaluated for symptoms of RLS and treated appropriately, often with dopaminergic agonists. Additionally, when a case of RLS is clinically suspected, it is helpful to check a complete blood count (CBC) for anemia and a comprehensive metabolic panel (CMP) for liver or kidney dysfunction. Iron studies, thyroid stimulating hormone, magnesium, vitamin B_{12}, and folate levels are also important as these deficiencies can exacerbate symptoms. Often, correcting these parameters can provide significant relief.

OTHER INTEGRATIVE MODALITIES FOR PAIN AND SLEEP

Isolated attempts to treat one aspect of this constellation of comorbidities often give rise to inadequate treatment, overmedication, or exacerbation of the overlooked entity. For this reason, comprehensive screening methods must be used to identify the root of the problem as described in the preceding sections. Apart from the aforementioned treatment strategies, a number of complementary modalities can help ameliorate the debilitating symptom cluster that accompanies these interrelated conditions. In particular, yoga, acupuncture, massage, and tai chi have been shown to improve overall sleep quality in patients with depression or pain. One pilot study with 55 participants noted improved overall sleep quality, reduced depression, less daytime dysfunction, and fewer sleep disturbances in those who practiced a 70-minute yoga routine three times weekly for 6 months.[38,39] A reduction in pain associated with fibromyalgia and Substance P was noted in a small sample of 22 patients who underwent massage; this was also accompanied by increases in total sleep time. Tai chi has also been shown to decrease sleep latency and increase overall sleep time in elderly individuals.[40] A cost-effectiveness study conducted in the United Kingdom endorsed acupuncture for disabling migraines, a modality that has also significant benefit toward improving mood and reducing pain.[41]

A recent study revealed that vitamin D deficiency is correlated with heightened systemic inflammation and can also impair sleep quality. Screening for vitamin D deficiency and replenishing to optimal levels via supplementation or sunlight exposure is a mainstay of treatment for any patient with both chronic pain and poor sleep.[42]

Other Considerations for Sleep Loss Due to Chronic Pain

CONFOUNDED BY CAFFEINE

Caffeine is known to have some analgesic properties. However, patients with chronic pain adversely impacting sleep quality often use caffeine to cope with the accompanying fatigue. While this can further exacerbate a cycle of poor sleep quality, Scott and colleagues found that in patients with fibromyalgia who are taking opioid medication, caffeine had a favorable synergistic and pain-relieving effect.[43] Furthermore, a green tea polyphenol known as EpiGalloCatechin-3-Gallate, widely recognized for its powerful antioxidant and anti-inflammatory properties, is being studied in animal models of pain related to spinal cord injury, bone metastasis, and peripheral neuropathy.[44] For this reason, clinicians may find it useful to encourage organic green tea in place of coffee in patients who are overly reliant on high doses of caffeine to perform daily duties.

HERBS FOR PAIN

Wisdom of ancient healing traditions from all over the world provide the practitioner of integrative medicine many useful adjuncts in the treatment of patients with chronic pain and poor sleep quality. A dialogue of integrative approaches for the treatment of this symptom cluster would be incomplete without mention of a few key flowering plants. *Arnica montana* has long been used in Native American cultures to address pain and inflammation that result from soft tissue injury. The topical application of arnica gel and even internal ingestion of arnica formulations have been evaluated in pilot trials and showed promise in reducing postoperative ecchymosis, seroma formation, and bleeding.[45] Topical arnica may be preferred for pain management in the context of treatment for soft tissue injuries or after surgery or blunt trauma. Topical capsaicin is useful for peripheral neuropathy and degenerative joint conditions through a mechanism known as *defunctionalization* of pain transmitting neurons.[46] These topical remedies should be used along with acupuncture, massage, and other manual treatments as part of any regimen to reduce reliance on opioid medications for pain.

Cannabinoids have also demonstrated opioid-sparing properties through what are thought to be anti-inflammatory processes. High cannabidiol (CBD) concentrations, derived largely from the hemp flower, are currently being researched in palliative care settings, and a synthetic cannabinoid available in Canada, known as nabilone, was found to improve sleep in patients with fibromyalgia.[47] The use of anxiolytic chamomile and passionflower herbal teas made from the flowers of these plants can be part of a bedtime routine that helps promote sleep.

Case Resolution

Stef was referred for a split-night sleep study given her high risk of OSA (hypertension, obesity, snoring, and daytime fatigue). She declined visits with a physiatrist and a psychiatrist, although she did consider seeing a psychologist. She received CPAP treatment and was prescribed mindfulness, an exercise routine to include 30 minutes of walking 5 days per week, and a 1-hour yoga class weekly. Her vitamin D and magnesium levels were found to be suboptimal, and these were replenished. She was referred to acupuncture for her fatigue and neuropathy. An anti-inflammatory diet was recommended along with a protein supplement and green tea in place of coffee. Her cognitive impairment has improved with better sleep hygiene that contributed to better subjective sleep quality. One year later, her BMI is now 29 and her mood is markedly improved. Her pain is resolved, and she continues to adhere to a regular mindfulness and exercise plan.

Conclusion

In summary, nutritional guidance, an exercise plan, and mindfulness practice is at the very core of addressing the clinical challenge posed by chronic pain and its associated effect on sleep. Educating patients on how to incorporate these positive health behaviors provides the best chance of reducing the overall health burden these entities incur. Policy changes at both state and federal levels to address the opioid epidemic have created opportunities to innovate strategies that encompass multimodal, integrative treatment plans to address the conundrum of chronic pain and poor sleep quality. More research needs to be done to evaluate the cost-effectiveness of using this integrative approach to address this cluster of conditions so that third-party payers, such as insurance companies and government entities, can increase reimbursement for the provision of truly comprehensive care.

Let us labor for an inward stillness—
An inward stillness and an inward healing.
                    —Henry Wadsworth Longfellow

Resources

- Mindfulness:
  - www.kaiserpermanente.org/audio
- Nutrition:
  - http://www.drweil.com/drw/u/ART02995/Dr-Weil-Anti-Inflammatory-Food-Pyramid.html
- Sleep:
  - http://www.sleepfoundation.org/
- Exercise:
  - http://exerciseismedicine.org/

REFERENCES

1. Diaz-Piedra C, Catena A, Miro E, Martinez MP, Sanchez AI, Buela-Casal G. The impact of pain on anxiety and depression is mediated by objective and subjective sleep characteristics in fibromyalgia patients. *Clin J Pain.* 2014 Oct;30(10):852–859.
2. McCarter SJ, St Louis EK, Sandness DJ, et al. Antidepressants increase REM sleep muscle tone in patients with and without REM sleep behavior disorder. *Sleep.* 2015;38(6):907917.

3. Siegel JM. Sleep viewed as a state of adaptive inactivity. *Nat Rev Neurosci.* Oct 2009;10(10):747–753.

4. Campbell P, Tang N, McBeth J, et al. The role of sleep problems in the development of depression in those with persistent pain: A prospective cohort study. *Sleep.* Nov 2013;36(11):1693–1698.

5. Banks S, Dinges DF. Behavioral and physiological consequences of sleep restriction. *J Clin Sleep Med. JCSM.* Aug 15 2007;3(5):519–528.

6. Artner J, Cakir B, Spiekermann JA, et al. Prevalence of sleep deprivation in patients with chronic neck and back pain: A retrospective evaluation of 1016 patients. *J Pain Res.* 2013;6:1–6.

7. Koffel E, Kroenke K, Bair MJ, Leverty D, Polusny MA, Krebs EE. The bidirectional relationship between sleep complaints and pain: Analysis of data from a randomized trial. *Health Psychol.* 2016;35(1):41–49.

8. Alsaadi SM, McAuley JH, Hush JM, et al. Prevalence of sleep disturbance in patients with low back pain. *Eur Spine J.* 2011;20:737–743.

9. Wong PM, Manuck SB, DiNardo MM, Korytkowski M, Muldoon MF. Shorter sleep duration is associated with decreased insulin sensitivity in healthy white men. *Sleep.* 2015;38(2):223–231.

10. Field T, Diego M, Cullen C, Hernandez-Reif M, Sunshine W, Douglas S. Fibromyalgia pain and substance P decrease and sleep improves after massage therapy. *J Clin Rheumatol.* Apr 2002;8(2):72–76.

11. Finan PH, Smith MT. The comorbidity of insomnia, chronic pain, and depression: Dopamine as a putative mechanism. *Sleep Med Rev.* Jun 2013;17(3):173–183.

12. Nicassio PM, Ormseth SR, Kay M, et al. The contribution of pain and depression to self-reported sleep disturbance in patients with rheumatoid arthritis. *Pain.* Jan 2012;153(1):107–112.

13. Phillips B, Mannino DM. Do insomnia complaints cause hypertension or cardiovascular disease? *J Clin Sleep Med.* Aug 15 2007;3(5):489–494.

14. Sarsour K, Morin CM, Foley K, Kalsekar A, Walsh JK. Association of insomnia severity and comorbid medical and psychiatric disorders in a health plan-based sample: Insomnia severity and comorbidities. *Sleep Med.* Jan 2010;11(1):69–74.

15. Chan WS, Levsen MP, Puyat S, Robinson ME, Staud R, Berry RB, McCrae CS. Sleep discrepancy in patients with comorbid fibromyalgia and insomnia: Demographic, behavioral, and clinical correlates. *J Clin Sleep Med.* 2018 Nov 15;14(11):1911–1919. Published 2018 Nov 15. doi:10.5664/jcsm.7492

16. Bakke Johnsen, M, Heuch I, Grotle M, Zwart J, Nilsen K. The association between insomnia, c-reactive protein, and chronic low back pain: Cross-sectional analysis of the HUNT study, *Norway, Scand J Pain.* 2019;19(4):765–777.

17. Hohagen F, Kappler C, Schramm E, Riemann D, Weyerer S, Berger M. Sleep onset insomnia, sleep maintaining insomnia and insomnia with early morning awakening: Temporal stability of subtypes in a longitudinal study on general practice attenders. *Sleep.* Sep 1994;17(6):551–554.

18. McCrae CS, Williams J, Roditi D, et al. Cognitive behavioral treatments for insomnia and pain in adults with comorbid chronic insomnia and fibromyalgia: Clinical outcomes from the SPIN randomized controlled trial. *Sleep*. 2019 Mar;42(3):zsy234. doi: 10.1093/sleep/zsy234. PMID: 30496533; PMCID: PMC6424087.

19. Baron KG, Reid KJ, Zee PC. Exercise to improve sleep in insomnia: Exploration of the bidirectional effects. *J Clin Sleep Med*. 2013;9(8):819–824.

20. Mustian KM, Sprod LK, Janelsins M, Peppone LJ, Mohile S. Exercise recommendations for cancer-related fatigue, cognitive impairment, sleep problems, depression, pain, anxiety, and physical dysfunction: A review. *Oncol Hematol Rev*. 2012;8(2):81–88.

21. Cheville AL, Kollasch J, Vandenberg J, et al. A home-based exercise program to improve function, fatigue, and sleep quality in patients with Stage IV lung and colorectal cancer: A randomized controlled trial. *J Pain Sympt Mgmt*. May 2013;45(5):811–821.

22. Zou L, Yeung A, Quan X, Boyden SD, Wang H. A systematic review and meta-analysis of mindfulness-based (baduanjin) exercise for alleviating musculoskeletal pain and improving sleep quality in people with chronic diseases. *Int J Environ Res Public Health*. 2018;15(2):206.

23. Kwekkeboom KL, Cherwin CH, Lee JW, Wanta B. Mind-body treatments for the pain-fatigue-sleep disturbance symptom cluster in persons with cancer. *J Pain Sympt Mgmt*. Jan 2010;39(1):126–138.

24. Garland SN, Carlson LE, Antle MC, Samuels C, Campbell T. I-CAN SLEEP: Rationale and design of a non-inferiority RCT of Mindfulness-based Stress Reduction and Cognitive Behavioral Therapy for the treatment of Insomnia in CANcer survivors. *Contemp Clin Trials*. Sep 2011;32(5):747–754.

25. Wang LN, Tao H, Zhao Y, Zhou YQ, Jiang XR. Optimal timing for initiation of biofeedback-assisted relaxation training in hospitalized coronary heart disease patients with sleep disturbances. *J Cardiovasc Nurs*.2014 Jul;29(4):367–376.

26. Garland EL, Howard MO. Mindfulness-oriented recovery enhancement reduces pain attentional bias in chronic pain patients. *Psychother Psychosom*. 2013;82(5):311–318.

27. Brown CA, Jones AK. Psychobiological correlates of improved mental health in patients with musculoskeletal pain after a mindfulness-based pain management program. *Clin J Pain*. Mar 2013;29(3):233–244.

28. Sabanayagam C, Zhang R, Shankar A. Markers of sleep-disordered breathing and metabolic syndrome in a multiethnic sample of US adults: Results from the National Health and Nutrition Examination Survey 2005–2008. *Cardiol Res Pract*. 2012;2012:630802.

29. Hornyak M, Voderholzer U, Hohagen F, Berger M, Riemann D. Magnesium therapy for periodic leg movements-related insomnia and restless legs syndrome: An open pilot study. *Sleep*. Aug 1 1998;21(5):501–505.

30. James FO, Cermakian N, Boivin DB. Circadian rhythms of melatonin, cortisol, and clock gene expression during simulated night shift work. *Sleep*. Nov 2007;30(11):1427–1436.

31. Taavoni S, Nazem Ekbatani N, Haghani H. Valerian/lemon balm use for sleep disorders during menopause. *Compl Ther Clin Pract*. Nov 2013;19(4):193–196.

32. Ancoli-Israel S, DuHamel ER, Stepnowsky C, Engler R, Cohen-Zion M, Marler M. The relationship between congestive heart failure, sleep apnea, and mortality in older men. *Chest*. Oct 2003;124(4):1400–1405.

33. Parish JM, Somers VK. Obstructive sleep apnea and cardiovascular disease. *Mayo Clin Proc*. Aug 2004;79(8):1036–1046.

34. Hrubos-Strom H, Einvik G, Nordhus IH, et al. Sleep apnoea, anxiety, depression and somatoform pain: A community-based high-risk sample. *Eur Resp J*. Aug 2012;40(2):400–407.

35. Troitino A, Labedi N, Kufel T, El-Solh AA. Positive airway pressure therapy in patients with opioid-related central sleep apnea. *Sleep Breathing/Schlaf Atmung*. 2014 May;18(2):367–373.

36. Clemens S, Rye D, Hochman S. Restless legs syndrome: Revisiting the dopamine hypothesis from the spinal cord perspective. *Neurology*. Jul 11 2006;67(1):125–130.

37. Edwards RR, Quartana PJ, Allen RP, Greenbaum S, Earley CJ, Smith MT. Alterations in pain responses in treated and untreated patients with restless legs syndrome: Associations with sleep disruption. *Sleep Med*. Jun 2011;12(6):603–609.

38. Chen KM, Chen MH, Lin MH, Fan JT, Lin HS, Li CH. Effects of yoga on sleep quality and depression in elders in assisted living facilities. *J Nurs Res*. Mar 2010;18(1):53–61.

39. Vera FM, Manzaneque JM, Maldonado EF, et al. Subjective sleep quality and hormonal modulation in long-term yoga practitioners. *Biol Psychol*. Jul 2009;81(3):164–168.

40. Li F, Fisher KJ, Harmer P, Irbe D, Tearse RG, Weimer C. Tai chi and self-rated quality of sleep and daytime sleepiness in older adults: A randomized controlled trial. *J Am Geriatr Soc*. Jun 2004;52(6):892–900.

41. Taylor P, Pezzullo L, Grant SJ, Bensoussan A. Cost-effectiveness of acupuncture for chronic nonspecific low back pain. *Pain Pract*. 2014 Sep;14(7):599–606.

42. McCarty DE, Chesson AL Jr, Jain SK, Marino AA. The link between vitamin D metabolism and sleep medicine. *Sleep Med Rev*. 2014 Aug;18(4):311–319. doi:10.1016/j.smrv.2013.07.001.

43. Scott JR, Hassett AL, Brummett CM, Harris RE, Clauw DJ, Harte SE. Caffeine as an opioid analgesic adjuvant in fibromyalgia. *J Pain Res*. 2017 Jul 28;10:1801–1809.

44. Bimonte S, Cascella M, Schiavone V, Mehrabi-Kermani F, Cuomo A. The roles of epigallocatechin-3-gallate in the treatment of neuropathic pain: An update on preclinical in vivo studies and future perspectives. *Drug Des Devel Ther*. 2017;11:2737–2742.

45. Sorrentino L, Piraneo S, Riggio E, Basilicò S, Sartani A, Bossi D, Corsi F. Is there a role for homeopathy in breast cancer surgery? A first randomized clinical trial on treatment with Arnica montana to reduce post-operative seroma and bleeding in patients undergoing total mastectomy. *J Intercult Ethnopharmacol.* 2017 Jan 3;6(1):1–8.

46. Gagnier JJ, Oltean H, van Tulder MW, Berman BM, Bombardier C, Robbins CB. Herbal medicine for low back pain: A Cochrane review. *Spine (Phila Pa 1976).* 2016 Jan;41(2):116–133.

47. Ware MA, Fitzcharles MA, Joseph L, Shir Y. The effects of nabilone on sleep in fibromyalgia: Results of a randomized controlled trial. *Anesth Analg.* 2010 Feb 1;110(2):604–610.

28

Sleep and Mental Health Disorders

SUTAPA DUBE, CLAIRE E. WHEELER, AND NOSHENE RANJBAR

Introduction

Sleep disorders are common ailments that affect a sizeable number of patients. Between 10% and 20% of the population suffer from clinically significant sleep disorders in the United States alone.[1,2] These disorders result in loss of productivity and worsened health outcomes and are therefore a public health concern.[2,3] To better understand how sleep disturbance affects health and productivity, a basic understanding of sleep psychophysiology is fundamental.

Sleep health is crucial to well-being, resiliency, and optimal function. Individuals spend an average of one-third of each day sleeping, with sufficient sleep for adults being defined as 7–9 hours per night.[2,4] Sleep is composed of a specific set of behavioral criteria (unconscious state, reduced cognitive function, often recumbent posture, and decreased responsiveness to external stimuli) and physiological criteria (overall reduction in blood pressure, respiratory rate, temperature, and arousal).[5] While a complete understanding of the biological basis for sleep has not been delineated, research shows that sleep is imperative for overall functioning. Sleep affects every system in the body, including neuronal, cardiac, respiratory, and immune systems, as well as the regulation of affect.[4] Insufficient sleep is linked to increased risk of diabetes, hypertension, obesity, and all-cause mortality.[2]

Bidirectional Relationships with Sleep

Sleep (duration and quality) can affect other body systems, and these systems, in turn, can affect sleep. Specifically, sleep deprivation can adversely affect the function of the hypothalamus-pituitary-adrenal-axis (HPA-axis). HPA-axis functioning is central to stress responses as it directs cortisol levels to increase or decrease to facilitate coping with stressors in the environment.[6] The release of cortisol and adrenaline prepare the body to fight or flee. HPA dysregulation has a profound effect not only on the body's physiologic state, but also on mood. In HPA dysregulation, stress becomes chronic rather than transient and diminishes the ability to distinguish actual from perceived danger. This can lead to hypercortisolism, with ongoing mood symptoms, such as low mood, anxiety, dysphoria, etc. Constant hypercortisolism can lead to development of chronic fatigue, posttraumatic stress disorder (PTSD), depression, and fibromyalgia—all of which can then negatively affect sleep.[7]

Additionally, stress can have a marked impact on sleep duration and quality. In a 1981 study, 74% of subjects with chronic insomnia reported that their insomnia was associated with life stressors at the time of onset.[8] Further studies have shown that experiencing stress and negative emotion states is associated with changes in sleep quality and quantity, often leading to fragmentation of sleep.[9] The effect of stress on sleep can lead to seemingly disparate sleep responses—one in which a person is hypervigilant and unable to sleep and, conversely, another where a person may feel exhausted and try to conserve energy with extended sleep.[10] In both situations, the experience of stress directly affects the individual's experience of sleep.

Similar to the relationship between stress and sleep, the relationship between sleep and psychiatric disorders is bidirectional. Among the criteria of the *Diagnostic and Statistical Manual of Mental Disorders* (DSM-5) for psychiatric disorders there is often a criterion associated with sleep patterns.[11–14] This association is thought to be primarily due to the fact that emotion processing and sleep are influenced by several common overlying structures in the brain. Specifically, structural and chemical changes in the brain during rapid eye movement (REM) sleep appear similar to emotion regulation and reactivity during wake times. During REM sleep there is increased activity in the areas of the amygdala, striatum, hippocampus, insula, and medial prefrontal cortex—areas that are also associated with emotion.[15] In their model of "sleep to remember, sleep to forget," Walker and van der Helm posit that memories that have an emotional component are formed in an environment of increased adrenergic response and are better remembered. During REM sleep, the emotional tone is reduced through a decrease in emotional reactivity of the amygdala to the memory, and the hippocampus preserves the core information of the memory.[16] Several studies illustrate this connection between sleep and psychiatric disorders.

In one such study, 62% of college students ($N = 7,626$) aged 18–29 years met the criteria for poor sleep. The study reveals that symptoms of anxiety, depression, and attention deficit hyperactivity disorder (ADHD) are associated with disruption in sleep domains defined by the Pittsburgh Sleep Quality Index (PSQI).[17]

Other studies focusing on older adults also have found an association between sleep disturbances and mental illness. Reid et al. found a correlation between the number and types of sleep disturbances reported by participants and their mental health, physical health, and quality of life.[18] This correlation is also confirmed by the finding in the Nadorff et al. 2017 literature review that "sleep disorders are robustly associated with anxiety, depression, dementia, and suicidal behavior later in life."[19]

Psychiatric Illnesses and Sleep

Given the associations between sleep and mental health, patients should be assessed and treated for sleep disturbances as part of their psychiatric care. In most cases, addressing sleep problems will help with the mental health condition, and sleep treatment should be part of the course of care from the beginning. To successfully address mental health issues, sleep disorders need to be tackled, and treating sleep disorders in many psychiatric patients necessitates addressing mental health issues. The relationships between sleep disturbances and common psychiatric illnesses including depressive, bipolar, anxiety, obsessive compulsive, posttraumatic stress, psychotic, and attention deficit-hyperactivity disorders are explored here.

Depression

Major depressive disorder has an estimated lifetime prevalence of up to 17% in the United States, with an estimated loss of up to $44 billion per year in productivity.[20,21] Sleep disturbance is included among the nine major symptoms used to diagnose depression. The criteria for a diagnosis of major depressive disorder are met if five of nine symptoms are present—depressed mood, loss of interest/pleasure, change in appetite, psychomotor agitation or retardation, fatigue, feelings of worthlessness or guilt, poor concentration and difficulty making decisions, suicidal ideation, and insomnia or hypersomnia—over a 2 -week time frame, with one of the five symptoms being either depressed mood or loss of interest/pleasure. Various studies state that nearly 70–90% of individuals with major depressive disorder report concurrent sleep disturbances.[12,22]

The types of sleep disturbances associated with major depressive disorder vary from poor sleep quality and difficulties falling asleep to increased daytime sleepiness and frequent awakenings.[12,22] There is a bidirectional relationship between insomnia and depression.[23] Yates et al. found that up to 88% of patients with major depressive disorder report symptoms of insomnia, and 27% report symptoms of hypersomnia.[24] Moreover, having sleep disturbances increases the risk of developing major depressive disorder: patients with insomnia are two to three times more likely to develop major depressive disorder in comparison to the general population.[25,26] In a study on older adults, not only did sleep disturbances increase the risk of depression and the risk of recurrence and worsening of depression, but depression also increased the risk of both developing and worsening symptoms of sleep disturbances.[27] In addition, major depressive disorder is associated with higher incidence of obstructive sleep apnea, restless legs syndrome, and narcolepsy than in the general population.[22]

Bipolar Disorder

Bipolar I and II disorders have a lifetime prevalence of 1% and 0.5%, respectively, and approximately 20% of individuals with this diagnosis complete suicide.[28] Bipolar I disorder consists of having a manic or mixed episode and bipolar II disorder consists of at least one hypomanic episode and one depressive episode.[11] A manic episode consists of a period of abnormally elevated or irritable mood with consistent increased energy or goal-directed activity for a duration of 1 week or requiring hospitalization. Additionally, three or four (if mood is primarily irritable) or more of the following symptoms need to be present for this diagnosis: grandiosity, pressured speech, racing thoughts/flight of ideas, increased distractibility, increased goal-directed activity or psychomotor agitation, impulsivity/involvement in high-risk activities, and a decreased need for sleep.[11,12] A hypomanic episode has the same symptom criterion as a manic episode except for being of shorter duration (4 days rather than 1 week).[11] Given the bidirectional relationship between sleep and affect dysregulation, it is not surprising that sleep disturbances are found to be the most common prodrome of a manic episode and the sixth most common prodrome of a depressive episode.[29–31] In fact, 69–99% of individuals experience a reduced need for sleep during a manic episode.[30]

Sleep disturbances commonly seen in the manic or hypomanic phase of bipolar disorder include shortened REM latency, shortened total sleep time, increased latency to sleep onset, poor sleep efficiency, increased sleep fragmentation, and greater variability in sleep duration.[32] During the depressive episodes of bipolar disorder, there is evidence showing sleep disturbances similar to those reported in unipolar depression, though there are some data indicating that bipolar depression may have a greater risk for increased REM density and early morning awakenings. There may be more reports of hypersomnia as opposed to insomnia in bipolar depression.[31] Giglio et al. assert that treatment of sleep disturbance in bipolar disorder is important for three primary reasons: (1) a large portion of patients with bipolar disorder can be induced into a manic or hypomanic episode by exposure to sleep deprivation, (2) sleep disturbances are common prodromes for manic and depressive episodes (as noted earlier), and (3) the sleep–wake cycle is thought to be an integral part of understanding bipolar disorder.[31] Furthermore, sleep disturbance is thought not only to induce manic episodes, but also to be exacerbated by presence of a manic episode.[31,32]

Anxiety

Anxiety disorders have been separated into three categories in the DSM-5: anxiety disorders, obsessive compulsive disorders, and trauma- and stressor-related disorders.[11] The anxiety disorders include separation anxiety disorder, selective mutism, specific phobia, social phobia, panic disorder, agoraphobia, and generalized anxiety disorder (GAD).[11,33] According to the National Institute of Mental Health, data collected in 2001 through 2003 indicate that approximately 19.1% of adults in the United States have an anxiety disorder, with a prevalence of insomnia for these individuals ranging from 70% to 90%.[34] In a large European study ($N = 14,915$), anxiety and insomnia appeared together approximately 40% of the time in anxious subjects, and in another 40% of anxious subjects, insomnia developed after anxiety.[35] In fact, even for those subjects whose daytime anxiety decreases, sleep disturbances have been shown to continue without much improvement.[36] Sleep problems in childhood may predict anxiety in adulthood although the mechanisms in this association need to be further explored.[37]

Among the anxiety disorders, insomnia and GAD have the highest comorbidity.[36] The prevalence of GAD in the United States adult population is 3.1%.[36] GAD is defined as having excessive worries for at least 6 months in addition to at least three of the following six symptoms: increased irritability, difficulty with concentration, muscle tension, restlessness, easily fatigued, and/or a disturbance of sleep.[11,33] Boland and Ross note how insomnia and anxiety are intimately related and that 50–70% of patients who have GAD also report having sleep disturbances.[36] In a comprehensive review of anxiety and sleep disturbances, patients with a diagnosis of GAD exhibited decreased total sleep time, with some evidence for poor sleep efficiency, increased latency to sleep onset, and increased percentage of time in stage 2 of sleep.[38] Another anxiety disorder that illustrates a bidirectional relationship with sleep is panic disorder. A common symptom for patients with panic disorder is sleep panic attacks. During such events, an individual may experience a panic attack while asleep, which awakens the individual from sleep. Polysomnography changes in subjects who experience sleep panic attacks indicate difficulty with sleep onset and maintenance. Data illustrate that between 33% and 71% of individuals with a panic disorder report having sleep panic attacks, which may contribute to latency of sleep onset due to patient apprehension of experiencing a panic episode while sleeping.[36,39] Furthermore, Mellman reports that, in comparison to patients who have daytime panic, individuals with sleep panic attacks have more severe symptoms that are associated with suicidal ideation, depression, and earlier onset of disorder.[39]

Obsessive-Compulsive Disorder

Obsessive-compulsive disorder (OCD), previously categorized in the DSM as an anxiety disorder, has more recently been placed in a separate category with body dysmorphic disorder, hoarding disorder, trichotillomania, and excoriation disorder.[11] The primary symptoms of OCD comprise obsessions (repetitive, intrusive, uncontrolled, undesired images, thoughts, impulses, and/or feelings) and compulsions (repetitive behaviors aimed at reducing the anxiety of the obsessions).[11,36,40] Individuals with a diagnosis of OCD have worsened sleep efficiency, more frequent awakenings after onset of sleep, and spend less total time asleep.[36,38,39,41] Data indicate a relationship between OCD and sleep disturbances, but the results are mixed with regards to which specific sleep abnormalities are associated with OCD. This is in part due to the comorbidity of OCD with depression as a confounding factor.[39] Researchers have found that the sleep disturbances associated with OCD appear to be influenced more strongly by obsessions than by compulsions, and individuals with OCD have higher incidence of circadian rhythm abnormalities.[36] In fact, several studies have found that patients with a diagnosis of OCD exhibit delayed sleep phase in comparison to healthy individuals, even when controlled for comorbid depression diagnosis.[36,41-43] Further studies are indicated to explore the specific relationship between OCD and sleep disturbances.

Posttraumatic Stress Disorder

PTSD, similar to OCD, has recently been removed from the DSM anxiety disorder category and placed in the trauma- and stress-related disorders along with the diagnoses of acute stress disorder, reactive attachment disorder, disinhibited social engagement disorder, and adjustment disorder.[11] The lifetime prevalence for PTSD is between 5% and 10% in the general population.[44] PTSD is characterized by the exposure to a traumatic event (either death, serious injury, sexual violence, or threat of death) and the patient's subsequent reaction to experiencing such an event that causes distress for the patient and has lasted more than 1 month. Criteria for PTSD include re-experiencing the event; avoidance of trauma-related stimuli; and experiencing worsening of at least two of the following: inability to recall trauma details, overly negative thoughts about oneself/surroundings, exaggerated self-blame for causing the trauma, negative affect, apathy, feeling isolated, or having difficultly experiencing positive affect. Furthermore, two of the following worsening arousal symptoms also must be present: increased irritability/aggression, becoming involved in risky behaviors, hypervigilance, being easily startled, poor concentration, and difficulty with sleep.[11,45,46] The most common sleep disturbances seen in PTSD are nightmares (re-experiencing the traumatic event) and insomnia (hyperarousal), with up to 70% and 90% of PTSD patients reporting these symptoms, respectively.[44,45]

Trauma exposure and sleep disturbance have a bidirectional relationship in which sleep disturbance can worsen responses to trauma and increase the risk for poor psychiatric outcomes, and trauma exposure can increase the risk for sleep disturbances.[44] Assessment and treatment of persistent sleep disturbances after a traumatic event are warranted as they may be early indicators of PTSD.[47] In fact, the use of treatments aimed at reducing sleep disturbances may result in improvement in daytime PTSD symptoms.[44] In a review of the underlying sleep architecture changes in patients with PTSD, alterations in REM sleep were identified as most significant.[36] As noted earlier, REM sleep is involved with processing emotion-laden memories and might have a role in both consolidating fear memories and aiding with discrimination between cues that signal threat or safety through the activation of the amygdala.[16,36,44]

Psychosis

Psychotic disorders (including schizophreniform disorder, schizophrenia, schizoaffective disorder, delusional disorder, and unspecified psychotic disorders) do not have a specific criterion for abnormal sleep symptoms. "Negative" symptoms of psychotic disorders include lack of motivation, apathy, and social isolation. "Positive" symptoms of psychotic disorders include perceptual disturbances (hallucinations), delusions, and disordered thoughts.[11] Sleep disturbances (primarily poor sleep efficiency and quality) are reported in 30–80% of individuals with schizophrenia, with an increase in both negative and positive symptoms of schizophrenia.[48,49] Additionally, disordered sleep (such as delayed sleep onset, frequent awakenings) and decreased slow wave sleep (SWS) can present in prodromal patients who are considered at high risk for developing a psychotic disorder when compared to healthy peers.[49,50] Other changes, such as increased REM density or decreased REM latency, have been reported. However, these changes have not been consistently observed.[50]

Attention Deficit Hyperactivity Disorder

ADHD is one of the most common neurodevelopmental disorders and affects an estimated 7% of youth globally.[51] In the United States, approximately 11% of youth have been diagnosed with ADHD, with 60–80% of those diagnosed having symptoms that last into adulthood.[52,53] Criteria for ADHD include onset of symptoms prior to the age of 12 years with pervasive (present in at least two settings) symptoms persisting for more than 6 months. For the diagnosis of

ADHD, the patient must display either five of nine inattentive symptoms, five of nine impulsive/hyperactive symptoms, or both, depending on which ADHD sub-type is predominant.[11,53] Per Corkum et al., 25–55% of the parents of children with ADHD report concerns regarding poor sleep.[54]

As with many of the psychiatric disorders just discussed, the relationship between sleep and ADHD is also bidirectional, with treatment of sleep im-proving ADHD symptoms and vice versa.[55] There are several changes in sleep associated with an ADHD diagnosis in youth and children, including delayed sleep onset, poor sleep quality and efficiency, decreased total sleep time, fre-quent awakenings from sleep, and more periodic limb movements.[52] In adults with ADHD, only sleep onset latency and poor sleep efficiency are consistent.[56] In addition to sleep disturbances associated with an ADHD diagnosis, there are also mixed findings regarding sleep disturbances in subjects diagnosed with ADHD who are being treated with stimulant medication. Some data indicate that controlling ADHD symptomatology with stimulants can actually improve sleep by improving bedtime resistance. However, other data suggest that stim-ulant medication disrupts sleep by causing insomnia, reducing total sleep time, contributing to poor sleep efficiency, and increasing sleep onset latency.[52] A sys-tematic review regarding sleep disturbances in adolescents with ADHD noted three likely areas where the bidirectionality of the relationship between ADHD and sleep disturbances is observable.[52] Evidence shows that adolescents with an ADHD diagnosis have delays in neuromaturation, which may interfere with the normal decline of SWS associated with puberty; the disrupted SWS trajectory then may impede neuromaturation, which in turn would continue to interfere with normal SWS changes of adolescence in a positive feedback loop.[52] Second, poor sleep can cause impairment due to interfering with memory, emotional reg-ulation, executive functioning, and reward-based decision-making across all ages of healthy individuals, which then may become amplified in individuals who also have an ADHD diagnosis.[52] Finally, ADHD symptoms and disordered sleep may also work synergistically to increase psychosocial stress for adolescents with an ADHD diagnosis in that impairment with executive functioning can lead to poor academic and social achievements.[52]

Assessment of Psychiatric Disorders and Sleep Disturbances

The evaluation of individuals for sleep disturbances and psychiatric disorders begins with an interview. One of the most important aspects of assessing either of these concerns is to remember to ask about them, most preferably with open-ended questions. A widely used screening tool is the PSQI, a 19-item, self-report questionnaire that looks at sleep and sleep disturbances over a 1-month period.[55] When interviewing patients with potential psychiatric disorders, it is important to assess for anxiety, psychosis, executive function, trauma, and mood symptoms as detailed for each disorder earlier.[11,57] Additionally, a good history and physical examination will aid in making a well-rounded differential diagnosis. While polysomnography may be the gold standard with regard to sleep architecture, it is not always necessary. A completed sleep diary from the patient and a thorough history will best aid in developing a plan for treatment.

It is important to attempt to determine whether ongoing sleep problems precipitated the mental health issue or whether the mental health problem led to sleep problems. If poor sleep is an instigating factor, that may warrant an initial focus on addressing sleep issues through some of the approaches described here. If sleep problems are secondary to the psychiatric disturbance, then it may be best to focus on the psychiatric issue in the first instance.

Treatments for Psychiatric Disorders and Sleep Disturbances

This section reviews a selected number of treatments to consider for sleep disturbances within the context of psychiatric conditions. Because there is a bidirectional relationship between many psychiatric disorders and sleep disturbances, it is important to treat both simultaneously. The particular treatment recommended depends on the sleep issues the patient presents with, how receptive they are to certain types of treatment, and any drug interactions that should be avoided. Needs should be addressed according to the individual patient, and it is important to meet the patient where they are. Integrative sleep treatments are discussed in depth in other chapters this volume.

PHARMACOLOGIC APPROACHES

Several pharmacological agents are available to aid with sleep induction, the most well-known of which are the benzodiazepine receptor agonists. These agents include benzodiazepines and nonbenzodiazepine medications. These work via binding with variable affinity to benzodiazepine receptors 1 and 2.[58] These medications are not indicated for long-term use due to concerns regarding memory impairment.[58] Tiagabine and sodium oxybate are gamma-aminobutyric acid-ergic (GABA-ergic) compounds that have been shown to improve SWS, which in turn can improve alertness and performance.[58] However, the use of tiagabine is off-label and associated with an increased risk of new-onset seizures and suicidal thoughts/behaviors, and these have led to a warning from the US Food and Drug Administration (FDA).[58] This may limit its use in patients with psychiatric disorders. Another pharmacologic class of medications, hypocretin/orexin receptor agonists, is under investigation for the ability to reduce sleep latency and improve sleep efficiency. In addition to the available pharmacologic agents just discussed, clinical trials for newly developing medications are ongoing.

Patient consumption of caffeine and alcohol should also be evaluated for their potential contribution to sleep disturbances and mental health problems. While caffeine has been shown to have a mildly inverse relationship to depressive disorders, it can exacerbate anxiety as well as psychosis and manic symptoms, in addition to interfering with sleep.[59-62] Drug and alcohol use often correlate with sleep disturbances and appear to have a bidirectional relationship.[63] For patients with bipolar disorder, avoidance of caffeine and alcohol, together with sleep association and sleep hygiene, is preferred to sleep restriction, given that sleep restriction can precipitate a manic episode.

Micronutrient assessments are recommended when treating patients with sleep and psychiatric disorders.[64] Resources that can help with making an assessment are readily available, such as www.mytavin.com and www.drugbank.ca. These sites provide information about the deficiencies that are most likely to arise when a patient is taking a certain medication. Broad-spectrum micronutrients may be beneficial in treating some psychiatric illnesses. In many cases, the utilization of these formulas can help reduce the doses of psychotropic medications needed, thereby reducing medication side effects.[65,66] There also appears to be a link between trace elements, vitamins, and minerals and sleep patterns.[64] Antipsychotic medications can sometimes lead to unfavorable changes to the gut microbiome,[67,68] as well as to micronutrient imbalances, possibly resulting in serious side effects such as tardive dyskinesia; such imbalances therefore warrant assessing micronutrients when a patient presents with psychiatric disorders.[69] Addressing the relationships between sleep, psychiatric problems, and micronutrients requires training and experience.

COGNITIVE-BEHAVIORAL APPROACHES

Given the potential for adverse effects and dependency on pharmacological agents commonly used for insomnia, it is important to explore other modalities for treatment. Cognitive-behavioral theory posits that negative thoughts generate negative emotional responses, which in turn provoke a physiological stress response that alters endocrine, digestive, and immune function, among others. By reining in one's habitually busy and negative thought patterns and practicing replacing them with an attitude of equanimity and gratitude, one can experience fewer episodes of stress and its attendant physiological arousal.

There are several cognitive and/or behavioral approaches to treatment of sleep within mental health settings. *Sleep hygiene therapy* consists of educating patients regarding general health-related interventions, as well as having patients learn and commit to sleep stimulus control guidelines. Other behavioral approaches include *sleep restriction therapy, relaxation therapy,* and *paradoxical intention setting.*[70] An additional cognitive and behavioral approach to sleep and psychiatric disorders is *cognitive-behavioral therapy for insomnia* (CBT-I). This approach has been found to be effective not only in the treatment of insomnia but also in addressing worrying, rumination, and negative thought patterns associated with anxiety and depression.[71] Some patients may not be ready for CBT-I. In these cases, *motivational interviewing* is suggested as an initial approach. Sleep hygiene, CBT-I, and other behavioral approaches to treatment of sleep within mental health settings are discussed in elsewhere in this volume.

MIND–BODY MEDICINE

Various mind–body techniques have been studied for their potential efficacy in improving sleep patterns in people with a variety of diagnoses.[72] While the research in this area is still relatively scant, there have been promising results from the use of breath work, autogenic training, and mindfulness body scan to improve sleep duration and quality.[73]

Breath Work

Relaxation is a cornerstone of behavioral treatment of insomnia, and the voluntary regulation of breathing is central to relaxation. Most relaxation techniques begin with a focus on the breath, with an intention to make it deeper and slower. A special emphasis should be placed on the balance between inhalation and exhalation.[74] During exhalation, the vagus nerve is stimulated, leading to a reduction in heart rate and blood pressure. This phenomenon is referred to as heart rate variability (HRV). As HRV increases, so does one's subjective sense of relaxation, along with myriad other effects of vagal activity: muscle relaxation, increased perfusion of the gastrointestinal system, and a quieting of thoughts. Breathing techniques have been used in some insomnia research, but they are most often integrated into studies of other relaxation skills for better sleep.[75-77] Some studies have found breath regulation effective for several diagnoses, including stress-related conditions, but a need for controlled studies of the efficacy for breath work alone in the management of insomnia has been noted.[78,79] Although further study is needed, given what is known about the impact of mindful, deep breathing on autonomic nervous system balance, especially with an increased exhale-to-inhale ratio, it seems reasonable to consider this a viable first step in the nonpharmacological treatment of insomnia.

Autogenic Training

Autogenic training (AT) develops the skill of generating a state of greater relaxation for oneself, marked by a shift in autonomic nervous system function to a more vagal- (parasympathetic) dominant state. The process begins with assuming a comfortable position and quietly or silently repeating a series of phrases to oneself. Each phrase, such as "my arms are heavy and warm" addresses a different somatic aspect of the relaxation response. Over time, with practice, individuals are able to activate that response with increasing ease and efficiency.

Several reviews of nonpharmacological approaches to insomnia treatment include mention of AT as one of many relaxation techniques that may be useful.[80,81] In a study of the utility of AT as a treatment for people with anxiety and depression, 39% of participants reported shorter sleep latency times while 30% reported fewer night-time awakenings. Thirty-seven percent reported getting more hours of sleep per night, with 61% reporting they more often felt refreshed upon awakening.[82] A very small trial (n = 28) of a 12-week behavioral intervention for insomnia entailed weekly sessions during which a variety of relaxation techniques, including AT, were taught. The researchers used the Insomnia Severity Index (ISI) to evaluate what changes, if any, occurred in participants' sleep patterns. They found statistically significant reductions in insomnia severity using the ISI, from "moderate" to "mild," along with self-reports of increased satisfaction with sleep and better daytime performance among participants.[83] These results suggest that further research into AT as a safe, nontoxic remedy for insomnia is warranted.

Mindfulness-Based Stress Reduction

Mindfulness and mindfulness-based stress reduction (MBSR) have been found to be effective in the prevention and management of a wide array of stress-related conditions,[84] after being introduced as a clinical tool by Jon Kabat-Zinn of the University of Massachusetts in the early 1990s. MBSR has been characterized as a "third-wave therapy" for insomnia, one that goes beyond traditional cognitive-behavioral approaches to induce "metacognitive shifts" and "experiential change strategies."[85] These shifts and strategies may offer an alternative to, or enhancement of, techniques that involve focusing on sleep behaviors and thoughts about sleep behavior to a broader perspective on life and one's relationship with one's mind, yielding benefits that go beyond better sleep. The essence of MBSR is the development of the ability to be attentive to oneself and one's thoughts, body, and surroundings without distraction and without judgment. Mindfulness is a process by which one learns to quiet the chatter of everyday thoughts, which are often self-deprecating, fearful, unrealistic, or otherwise negative, by focusing on the here and now and resisting the temptation to constantly evaluate one's experience as "bad" or "good." It is not difficult to imagine how this approach could be beneficial to those who have trouble relaxing into sleep, and several studies of MBSR for insomnia bear this out.[86–88] Interestingly, most interventions studied have resulted in improvements in subjective, but not objective, measures of sleep quality.

COMPLEMENTARY AND ALTERNATIVE APPROACHES

A variety of complementary and alternative medicine (CAM) interventions are used to address sleep and mental health concerns. Within the realm of herbal medicine, plants such as lemon balm, German chamomile, hops, passionflower, valerian, ashwagandha, and kava are utilized to improve sleep duration and decrease sleep latency.[89] While the mechanisms of action for these plants are still being explored, it is thought that they may modulate the actions of GABA and the 5-hydroxytryptophan (5-HT) receptors.[90] In their meta-analysis on herbal medicine for insomnia, Leach and Page (2015) found that while there was insufficient evidence to support the use of herbal medicine for the treatment of insomnia, the safety profile for kava, chamomile, and wuling was similar to placebo.[91] They noted, however, that valerian had a greater number of adverse events than placebo.[91] Table 28.1 summarizes some of the common herbs and supplements used in treating insomnia and symptoms of psychiatric illnesses.

Meditative movement is another broad area of integrative interventions for treatment of sleep. Some of the techniques encompassed in this category of interventions include but are not limited to yoga, tai chi, and qi gong. In their systematic review of meditative movement and sleep quality, Wang et al. found that "improvement in sleep quality was . . . often accompanied by improvements in quality of life, physical performance, and depression," though they concluded that further rigorous randomized control studies were needed to establish the efficacy of these interventions.[96] An exciting area of research is the exploration of *aromatherapy* for treatment of sleep disturbances and psychiatric disorders. In a small case series, lavender oil capsules (Lasea) used in conjunction with an antidepressant were helpful in reducing depressive and anxious symptoms and, in a few cases, aided in improving insomnia.[97] As with many CAM interventions, a more thorough exploration with a larger sample size would be beneficial in establishing the efficacy of this type of treatment.

Table 28.1 Herbs and supplements used to treat symptoms of psychiatric illness and sleep disturbances

Herb/Supplement	Symptoms treated	Dosage[a]	Notes
Hops (*Humulus lupulus*)	Insomnia Anxiety	0.5–1 dropper full of 5:1 ethanolic extract; taken 30–60 minutes before bedtime	Can help to reduce muscle tension Found to be effective when used in combination with valerian for a hypnotic effect Not for use with pregnant women
Kava (*Piper methysticum*)	Anxiety Insomnia	50–70 mg; taken three times daily	Caution when used with other sedative medications May cause extrapyramidal symptoms At extremely high doses (300–400 mg/d) can cause rash, difficulties with visual accommodation, ataxia, and redness of eyes Not recommended for use with patients with liver disease; case reports of idiopathic hepatotoxic hepatitis
Lemon balm (*Melissa officinalis*)	Insomnia Anxiety Mood	Crude herb: 500–1000 mg 2–3 times per day Tincture (1:5): 3–5 mL taken 2–3 times per day	Not recommended for use with pregnant or lactating women Can be used in aromatherapy
L-theanine	Insomnia Anxiety	50–400 mg; taken 30–60 minutes before bedtime	Not recommended for use with pregnant or lactating women Has an antihypertensive effect; caution when used with antihypertensives Studies in boys with ADHD and shown to improve sleep efficacy Does not usually cause increased sedation, rather likely works as an anxiolytic.

Table 28.1 Continued

Herb/Supplement	Symptoms treated	Dosage[a]	Notes
Melatonin	Insomnia	0.3–0.5 mg at 5 PM or 1–6 mg taken 30–60 minutes before bedtime	Sustained-release may be more effective to maintain adequate levels throughout the night Immediate-release formulations may be more helpful in treating frequent/early awakenings Works to regulate circadian rhythm and in some (taken at 1–6 mg dosage) as a hypnotic Not recommended for use with pregnant women
Valerian root (*Valeriana officinalis*)	Insomnia Anxiety	For Insomnia: 300–900 mg standardized extract of 0.8% extract or tea made of 2–3 g of dried root; taken 30 minutes to 2 hours before bedtime For Anxiety: 100–150 mg, taken thrice daily	Assess efficacy in 2–4 weeks May cause increased sedation Use with caution in pregnant women and patients with liver disease May be used in combination with hops (*Humulus lupulus*) or lemon balm (*Melissa officinalis*)
Vitamin D	Mood Insomnia	400–800 IUI; taken daily	Caution regarding side effects at extremely high doses (4,000 IU+) Caution recommended when using with a patient already taking multiple medications due to possible interactions

[a]Dose based on traditional use and modern clinical studies. Long-term studies have not been conducted to determine safety.

Sources: Plante DT, Winkelman JW. Sleep Disturbance in bipolar disorder: Therapeutic implications. *Am J Psychiatry*. 2008;165(7):830–843; Kearney D et al. Post traumatic stress disorder. In D Rakel, ed. *Integrative medicine*. 4th ed. Philadelphia, PA: Elsevier; 2017: 86–93; Sawni A, Kemper K. Attention deficit disorder. In D Rakel, ed. *Integrative medicine*. 4th ed. Philadelphia, PA: Elsevier; 2017: 53–63; Schneider C, Wissink T. Depression. In D Rakel, ed. *Integrative medicine*. 4th ed. Philadelphia, PA: Elsevier; 2017: 36–45; Naiman R. Insomnia. In D Rakel, ed. *Integrative medicine*. 4th ed. Philadelphia, PA: Elsevier; 2017: 74–85; Sarris J. Herbal medicines in the treatment of psychiatric disorders: 10 year updated review. *Phytother Res*. 2018;32:1147–1162; Yeung K, et al. Herbal medicine for depression and anxiety: A systematic review with assessment of potential psycho-oncologic relevance. *Phytother Res*. 2018;32:865–891.

Conclusion

Psychiatric disorders and sleep disturbances have a bidirectional relationship, with each exacerbating the other. When assessing for either sleep disturbances or psychiatric disorders, it is important to inquire about both because of their comorbidity. Progress has been made with regard to understanding the multifactorial aspects (neurocircuitry, neurotransmitters, genetics, and circadian rhythms) involved in sleep and psychiatric disorders; however, further research must be done to explore the etiologies and bidirectional impact.

REFERENCES

1. Ram S, Seirawan RS, Kumar SKS, et al. Prevalence and impact of sleep disorders and sleep habits in the United States. *Sleep Breath*. 2010;14(1):63–70.
2. Losing sleep over your health. *EBioMedicine* 2017;24:1–2.
3. Institute of Medicine Sleep Disorders and Sleep Deprivation. *An unmet public health problem*. Washington DC: National Academies Press; 2006.
4. NIH National Institute of Neurological Disorders and Stroke. Understanding sleep. Patient Caregiver Education. 2017. https://www.ninds.nigh.gov/Disorders/Patient-Caregiver-Education/Understanding-Sleep
5. Rama AN, Zachariah R. Normal human sleep. In C. Kushida, ed. *Encyclopedia of sleep*. 1st ed. London: Elsevier; 2013: 16–23.
6. Zorn JV et al. Cortisol stress reactivity across psychiatric disorders: A systematic review and meta-analysis. *Psychoneuroendocrinology*. 2017;77:25–36.
7. Gottfried S. The hypothalamic-pituitary-adrenal-axis in mood disorder. In JM Greenblatt, K Brogan, eds. *Integrative therapies for depression: Redefining models for assessment, treatment, and prevention*. Boca Raton, FL: CRC; 2016: 171–187.
8. Healy ES et al. Onset of insomnia: Role of life-stress events. *Psychosomatic Med*. 1981;43:439–451.
9. Mezick EJ et al. Intra-individual variability in sleep duration and fragmentation: Associations with stress. *Psychoneuroendocrinology*. 2009;34(9):1346–1354.
10. Sadeh A et al. Effects of stress on sleep: The moderating role of coping style. *Health Psychol*. 2004;23(5):542–545.
11. American Psychiatric Association. *Diagnostic and statistical manual of mental disorders*. 5th ed. Arlington, VA: Author; 2013.
12. Krystal AD. Psychiatric disorders and sleep. *Neurology Clin*. 2012;30:1389–1413.
13. Baglionil C et al. Sleep and mental disorders: A meta-analysis of polysomnographic research. *Psychol Bull*. 2016;142(9):969–990.
14. Lee EK, Douglass AB. Sleep in psychiatric disorders: Where are we now? *Can J Psychiatry*. 2010;55(7):403–412.

15. Goldstein AN, Walker MP. The role of sleep in emotional brain function. *Annu Rev Clin Psychol.* 2014;10:679–708.

16. Walker MP, van der Helm E. Overnight therapy? The role of sleep in emotional brain processing. *Psychological Bull.* 2009;135(5):731–748.

17. Becker S et al. Sleep in a large, multi-university sample of college students: Sleep problem prevalence, sex differences, and mental health correlates. *J Natl Sleep Foundation.* 2018;4(2):174–181.

18. Reid KJ et al. Sleep: A marker of physical and mental health in the elderly. *Am J Geriatr Psychiatry.* 2006;14(10):860–866.

19. Nadorff MR et al. Psychiatric illness and sleep in older adults. *Sleep Med Clin.* 2018;13(1);81–91.

20. Stewart WF, Ricci JA, Chee E, et al. Cost of lost productive work time among US workers with depression. *JAMA.* 2003;289(23):3135–3144.

21. Murphy M, Peterson MJ. Sleep disturbances in depression. *Sleep Med Clin.* 2015;10(1):17–23.

22. Medina AB et al. Update of sleep alterations in depression. *Sleep Science.* 2014;7:165–169.

23. Jansson-Frojmark M, Lindblom K. A bidirectional relationship between anxiety and depression and insomnia? A prospective study in the general population. *J Psychosom Res.* 2008;64:443–449.

24. Yates WR et al. Clinical features of depressed outpatients with and without co-occurring general medical conditions in STAR*D. *Gen Hosp Psychiatry.* 2004;26(6):421–429.

25. Johnson EO et al. The association of insomnia with anxiety disorders and depression: Exploration of the direction of risk. *J Psychiatry Res.* 2006;40(8):700–708.

26. Baglioni C et al. Insomnia as a predictor of depression: A meta-analytic evaluation of longitudinal epidemiological studies. *J Affect Dis.* 2011;135:10–19.

27. Bao Y-P et al. Co-occurence and bidirectional prediction of sleep disturbances and depression in older adults: Meta-analysis and systematic review. *Neurosci Biobehav Rev.* 2017;75:257–273.

28. Harvey AG et al. Interventions for sleep disturbance in bipolar disorder. *Sleep Med Clin.* 2015;10(1):101–105.

29. Harvey AG et al. Sleep-related functioning in euthymic patients with bipolar disorder, patients with insomnia and subjects without sleep problems. *Am J Psychiatry.* 2005;162:50–57.

30. Harvey AG. Sleep and circadian rhythms in bipolar disorder: Seeking synchrony, harmony, and regulation. *Am J Psychiatry.* 2008;165(7):820–829.

31. Giglio LMF et al. Sleep in bipolar patients. *Sleep Breath.* 2009;13:169–173

32. Plante DT, Winkelman JW. Sleep Disturbance in bipolar disorder: Therapeutic implications. *Am J Psychiatry.* 2008;165(7):830–843.

33. Lee R. Anxiety. In D Rakel, ed. *Integrative medicine.* 4th ed. Philadelphia, PA: Elsevier; 2017: 46–52.

34. NIH National Institutes of Mental Health. Any anxiety disorder. Statistics. 2017. www.nimh.nih.gov/health/statistics/any-anxiety-disorder.shtml.

35. Ohayon MM, Roth T. Place of chronic insomnia in the course of depressive and anxiety disorders. *J Psychiatric Res.* 2003;27:9–15.

36. Boland EM, Ross RJ. Recent advances in the study of sleep in the anxiety disorders, obsessive-compulsive disorder, and posttraumatic stress disorder. *Psychiatric Clin N Am.* 2015;38:761–776.

37. Gregory AM et al. Prospective longitudinal associations between persistent sleep problems in childhood and anxiety and depression disorders in adulthood. *J Abnorm Child Psychol.* 2005;33(2):157–163.

38. Cox RC, Olatunji BO. A systematic review of sleep disturbance in anxiety and related disorders. *J Anxiety Dis.* 2016;37:104–129.

39. Mellman TA. Sleep and anxiety disorders. *Sleep Med Clin.* 2008;3:261–268.

40. Shen J, Shapiro CM. Obsessive-compulsive disorder and sleep. In C Kushida, ed. *Encyclopedia of sleep.* 1st ed. London: Elsevier; 2013: 272–274.

41. Paterson JL et al. Sleep and obsessive compulsive disorder (OCD). *Sleep Med Rev.* 2013;17:465–474.

42. Nesbit AD, Dijk DJ. Out of synch with society: An update on delayed sleep phase disorder. *Curr Opin Pulm Med.* 2014;20(6):581–587.

43. Nola JA et al. Sleep, arousal, and circadian rhythms in adults with obsessive compulsive disorder: A meta-analysis. *Neurosci Biobehav Rev.* 2015;51:100–107.

44. Germain A et al. Sleep in PTSD: Conceptual model and novel directions in brain-based research and interventions. *Curr Opin Psychol.* 2017;14:84–89

45. Filippone AB et al. Trauma exposure and postraumatic stress disorder. In C Kushida, ed. *Encyclopedia of sleep.* 1st ed. London: Elsevier; 2013: 390–394.

46. Kearney D et al. Post traumatic stress disorder. In D Rakel, ed. *Integrative medicine.* 4th ed. Philadelphia, PA: Elsevier; 2017: 86–93.

47. Belleville G et al. Impact of sleep disturbance on PTSD symptoms and perceived health. *J Nerv Ment Dis.* 2009;197(2):126–132.

48. Ered A et al. Sleep quality, psychological symptoms, and psychotic-like experiences. *J Psychiatric Res.* 2018;98 95–98.

49. Lunsford-Avery JR, Mittal VA. Sleep dysfunction prior to the onset of schizophrenia: A review and neurodevelopmental diathesis–stress conceptualization. *Clin Psychol.* 2013;20:291–320.

50. Manoach DS, et al. Schizophrenia, other neuropsychiatric disorders, and sleep. In C Kushida, ed. *Encyclopedia of sleep.* 1st ed. London: Elsevier; 2013: 390–394.

51. Lunsford-Avery J et al. Sleep disturbances in adolescents with ADHD: A systematic review and framework for future research. *Clin Psychol Rev.* 2016;50:159–174.

52. Division of Human Development and Disability, National Center on Birth Defects and Developmental Disabilities, Centers for Disease Control and Prevention. Data and Statistics. Attention-deficit/hyperactivity disorder (ADHD). 2018. www.cdc.gov/ncbddd/adhd/data.html.

53. Sawni A, Kemper K. Attention deficit disorder. In D Rakel, ed. *Integrative medicine.* 4th ed. Philadelphia, PA: Elsevier; 2017: 53–63.
54. Corkum P, Tannock R, Moldofsky H: Sleep disturbances in children with attention-deficit/hyperactivity disorder. *J Am Acad Child Adolesc Psychiatry* 1998;37:637–646.
55. Tsai MH et al. Attention-deficit/hyperactivity disorder and sleep disorders in children. *Med Clin N Am* 2010;94(3):615–632.
56. Diaz-Roman A et al. Sleep in adults with ADHD: Systematic review and meta-analysis of subjective and objective studies. *Neurosci Behav Rev.* 2018;S0149–7634(18):30013–30017.
57. Schoenberg MR, Kilgore, WDS. Psychologic and psychiatric assessment. In C Kushida, ed. *Encyclopedia of sleep.* 1st ed. London: Elsevier; 2013:390–394.
58. Wesensten NJ. Role of pharmacological interventions for sleep deprivation. In C Kushida, ed. *Encyclopedia of sleep.* 1st ed. London: Elsevier; 2013:366–370.
59. Lucas N, Mirzaei F, Pan A, et al. Coffee, caffeine, and the risk of depression among women. *Arch Intern Med.* 2015;171(17):1571–1577.
60. Lara DR. Caffeine, mental health, and psychiatric disorders. *J Alzheimer's Dis.* 2010;20:S239–S248.
61. Winston AP, Hardwick E, Jaberi N. Neuropsychiatric effects of caffeine. *Adv Psychiatric Treatm.* 2005;11:432–439.
62. Wang HR, Woo YS, Bahk, W-M. Caffeine-induced psychiatric manifestations: A review. *Int Clin Psychopharmacol.* 2015;30(4):179–182.
63. Angarita GA, Emadi N, Hodges S, Morgan PT. Sleep abnormalities associated with alcohol, cannabis, cocaine, and opiate use: A comprehensive review. *Addict Sci Clin Pract.* 2016;11(1):9.
64. Ji X, Grandner M, Liu J. The relationship between micronutrient status and sleep patterns: A systematic review. *Public Health Nutrition.* 2016;20(4):687–701.
65. Cornish S, Mehl-Madrona L. The role of vitamins and minerals in psychiatry. *Integr Med Insights.* 2008;3:33–42.
66. Rucklidge JJ, Kaplan BJ. Broad-spectrum micronutrient formulas for the treatment of psychiatric symptoms: A systematic review. *Exp Rev Neurotherapeut.* 2013;13(1):49–73.
67. Bahr SM, Weidemann BJ, Castro AN, Walsh JW, et al. Risperidone-induced weight gain is mediated through shifts in the gut microbiome and suppression of energy expenditure. *EBioMedicine.* 2015;2(11):1725–1734.
68. Flowers SA, Evans SJ, Ward KM et al. Interaction between atypical antipsychotics and the gut microbiome in a bipolar disease cohort. *Pharmacotherapy.* 2017;37(3):261–267.
69. Lerner V. Antioxidants as a treatment and prevention of Tardive Dyskinesia. In M Ritsner, ed. *Handbook of schizophrenia spectrum disorders, vol. 3: Therapeutic approaches, comorbidity, and outcomes.* Dordrecht, Netherlands: Springer Netherlands; 2011: 109–134.
70. Sanchez-Ortuno MM, Edinger JD. Behavioral treatment of insomnia. In C Kushida, ed. *Encyclopedia of sleep.* 1st ed., vol. 2 London: Elsevier; 2013: 283–289.

71. Soehner A et al. Cognitive therapy for insomnia. In C Kushida, ed. *Encyclopedia of sleep*. 1st ed., vol. 2 London: Elsevier; 2013: 290–295.

72. Ebben MR, Narizhnaya M. Cognitive and behavioral treatment options for insomnia. *Mt Sinai J Med.* 2012;79(4):512–523.

73. Zhou ES, Gardiner P, Bertisch SM. Integrative medicine for insomnia. *Med Clin.* 2017;101(5):865–879.

74. Van Diest I, Verstappen K, Aubert AE, Widjaja D, Vansteenwegen D, Vlemincx E. Inhalation/exhalation ratio modulates the effect of slow breathing on heart rate variability and relaxation. *Appl Psychophysiol Biofeedback.* 2014;39(3–4):171–180.

75. Bertisch SM, Wells RE, Smith MT, McCarthy EP. Use of relaxation techniques and complementary and alternative medicine by American adults with insomnia symptoms: Results from a national survey. *J Clin Sleep Med.* 2012;8(06):681–691.

76. Konsta A, Dikeos D, Bonaki A, Economou N, Chrousos G, Darviri C. Stress management techniques in primary insomnia: A randomized controlled trial. *Sleep Med.* 2013;14:e173.

77. Pigeon WR, Bishop TM, Marcus JA. Current pharmacological and nonpharmacological options for the management of insomnia. *Clin Med Insights: Therapeutics.* 2013;5:CMT-S10239.

78. Brown RP, Gerbarg PL, Muench F. Breathing practices for treatment of psychiatric and stress-related medical conditions. *Psychiatric Clin.* 2013;36(1):121–140.

79. Jerath R, Beveridge C, Barnes VA. Self-regulation of breathing as an adjunctive treatment of insomnia. *Front Psychiatry.* 2018;9.

80. De Niet GJ, Tiemens BG, Kloos MW, Hutschemaekers GJ. Review of systematic reviews about the efficacy of non-pharmacological interventions to improve sleep quality in insomnia. *Int J Evidence-Based Healthc.* 2009;7(4):233–242.

81. Siebern AT, Suh S, Nowakowski S. Non-pharmacological treatment of insomnia. *Neurotherapeutics.* 2010;9(4):717–727.

82. Bowden A, Lorenc A, Robinson N. Autogenic training as a behavioural approach to insomnia: A prospective cohort study. *Primary Health Care Res Dev.* 2012;13(2):175–185

83. Pinheiro M, Mendes D, Pais J et al. Sleep quality–impact of relaxation techniques and autogenic training in patients diagnosed with insomnia. *Eur Psychiatry.* 2015;30:1781.

84. Baer RA. Mindfulness training as a clinical intervention: A conceptual and empirical review. *Clin Psycholl Sci Pract.* 2003;10:125–143.

85. Taylor HL, Hailes HP, Ong J. Third-wave therapies for insomnia. *Curr Sleep Med Rep.* 2015;1(3):166–176.

86. Ong JC, Smith CE. Using mindfulness for the treatment of insomnia. *Curr Sleep Med Rep.* 2017;3(2):57–65.

87. Cincotta AL, Gehrman P, Gooneratne NS, Baime MJ. The effects of a mindfulness-based stress reduction programme on pre-sleep cognitive arousal and insomnia symptoms: A pilot study. *Stress Health.* 2011;27(3):e299–e305.

88. Wong MY, Ree MJ, Lee CW. Enhancing CBT for chronic insomnia: A randomised clinical trial of additive components of mindfulness or cognitive therapy. *Clin Psychol Psychother.* 2016;23(5):377–385.

89. Sanchez-Ortuno MM et al. The use of natural products for sleep: A common practice? *Sleep Med.* 2009;10:982–987.

90. Cho S et al. Hypnotic effects and binding studies for GABA(A) and 5-HT(2C) receptors of traditional medicinal plants used in Asia for insomnia. *J Ethnopharmacol.* 2010;132(1):225–232.

91. Leach MJ, Page AT. Herbal medicine for insomnia: A systematic review and meta-analysis. *Sleep Med Rev.* 2015;24:1–12.

92. Schneider C, Wissink T. Depression. In D Rakel, ed. *Integrative medicine.* 4th ed. Philadelphia, PA: Elsevier; 2017: 36–45.

93. Naiman R. Insomnia. In D Rakel, ed. *Integrative medicine.* 4th ed. Philadelphia, PA: Elsevier; 2017: 74–85.

94. Sarris J. Herbal medicines in the treatment of psychiatric disorders: 10 year updated review. *Phytother Res.* 2018;32:1147–1162.

95. Yeung K, et al. Herbal medicine for depression and anxiety: A systematic review with assessment of potential psycho-oncologic relevance. *Phytother Res.* 2018;32:865–891.

96. Wang F et al. The effect of meditative movement on sleep quality: A systematic review. *Sleep Med Rev.* 2016;30:43–52.

97. Fibler M, Quante A. A case series on the use of lavendulan oil capsules on patients suffering from major depressive disorder and symptoms of psychomotor agitation, insomnia and anxiety. *Compl Ther Med.* 2014;22:63–69.

29

Sleep and Women

NICOLA FINLEY

Introduction

The incidence of sleep problems is greater in women than in men, and there are features of sleep that are unique to women. Women are 1.4 times more likely than men to report insomnia,[1] yet the topic of sleep disturbances in women has only recently been more widely addressed by physicians. Research has consistently demonstrated that women report more sleep initiation and maintenance problems and are at greater risk for a diagnosis of insomnia as compared to men.[2] This gender difference can be observed over the life span of women. Changes in sleep patterns can be observed during a woman's menstrual cycle, during pregnancy, and during menopause. Furthermore, sleep problems can worsen in the postmenopausal years, and the incidence of sleep apnea in women increases with age. Also, social and psychological factors can impact a woman's sleep. For example, the snoring of a woman's bed partner can adversely impact her sleep. Juggling the demands placed on women from immediate family, extended family, friends, and work, as well as the expectations that she has for herself, can all adversely impact sleep. Women may also have primary sleep disorders such as obstructive sleep apnea (OSA) and restless legs syndrome (RLS), which can disturb sleep. Differences in sleep behavior and sleep disorders may be driven not only by biological factors but also by gender differences in the way women and men report symptoms.[3] Interestingly, a number of studies report that women have no clear-cut differences from men in sleep architecture when assessed with objective methods such as polysomnography.[4] This chapter highlights how sleep disturbances in women are unique.

Insomnia in Women

Sleep duration impacts the risk of heart disease for women similarly to men. A study conducted among 71,617 middle-aged women in the Nurses' Health Study showed an increased risk for any coronary event that was associated with both long (>9 hours) and short (<5 hours) sleep duration,[5] highlighting insomnia as an important indicator of wellness for women. Of note, there are gender differences in the pharmacological treatment of sleep disturbances that should be recognized. In 2013, the US Food and Drug Administration (FDA) reduced the recommended dose of zolpidem (Ambien) for women by 50%, making it the first time that the FDA has issued a gender-specific guideline for any drug.[3] This change in dosing was based on the discovery that women metabolized the same dose of zolpidem more slowly than men, resulting in 50% higher serum levels[3] and thus making zolpidem the only medication for any medical condition that has a different dosing recommendation for women than men.

Insomnia is linked to depression, and the prevalence of both depression and insomnia is higher in women than in men.[3] When taking an integrative approach, a woman's emotional state is a significant contributor to managing sleep disturbances. Some women may experience cyclical or continuous depressed mood symptoms at times of high hormone fluxes such as menopause, menstrual cycle phases, and pregnancy, which have been profiled as a window of vulnerability to depressed mood.[6] The hypothalamic-pituitary-ovarian hormone fluctuations contribute to the connection between hormones and mood. However, it can be challenging to distinguish if depression is causing the sleep disturbances or if the sleep disturbance is causing the depression. Additionally, women may have ruminative thoughts and anxiety that can disrupt sleep. Similar to many other conditions in medicine, the underlying cause can vary from woman to woman.

Women, especially those who are married with children, spend more time than men doing unpaid work even if they are employed and have less leisure time.[7] More women are in the workforce, yet many still have to fulfill household and family obligations. Women who do not work outside the home are often expected to take on more family responsibilities such as childcare and planning the family calendar. Also, family circumstances can influence the prevalence of sleep disturbances, as in the increased demands placed on women who are single parents. In addition, women often have multiple other tasks to complete, such as staying connected with friends and extended family. These scenarios illustrate why women may feel overwhelmed, and many women will preferentially take care of others before taking care of themselves. An integrative approach encourages women to prioritize self-care activities by carving out time for themselves.

INTEGRATIVE APPROACHES TO TREATING INSOMNIA

Although a comprehensive discussion of insomnia is beyond the scope of this chapter and is covered elsewhere, it is well-established that *cognitive-behavioral therapy for insomnia* (CBT-I) is beneficial for both men and women, and CBT-I is considered first-line treatment for chronic insomnia. Behavioral treatments such as CBT-I offer longer lasting improvements in sleep quality without the side effects that are often accompanied by medications.[8] Other strategies to help with insomnia include *mindfulness meditation* and *mindfulness-based therapy for insomnia* (MBT-I). Mindfulness meditation practice involves being in the present moment without judgment, and MBT-I utilizes mindfulness and behavioral therapy for the treatment of insomnia. Decreasing alcohol consumption can improve sleep, as can relaxation and other mind–body techniques such as progressive muscle relaxation, reflexology, massage, and yoga. Women may benefit from sleep hygiene therapy as well as developing a bedtime ritual. Some women may have racing thoughts, and one method to overcome this is to journal thoughts prior to bedtime. In short, self-care is an important part of treating insomnia for women.

For both women and men, exercise can reduce insomnia. Compared to men, women in general are less active in recreational physical activity but similarly active when physical activity related to household and caregiving duties is considered.[9] Most of the research on the impact of exercise on sleep looks specifically at recreational activity, like participation in sports. Higher levels of recreational physical activity but not lifestyle—or household-related/caregiving activity—are associated with better sleep in midlife women.[9] One of the proposed reasons for this difference is the higher intensity of exercise that can be achieved with recreational activity.

Menstruation and Sleep

During the years when a woman is menstruating, sleep can be affected for a variety of reasons. Studies have shown differences in sleep quality between the menstrual cycle phases, with poorer subjective sleep reported by women in their premenstrual phase than either during the days of their menses or the midcycle phase.[4] Specifically, recent studies have shown that women experience various sleep disturbances during the late luteal phase of the menstrual cycle, influencing stage 2 and rapid eye movement (REM) sleep.[10] Factors involved in the connection between menstrual cycles and sleep include temperature changes and variations in ovarian hormones, pituitary hormones, melatonin, and cortisol.[4] One-third of women complain of sleep disturbances and related symptoms such as cramps, bloating, and headaches as reasons for disrupted sleep during the premenstrual week or during menses.[3] Painful menstrual cramps can play a significant role in sleep disturbances. Sleep onset latency was longer and sleep efficiency was found to be lower in women with severe dysmenorrhea than in those with mild dysmenorrhea.[11] Also, women's emotional health, such as irritability during the premenstrual period, can lead to insomnia. Women with premenstrual syndrome/premenstrual dysphoric disorder typically report sleep-related complaints such as insomnia, frequent awakenings, nonrestorative sleep, unpleasant dreams or nightmares, and poor sleep quality associated with their symptoms.[8] In short, there are multiple variables that influence sleep for menstruating women. The integrative medicine approach as described for insomnia can be used to manage the sleep disturbances of menstruating women because there are no specific studies on treating sleep disturbances in these women.

Sleep Apnea

Previously, sleep apnea was a "man's disease"; however, recent research has been focusing on sleep apnea in women. Sleep apnea is more common in postmenopausal than premenopausal women. Among younger adults, the prevalence of sleep-disordered breathing in men is roughly twice the prevalence in women, but, among older adults, women's prevalence of sleep apnea approaches that of men's.[12] In postmenopausal women, hormonal shifts contribute to the changes in fat distribution that in turn may contribute to the higher prevalence of sleep apnea in this age group. The presence of more airway fat, greater neck circumference, and susceptibility of the airway to collapse is greater in men as compared with women.[3] The anatomical difference between women and men is an important reason why sleep apnea presents differently between genders. In addition, differences exist in how men and women report symptoms of OSA; men frequently report snoring, snorting, gasping, and sleepiness, while women report unrefreshing sleep, fatigue, insomnia, and depression.[3] Furthermore, women may have less astute bed partners who are less likely to report snoring and snorting due to social awkwardness.[3] Recent literature suggests a gender bias against diagnosing sleep apnea as well as a delay in treatment among women who presented to sleep clinics.[3] One potential contributor to this gender bias is that healthcare providers may misdiagnose a woman who reports she is having sleep disruption, especially if she does not present with classic sleep apnea symptoms. The different manner in which women present with sleep apnea as compared to men may also lead to the underdiagnosis of this disorder.

Pregnancy and Sleep

Sleep during pregnancy is another unique aspect of women's sleep. Studies indicate that approximately 50% of women experience insomnia during pregnancy.[13] Pregnant women can experience a variety of sleep issues from poor sleep quality, disrupted sleep, and insufficient nighttime sleep to daytime sleepiness. Progesterone, while promoting daytime sleepiness, also causes nocturnal sleep fragmentation, and oxytocin, the hormone responsible for uterine contractions, peaks at night and may cause sleep fragmentation in late pregnancy.[14] Conditions of sleep loss such as short sleep duration, poor sleep quality, and poor sleep efficiency along with an increase in insomnia and wake time at night characterize the sleep of pregnant women.[15] Sleep is important at any stage of life, but it is particularly important for pregnant women as sufficient sleep nourishes the development of the fetus.

Poor and insufficient sleep has been associated with adverse maternal and fetal outcomes as depicted in Figure 29.1. In addition, sleeping less than 6 hours during the last month of pregnancy has been associated with longer labor and greater risk for cesarean deliveries compared to women getting more than 6 hours of sleep.[14] It has been postulated that inflammatory cytokines may play a key role in the association of preterm delivery and sleep deprivation.[16] Short nocturnal sleep duration (<6 hours) has been associated with gestational diabetes in research studies in ethnically diverse populations.[17] One large-scale survey of sleep patterns of pregnant women (>20,000 women) showed that all the pregnant women reported at least one nighttime awakening per night, with an average of 2.7 awakenings for 70 minutes.[13] Interestingly, pre-pregnancy body mass index (BMI) might be a determinant for sleep disturbance in pregnant women. As the pregnancy progresses, high fluid volume and engorged capillaries cause nasal congestion, and high BMI

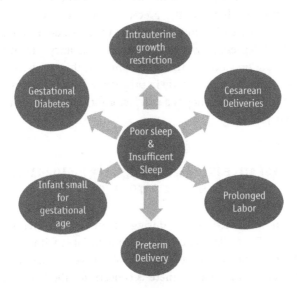

FIGURE 29.1 Poor sleep and insufficient sleep during pregnancy is associated with intrauterine growth restriction, preterm delivery, prolonged labor, gestational diabetes, cesarean deliveries, and having an infant small for gestational age.
From Nowakowski S, Meers J, Heimback E 2013 and Cai, S, Tan S, Gluckman P et al 2017.

and excess gestational weight gain may further increase the likelihood of snoring, sleep-disordered breathing, and OSA.[18] These same mechanisms could also lead to sleep disruption and insomnia.

During late pregnancy, numerous sleep-related conditions surface. During the third trimester of pregnancy, women have increased nocturia, which can adversely impact sleep. Also, as the expectant woman increases in size, she may have increased discomfort, like back or pelvic pain, that can make it difficult for her to find a comfortable sleeping position. Other symptoms that can increase during pregnancy are anxiety, leg cramps, breast tenderness, abdominal discomfort, and gastroesophageal reflux. Another factor that influences sleep is increased fetal activity later in pregnancy. Not only does the movement of the baby disturb sleep but there may also be an increase in worry if a women does not feel movement. Other worries that may adversely impact pregnant women's sleep include distress about the pregnancy in general as well as the upcoming labor and delivery. Sleep late in the third trimester is especially valuable because pregnant women need to ensure that they have energy for the labor and delivery process.

Though pregnancy is a joyous time, it can also be stressful if the pregnant woman is worrying about labor and delivery, her health, or her baby's health. There might also be worry about the increased responsibilities imposed by parenthood. These concerns are common and understandable for pregnant women. However, worry can lead to anxiety, which can adversely impact sleep. Of note, subjective and objective sleep measures during pregnancy correlate differently with a women's mood. For pregnant women, sleep problems not only affect their mood at that given time but may also precede mood problems. There is evidence that poor sleep quality earlier in pregnancy may contribute to the development of higher levels of depressive symptoms later in pregnancy.[19] Even though sleep disturbance is more prevalent in the third trimester, this research highlights the importance of screening women early in pregnancy for sleep issues. Also, studies show sleep loss during pregnancy is a risk factor for the subsequent development of postpartum depression.[20]

INTEGRATIVE TREATMENTS FOR SLEEP DISTURBANCES DURING PREGNANCY

Treating women with medications during pregnancy involves evaluating the risk–benefit ratio. Benzodiazepines have been associated with an increased risk of preterm births, cesarean delivery, and small-for-gestational-age and/or low-birth-weight infants.[21] In addition, there is concern for the teratogenic effects of sleep-promoting medications. As a result, an integrative approach for treating sleep disturbances is often preferred for pregnant women. Nonpharmacologic treatment options for sleep complaints in pregnant women may include exercise, meditation, and/or cognitive-behavioral therapy as previously described.

In general, there is a paucity of evidence researching treatment options for insomnia for pregnant women. However, some studies suggest a benefit from acupuncture, exercise, massage, relaxation therapy, mindfulness meditation, and prenatal yoga.[22] In an 8-week prospective control study looking at the effects of traditional acupuncture versus no acupuncture in pregnant women with insomnia, researchers discovered a 50% decrease in the average insomnia score in a majority of the subjects compared to controls.[23] There is research supporting the benefits of moderate exercise and yoga for pregnant women. One study specifically examined water exercise and found that supervised water exercises improved subjective sleep in pregnant women.[24] Another approach could be daytime napping, although the data are sparse and one study found that daytime naps only modestly impact nocturnal sleep in pregnant women.[25]

Restless Leg Syndrome in Pregnancy

RLS is a sleep-related condition commonly seen during pregnancy. RLS is characterized by a compelling urge to move the legs that often begins or worsens at night and is frequently accompanied by uncomfortable sensations in the legs.[26] For the general population in the United States, the prevalence of RLS is estimated at 5–15% but in pregnancy, the prevalence is estimated at 12–20%.[27] Not only is RLS more common during pregnancy but the number of pregnancies can influence the likelihood of developing RLS. Studies have shown that women who have been pregnant before are affected by RLS up to three times more often than women who have never been pregnant.[28]

RLS symptoms are worse during the third trimester. During this period, iron consumption by the developing fetus contributes to the development or worsening of symptoms in predisposed women.[29] In addition to reduced iron, there are other contributors to RLS that are unique to pregnancy, such as folate metabolism and hormonal changes. Also, prolactin and progesterone have been shown to contribute to RLS. Often, RLS symptoms that arise during pregnancy resolve after the delivery of the baby. As with any medical condition being treated during pregnancy, it is important to evaluate the benefits versus risks of medications during pregnancy and the lactation period. Shared decision-making is the ideal approach, and often pregnant women will prefer to use nonpharmacological treatment options first, like leg massages. Reassurance, moderate exercise, elastic stockings or pneumatic compression devices, and avoidance of caffeinated and alcoholic beverages may be beneficial. For pregnant women, first-line supplement treatment options include iron, if ferritin levels are low, and folate. The safety of using pharmacologic treatment options for RLS during pregnancy has not been established.

Sleep-Disordered Breathing in Pregnancy

Sleep-disordered breathing is common during pregnancy, and it worsens as the pregnancy progresses. One study of 500 women who completed surveys during their first and third trimesters found that snoring increased from 7.9% to 21.2%.[13] Moderate to severe sleep-disordered breathing is associated with an increased risk of maternal and fetal complications, and OSA can lead to hypoxia in the fetoplacental circulation. Natural physiological changes of pregnancy like upper airway edema and capillary engorgement lead to higher airway resistance, and high progesterone levels stimulate an increase in oxygen consumption.[30] These changes, as well as maternal weight gain, all contribute to the higher risk of OSA during pregnancy. OSA is also associated with increased pregnancy-related morbidity like preeclampsia and eclampsia, pulmonary embolism, and cardiomyopathy.[31] Moderate to severe sleep-disordered breathing is associated with gestational diabetes, pregnancy-related hypertension, preterm delivery, low birth weight, intrauterine growth restriction, and low Apgar scores.[13] Ongoing research is evaluating if treatment with continuous positive airway pressure (CPAP) can prevent adverse pregnancy outcomes in pregnant women with OSA. CPAP has demonstrated safety and good compliance in pregnancy and is the treatment of choice.[30]

Postpartum

Postpartum depression is a significant health condition that can lead to increased morbidity and mortality. As a result, postpartum depression is being increasingly discussed in clinical practice, but its connection to sleep is discussed less. Postpartum depression starts within 4 weeks of delivery and can last up to 6 months in duration. Poor postpartum sleep may serve as not only a marker of impending depression but also as a contributing cause.[32] Postpartum women sleep less during the early weeks following delivery compared to during pregnancy or during other periods of reproductive age, and these women are at an increased risk of depression.[33] There are unique contributory causes of insomnia in the postpartum period such as the care of a newborn infant. Breastfeeding and co-sleeping can disrupt the pattern of maternal sleep as infants often have night awakenings, short sleep periods, and frequent feedings in the first months of life. The temperament of the infant can also negatively or positively impact maternal sleep.

Maternal sleep also is affected by factors in addition to the infant. Research has shown that the regularity of the home environment appears to contribute to maternal sleep, depression, and fatigue.[34] Furthermore, hormonal changes can lead to interrupted sleep, fatigue, and sleep deprivation. Difficulty sleeping and sleep deprivation are associated with greater depressed moods in the postpartum period.[16]

Fortunately there is increased awareness about the seriousness of postpartum depression not only among physicians but also within society as a whole.

INTEGRATIVE APPROACHES TO THE POSTPARTUM PERIOD

Similar to when women are pregnant, many women in the postpartum period attempt to minimize the use of sleep aids when they are breastfeeding. Clinicians need to be aware of which medications are excreted via breast milk. For this reason, exploring alternatives to pharmacologic interventions is preferred. Some options include psychotherapy, aromatherapy with lavender, and exercise. Data support exercise as an effective approach for improving sleep in postpartum women. One study examined the effects of an 8-week Pilates program for postpartum sleep and found that the intervention group showed a significant improvement in subjective sleep quality, sleep latency, and daytime dysfunction.[35] Another study demonstrated that inhaling lavender essential oil every 8 hours for 4 weeks resulted in statistically significant lower rates of stress, anxiety, and depression in postpartum women compared to the control group.[36]

Some ways of creating regularity in the home include having a schedule for bedtime and mealtimes, and having less variability promotes stable sleep patterns. In addition, good sleep hygiene and behavioral modifications for the mother are helpful strategies. Recommendations might include limiting the amount of wake time in bed and getting out of the bed when not sleepy. This allows the woman to reset her sleep schedule and strengthen the bed as a cue for sleep. If the mother naps during the day and is having difficulty sleeping at night, she should consider avoiding daytime naps. On the other hand, some mothers find that napping when their infant naps is an effective strategy that does not adversely impact nighttime sleeping.

Menopause and Sleep

Difficulties with sleep increase as a women age, and research shows that the prevalence of insomnia increases from 33% to 36% in premenopausal women to 44% to 61% in postmenopausal women.[3] Menopause, defined as the cessation of a woman's menstrual period for 12 continuous months, reflects the cessation of ovulation, which leads to reduced ovarian production of estradiol. Spontaneous menopause occurs at a mean age of 51–52 years.[37] Symptoms of menopause include sleep disturbance, hot flashes, and irritability. Of those symptoms, hot flashes are the most common. Depending on how long a woman lives, she could spend up to a third of her life in the postmenopausal period.

Women's Health Initiative study data show that aging is not the sole cause of insomnia, and the context of physical impairment and psychological influences should be considered as well.[38] Other contributors that may occur concurrent with menopause include caring for aging parents and being an empty-nester. As a result, it may be difficult to determine if the cause of sleep difficulties in post-menopausal women is due to hormonal changes, effects of normal aging on sleep, life changes or role transitions, other physical and medical conditions that are acquired with advanced age, or other comorbid sleep disorders such as periodic limb movements or sleep apnea.[2] There may be a link between hormonal changes and mood changes in women entering menopause, but this may vary individually. The symptoms reported during menopause could be caused by hormonal changes as well as by undiagnosed depression or dysthymia. For this reason, an integrative approach embodies an individualized treatment plan for every female patient.

PERIMENOPAUSE

Perimenopause is the window of time during the menopause transition. Women in perimenopause have the greatest fluctuations in sex steroid hormones and may report menopausal symptoms that worsen their sleep quality, yet some women transition through menopause without symptoms. Some women have hot flashes that adversely impact their sleep as well as sleep disturbances independent of their hot flashes. In polysomnography studies, nocturnal hot flashes are more common during the first 4 hours of sleep, whereas subsequent REM sleep suppresses hot flashes, arousals, and awakenings.[39] The prevalence of chronic insomnia dramatically increases with the severity of the hot flashes, affecting more than 80% of women with severe hot flashes.[40] There is no consensus about whether hot flashes cause a disruption in sleep or whether hot flashes happen to occur concurrently with sleep disturbances. Furthermore, some women may perceive their vasomotor symptoms as being more severe and bothersome than other women with similar symptoms.

HORMONAL TREATMENT OF HOT FLASHES

Hot flashes are more likely to occur during the perimenopausal period and early postmenopause. It is during this menopausal transition that treatment of hot flashes may positively impact sleep. The most effective treatment of menopausal hot flashes is hormone therapy, specifically estrogen. Hormone therapy given in the context of the menopause transition is said to improve sleep quality and sleep patterns.[6] Emerging research is showing that hormone therapy not only improves hot flashes, but also may have a direct effect on improving sleep disturbances.[40] Women have reported that their sleep improves while on hormone therapy during menopause even if they do not have hot flashes.

The ideal approach to hormone therapy is achieved through shared decision-making between the patient and her healthcare provider, and the benefits versus risks should be reviewed with all patients. The risks associated with hormone therapy include increased risk of breast cancer, cardiovascular disease, strokes, and thromboembolic events. However, the benefits are more likely to outweigh risks when hormone therapy is initiated before age 60 or within 10 years of menopause.[41] Numerous randomized controlled trials have demonstrated that estrogen represents the most effective treatment for menopausal vasomotor symptoms and related issues including impaired sleep, irritability, and decreased quality of life.[37] The bioidentical form of estrogen is estradiol, and this is becoming an increasingly popular option because some women prefer estradiol, which is viewed as more natural than synthetic estrogen or conjugated estrogen from pregnant horse urine. Estradiol can be compounded or FDA-approved, and both of those options are bioidentical. Compounded bioidentical hormone preparations have the same chemical and molecular structure as the estrogens and progesterone produced within the human body. They are plant-derived and specifically compounded for an individual patient.[42] However, there are no studies to show compounded hormones are more effective or safer than the FDA-approved hormone replacement. The transdermal route of delivery of estradiol is commonly prescribed. If a woman decides to use hormone therapy, then a yearly discussion of the benefits and harms of hormone therapy allows for personalized care. This approach of shared decision-making empowers women to make informed decisions.

INTEGRATIVE APPROACHES TO THE TREATMENT OF HOT FLASHES

Mind–body approaches like mindfulness have been shown to improve sleep in peri- and postmenopausal women with hot flashes. One study showed that the mindfulness-based stress reduction program of listening to a CD 45 minutes per day not only improved hot flashes but also improved subjective sleep quality.[43] Research also found hypnosis to be beneficial for sleep in women experiencing hot flashes.[44] An added benefit of these integrative approaches is that there are relatively no adverse side effects.

Supplements can also be used to treat menopausal symptoms, and these may be an option for improving sleep in postmenopausal women. Limited data exist for the effects of black cohosh on sleep; one study found that taking black cohosh daily (2.5 mg extract) reduced the time of being awake after sleep onset in early postmenopausal women based on polysomnography and subjective data.[45] Research suggests that melatonin is a reasonable option for sleep onset difficulties in both peri- and postmenopausal women.[46] In addition, complementary therapies such as cooling techniques, avoiding triggers, exercise, yoga, hypnosis, mindfulness, and relaxation can be helpful in reducing hot flashes and night sweats that can adversely impact sleep.[47]

POSTMENOPAUSE AND SLEEP

Older postmenopausal women may also have sleep disturbances beyond having hot flashes. For this age group, age-related medical conditions like arthritis, chronic pain problems, urinary problems, side effects of medications, and gastrointestinal problems can contribute to sleep problems. A common complaint of older women includes frequent nighttime awakening. In one study, half of the women aged 60 and older reported more than three nighttime awakenings,[48] though the exact reason for this occurrence is not clear. Similar to other age groups, a women's mood impacts her sleep as well as her physical activity level. In one study of women with an average age of 66, moderate-intensity aerobic exercise improved exercise quality by lowering wake time after sleep onset and number of awakenings.[49] In the same study, light-intensity exercise did not significantly impact sleep. For many women older than 60, changes in sleep patterns occur with age.

Postmenopausal women can consider other integrative options to help with their sleep. CBT-I is one approach for sleep that has been shown to be effective for menopausal women. Studies have shown that CBT-I produced the greatest reduction in insomnia symptoms and increase in sleep quality ratings in postmenopausal women as compared to physical exercise, venlafaxine, escitalopram, yoga, and estradiol.[50] Another study found improvement in sleep quality, sleep duration, and sleep disturbance in menopausal women with acupressure.[51] In that study, women self-administered a circular massage to four specific acupoints that were located on the wrist, feet, occipital area of head, and between the eyebrows. One of the benefits of using acupressure is that it is not difficult to learn. A few small studies show that yoga, therapeutic massage, and exercise may be helpful for insomnia in postmenopausal women.[52] Additional research showed that the herbal supplement of valerian used twice a day improved insomnia in postmenopausal women.[53]

Conclusion

Research has shown that women experience greater subjective complaints of insufficient or nonrestorative sleep. They also have an increased need for sleep compared to men.[54] Women have fluctuations in hormone levels throughout their life span, from menarche to menopause and during pregnancy, and women face unique challenges to obtaining sufficient quantity and quality of sleep throughout their lives. During pregnancy, poor sleep is a risk factor for obstetric complications. The postmenopausal woman has sleep challenges due to declining hormone levels and age-related health conditions. Sleep can be low on the priority list for women who are often balancing work, family, social obligations, and caregiver responsibilities for their families. Furthermore, a woman's emotional state, perceived stress, and social support impact her quality and quantity of sleep. The unique interplay of a woman's mind, body, and social relationships determines how sleep issues impact her, and an integrative approach to treatment can best address these multifaceted issues.

REFERENCES

1. Lind MJ, Aggen SH, Kirkpatrick RM, et al. A longitudinal twin study of insomnia symptoms in adults. *Sleep.* 2015;38(9):1423–1430.
2. Grandner M, Nowakowski S, Kloss J, et al. Insomnia symptoms predict physical and mental impairments among postmenopausal women. *Sleep Med.* 2015;16:317–318.
3. Mallampali M, Carter C. Exploring sex and gender differences in sleep health: A Society for Women's Health research report. *J Women's Health.* 2014;23(7):553–562.
4. Romans SE, Kreindler D, Einstein G. Sleep quality and the menstrual cycle. *Sleep Med.* 2015;16:489–495.
5. Sands-Lincoln M, Loucks E, Lu B. Sleep duration, insomnia, and coronary heart disease among postmenopausal women in the Women's Health Initiative. *J Women's Health.* 2013;22(6):477–486.
6. Shaver J, Woods N. Sleep and menopause: A narrative review. *Menopause.* 2015 Aug;22(8):899–915.
7. Burgard SA, Ailshire JA. Gender and time for sleep among US adults. *Am Sociol Rev.* 2013 February;78(1):51–69.
8. Nowakowski S, Meers J, Heimback E. Sleep and women's health. *Sleep Med Res.* 2013;4(1):1–22.
9. Kline C, Irish L, Krafty R, et al. Consistently high sports/exercise activity is associated with better sleep quality, continuity and depth in midlife women: The SWAN sleep study. *Sleep.* 2013 Sep 1;36(9):1279–1288.
10. Jehan S, Auguste E, Hussain M, et al. Sleep and premenstrual syndrome. *J Sleep Med Disord.* 2016;3(5):1061.
11. Woosley J, Lichstein K. Dysmenorrhea, the menstrual cycle, and sleep. *Behav Med.* 2014;40:14–21.
12. Mirer A, Peppard P, Palta M, et al. Menopausal hormone therapy and sleep-disordered breathing: Evidence for a healthy user bias. *Ann Epidemiol.* 2015;25:779–784.

13. Mindell J, Cook R, Nikolovski J. Sleep patterns and sleep disturbances across pregnancy. *Sleep Med.* 2016;16:483–488.

14. Won C. Sleeping for two: The great paradox of sleep in pregnancy. *J Clin Sleep Med.* 2015;11(6):593–594.

15. Palagini L, Gemignani A, Banti S. Chronic sleep loss during pregnancy as a determinant of stress: Impact on pregnancy outcome. *Sleep Med.* 2014;15:853–859.

16. Chang J, Pien G, Duntley S, et al. Sleep deprivation during pregnancy and maternal and fetal outcomes: Is there a relationship? *Sleep Med Rev.* 2010 April;14(2):107–114.

17. Cai S, Tan S, Gluckman P, et al. Sleep quality and nocturnal sleep duration in pregnancy and risk of gestational diabetes mellitus. *Sleep.* 2017;40(2). doi:10.1093/sleep/zsw058. PMID: 28364489.

18. Gay C, Richoux S, Beebe K. Sleep disruption and duration in late pregnancy is associated with excess gestational weight gain among overweight and obese women. *Birth.* 2017;44:173–180.

19. Skouteris H, Wertheim E, Germano C, et al. Assessing sleep during pregnancy: A study across two time points examining the Pittsburgh Sleep Quality Index and associations with depressive symptoms. *Women's Health Iss.* 2009;19:45–51.

20. Abbot S, Attarian H, Zee P, et al. Sleep disorders in perinatal women. *Best Pract Res Clin Obstet Gynaecol.* 2014;28:159–168.

21. Okun M, Ebert R, Saini B. A review of sleep-promoting medications used in pregnancy. *Am J Obstet Gynecol.* April 2015;212(4):428–441.

22. Reichner C. Insomnia and sleep deficiency in pregnancy. *Obstet Med* 2015;8(4):168–171.

23. Hollenbach D, Broker R, et al. Non-pharmacological interventions for sleep quality and insomnia during pregnancy: A systematic review. *J Can Chiropr Assoc.* 2013;57:260–270.

24. Rodriguez-Blanque R, Sanchez-Garcia JC, Sanchez-Lopez AM, et al. The influence of physical activity in water on sleep quality in pregnant women: A randomised trial. *Women Birth.* 2018;31(1):e51–358.

25. Ebert R, Wood A, Okun M, et al. Minimal effect of daytime napping behavior on nocturnal sleep in pregnant women. *J Clin Sleep Med.* 2015;11(6):635–643.

26. Innes K, Kandati S Flack K, et al. The relationship of restless legs syndrome to history of pregnancy-induced hypertension. *J Women's Health.* 2016;25(4):397–408.

27. Grover A, Clark-Bilodeau C, D'Ambriosio C. Restless leg syndrome in pregnancy. *Obstet Med.* 2015;8(3):121–125.

28. Dunietz GL, Lisabeth LD, Shedden K, et al. Restless legs syndrome and sleep-wake disturbances in pregnancy. *J Clin Sleep Med.* 2017;13(7):863–870.

29. Minar M, Kosutzka Z, Habanova H. Restless legs syndrome in pregnancy is connected with iron deficiency. *Sleep Med.* 2015;16:589–592.

30. Booth J, Tonidanel A. Peripartum management of obstructive sleep apnea. *Clin Obstet Gynecol.* 2017;60(2):405–417.

31. Jehan S, Auguste E, Zizi F, et al. Obstructive sleep apnea: Women's perspective. *J Sleep Med Disord.* 2016;3(6):1064.

32. Park E, Meltzer-Brody S, Stickgold R. Poor sleep maintenance and subjective sleep quality are associated with postpartum maternal depression symptom severity. *Arch Womens Ment Health.* 2013;16:539–547.

33. Dørheim SK, Bondevik GT, Eberhard-Gran M, Bjorvatn B. Sleep and depression in postpartum women: A population-based study. *Sleep.* 2009;32(7):847–855.

34. Thomas K, Spieker S. Sleep, depression, and fatigue in late postpartum. *MCN Am J Matern Child Nurs.* 2016;41(2):104–109.

35. Ashrafina F, Mirmohammadali M, Rajabi H, et al. The effects of Pilates exercise on sleep quality in postpartum women. *J Bodywork Movement Ther.* 2014;18:190–199.

36. Kianpour M, Mansouri A, Mehrabi T, et al. Effect of lavender scent inhalation on prevention of stress, anxiety and depression in the postpartum period. *Iran J Nurs Midwif Res.* 2016;21(2):197–201.

37. Kaunitz A., Manson J. Management of menopausal symptoms. *Obstet Gynecol.* 2015;126:859–876.

38. Zaslavky O, LaCriox A, Hale L, et al. Longitudinal changes in insomnia status and incidence of physical, emotional, or mixed impairment in postmenopausal women participating in the Women's Health Initiative (WHI) study. *Sleep Med.* 2015;16:364–371.

39. Stuenkel C, Davis S, Gompel A, et al. Treatment of symptoms of the menopause: An Endocrine Society clinical practice guideline. *J Clin Endocrinol Metab.* 2015 Nov;100(11):3975–4011.

40. Pinkerton J, Abraham L, Bushmakin A., et al. Relationship between changes in vasomotor symptoms and changes in menopause-specific quality of life and sleep parameters. *Menopause.* 2016;23(10):1060–1066.

41. Lipold L, Batur P, Kagan R. Is there a time limit for systemic menopausal hormone therapy? *Cleve Clin J Med.* Aug. 2016;83(8):605–612.

42. Files J, Ko M, Pruthi S. Bioidentical hormone therapy. *Mayo Clin Proc.* 2011;86(7):673–680.

43. Carmody J, Crawfod S, Salmoirago-Blotcher E, et al. Mindfulness training for coping with hot flashes: Results of a randomized trial. *Menopause.* 2011;18(6):611–620.

44. Elkins GR, Fisher WI, Johnson AK, et al. Clinical hypnosis in the treatment of post-menopausal hot flashes: A randomized controlled trial. *Menopause.* 2013 March;20(3):291–298.

45. Jiang K, Huang L, Feng X, et al. Black cohosh improves objective sleep in postmenopausal women with sleep disturbance. *Climacteric.* 2015;18:559–567.

46. Jehan S, Jean-Louis G, Zizi F, et al. Sleep, melatonin and the menopausal transition: What are the links? *Sleep Sci.* 2017;10(1):11–18.

47. NAMS Statement. Non-hormonal management of menopause-associated vasomotor symptoms: 2015 position statement of The North American Menopause Society. *Menopause.* 2015;22(11):1155–1172.

48. Seib C, Anderson D, Lee K. Prevalence and correlates of sleep disturbance in postmenopausal women: The Australian Healthy Aging of Women (HOW) study. *J Women's Health.* 2014;23(2):151–158.

49. Wang X, Yongstedt S. Sleep quality improved following a single session of moderate-intensity aerobic exercise in older women: Results from a pilot study. *J Sport Health Sci.* 2014 December 1;3(4):338–342.

50. Guthrie KA, Larson JC, Ensrud KE, et al. Effects of pharmacologic and nonpharmacologic interventions on insomnia symptoms and self-reported sleep quality in women with hot flashes: A pooled analysis of individual participant data from four MsFLASH Trials. *Sleep.* 2018;41(1):zsx190.

51. Adedian Z, Eskandari L, Abdi H, et al. The effect of acupressure on sleep quality in menopausal women: A randomized control trial. *Iran J Med Sci* July 2015;40(4):328–334.

52. Tal J, Suh S, Dowdle C, et al. Treatment of Insomnia, insomnia symptoms, and obstructive sleep apnea during and after menopause: Therapeutic approaches. *Curr Psychiatry Rev.* 2015;11(1):63–83.

53. Taawoni S, Ekbstani N, Kashaniyan M. Effect of valerian on sleep quality in postmenopausal women: A randomized placebo-controlled clinical trial. *Menopause.* 2011;18(9):951–955.

54. Sibern A, Suh S, Nowakowski S. Non-pharmacological treatment of insomnia. *Neurotherapeutics.* 2012;9:717–727.

30

Diagnosis and Treatment of the Central Disorders of Hypersomnolence

CAROLINE MANESS AND LYNN MARIE TROTTI

Introduction to the Central Disorders of Hypersomnolence

The central disorders of hypersomnolence (CDH) are a group of eight disorders, as defined by the *International Classification of Sleep Disorders—Third Edition* (ICSD-3), that are centered around hypersomnolence, or the "inability to stay awake and alert during the major waking episodes of the day, resulting in periods of irrepressible need for sleep or unintended lapses into drowsiness or sleep."[1] This hypersomnolence, which can also be referred to as excessive daytime sleepiness (EDS), may occur as primary disorders or secondarily as the result of medications or other conditions (Figure 30.1).

This chapter focuses on the clinical features and management of the primary central disorders of hypersomnolence, specifically narcolepsy type 1 (NT1), narcolepsy type 2 (NT2), and idiopathic hypersomnia (IH). Kleine-Levin syndrome (KLS), which is also considered a primary central disorder of hypersomnolence, will not be included. Patients with KLS experience recurrent episodes of EDS accompanied by cognitive dysfunction, altered perception, eating disorders, and disinhibited behavior.[1] Sleep propensity, alertness, behavior, and cognition return to normal between episodes of hypersomnia.[1] Given the rarity of KLS (estimated prevalence of 1–5 cases per million individuals[2]) and dramatically different symptom presentation, KLS is excluded from review in this chapter.

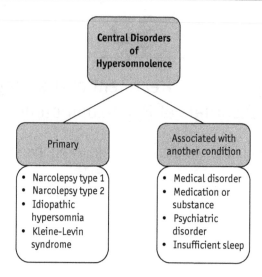

FIGURE 30.1 Classification of the central disorders of hypersomnolence.

Narcolepsy Type 1

Narcolepsy was first described by Jean Baptiste Gélineau in an article published in 1880, describing a patient who experienced more than 200 attacks of sleepiness per day.[3] It is a chronic disorder with a global prevalence about 20–55 cases per 100,000 individuals.[4-8] Among studied populations, prevalence appears to be lowest in Israel[9] and highest in Japan.[10] Age of onset of NT1 is thought to be bimodal, with the highest incidence of new cases presenting in the second decade of life and a smaller peak of patients with new onset sleepiness in the fourth decade.[4,11,12] Though symptom severity can vary patient-to-patient and throughout the course of the disease, NT1 carries a considerable disease burden that extends beyond health-related costs to impact social, professional, and interpersonal aspects of patients' lives.[13,14]

CLINICAL FEATURES OF NARCOLEPSY TYPE 1

Narcolepsy is characterized by EDS, accompanied by rapid eye movement (REM) sleep dysregulation.[1] The classic symptom tetrad of NT1 includes EDS, cataplexy, sleep paralysis, and hypnagogic or hypnopompic hallucinations (hallucinations at sleep onset and sleep offset, respectively).

EDS is considered to be the cardinal symptom of NT1. Patients will experience numerous daily episodes of an irrepressible need for sleep. Sleepiness most often occurs in monotonous situations, and physical activity may suppress the urge to sleep. Most patients with NT1 will feel refreshed after episodes of sleep, but the feeling of sleepiness often returns.

Cataplexy manifests as an abrupt decrease or loss of muscle tone in response to strong, generally positive, emotions such as laughter.[15] The weakness usually lasts seconds to minutes and can be generalized or limited to specific muscle groups, often the face or the neck.[16] These episodes of weakness reflect the abnormal intrusion of REM-like periods of muscle atonia during wakefulness.[17] The presence of cataplexy is pathognomonic for NT1. In roughly half of patients, onset of EDS and cataplexy are simultaneous, but in some cases onset of cataplexy may be delayed by weeks, months, or even years.[18]

Hypnagogic or hypnopompic hallucinations occur in 63% of patients of narcolepsy type 1, and sleep paralysis occurs in 53% of patients.[18] However, the presence of sleep paralysis must be interpreted carefully as it can present as an isolated phenomenon in about 25% of healthy subjects.[19] Despite the consideration of aforementioned four symptoms as the classic tetrad of narcolepsy, only about 40% will exhibit the entire tetrad when cases are viewed retrospectively.[18]

While NT1 is characterized by excessive sleepiness during the day, most patients do not necessarily sleep more than healthy persons in a 24-hour period, often averaging about 7 hours.[20,21] However, a small number of patients with NT1 have "long sleep time" as part of their phenotype and will sleep an excess of 10 hours per night.[21] About 18% of all patients with narcolepsy exhibit this phenotype—only 13% of those are patients with NT1.[21]

Metabolic alterations are also associated with NT1. Hypocretin, which is involved in the pathophysiology of excessive sleepiness (discussed in the following section) is also thought be involved in the regulation of feeding behavior and energy balance.[22]

A case-control study comparing patients with NT1 to those with IH showed that patients with NT1 display significant increases in body mass index and waist circumference despite significantly smaller caloric intake.[23] This was accompanied by pathologic total cholesterol, HDL, and measures of insulin resistance in patients with NT1.[23]

PATHOPHYSIOLOGY OF NARCOLEPSY TYPE 1

Hypocretin (also called orexin) is a neuropeptide produced in the lateral hypothalamus that maintains sleep and wakefulness states through action on the histaminergic, noradrenergic, serotonergic, and cholinergic systems.[22] Cerebrospinal fluid (CSF) hypocretin has been found to be decreased in about 90–95% of patients with narcolepsy and typical cataplexy (defined as <110 pg/mL),[24] with lower hypocretin levels correlating with more sleep–wake instability.[25] Loss of hypocretin is thought to be secondary to autoimmune destruction of the hypocretin-producing neurons in genetically susceptible individuals. In the early 1980s, several human leukocyte antigen (HLA) loci were identified in patients from various ethnic backgrounds.[26-29] HLA DQB1*0602 is the allele most tightly associated with NT1 across all ethnic groups and is present in approximately 98% of patients with NT1 compared to 18% of healthy controls.[30,31] HLA DQB1*0602 is more commonly present in patients with clear-cut cataplexy than those with atypical or doubtful cataplexy, with a 83–93% HLA DQB1*0602 positivity rate in patients with typical cataplexy versus 35–55% positivity in patients atypical cataplexy.[30,32] HLA DQB1*0602 positivity also correlates with a decrease in CSF hypocretin, with about 91–97% of patients with a CSF hypocretin level of less than 110 pg/mL testing positive for the HLA allele.[24,32]

Although the HLA DQB1*0602 allele is more often present in individuals with NT1, it is commonly present in healthy individuals, indicating that genetic predisposition alone does not account for the development of narcolepsy. In fact, in twin studies, only 25–31% of identical twins are concordant for the disease.[33] It is thought that in cases of NT1 there is an environmental trigger, such as infection, that leads to immune destruction of hypocretin producing neurons.[26] This hypothesis is supported by the documented association between the increased presence of anti-streptococcal antibodies in patients with newly diagnosed narcolepsy (within 1 year) compared to age-matched controls (65% vs. 26%).[34] Furthermore an increased incidence of NT1 has been seen in China following the 2009 H1N1 pandemic winter flu and in Europe following pandemic H1N1 flu vaccination with a specific adjuvant vaccine.[35,36]

NARCOLEPSY TYPE 1 DIAGNOSTIC TESTING

Given lifelong need for treatment with potentially habit-forming medications, it is imperative to assess several subjective and objective clinical markers in order to make a diagnosis of NT1. Diagnosing NT1 requires a thorough clinic history along with overnight polysomnography (PSG), multiple sleep latency testing (MSLT), plus/minus actigraphy and lumbar puncture with CSF analysis. The ICSD-3 diagnostic criteria for NT1 are shown in Figure 30.2.

The key objective findings on MSLT are a mean sleep latency (MSL) of 8 minutes or less and two or more sleep onset REM periods (SOREMPs).[1] Patients with NT1 will generally have a MSL around 3.92 ± 3.03 minutes.[18] If a SOREMP occurred during the nocturnal PSG in the night preceding the MSLT, this may be counted toward the two SOREMPs necessary to diagnose NT1. It is necessary that the nocturnal PSG be performed during the night immediately preceding the MSLT. Additionally, it is recommended that 1 week of actigraphy be performed in the preceding week to rule out insufficient sleep or other circadian disorders. Ideally, the patient has also been free of drugs that influence sleep for 2 weeks, and absence of exogenous agents has been confirmed by urine drug screen.

ICSD-3 Diagnostic Criteria for CDH[1]

Narcolepsy Type 1

A. The patient must have at least 3 months of EDS.
B. Presence of at least one of the following:
   1. Cataplexy and a mean sleep latency of ≤8 minutes with two or more SOREMPs* on MSLT.
   2. CSF hypocretin-1 levels of ≤110 pg/mL.

Narcolepsy Type 2[†]

A. The patient must have at least 3 months of EDS.
B. A mean sleep latency of ≤8 minutes and two or more SOREMPs* on MSLT.
C. Cataplexy is absent.
D. CSF hypocretin-1 concentration has not been measured or is > 110 pg/mL.

Idiopathic Hypersomnia[†]

A. The patient must have at least 3 months of EDS.
B. Cataplexy is absent.
C. MSLT with ≤1 SOREMP* or no SOREMP* if REM latency on PSG ≤15 minutes.
D. Presence of at least one of the following:
   1. MSL of ≤8 minutes.
   2. Total 24-hour sleep is ≥660 minutes on 24-hour PSG.
   3. Total 24-hour sleep is ≥660 minutes by wrist actigraphy.

FIGURE 30.2 *International Classification of Sleep Disorders* (ICSD-3) diagnostic criteria for the central disorders of hypersomnolence. SOREMP is the combined number of sleep onset REM periods from the MSLT and preceding night PSG. Hypersomnolence and objective data from PSG/MSLT must not be better explained by obstructive sleep apnea, insufficient sleep, a sleep phase disorder, or the use of, or withdrawal from, a substance or medication.

CDH, central disorders of hypersomnolence; CSF, cerebrospinal fluid; EDS, excessive daytime sleepiness; MSLT, multiple sleep latency testing; PSG, polysomnography; SOREMP, sleep onset REM period.

From International classification of sleep disorders. 3rd ed. Darien, IL: American Academy of Sleep Medicine; 2014.

PSG with MSLT has a sensitivity of 86%,[32] missing a portion of patients who otherwise fit the clinical picture of NT1. As a result, it may be necessary to measure a CSF hypocretin level via lumbar puncture in order to diagnosis NT1, or to differentiate NT1 from NT2. A cutoff of less than 110pg/mL of hypocretin in the CSF is used to diagnose narcolepsy. This threshold yields a 87% sensitivity and a 99% specificity in patients with clear cataplexy.[32]

HLA DQB1*0602 genetic testing can be a helpful adjunct when diagnosing narcolepsy. HLA testing may be most appropriate when deciding whether to perform a diagnostic lumbar puncture as a negative HLA indicates that CSF hypocretin is likely normal. However, as discussed earlier, positive genetic testing must be interpreted in context of the entire clinical picture as HLA DQB1*0602 can be positive in up to 18% percent of healthy controls and 36–56% of patients with NT2.[20,31,32] Positive genetic testing in the context of clear-cut cataplexy however, increases pretest probability of finding low CSF hypocretin before performing a lumbar puncture.[24]

Diagnostic delay is a significant problem among patients with NT1. On average, the time between symptom onset and diagnosis is nearly a decade.[37] Patients are referred to an average of three physicians prior to correct diagnosis, reflecting that many providers in the healthcare community are not trained to recognize the signs and symptoms of NT1.[37] Independent predictors of a longer diagnostic delay are older age of symptom onset, delayed onset of cataplexy, and female gender.[18,37]

Narcolepsy Type 2

NT2 is characterized by EDS and abnormal REM phenomena. However, in contrast to NT1, cataplexy is not present and CSF hypocretin levels are normal. In the previous iteration of the ICSD, narcolepsy was divided into narcolepsy with cataplexy and narcolepsy without cataplexy.[38] This nomenclature was changed in ICSD-3 to narcolepsy type 1 and narcolepsy type 2 to more clearly reflect the differences in etiology between the two conditions, as opposed to their symptomatology. The new definition delineated the two diseases into NT1, which was due to hypocretin deficiency and often accompanied by cataplexy, and NT2, which has a separate pathophysiology and lacks cataplexy as a part of the phenotype.

The population prevalence of NT2 is not as well-characterized. Narcolepsy lacking cataplexy has been documented to make up about 17% patients who present with EDS symptomatology consistent with narcolepsy.[30,32] The estimated population prevalence of NT2 is 20.5 in 100,000.[1] From studies with small numbers of patients, NT2 may be more common in men than women. The age of onset appears to be similar to that of NT1, with many cases emerging in the second or third decade of life.[39,40] In about one-fourth of patients, cataplexy will present later in life and the patient's diagnosis will be changed at that time to NT1.[41]

CLINICAL FEATURES OF NARCOLEPSY TYPE 2

NT2 is characterized by EDS along with evidence of REM sleep instability on PSG/MSLT.[1] EDS in NT2 can also be accompanied by sleep paralysis, hypnagogic/

hypnopompic hallucinations, or automatic behaviors. However, as in NT1, these features are neither sensitive nor specific for NT2, with hypnagogic hallucinations and sleep paralysis occurring only in about half of patient with NT2.[20]

Like patients with NT1, patients with NT2 also experience daily irresistible unwanted naps. However, unlike patients with NT1, those with NT2 are less likely to feel refreshed after awakening from an episode of sleep and will have greater difficulty awakening from a nap.[40] The phenotype of long sleep time also occurs in NT2 and is more commonly seen in these patients than those with NT1.[21]

PATHOPHYSIOLOGY OF NARCOLEPSY TYPE 2

The pathophysiology of NT2 is largely unknown, and the phenotypic presentation may be the result of a heterogenous group of etiologies. Some patients with NT2 have CSF hypocretin levels in the intermediate range (>110 pg/mL but ≤200 pg/mL),[32,39] but the majority have normal hypocretin levels if tested. Though hypocretin levels are generally normal, analysis of CSF from patients with NT2 has shown enhanced activity of gamma-aminobutyric acid $(GABA)_A$ receptors in vitro compared to CSF from control subjects.[42] While this in vitro enhancement has not been demonstrated to be casual to symptoms of EDS, a GABAergic etiology is plausible given the known role of $GABA_A$ receptor agonists as anesthetics to produce pharmacologic sleep.[43,44] This mechanism is further supported by the fact that flumazenil, a $GABA_A$ receptor modulator, reverses the in vitro enhancement of $GABA_A$ signaling produced by the CSF of patients with NT2.[42] Furthermore, some patients report symptomatic improvement following administration of flumazenil.[42]

NARCOLEPSY TYPE 2 DIAGNOSTIC TESTING

Similar to testing for NT1, the diagnostic workup for NT2 requires a thorough patient history, along with in-lab PSG/MSLT. Actigraphy in the week preceding the patient's overnight testing also provides supportive evidence that the patient is not suffering from insufficient sleep or a circadian disorder. The PSG/MSLT findings required to diagnose NT2 are identical to the requirements for NT1: the patient's mean sleep latency must be 8 minutes or less, with two or more SOREMPs during the five daytime naps, or one SOREMP in a daytime nap and a SOREM on PSG on the night prior. Although a mean sleep latency of less than 8 minutes is required for diagnosis, patients with NT2 on average have a mean sleep latency of about 4.5 minutes.[40] In contrast to NT1, the symptom of hypersomnolence in NT2 must not be better explained by insufficient sleep, obstructive sleep apnea, delayed sleep phase, or medications/medication withdrawal.[1] Figure 30.2 displays the ICSD-3 diagnostic criteria for NT2.

HLA DQB1*0602 genetic testing can be considered as part of the workup of NT2 as a test to rule out hypocretin deficiency as the culprit pathophysiology. Roughly half of patients with NT2 will test positive for the allele, which will not aid in differentiating between the two types of narcolepsy. However, a negative result, together with the absence of cataplexy, will argue strongly against NT1.

Idiopathic Hypersomnia

The term "idiopathic hypersomnia" was first coined by Roth, in a 1976 paper that distinguished hypersomnia from narcolepsy.[45] Roth and colleagues proposed that "idiopathic hypersomnia" was made up of two phenotypes: monosymptomatic and polysymptomatic.[46] The monosymptomatic form presented as purely excessive daytime sleepiness, and the polysymptomatic form also included sleep of an "abnormally long duration" and "sleep drunkenness" after awakening.[46] Since that time, diagnostic criteria, required ancillary features, and subclassifications have continued to evolve throughout the three iterations of the ICSD.[47] Generally, however, the disorder is characterized by EDS that occurs in the absence of cataplexy or REM instability as seen on PSG/MSLT.[1]

The prevalence of IH is unknown, but the available literature estimates the prevalence to be between 0.002% and 0.010%.[48,49] These numbers may be an underestimation as population studies reveal that 1.6% of subjects report sleep durations of greater than 9 hours in a 24-hour period that lead to functional impairment or distress.[50] Published data on gender predilection in IH are limited, but a small study of 28 patients showed a female to male ratio of 1.8:1.[48,49] Age of onset is usually in a patient's early 20s, but delays in diagnosis are common.[49]

CLINICAL FEATURES OF IH

The hallmark feature of IH is EDS that occurs with no signs of cataplexy or REM dysregulation.[1] EDS may or may not be accompanied by abnormally long sleep durations (>11 hours per night).[1] In fact, some patients may present with prolonged nighttime sleep alone, with only mild EDS. IH patients with prolonged nighttime sleep have a significantly longer MSL compared to those without long sleep (9.6 ± 0.7 vs. 5.6 ± 0.3 minutes).[51]

The long-sleeping phenotype was reflected in the prior iteration of the ICSD (ICSD-2), as IH was divided into the subtypes "IH with long sleep time" and "IH without long sleep"; however, these conventions were abandoned in the more recent ICSD-3.[47]

Hypnagogic/hypnopompic hallucinations and sleep paralysis are present in about a quarter of patients with IH,[51] but neither is required for the diagnosis or specific for the condition.[1] Unlike NT1, patients with IH are less likely to find daytime napping refreshing and experience great difficulty when awakening from naps.[40,52,53]

A key feature of IH, though not required for diagnosis, is sleep inertia or "sleep drunkenness." Sleep drunkenness is a prolonged difficulty awakening from sleep that is accompanied by automatic behavior, confusion, and relapses into sleep.[52] Of patients with IH, about half endorse feelings of sleep drunkenness upon awakening.[53] In some cases, patients report sleep drunkenness to be the more profound and disabling feature of the disease.[45,54] Sleep drunkenness becomes particularly problematic in the management of IH because patients may have difficulty waking up sufficiently to take medications that combat sleepiness.

Patients with IH will also often report cognitive problems as part of their disease phenotype. Most frequently, patients will report memory problems (79% of patients) and attention deficit (55% of patients).[52]

PATHOPHYSIOLOGY OF IH

As the name implies, the exact pathophysiology of IH remains unknown, but the diagnosis likely captures patients with similar symptomatology stemming from heterogeneous etiologies. HLA DQB1*0602 genetic predisposition is not thought to play a role in the development of IH as the allele occurs with equal frequency in those with IH and healthy controls.[51] Additionally, CSF hypocretin-1 levels are normal in IH patients.[32] As with patients with NT2, analysis of CSF from some with patients with IH reveals abnormal enhancement of $GABA_A$ receptors, suggesting that endogenous overactivation of GABAergic pathways may contribute to excessive sleepiness.[42]

Although there is no association with the HLA DQB1*0602 and IH, about one-third of patients have a positive family history, suggesting that some people may have a genetic predisposition to develop the disease.[55] A case report of a family with a parent and multiple children with IH suggest that there could be an autosomal dominant pattern of inheritance in some cases.[56]

In many patients IH is a lifelong disease, but spontaneous remission is seen in 14–33% of cases.[48,57,58]

IDIOPATHIC HYPERSOMNIA DIAGNOSTIC TESTING

Diagnosing IH requires a thorough clinical history, PSG, and at least one of three objective tests: MSLT, extended (24-hour) PSG, or 7+ day actigraphy. Patients must endorse 3 months or more of "daily periods of irrepressible need to sleep or daytime lapses into sleep" without reports of cataplexy.[1] MSLT must show no more than one sleep onset REM periods.[1] Additionally, MSLT must show a short MSL (≤8 minutes), or 24-hour PSG or actigraphy must show a sleep time for 660 minutes or more. MSL for patients with IH is generally around 7.8 ± 0.5 minutes and total nighttime sleep is 579 ± 90 minutes.[51] Complete ICSD-3 diagnostic criteria for IH are in Figure 30.2.

One diagnostic challenge that often arises when assessing a patient for IH is distinguishing IH from hypersomnia associated with a psychiatric disorder, as hypersomnolence is often present in mental disorders and may even predict the development of subsequent mood episodes.[59] Further clouding the picture, patients with IH have been shown to rate higher levels of anxiety and depression compared to healthy controls.[52] Though the ICSD-3 specifies that hypersomnolence and sleep study findings must not be better explained by a psychiatric disorder, it is often difficult to parse out whether the primary disorder is psychiatric or IH. Determination is left to the physician as to whether he or she believes the hypersomnolence is associated with a primary psychiatric disorder or if the patient has IH with a comorbid mood disorder.

Treatment of Central Disorders of Hypersomnolence

Unfortunately, at this time, there are no curative or disease-modifying agents for the central disorders of hypersomnolence. Therapies are thus aimed at symptom management and are usually needed lifelong.

When determining how best to manage patients with CDH, it is first important to ensure appropriate management of comorbid conditions that could be contributing to hypersomnolence. For example, if a patient also has a mood disorder, careful assessment should be made of whether therapy for a psychiatric condition is sufficient or if a currently prescribed psychiatric medication is leading to EDS.[60] Additionally, patients with comorbid obstructive sleep apnea should be treated with positive airway pressure therapy or oral appliance therapy to ensure appropriate disease control. Once comorbidities are effectively managed and medication regimens have been optimized, attention can be turned to symptom-directed therapy.

NONPHARMACOLOGIC TREATMENT OPTIONS

Most patients with CDH endorse using nonpharmacologic strategies to help control their symptoms.[61] Though personal effectiveness may vary, survey data of patients with CDH have shown that patients with narcolepsy find nonpharmacologic treatment strategies more effective than patients with IH.[61]

Dietary Considerations

Although data are currently very limited, intentional dietary practices may aid in decreasing sleepiness and increasing alertness in patients with CDH. Three-fourths of patients with CDH report using caffeine to aid alertness.[61,62] Most data for the helpful effects of caffeine come from studies of healthy volunteers, but caffeine can provide a moderate benefit for patients with CDH.[61] For best effect, caffeinated beverages should be consumed with consistent preparations and consistent times.[62] Caffeine consumption directly before a short nap has also been shown to be particularly effective for reducing sleepiness prior to driving.[63] Caffeine gum is also available and, when chewed upon awakening, has been shown to reduce sleep inertia, a symptom that often accompanies IH.[64]

The effect of meal size and content has been studied in patients with narcolepsy, but fewer data are available for patients with IH. Patients with narcolepsy are more likely to have an irresistible urge to nap after a meal as opposed to before a meal, with lunch being the most common meal to proceed a nap.[65] Meal size and macronutrient composition do not appear to have an effect on propensity for a post-meal nap.[65] While randomized controlled trials (RCT) have not demonstrated an effect of macronutrient intake on EDS, some patients with narcolepsy find it helpful to avoid carbohydrates, and especially simple sugars, during morning and midday meals in order to increase alertness.[62] In a pilot study, nine patients with narcolepsy (type 1 or 2) with persistent sleepiness despite medications were started on an Atkins-type low-carbohydrate diet. After excluding one dropout due to difficulty with the diet, remaining participants demonstrated an 18% reduction in a composite scale of narcolepsy symptoms, including sleepiness, although Epworth Sleepiness Scale scores did not change.[93]

Scheduled Sleep Time and Naps

Many patients with CDH report using daytime naps and scheduled nocturnal sleep to help relieve EDS symptoms. Despite the fact that 86% of patients with CDH report using daytime napping as a method to combat sleepiness, patients with narcolepsy tend to find napping far more effective than those with IH,[40] rating its effectiveness 5.0 on a scale of 1–10 (ten being most effective) versus a 2.7 in patients with IH.[61] This difference is likely due in part to sleep inertia or difficulty awakening, which is prominent in IH but seen less commonly in narcolepsy. Scheduling nighttime sleep is also endorsed by three-fourths of patients with CDH.[61] However, this method is also only moderately helpful, with patients on average rating scheduled night sleep a 4.0 out of 10 in effectiveness.[61] Studies of patients with narcolepsy have shown increased benefit in terms of daytime alertness when pairing daytime naps and a regularly scheduled bedtime with pharmacotherapy.[66]

Safety and Other Tools for Reducing Daytime Sleepiness and Sleep Inertia

Simple exposure to light has not been shown to be helpful in decreasing sleep inertia and increasing alertness. However, dawn simulators, which emit progressively brighter light prior to awakening, have been shown in healthy volunteers to decrease sleep inertia upon awakening.[67] Bright light therapy may also be helpful in patients with comorbid mood disorders. A randomized crossover study demonstrated that patients with seasonal affective disorder with associated hypersomnia responded more favorably in terms of mood improvement when exposed to morning light.[68]

Body temperature manipulation can also be an effective method to maintain alertness. Fronczek et al. demonstrated that patients with narcolepsy are better able to maintain vigilance with increases in core body temperature, suggesting that simply altering the temperature of food and beverages or clothing choices can be leveraged to improve alertness.[69] Additionally, the same study showed that cooling the distal skin (i.e., hands and feet) increased sleep onset latency during the Maintenance of Wakefulness Test (MWT).[69] Alterations in body temperature can also help to combat sleep inertia when awakening from sleep. Patients can try applying cold wet towels or sitting near a fan—both have been shown to improve post-nap alertness in healthy subjects.[70]

To optimize productivity and daily functioning, patients should try to work with employers or schools to accommodate the need for daytime napping. If feasible, patients may benefit from working from home so that they can work when alert and sleep when needed. Also, if possible, patients should find work or courses of study that are active and engaging as daytime sleepiness is more likely to occur in passive settings.

Cognitive-behavioral therapy (CBT) has also been shown to be a helpful adjunct therapy in the treatment of CDH. CBT for sleep disorders should take multiple approaches to manage the patient's experience with their disease. These approaches include a behavioral component (sleep and nap scheduling), cognitive component (modifying beliefs and emotions associated with the disease), and educational component (understanding the nature of disease and therapy).[70]

This multicomponent approach has been shown in a RCT to significantly improve patients' quality of life and decrease subjective and objective measures of sleepiness.[71]

Patients should also be counseled on appropriate safety measures given their propensity for daytime sleepiness. Those with CDH should take care not to drive or operate heavy machinery when drowsy. Pathologically short sleep latencies on MWT have been shown to be predictive of driving impairment in patients with CDH and thus may be a helpful adjunct test to assess a patient's safety to drive.[72]

Pharmacologic Treatment of the Central Disorders of Hypersomnolence

As noted previously, there are no curative therapies for CDH. Thus, treatment is directed at specific symptoms. Currently, there are no medications approved by the US Food and Drug Administration (FDA) for the treatment of IH, so medications approved for the treatment of narcolepsy are used off-label for these patients. A few RCTs have emerged in the past few years that evaluate the efficacy of various treatments IH, but most of the data regarding effectiveness of wake-promoting agents have been evaluated in the context of narcolepsy.

TRADITIONAL THERAPIES FOR THE CENTRAL DISORDERS OF HYPERSOMNOLENCE

Modafinil or the longer acting, r-enantiomer armodafinil should be used as first-line agents for the treatment of EDS in the narcolepsies and IH.[73,74] Both drugs have been approved by the FDA for the treatment of NT1 and NT2 and are often used off-label to treat IH. Multiple RCTs have demonstrated the efficacy of modafinil in doses of 200–400 mg/d in reducing EDS by subjective assessment (Epworth Sleepiness Scale[75] [ESS]) and objective assessment (MSLT, MWT).[76–78] Fewer data are available for the effect of modafinil on EDS in IH, but the RCTs that are available demonstrate a significant reduction on daytime sleepiness based on the ESS.[79,80]

Sodium oxybate is also considered a first-line agent in the treatment of narcolepsy.[73] The medication is taken at night prior to sleep and improves cataplexy, EDS, and disturbed nighttime sleep.[74,81] Though somewhat counterintuitive, as sodium oxybate is a sleep-producing agent, the drug has been reported to be beneficial in patients with IH by reducing subjective sleepiness and improving sleep inertia upon awakening.[82]

Methylphenidate may be used as a second-line agent for NT1, NT2, and IH.[74,83] However, side effects such as tachycardia, hypertension, sweating, palpitations, and anorexia may develop with use. Additionally, patients often develop tolerance to methylphenidate over time.[84] Pitolisant has been shown in several RCTs to be effective in decreasing ESS scores in patients with narcolepsy.[85] A large case series also demonstrated pitolisant to be beneficial in some patients with IH, though the benefit is modest compared to that seen in patients with narcolepsy.[86] Pitolisant is currently available in the United States it was approved previously for narcolepsy treatment only in Europe.[74] Solriamfetol, a selective norepinephrine-dopamine reuptake inhibitor is another approved medication for the treatment of EDS in narcolepsy.[94] Amphetamine, methamphetamine, and dextroamphetamine are also effective treatments for EDS, but have more limited data available about their risk-to-benefit ratio.[73,74]

First-line treatment therapy for cataplexy includes the use of either sodium oxybate or venlafaxine.[74] Clinical judgment should be used to assess comorbidities or presence of disturbed nighttime sleep when deciding which therapy to initiate. Selective serotonin reuptake inhibitors may be used as alternate agents in the treatment of cataplexy, but data supporting their efficacy are limited.[74]

NOVEL APPROACHES TO THE TREATMENT OF CENTRAL DISORDERS OF HYPERSOMNOLENCE

Many patients with CDH respond well to first- and second-line therapies for CDH. A little over of half of patients with NT1 or NT2 are "good responders" when treated with modafinil monotherapy,[76] and about the same percentage of patients with IH report complete response to pharmacotherapy.[83] However, there is a subset of patients that require multiple medications to control their symptoms or report inadequate control of symptoms despite multiple medications. In these cases of patients with treatment-refractory symptoms or patients who are unable to tolerate standard therapies due to side effects, alternate pharmacologic options are needed to control symptoms.

Based on the discovery that CSF from some patients with CDH potentiates $GABA_A$ receptor activity,[42] medications that act as negative allosteric modulators at the $GABA_A$ receptor have been trialed to combat sleepiness. One of these agents is the antibiotic clarithromycin. In a randomized crossover trial of patients with NT2 and IH, a 2-week course of clarithromycin significantly improved subjective sleepiness.[87] The improvement of sleepiness seen in patients in the clarithromycin trial was of clinically significant magnitude, similar to that seen in clinical trials of other wake-promoting medications.[87,88]

Flumazenil is another $GABA_A$ receptor modulator that may be helpful in treating patients with CDH. The effect of flumazenil was initially demonstrated in vitro: adding the drug reversed endogenous enhancement of $GABA_A$ signaling caused by the CSF of patients with IH.[42] A subsequent large case series showed administration of flumazenil either transdermally or sublingually to provide symptomatic benefit in about 60% of patients undergoing therapy.[89] However, therapy with flumazenil is complicated by difficulties in drug delivery. Due to significant hepatic first-pass metabolism, the oral bioavailability of flumazenil is only 16%.[90] Therefore, to support sustainable, long-term use, the drug can be compounded into a cream or sublingual lozenge to bypass first-pass metabolism.[89] Also physicians and patients should be cautioned, as historically flumazenil has only been used short-term in the termination of anesthesia, and little is known about long-term use of the medication for management of chronic condition.

Melatonin, which is available over the counter, can also be tried to alleviate sleep inertia.[51] When administered exogenously, the hormone can shift the phase of the circadian clock to earlier or later depending on time of administration.[91] A small unpublished study of a series of patients with IH showed giving slow-release melatonin at bedtime decreased sleep drunkenness upon awakening.[92]

Levothyroxine or other thyroid supplementation can be tried to combat EDS. In a small series of patients with IH but normal thyroid function, low-dose levothyroxine significantly decreased subjective sleepiness.

Conclusion

CDH include NT1, NT2, and IH. Each condition is associated with excessive sleepiness during the day and can be accompanied by prolonged sleep durations, sleep paralysis, sleep drunkenness, or hypnagogic/hypnopompic hallucinations. To differentiate between the disorders within the CDH category, a careful clinical history must be taken in order to elicit information about presence of cataplexy, prolonged sleep durations, metabolic disturbances, family history, and comorbid mood conditions. Evaluation with PSG/MSLT is critical for determining diagnosis. Although there are rare cases of remission,[57] treatment for the CDH is often required lifelong. Dietary and other lifestyle interventions can play a role in the management of CDH. For patients requiring pharmacologic therapy, modafinil and sodium oxybate are first-line treatments. In cases of treatment failure, stimulant medications should be used, or patients can be trialed on novel agents such as clarithromycin or flumazenil.

REFERENCES

1. American Academy of Sleep Medicine. *International classification of sleep disorders.* 3rd ed. Darien, IL: American Academy of Sleep Medicine; 2014.

2. Frenette E, Kushida CA. Primary hypersomnias of central origin. *Semin Neurol.* 2009;29(4):354–367. doi:10.1055/s-0029-1237114.

3. Schenck CH, Bassetti CL, Arnulf I, Mignot E. English translations of the first clinical reports on narcolepsy and cataplexy by Westphal And Gélineau in the late 19th century, with commentary. *J Clin Sleep Med.* 2007;3(3):301–311.

4. Silber MH, Krahn LE, Olson EJ, Pankratz VS. The epidemiology of narcolepsy in Olmsted County, Minnesota: A population-based study. *Sleep.* 2002;25(2):197–202. doi:10.1093/sleep/25.2.197.

5. Heier MS, Evsiukova T, Wilson J, Abdelnoor M, Hublin C, Ervik S. Prevalence of narcolepsy with cataplexy in Norway. *Acta Neurol Scand.* 2009;120(4):276–280. doi:10.1111/j.1600-0404.2009.01166.x.

6. Hublin C, Partinen M, Kaprio J, Koskenvuo M, Guilleminault C. Epidemiology of Narcolepsy. *Sleep.* 1994;17(suppl_8):S7–S12. doi:10.1093/sleep/17.suppl_8.S7.

7. Hublin C, Kaprio J, Partinen M, et al. The prevalence of narcolepsy: An epidemiological study of the Finnish Twin Cohort. *Ann Neurol.* 1994;35(6):709–716. doi:10.1002/ana.410350612.

8. Ohayon MMM, Priest RGM, Zulley J, Smirne S, Paiva T. Prevalence of narcolepsy symptomatology and diagnosis in the European general population. *Neurology.* 2002;58(12):1826–1833. doi:10.1212/WNL.58.12.1826.

9. Lavie P, Peled R. Narcolepsy is a rare disease in Israel. *Sleep.* 1987;10(6):608–609. doi:10.1093/sleep/10.6.608.

10. Wing Y-K, Li RH-Y, Lam C-W, Ho CK-W, Fong SY-Y, Leung T. The prevalence of narcolepsy among Chinese in Hong Kong. *Ann Neurol.* 2002;51(5):578–584. doi:10.1002/ana.10162.

11. Dauvilliers Y, Montplaisir J, Molinari N, et al. Age at onset of narcolepsy in two large populations of patients in France and Quebec. *Neurology.* 2001;57(11):2029–2033. doi:10.1212/WNL.57.11.2029.

12. Rye DB, Dihenia B, Weissman JD, Epstein CM, Bliwise DL. Presentation of narcolepsy after 40. *Neurology.* 1998;50(2):459–465.

13. Dodel R, Peter H, Spottke A, et al. Health-related quality of life in patients with narcolepsy. *Sleep Med.* 2007;8(7-8):733–741. doi:10.1016/j.sleep.2006.10.010.

14. Jennum P, Ibsen R, Petersen ER, Knudsen S, Kjellberg J. Health, social, and economic consequences of narcolepsy: A controlled national study evaluating the societal effect on patients and their partners. *Sleep Med.* 2012;13(8):1086–1093. doi:10.1016/j.sleep.2012.06.006.

15. Krahn LE, Lymp JF, Moore WR, Slocumb N, Silber MH. Characterizing the emotions that trigger cataplexy. *J Neuropsychiatry Clin Neurosci.* 2005;17(1):45–50. doi:10.1176/jnp.17.1.45.

16. Parkes JD, Chen SY, Clift SJ, Dahlitz MJ, Dunn G. The clinical diagnosis of the narcoleptic syndrome. *J Sleep Res.* 1998;7(1):41–52.

17. Saper CB, Cano G, Scammell TE. Homeostatic, circadian, and emotional regulation of sleep. *J Comp Neurol.* 2005;493(1):92–98. doi:10.1002/cne.20770.

18. Luca G, Haba-Rubio J, Dauvilliers Y, et al. Clinical, polysomnographic and genome-wide association analyses of narcolepsy with cataplexy: A European Narcolepsy Network study. *J Sleep Res.* 2013;22(5):482–495. doi:10.1111/jsr.12044.

19. Bell CC, Dixie-Bell DD, Thompson B. Further studies on the prevalence of isolated sleep paralysis in black subjects. *J Natl Med Assoc.* 1986;78(7):649–659.

20. Sasai T, Inoue Y, Komada Y, Sugiura T, Matsushima E. Comparison of clinical characteristics among narcolepsy with and without cataplexy and idiopathic hypersomnia without long sleep time, focusing on HLA-DRB1*1501/DQB*10602 finding. *Sleep Med.* 2009;10(9):961–966. doi:10.1016/j.sleep.2008.12.007.

21. Vernet C, Arnulf I. Narcolepsy with long sleep time: A specific entity? *Sleep.* 2009;32(9):1229–1235.

22. Inutsuka A, Yamanaka A. The physiological role of orexin/hypocretin neurons in the regulation of sleep/wakefulness and neuroendocrine functions. *Front Endocrinol.* 2013;4. doi:10.3389/fendo.2013.00018.

23. Poli F, Plazzi G, Di Dalmazi G, et al. Body mass index-independent metabolic alterations in narcolepsy with cataplexy. *Sleep.* 2009;32(11):1491–1497.

24. Bourgin P, Zeitzer JM, Mignot E. CSF hypocretin-1 assessment in sleep and neurological disorders. *Lancet Neurol.* 2008-7(7):649–662. doi:10.1016/S1474-4422(08)70140-6.

25. Hansen MH, Kornum BR, Jennum P. Sleep–wake stability in narcolepsy patients with normal, low and unmeasurable hypocretin levels. *Sleep Med.* 2017;34:1–6. doi:10.1016/j.sleep.2017.01.021.

26. Liblau RS, Vassalli A, Seifinejad A, Tafti M. Hypocretin (orexin) biology and the pathophysiology of narcolepsy with cataplexy. *Lancet Neurol.* 2015;14(3):318–328. doi:10.1016/S1474-4422(14)70218-2.

27. Juji T, Matsuki K, Tokunaga K, Naohara T, Honda Y. Narcolepsy and HLA in the Japanese. *Ann N Y Acad Sci.* 1988;540:106–114.

28. Seignalet J, Billiard M. Possible association between HLA-B7 and narcolepsy. *Tissue Antigens.* 1984;23(3):188–189.

29. Langdon N, Welsh KI, van Dam M, Vaughan RW, Parkes D. Genetic markers in narcolepsy. *Lancet Lond Engl.* 1984;2(8413):1178–1180.

30. Mignot E, Hayduk R, Black J, Grumet FC, Guilleminault C. HLA DQB1*0602 is associated with cataplexy in 509 narcoleptic patients. *Sleep.* 1997;20(11):1012–1020. doi:10.1093/sleep/20.11.1012.

31. Tafti M, Hor H, Dauvilliers Y, et al. DQB1 locus alone explains most of the risk and protection in narcolepsy with cataplexy in Europe. *Sleep.* 2014;37(1):19–25. doi:10.5665/sleep.3300.

32. Mignot E, Lammers GJ, Ripley B, et al. The role of cerebrospinal fluid hypocretin measurement in the diagnosis of narcolepsy and other hypersomnias. *Arch Neurol.* 2002;59(10):1553-1562. doi:10.1001/archneur.59.10.1553.

33. Mignot E. Genetic and familial aspects of narcolepsy. *Neurology.* 1998;50(2 Suppl 1):S16–22.

34. Aran A, Lin L, Nevsimalova S, et al. Elevated anti-streptococcal antibodies in patients with recent narcolepsy onset. *Sleep.* 2009;32(8):979–983.

35. Han F, Lin L, Mignot E. Decreased incidence of childhood narcolepsy 2 years after the 2009 H1N1 winter flu pandemic. *Ann Neurol.* 2013;73(4):560. doi:10.1002/ana.23799.

36. Ahmed SS, Schur PH, MacDonald NE, Steinman L. Narcolepsy, 2009 A(H1N1) pandemic influenza, and pandemic influenza vaccinations: What is known and unknown about the neurological disorder, the role for autoimmunity, and vaccine adjuvants. *J Autoimmun.* 2014;50:1–11. doi:10.1016/j.jaut.2014.01.033.

37. Taddei RN, Werth E, Poryazova R, Baumann CR, Valko PO. Diagnostic delay in narcolepsy type 1: Combining the patients' and the doctors' perspectives. *J Sleep Res.* 2016;25(6):709–715. doi:info:doi/10.1111/jsr.12420.

38. American Academy of Sleep Medicine. *ICSD-2: International Classification of Sleep Disorders,* 2nd ed. Darien, IL: American Academy of Sleep Medicine; 2005.

39. Oka Y, Inoue Y, Kanbayashi T, et al. Narcolepsy without cataplexy: 2 Subtypes based on CSF hypocretin-1/orexin-a findings. *Sleep.* 2006;29(11):1439–1443. doi:10.1093/sleep/29.11.1439.

40. Šonka K, Šusta M, Billiard M. Narcolepsy with and without cataplexy, idiopathic hypersomnia with and without long sleep time: A cluster analysis. *Sleep Med.* 2015;16(2):225–231. doi:10.1016/j.sleep.2014.09.016.

41. Sours JA. Narcolepsy and other disturbances in the sleep-waking rhythm: A study of 115 cases with review of the literature. *J Nerv.* 1963;137(6):525–542.

42. Rye DB, Bliwise DL, Parker K, et al. Modulation of vigilance in the primary hypersomnias by endogenous enhancement of GABAA receptors. *Sci Transl Med.* 2012;4(161):161ra151. doi:10.1126/scitranslmed.3004685.

43. Franks NP, Zecharia AY. Sleep and general anesthesia. *Can J Anesth Can Anesth.* 2011;58(2):139–148. doi:10.1007/s12630-010-9420-3.

44. Franks NP. General anaesthesia: From molecular targets to neuronal pathways of sleep and arousal. *Nat Rev Neurosci.* 2008;9(5):370–386. doi:10.1038/nrn2372.

45. Roth B. Narcolepsy and hypersomnia: Review and classification of 642 personally observed cases. *Schweiz Arch Neurol Neurochir Psychiatr Arch Suisses Neurol Neurochir Psychiatr.* 1976;119(1):31–41.

46. Billiard M, Dauvilliers Y. Idiopathic hypersomnia. *Sleep Med Rev.* 2001;5(5):349–358. doi:10.1053/smrv.2001.0168.

47. Saini P, Rye DB. Hypersomnia: Evaluation, treatment, and social and economic aspects. *Sleep Med Clin.* 2017;12(1):47–60. doi:10.1016/j.jsmc.2016.10.013.

48. Bassetti C, Aldrich MS. Idiopathic hypersomnia. A series of 42 patients. *Brain.* 1997;120(8):1423–1435. doi:10.1093/brain/120.8.1423.

49. Sowa NA. Idiopathic hypersomnia and hypersomnolence disorder: A systematic review of the literature. *Psychosomatics.* 2016;57(2):152–164. doi:10.1016/j.psym.2015.12.006.

50. Ohayon MM, Reynolds CF, Dauvilliers Y. Excessive sleep duration and quality of life. *Ann Neurol.* 2013;73(6):785–794. doi:10.1002/ana.23818.

51. Vernet C, Arnulf I. Idiopathic hypersomnia with and without long sleep time: A controlled series of 75 patients. *Sleep*. 2009;32(6):753–759.

52. Vernet C, Leu-Semenescu S, Buzare M-A, Arnulf I. Subjective symptoms in idiopathic hypersomnia: Beyond excessive sleepiness. *J Sleep Res*. 2010;19(4):525–534. doi:10.1111/j.1365-2869.2010.00824.x.

53. Trotti LM. Waking up is the hardest thing I do all day: Sleep inertia and sleep drunkenness. *Sleep Med Rev*. doi:10.1016/j.smrv.2016.08.005.

54. Roth B, Nevsimalova S, Rechtschaffen A. Hypersomnia with sleep drunkenness. *Arch Gen Psychiatry*. 1972;26(5):456–462. doi:10.1001/archpsyc.1972.01750230066013.

55. Billiard M, Sonka K. Idiopathic hypersomnia. *Sleep Med Rev*. 2016;29:23–33. doi:10.1016/j.smrv.2015.08.007.

56. Janáčková S, Motte J, Bakchine S, Sforza E. Idiopathic hypersomnia: A report of three adolescent-onset cases in a two-generation family. *J Child Neurol*. 2011;26(4):522–525. doi:10.1177/0883073810384865.

57. Anderson KN, Pilsworth S, Sharples LD, Smith IE, Shneerson JM. Idiopathic hypersomnia: A study of 77 cases. *Sleep*. 2007;30(10):1274–1281.

58. Kim T, Lee JH, Lee CS, Yoon IY. Different fates of excessive daytime sleepiness: Survival analysis for remission. *Acta Neurol Scand*. 2016;134(1):35–41. doi:10.1111/ane.12504.

59. Kaplan KA, Harvey AG. Hypersomnia across mood disorders: A review and synthesis. *Sleep Med Rev*. 2009;13(4):275–285. doi:10.1016/j.smrv.2008.09.001.

60. Barateau L, Lopez R, Franchi JAM, Dauvilliers Y. Hypersomnolence, hypersomnia, and mood disorders. *Curr Psychiatry Rep*. 2017;19(2):13. doi:10.1007/s11920-017-0763-0.

61. Neikrug AB, Crawford MR, Ong JC. Behavioral sleep medicine services for hypersomnia disorders: A survey study. *Behav Sleep Med*. 2017;15(2):158–171. doi:10.1080/15402002.2015.1120201.

62. Garma L, Marchand F. Non-pharmacological approaches to the treatment of narcolepsy. *Sleep*. 1994;17(suppl_8):S97–S102. doi:10.1093/sleep/17.suppl_8.S97.

63. Reyner LA, Horne JA. Suppression of sleepiness in drivers: Combination of caffeine with a short nap. *Psychophysiology*. 1997;34(6):721–725.

64. Newman RA, Kamimori GH, Wesensten NJ, Picchioni D, Balkin TJ. Caffeine gum minimizes sleep inertia. *Percept Mot Skills*. 2013;116(1):280–293. doi:10.2466/29.22.25.PMS.116.1.280-293.

65. Pollak CP, Green J. Eating and its relationships with subjective alertness and sleep in narcoleptic subjects living without temporal cues. *Sleep*. 1990;13(6):467–478. doi:10.1093/sleep/13.6.467.

66. Rogers AE, Aldrich MS, Lin X. A comparison of three different sleep schedules for reducing daytime sleepiness in narcolepsy. *Sleep*. 2001;24(4):385–391. doi:10.1093/sleep/24.4.385.

67. Giménez MC, Hessels M, van de Werken M, de Vries B, Beersma DGM, Gordijn MCM. Effects of artificial dawn on subjective ratings of sleep inertia and dim light melatonin onset. *Chronobiol Int*. 2010;27(6):1219–1241. doi:10.3109/07420528.2010.496912.

68. Avery DH, Khan A, Dager SR, Cohen S, Cox GB, Dunner DL. Morning or evening bright light treatment of winter depression? The significance of hypersomnia. *Biol Psychiatry*. 1991;29(2):117–126.

69. Fronczek R, Raymann RJEM, Romeijn N, et al. Manipulation of core body and skin temperature improves vigilance and maintenance of wakefulness in narcolepsy. *Sleep*. 2008;31(2):233–240.

70. Marín Agudelo HA, Jiménez Correa U, Carlos Sierra J, Pandi-Perumal SR, Schenck CH. Cognitive behavioral treatment for narcolepsy: Can it complement pharmacotherapy? *Sleep Sci*. 2014;7(1):30–42. doi:10.1016/j.slsci.2014.07.023.

71. Agudelo HAM. M-N-123 multicomponent cognitive behavioral treatment efficacy for narcolepsy (MCBT-N). *Sleep Med*. 2011;12:S55. doi:10.1016/S1389-9457(11)70203-9.

72. Philip P, Chaufton C, Taillard J, et al. Maintenance of wakefulness test scores and driving performance in sleep disorder patients and controls. *Int J Psychophysiol Off J Int Organ Psychophysiol*. 2013;89(2):195–202. doi:10.1016/j.ijpsycho.2013.05.013.

73. Morgenthaler TI, Kapur VK, Brown T, et al. Practice parameters for the treatment of narcolepsy and other hypersomnias of central origin: An American Academy of Sleep Medicine report. *Sleep*. 2007;30(12):1705–1711.

74. Kallweit U, Bassetti CL. Pharmacological management of narcolepsy with and without cataplexy. *Expert Opin Pharmacother*. May 2017:1–9. doi:10.1080/14656566.2017.1323877.

75. Johns MW. A new method for measuring daytime sleepiness: The Epworth sleepiness scale. *Sleep*. 1991;14(6):540–545.

76. Billiard M, Besset A, Montplaisir J, et al. Modafinil: A double-blind multicentric study. *Sleep*. 1994;17(8 Suppl):S107–112.

77. Moldofsky null, Broughton null, Hill null. A randomized trial of the long-term, continued efficacy and safety of modafinil in narcolepsy. *Sleep Med*. 2000;1(2):109–116.

78. US Modafinil in Narcolepsy Multicenter Study Group. Randomized trial of modafinil as a treatment for the excessive daytime somnolence of narcolepsy: US Modafinil in Narcolepsy Multicenter Study Group. *Neurology*. 2000;54(5):1166–1175.

79. Mayer G, Benes H, Young P, Bitterlich M, Rodenbeck A. Modafinil in the treatment of idiopathic hypersomnia without long sleep time: A randomized, double-blind, placebo-controlled study. *J Sleep Res*. 2015;24(1):74–81. doi:10.1111/jsr.12201.

80. Philip P, Chaufton C, Taillard J, et al. Modafinil improves real driving performance in patients with hypersomnia: A randomized double-blind placebo-controlled crossover clinical trial. *Sleep*. 2014;37(3):483–487. doi:10.5665/sleep.3480.

81. Mamelak M, Swick T, Emsellem H, Montplaisir J, Lai C, Black J. A 12-week open-label, multicenter study evaluating the safety and patient-reported efficacy of sodium oxybate in patients with narcolepsy and cataplexy. *Sleep Med*. 2015;16(1):52–58. doi:10.1016/j.sleep.2014.10.004.

82. Leu-Semenescu S, Louis P, Arnulf I. Benefits and risk of sodium oxybate in idiopathic hypersomnia versus narcolepsy type 1: A chart review. *Sleep Med*. 2016;17(Supplement C):38–44. doi:10.1016/j.sleep.2015.10.005.

83. Ali M, Auger RR, Slocumb NL, Morgenthaler TI. Idiopathic hypersomnia: Clinical features and response to treatment. *J Clin Sleep Med.* 2009;5(6):562–568.

84. Mitler MM, Shafor R, Hajdukovich R, Timms RM, Browman CP. Treatment of narcolepsy: Objective studies on methylphenidate, pemoline, and protriptyline. *Sleep.* 1986;9(1 Pt 2):260–264.

85. Calik MW. Update on the treatment of narcolepsy: Clinical efficacy of pitolisant. *Nat Sci Sleep.* 2017;9:127–133. doi:10.2147/NSS.S103462.

86. Leu-Semenescu S, Nittur N, Golmard J-L, Arnulf I. Effects of pitolisant, a histamine H3 inverse agonist, in drug-resistant idiopathic and symptomatic hypersomnia: A chart review. *Sleep Med.* 2014;15(6):681–687. doi:10.1016/j.sleep.2014.01.021.

87. Trotti LM, Saini P, Bliwise DL, Freeman AA, Jenkins A, Rye DB. Clarithromycin in γ-aminobutyric acid-Related hypersomnolence: A randomized, crossover trial. *Ann Neurol.* 2015;78(3):454–465. doi:10.1002/ana.24459.

88. Erman MK, Rosenberg R, for the US Modafinil Shift Work Sleep Disorder Study Group. Modafinil for excessive sleepiness associated with chronic shift work sleep disorder: Effects on patient functioning and health-related quality of life. *Prim Care Companion J Clin Psychiatry.* 2007;9(3):188–194.

89. Trotti LM, Saini P, Koola C, LaBarbera V, Bliwise DL, Rye DB. Flumazenil for the treatment of refractory hypersomnolence: Clinical experience with 153 patients. *J Clin Sleep Med.* 2016;12(10):1389–1394. doi:10.5664/jcsm.6196.

90. Roncari G, Ziegler WH, Guentert TW. Pharmacokinetics of the new benzodiazepine antagonist Ro 15-1788 in man following intravenous and oral administration. *Br J Clin Pharmacol.* 1986;22(4):421–428.

91. Arendt J, Skene DJ. Melatonin as a chronobiotic. *Sleep Med Rev.* 2005;9(1):25–39. doi:10.1016/j.smrv.2004.05.002.

92. Montplaisir J, Fantini L. Idiopathic hypersomnia: A diagnostic dilemma. A commentary of "Idiopathic hypersomnia" (M. Billiard and Y. Dauvilliers). *Sleep Med Rev.* 2001;5(5):361–362. doi:10.1053/smrv.2001.0216.

93. Husain AM, Yancy WS, Jr., Carwile ST, Miller PP, Westman EC (2004) Diet therapy for narcolepsy. Neurology 62 (12):2300–2302.

94. Subedi S, Singh R, Thakur RK, et al. Efficacy and safety of solriamfetol for excessive daytime sleepiness in narcolepsy and obstructive sleep apnea: a systematic review and meta-analysis of clinical trials. *Sleep Medicine.* 2020; 75:510–521,

31

Introduction to Sleep-Disordered Breathing and Treatment

JOANNE S. MARTIRES, REUBEN RAM, AND JEANNE WALLACE

Introduction

Sleep-disordered breathing encompasses a wide range of breathing disorders that occur during sleep and include obstructive sleep apnea (OSA), central sleep apnea (CSA), and sleep-related hypoventilation. Patients with sleep-disordered breathing can suffer from frequent nocturnal awakenings, unrefreshing sleep, and excessive daytime sleepiness (EDS), which can lead to poor quality of life and long-term health consequences. Treatment of these conditions is often a form of noninvasive ventilation. For example, continuous positive airway pressure (CPAP) is often used for OSA. However, there are often barriers to adapting this form of treatment, and it is important for a clinician to be familiar with the pathophysiology of sleep-disordered breathing, be able to educate patients on the consequences of untreated sleep-disordered breathing, and offer guidance and unique approaches when there is poor treatment adherence or intolerance.

Obstructive Sleep Apnea Syndrome

BACKGROUND AND PREVALENCE

OSA is the most common sleep-related breathing disorder, one characterized by complete or partial occlusion of the airway resulting in transient interruption of breathing, oxygen desaturation, and fragmentation of sleep. OSA can lead to EDS, mood alterations, and cognitive impairment. OSA was first described in the medical literature by Dr. William Osler in 1918, and the first polygraphic studies of OSA were done in 1965 by Gastaut et al. Since the 1980s, widely accepted definitions of OSA have been established; there have been numerous studies on the health consequences of OSA and wide interest and resources dedicated to the diagnosis and treatment of this condition.

OSA with daytime impairment is estimated to occur in 1 out of 20 adults. The prevalence of mild OSA is even higher at 1 out of 5.[1] Therefore, OSA affects tens of millions in the United States, with prevalence rates comparable to diabetes or asthma. However, numerous cases are undiagnosed, perhaps due to lack of knowledge about this condition in the general population and poor recognition by clinicians. In the Wisconsin Sleep Cohort Study, which examined prevalence rates of OSA in working-class middle-aged adults in 1988–1994, moderate to severe OSA occurred at a rate of 9% in men and 4% in women.[2] Due to the ongoing obesity epidemic, the prevalence OSA has increased over the past couple of decades. Estimates of OSA prevalence have been updated using the Wisconsin Sleep Cohort in 2007–2011 and data from the National Health and Nutrition Examination Survey. Currently, the prevalence of moderate to severe OSA in persons aged 30–70 is approximately 13% in men and 6% in women.[3] Depending on the subgroup examined, prevalence rates increased by double-digit percentages, representing estimated increases in the millions of additional afflicted persons in the United States.

PATHOPHYSIOLOGY AND RISK FACTORS

The pathophysiology of OSA involves some degree of impairment of the collapsible upper airway during sleep. Craniofacial structural abnormalities that reduced the bony enclosure of the upper airway, excess or redundant tissue that can lower the threshold for airway collapsibility, and impaired pharyngeal dilator muscle activation can all impair the upper airway anatomy and predispose to OSA. Arousals from sleep occur in response to apnea, and often an exaggerated ventilatory response follows. These responses to apnea are also important contributors to the pathophysiology of OSA.[4]

The strongest risk factors for OSA are sex, obesity, and age. OSA is two to three times more prevalent in men than in women. Hormonal differences may play a role in this predisposition as postmenopausal women have a higher prevalence of OSA compared with premenopausal women.[5] The strongest risk factor for OSA across both sexes is obesity. Obesity may lead to increased adiposity and loss of caudal traction around the upper airway and greater pharyngeal collapsibility in obese patients.[6] About 70% of patients with OSA are obese, and the prevalence of OSA in obese patients is 40%.[7,8] In particular, large neck circumference (40 cm or greater) is a great predictor of OSA.[9] OSA prevalence increases with age, beginning in mid-life, but seems to plateau after 65 years.[1] The prevalence of OSA in older adults over 60 varies widely based on setting. However, the most recent prevalence estimates for community-based older adults aged 50–70 were higher than in middle-aged adults: 17.4% for men and 9.1% for women.[3]

OSA is more prevalent in African Americans than Caucasians.[10] A recent study found the prevalence of OSA in Hispanics to be similar to that of the general US population, but many had not been given a prior clinical diagnosis, suggesting the underdiagnosis of OSA in this population.[11] OSAS is common among Asians, in particular Chinese individuals, with the predisposition being more related to craniopharyngeal features, such as a crowded upper airway and retrognathia, rather than obesity.[12]

As eluded to previously, craniofacial characteristics including retrognathia, recessed maxilla and mandible, and high arched palate predispose to OSA.[13] Patients with congenital craniofacial abnormalities such as Down syndrome, Treacher Collins syndrome, and Pierre Robin syndrome are at increased risk for OSA.

Cigarette smoking and alcohol have been shown to be risk factors for OSA syndrome (OSAS). In the Wisconsin Sleep Cohort Study, smokers had a greater risk of moderate or greater OSAS (odds ratio 4.44) compared with never smokers,[2] possibly due to cigarette-induced airway inflammation and damage changing the properties of the upper airway and increasing the risk of collapsibility during sleep. Alcohol relaxes upper airway dilator muscles, thus increasing upper airway resistance and inducing OSAS in susceptible subjects. Furthermore, alcohol intake can prolong apnea duration, suppress arousals, increase frequency of occlusive episodes, and worsen the severity of hypoxemia.[14]

EVALUATION

During an evaluation for OSA, patients may complain of EDS, unrefreshing sleep, and morning headaches. However, classic symptoms such as loud snoring and apneas are often reported by family members. Other complaints may include nocturia, nocturnal chest pain, dry or sore throat, gastroesophageal reflux, sexual dysfunction, cognitive problems, and depression.

On physical exam, a normal or elevated body mass index (BMI) may be seen. Patients should be checked for any craniofacial abnormalities, an enlarged neck girth, or enlarged tonsils. Patients should be screened for medical conditions such as hypothyroidism or acromegaly, both of which can lead to macroglossia and redundant tissue in the posterior pharynx. A *Mallampati score* is frequently done to evaluate for risk of OSA. A Mallampati score is based on visualization of the upper airway structures and may range from Class I (soft palate, uvula, tonsillar fauces, and pillars visible) to Class IV (only hard palate visible). Mallampati III and IV scores indicate high OSA risk.[15]

DIAGNOSIS

The gold standard diagnostic test for OSA is overnight in-laboratory polysomnography (PSG). PSG is an attended study and consists of the recording through sensors of multiple physiologic signals: electroencephalography, electro-oculography, electromyography, electrocardiography, airflow, respiratory effort, oxygen saturation, snoring, and leg and sleep position. In addition to a variety of sleep disorders, PSG can identify different types of sleep-disordered breathing. An *apnea* is defined as the complete cessation of airflow for at least 10 seconds. A *hypopnea* is defined as a reduction in airflow followed by an arousal from sleep or a decrease in oxyhemoglobin saturation. OSA is diagnosed when the number of obstructive events is equal to or greater than 5 per hour in a patient who reports daytime sleepiness, unrefreshing sleep, waking with gasping or choking episodes, or has apneas witnessed by others or as a co-morbid condition such as:hypertension, coronary artery disease, congestive heart failure, atrial fibrillation, stroke, cognitive dysfunction, mood disorder or diabetes mellitus type 2. Another diagnostic criteria for OSA is 15 or more obstructive events per hour without the previously mentioned symptoms or co-morbid conditions. OSA severity is graded by the apnea-hypopnea index (AHI) or the number of apneas and hypopneas per hour of sleep: mild for an AHI of 5–15 per hour; moderate for an AHI of 16–30 per hour; and severe when the AHI is greater than 30 per hour.

The unattended home sleep apnea test (HSAT) may be used as an alternative to PSG for evaluating patients with high pretest probability for moderate to severe OSA.[16] Like PSG, an HSAT should be accompanied by a clinical assessment and administered under the supervision of sleep physician. At minimum, an adequate HSAT should include sensors for nasal pressure, chest and abdominal plethysmography, and oximetry. HSAT offers the benefits of comfort (administered at home), increased access to testing, and decreased cost, but patients with failed or equivocal home studies and those with negative studies but persistent symptoms should undergo a standard PSG because this remains the most sensitive for diagnosing OSA. Patients with significant cardiopulmonary disease, neuromuscular disorders, suspected sleep-related hypoventilation, chronic opioid use, or stroke or those with suspected comorbid sleep conditions are not appropriate for HSAT and should undergo PSG.

If a patient is found to have OSA, the preferred treatment is CPAP. An ideal pressure may be titrated in the sleep lab during a full titration study or split-night PSG (first half of the night diagnostic with an AHI greater than 20; second half CPAP titration). The goal is to find the lowest CPAP level needed to alleviate nearly all respiratory events. Certain auto-adjusting devices (or APAPs) may be used in an unattended setting to determine a fixed CPAP pressure for patients with uncomplicated OSA.[17]

CONSEQUENCES OF OSA

The consequences of untreated OSA are thought to result from the fragmented sleep, intermittent hypoxia and hypercapnia, intrathoracic pressure swings, and increased sympathetic nervous system activity that accompanies OSA. Patients with OSA may experience EDS, cognitive deficits, reduced driving competence, and impaired psychosocial well-being. These symptoms can lead to poor job performance and disability as well as a two to seven times higher risk of motor vehicle accidents.[18] Untreated OSAS can have particularly lethal consequences in those who operate commercial motor vehicles.[19] Therefore, it has been recommended that commercial drivers be prohibited from driving if they have moderate to severe untreated OSA, excessive sleepiness while driving, or a history of falling asleep while driving leading to a crash.[20]

OSA, when untreated, is associated with certain comorbid conditions such as hypertension and stroke and has been shown to increase mortality.[21,22] Peppard et al. published a landmark study in 2000 revealing OSA as an independent dose-dependent risk factor for hypertension.[23] Treatment with CPAP has been shown to improve blood pressure control even in resistant hypertension.[24] OSA has been identified as a treatable cause of cardiovascular disease. A large 10-year prospective study found that untreated severe OSA independently increased the odds of fatal and nonfatal cardiovascular events compared to patients without OSA, those with mild OSA, and those with severe OSA treated with CPAP.[25] Data from the Sleep Heart Health Study revealed that individuals with sleep-disordered breathing have two- to fourfold higher odds of complex arrhythmias such as atrial fibrillation and nonsustained ventricular tachycardia compared to those without sleep-disordered breathing.[26] CPAP has been shown to mitigate arrhythmias in patients with OSA.[27,28] Cerebrovascular disease is strongly and independently associated with OSA.[29,30] OSA is associated with a higher incidence of stroke and mortality in stroke,[31,32] and CPAP can reduce mortality in patients with OSA and stroke.[33]

OSA appears to be an independent risk factor for insulin resistance and the development of diabetes. The Sleep Heart Health Study showed that those with moderate to severe OSA were more likely to have an elevated fasting glucose level and 2-hour glucose tolerance.[34] The Wisconsin Sleep Cohort showed that those with severe OSA were more likely to have diabetes.[2] The effects of CPAP treatment on diabetes are unknown.

Unrecognized OSA may lead to perioperative complications including difficult intubations, exaggerated respiratory depressions from anesthetics, increased postoperative reintubations, cardiac dysrhythmias, and longer hospital stays. Therefore, the American Society of Anesthesiologists recommends screening and preoperative preparation for OSA.[35]

Undiagnosed OSA leads to high economic and healthcare costs due to decreased productivity, workplace accidents, motor vehicle accidents, increased cardiovascular comorbidities, and depression as well as increased healthcare utilization. Diagnosis and treatment of untreated OSA would likely add $49.5 billion to the healthcare system burden but is expected to lead to a savings of $100.1 billion.[36]

TREATMENT

CPAP is the first-line treatment for OSA and was first introduced into clinical practice in 1981.[37] A CPAP device delivers positive pressure to the upper airway via a mask and acts as a pneumatic splint, keeping the airway patent. CPAP can improve sleep architecture, improve sleep quality, reduce EDS, improve cognitive function, and decrease the risk for automobile accidents.[38-40]

CPAP can help to achieve modest improvements in blood pressure. However, the impact of CPAP in reducing cardiovascular risk is unclear. The long-term sequelae of mild to moderate OSA are not as well understood in severe OSA. However, there is evidence that effective CPAP treatment does improve well-being, quality of life, and daytime functioning in patients with mild to moderate OSA and significant daytime symptoms.[41]

Common side effects of CPAP treatment include discomfort, nasal congestion, abdominal bloating, and mask leak. There have been technical improvements in CPAP devices such as sleek design, the addition of humidification systems, and enhanced treatment monitoring, A wide variety of masks and interfaces geared toward better fit and comfort now exist. It is unclear whether these advances improve adherence to CPAP but they likely improve comfort and acceptance in those who are adherent to treatment. Automatically titrating CPAP (auto-CPAP) and bilevel positive airway pressure (BiPAP) may relieve discomfort in those requiring high treatment pressures, but they have not been shown to increase adherence.[42]

Other supportive interventions that would intuitively seem beneficial include electronic adherence monitoring systems that are currently included with most CPAP devices and CPAP mask desensitization techniques, in which the patient wears the disconnected mask for increasing periods of time while awake to allow sufficient acclimatization to allow sleep with the mask on at night. At this time, hard evidence showing that these interventions improve CPAP adherence or outcomes is not available.

Despite the significant quality of life and potential health benefits attributed to CPAP, adherence to treatment remains low. Adequate CPAP adherence has been proposed to be usage of least 4 hours per night, 70% of nights, but the optimal number of hours per night and frequency of usage to reap therapeutic benefits is not well established. Weaver et al. found that in severe OSA patients with subjective sleepiness at baseline, the greatest proportion normalized their subjective sleepiness with 4 hours per night of CPAP use and that there was a linear improvement in functional status up to 7 hours per night of use, implying that more CPAP usage results in better outcomes.[43] However, suboptimal CPAP usage may still provide some benefit. In a recent randomized controlled trial of patients with moderate to severe OSA who were at high risk for cardiovascular disease but without EDS, there were significant improvements in quality of life measures, especially body pain. These improvements were seen despite an average CPAP use of less than 4 hours per night.[44]

CPAP Treatment Adherence

Studies have indicated that 5–50% of patients recommended CPAP may simply reject treatment before even trying it, and a further 12–25% of patients abandon it within 3 years after initiation.[45] Using the adherence criteria of 4 or more hours of use nightly during 70% of nights, CPAP nonadherence has been reported in 46–83% of patients for whom it has been prescribed.[46]

Severity of OSA and daytime sleepiness are the most well-studied patient factors that may influence CPAP adherence. Patients who lack OSA symptoms may have larger initial rejection rates compared to those with symptoms. African American race and low socioeconomic status are associated with lower CPAP adherence.[47] More recently, increased nasal resistance has been associated with rejection of CPAP.[48] Those with comorbid insomnia may also have decreased adherence due to heightened awareness of CPAP discomfort. Patients with good social support and supportive partners tend to have higher CPAP adherence.

Early experiences with CPAP predict long-term adherence. Long-term CPAP adherence may be established as early as the first week of treatment.[49] Understanding the barriers to CPAP usage and employing early, cost-effective, multidisciplinary interventions are needed to increase CPAP acceptance and long-term adherence.

Increasing CPAP Adherence

Numerous studies have explored supportive measures, patient education, and behavioral interventions to improve CPAP adherence. Supportive measures involve early and intensive outreach to address barriers to and difficulties with CPAP treatment. Educational interventions impart knowledge about OSA and treatment with CPAP and are important since knowledge is a precondition for health behavior or change in health behavior. Behavioral interventions target modifiable constructs from psychological theories of health behavior change and preexisting health beliefs. Behavioral interventions include strategies to promote self-efficacy (the ability to make a behavior change during times when such a change is expected to be difficult), assess outcome expectations, and influence decisional balance toward CPAP.

A Cochrane Review examined the efficacy of supportive, educational, and behavioral interventions on increasing CPAP usage.[50] Thirty studies with a total of 2,047 adults with OSA were included. The vast majority of participants in these studies were new to CPAP and had severe OSA. All three interventions increased CPAP usage to varying degrees. Supportive interventions included telephone calls, CPAP machine downloads, and patient encounters. Supportive interventions increased CPAP usage by about 50 minutes per night. Educational interventions included videos, didactics, written materials, and telephone calls, and these increased average CPAP usage by about 35 minutes per night. Behavioral interventions, including motivational interviewing and cognitive-behavioral therapy, resulted in the largest increase in hours at 1.44 hours per night. The authors concluded that there was at least low to moderate evidence that these interventions improved CPAP usage. It is unclear whether any of these interventions led to meaningful improvements of daytime sleepiness or quality of life.

Significant limitations existed within the studies reviewed. The interventions were not blinded. Most of the participants had daytime sleepiness and may have already perceived a benefit to CPAP. The studies were of short duration and therefore it is unknown which interventions would have long-lasting effects. There were also no data on whether these interventions would improve use in patients who have already been shown to be nonadherent to CPAP. The supportive, educational, and behavioral interventions were carried out in a variety of ways, sometimes in combination, but all required time and resources, which may limit implementation in certain healthcare systems.

More recently, the addition of motivational enhancement programs to standard education and support has shown promise in increasing CPAP adherence. Lai et al. randomized newly diagnosed OSA patients to either usual care or a brief motivational enhancement and education program (BMEEP).[51] The usual care group received a 15-minute talk by a sleep center nurse to introduce the basic operation of the CPAP device before the start of in-laboratory CPAP titration and a 30-minute acclimatization to the CPAP device. The next day, patients met with a medical officer for an explanation of OSA and a discussion of the test results and the prescribed treatment, followed by further advice from a nurse regarding the importance of CPAP therapy and care of the accessories. In addition to usual care, the intervention group was shown a 25-minute video that included the real-life experience of a current CPAP user and given a booklet on OSA and CPAP the morning after CPAP titration. A 20-minute patient-centered face-to-face brief motivational interview followed that aimed to facilitate the subject's intrinsic motivation toward CPAP therapy. Two days later, a follow-up phone call was made by the individual who conducted the motivational enhancement. CPAP usage data were downloaded at 3 months. Compared to the usual care group, the intervention group had higher daily CPAP usage by 2 hours/day and a fourfold increase in the number using CPAP for 70% or more of days for at least 4 hours per day. In addition, the intervention group had greater improvements in Epworth sleepiness scores and treatment self-efficacy. This motivational enhancement program required only one face-to-face session and a follow-up phone call, making it feasible for healthcare systems with limited resources to administer.

Padilla et al. was able to adapt this motivational enhancement program in a Los Angeles County sleep center via a program entitled "CPAP Bootcamp."[52] The patients in this study were predominantly Hispanic with much higher BMIs but similar sleepiness scores as those in the study done by Lai et al. A dedicated face-to-face visit was done, during which a video containing a CPAP patient testimonial was shown followed by a motivational interview gauging the patients' perception of the importance of CPAP use and confidence that they would be able to use it. Similar to BMEEP, a positive summary statement at the end of the visit and negative message framing stressing the complications of not using CPAP were used. A separate face-to-face reinforcement visit was done sometimes several weeks after the initial encounter. Compared to patients who did not receive CPAP Bootcamp, adherence was similar at 1 month but significantly higher at 3 months, likely due to the delay of several weeks of the reinforcement visit and higher than average baseline CPAP adherence in this population.

Bakker et al. compared two groups of patients with moderate to severe OSA without excessive sleepiness but with or at risk for cardiovascular disease.[53] Both groups received standardized supportive and educational interventions that included a 14-day run-in before randomization wearing an unattached nasal mask and a 1-hour standardized educational session by a sleep technologist. The intervention group received, in addition, motivational enhancement delivered by a trained psychologist during two hour-long sessions, along with an initial educational video and six follow-up phone calls. CPAP adherence at 6 months was 3.3 hours per night in the standard group and 4.4 hours per night for the motivational enhancement group, a difference of 99 minutes per night. This difference in adherence remained intact for a subset of patients followed for more than a year, suggesting that motivational enhancement is a promising intervention for improving adherence in a group of relatively asymptomatic patients. The interventions undertaken in this study were time- and personnel-intensive and may not be feasible for healthcare systems with limited resources.

Adjunctive Treatment for OSA and Alternatives to CPAP

OSA is a chronic disease: treatment is long-term and requires a multidisciplinary approach. CPAP alone is not adequate to treat OSA. Behavioral modifications such as weight loss and exercise are integral to the treatment for OSA. When first-line treatment with CPAP fails, perhaps due to intolerance or nonadherence, alternatives, such as surgery or oral appliances, can be considered. All treatment decisions should involve the patient.

Behavioral and Lifestyle Modifications. Weight loss should be recommended for all overweight OSA patients. Although the effects of weight loss on OSA are variable, weight loss may improve AHI. Weight loss is not a primary treatment for OSA due to a low cure rate of OSA by dietary weight loss, and therefore a primary mode of treatment such as CPAP should be continued. After substantial weight loss (e.g., 10% or more of body weight), a follow-up PSG should be obtained to re-assess severity of OSA and to make CPAP pressure adjustments if needed.[17]

Bariatric surgery is considered in patients with a BMI of 40 kg/m^2 or more or in those with a BMI of 35 kg/m^2 or more who also have comorbidities and lack of success with conventional weight loss strategies. Bariatric surgery can result in significant weight loss and elimination of OSA. The remission rates for OSA in these patients is 40%, thus necessitating ongoing monitoring and follow-up testing.[54]

Avoidance of alcohol and tobacco products should be encouraged. Sedatives such as benzodiazepines and opioids should also be discouraged. These substances can lead to worsening OSA severity and are particularly hazardous when OSA is untreated.

Positional therapies that keep a patient in a non-supine position may be an adjunct in the treatment of OSA. Devices such as alarms, pillows, backpacks, or tennis balls can keep a patient on his or her side and dramatically reduce the severity of OSA. These treatments are often used in conjunction with primary therapy because patients may not completely normalize their AHI.

Oral Appliances. Oral appliances such as mandibular advance devices and tongue retaining devices are designed to maintain the mandible or tongue in a protruded position to prevent upper airway collapse during sleep. Oral appliances are the second most commonly used therapy to treat OSA after CPAP. Although generally regarded to be most efficacious in mild to moderate OSA, there is evidence that they can be effective in treating severe OSA by reducing AHI and improving symptoms in more severely affected patients. Although dental appliances have been less efficacious than CPAP in reducing upper airway obstruction, they appear to be tolerated better than PAP modalities. Short-term benefits from a mandibular advancing device, including a primary outcome of mean arterial pressure and several secondary outcomes, were found to be not inferior to that from CPAP.[55] A limiting factor for widespread dental appliance use is that the devices tend to be associated with more patient expense than CPAP and require fitting and oversight by a dental professional to avoid complications such as temporomandibular joint (TMJ) disease and dental malalignment.

Surgical Treatment. Surgical treatment for OSA can be considered in patients with mild OSA with obstructing anatomy that is surgically correctable or in those with more severe forms of OSA who are intolerant of CPAP therapy. Tracheostomy can eliminate OSA but is not often desirable for patients. Maxillary and mandibular advancement can provide treatment of OSA with similar efficacy to CPAP.[56] However, this procedure requires high surgical expertise and involves breaking and repositioning facial bones, often done in conjunction with advancement of the genioglossus muscle. Recovery can be prolonged and painful with this particular surgery. Most other surgeries for OSA, including uvulopalatoplasty, are less effective for the treatment of OSA.

Hypoglossal Nerve Stimulation. Hypoglossal nerve stimulation is achieved via a surgically implanted device. A stimulator is connected to the right hypoglossal nerve to activate the genioglossus muscle and protrude the tongue forward during stimulation. An effort sensor is placed within the intercostal muscles to sync nerve stimulation to respirations. Forward movement of the tongue and soft tissue palate creates enlargement of the retrolingual and retropalatal airways.

The Stimulation Therapy for Apnea Reduction (STAR) trial was a 12-month prospective multicenter cohort study of 126 participants with moderate to severe OSA with difficulty accepting or adhering to CPAP therapy.[57] The study included primarily middle-aged men with an average BMI of 28. Those who were screened underwent drug-induced sedation endoscopy, and those with complete collapse at the retropalatal airway were excluded from the study. Upper airway stimulation led to a 68% reduction in the AHI (29 to 9 events per hour) and a 70% reduction in the oxygen desaturation index (ODI) (25.4 to 7.4 events per hour). There were also significant improvements in daytime sleepiness and quality of life measures. In a randomized therapy withdrawal arm, a group of responders went off therapy for a week and regressed toward their baseline AHI compared to those who continued therapy.

It is important to note that 43 of the 126 (34%) participants did not respond to treatment, there is a high upfront cost associated with this therapy, and that those with morbid obesity, cardiovascular comorbidities, and concomitant CSA are unlikely to benefit from this therapy.

Myofunctional Therapy. The dilator muscles of the upper airway play a critical role in maintaining upper airway patency during sleep. Therefore, singing, didgeridoo, and other wind instrument playing have been explored as a potential treatment for OSA. Guimareaes et al. developed isotonic and isometric exercises to treat OSA.[58] These exercises target the soft palate, tongue, and facial muscles and involve exercises such as pronouncing vowels and moving the tongue along the superior and lateral surfaces of the teeth. Speech therapy often administers this therapy. Although a meta-analysis has shown a reduction in AHI of 50% in adults,[59] there are limited data for long-term efficacy beyond 6 months.

Nasal EPAP. Nasal expiratory positive airway pressure (EPAP) consists of a one-way resister valve placed over each nostril via a disposable adhesive device that uses the patient's own breathing to generate end expiratory pressure, thereby leading to upper airway dilatation. It is portable, has a minimal footprint, and does not require electricity. In a recent meta-analysis, nasal EPAP has been shown to reduce AHI by about 50%.[60] This device may be an effective treatment in patients with mild to moderate OSA. Although it is generally not adequate to treat severe OSA, it may improve quality of life and daytime sleepiness in patients who cannot tolerate CPAP.

Medical Cannabis. Medical cannabis has varying effects on sleep. Delta-9 tetrahydrocannabinol (THC) is the primary active component of cannabis that results in euphoria, hallucinations, and anxiety. Dronabinol, a synthetic THC, has been studied in OSA. In animal studies, it has been shown to improve respiratory stability through peripheral serotonergic antagonism. Prasad et al. reported a reduction in AHI of 32% at 3 weeks compared to baseline. A recent placebo-controlled randomized trial with patients with moderate to severe OSA found that dronabinol reduced AHI by 33%.[61] Side effects in both of these trials included sleepiness and drowsiness. It is important to note that these studies were limited due to small sample size and short duration (3–6 weeks).[62] Long-term treatment effects and side effects of cannabinoids such as THC on patients with OSA are unknown. In addition, medical cannabis contains highly variable compositions of cannabinoids and is unregulated, which may lead to variable treatment effects in OSA. Therefore, medical cannabis is not a currently recommended treatment for OSA. Further research in synthetic cannabis may lead to better targeted therapies for OSA with fewer side effects.

There are currently no medications specifically for the treatment of OSA. Hypnotic agents have been proposed to increase the arousal threshold in patients with OSA. However, these medications may ultimately reduce pharyngeal muscle activity and worsen OSA. Stimulants, such as modafinil, can improve daytime sleepiness associated with OSA but are unable to target the disease directly.

SUMMARY

OSA is a highly prevalent yet underdiagnosed disorder associated with EDS, impaired functioning, motor vehicle accidents, and cardiovascular disease. CPAP is the treatment of choice, but adherence remains poor. Support, education, and motivational enhancement show some promise in increasing CPAP adherence. Adjunctive and alternative therapies for OSA do exist but none has been proved as efficacious as CPAP. In the future, a personalized approach to the treatment of

OSA is needed, one that targets not just the anatomic aspect of this disease but also the other associated traits, such as low arousal threshold and poor muscle responsiveness. Perhaps in the future medication to target different aspects of OSA will be developed. For now, early and cost-effective interventions should be done to improve CPAP adherence.

Central Sleep Apnea

CSA is characterized by the repetitive cessation of breathing due to lack of respiratory effort during sleep. This is in contrast to OSA, where there is ongoing respiratory effort during periods of apnea. Like OSA, CSA can lead to increased nocturnal arousals and EDS. The prevalence of CSA is low in the general population. The most common associated conditions in patients with CSA are congestive heart failure (CHF), atrial fibrillation, stroke, and the chronic use of long-acting opioids.

Treatment of CSA may depend on the underlying condition. For instance, reductions in opioid dosage in patients with high opioid usage can improve CSA. In heart failure, optimizing medications, cardiac resynchronization therapy, and atrial overdrive pacing have led to improvements in CSA in these patients.

CPAP can be an effective treatment for CSA in some patients, but the mechanism for this is unclear. Some CSA patients do not respond to CPAP. The CANPAP trial proved that CPAP could attenuate CSA in heart failure patients. However, there was no beneficial effect on morbidity or mortality.[63] A post-hoc analysis showed that CSA was adequately treated and that there was a positive effect on both left ventricular ejection fraction and survival.[64] BiPAP, due to its ability to augment alveolar ventilation, can precipitate CSA and is therefore contraindicated as a treatment.

Adaptive servo-ventilation (ASV) is a form of bilevel ventilation that alleviates CSA by providing breath-to-breath adjustment of inspiratory pressure support with a back-up rate to normalize breathing patterns. It mitigates hyperventilation and associated hypocapnia. EPAP is used to stabilize upper airway obstruction. EPAP devices such as the Phillps-Respironics ASV deliver varying amounts pressure support (minimum and maximum is set) to target a peak flow based on peak flow values of preceding breaths. The ResMed ASV delivers varying amounts of pressure support based on minute ventilation from a preceding window of time. ASV can be used to treat varying forms of CSA and at one time was routinely used in the treatment of CSA associated with heart failure. In 2015, however, Cowie et al. published data on heart failure patients with an ejection fraction of 45% or less which showed that treatment with ASV led to an increase in all-cause and cardiovascular mortality in these patients.[65] It is thought that perhaps CSA is a compensatory mechanism in heart failure and that correcting it led to these findings.

Therefore, ASV is no longer recommended in CSA patients with heart failure and a low ejection fraction.

Cheyne-Stokes respirations is a pattern of CSA characterized by a central apnea followed by hyperventilation in a crescendo-decrescendo pattern. This occurs most often in patients with CHF and may signify poor prognosis. Oxygen therapy can attenuate Cheyne-Stokes respirations by reducing peripheral chemoresponsiveness and allowing CO_2 to rise above the apnea threshold.

CSA can arise in patients with primary OSA who begin treatment with CPAP. Complex sleep apnea or treatment-emergent sleep apnea occurs because CPAP reduces upper airway resistance, thereby improving the efficiency of CO_2 excretion and rendering the patient hypocapnic and thus leading to apnea. CPAP may also lead to increased lung volume, activation of stretch reflexes, and consequently the inhibition of ventilation. This is seen in patients who are overtitrated during CPAP titration studies. Complex sleep apnea has been minimally studied and there are no long-term data available. However, treatment-emergent central apneas are thought to frequently self-resolve with continued CPAP treatment since CSA is relatively uncommon among patients receiving stable CPAP.[66] There are studies that suggest ASV may lower the AHI in these patients.[67]

Sleep-Related Hypoventilation

Patients with chronic hypoventilation, also known has *chronic hypercapnic respiratory failure*, have diminished minute ventilation, elevations in $PaCO_2$ greater than 45, and evidence of metabolic compensation. Neuromuscular diseases and restrictive chest wall physiology, obesity hypoventilation syndrome, and chronic obstructive pulmonary disease (COPD) are common conditions leading to chronic hypoventilation, but these differ significantly in the pathophysiology leading to hypoventilation. Sleep-related hypoventilation may be the earliest manifestation of chronic hypoventilation because sleep is associated with a reduction of minute ventilation and a rise in CO_2 even in healthy persons. Symptoms of hypoventilation during sleep may include poor sleep quality, EDS, or morning headache, but the vast majority of patients report little to no symptoms. Sleep-related hypoventilation may be diagnosed on PSG using end-tidal CO_2 monitoring showing rises in CO_2 for greater than 10 minutes during sleep. Prolonged oxygen desaturations with low O_2 nadirs (<85%) are also suggestive of hypoventilation.

Due to the increasing prevalence of obesity, the respiratory consequences of extreme obesity, including *obesity hypoventilation syndrome* (OHS), are being recognized. OHS is defined when a patient exhibits a daytime PCO_2 greater than 45, a BMI of more than 30 (usually greater than 40), and other causes of hypoventilation have been excluded. The pathophysiology is not fully understood, but it is postulated that excess weight leads to pronounced decreases in lung volumes and increased work of breathing: CO_2 production increases due to a more rapid and shallow breathing pattern and blunted responses to hypercapnia and hypoxemia. Hormones like leptin (acts to suppress appetite and stimulate ventilation) and insulin-like growth factor-1 may lead to altered ventilatory control. OHS is associated with substantial morbidity and mortality including recurrent cardiorespiratory decompensation requiring intensive care management, mechanical ventilation, and prolonged hospital stays.

As one would expect, more than 90% of patients with OHS have OSA. Conversely, only about 10–20% of OSA patients have OHS. Patients with COPD may have comorbid OSA (overlap syndrome) which leads to more hypercapnia, pulmonary hypertension, and right heart failure. Even patients with neuromuscular disorders such as Duchenne muscular dystrophy may have breathing disturbances that begin with OSA. Therefore, part of the treatment for chronic hypoventilation disorders is addressing upper airway obstruction with adequate expiratory pressure (EPAP). The mainstay of treatment for hypoventilation, however, is countering elevated CO_2 with increased respiratory frequency and tidal volumes. Bilevel ventilation with a backup respiratory rate (BiPAP-ST) can generate enough pressure support (IPAP – EPAP) to augment ventilation. Volume-assured pressure support (VAPS) devices have been developed to automatically adjust pressure support from breath to breath in order to reach an adequate tidal volume or minute ventilation. Both devices have been used to successfully treat nocturnal hypoventilation. VAPS has been associated with lower CO_2 levels than BiPAP-ST but not necessarily better outcomes.

Conclusion

The most commonly encountered sleep-related breathing disorder is OSA. It is increasingly prevalent, underdiagnosed, can lead to significant daytime sleepiness and disability, and has been associated with a number of cardiovascular diseases. CPAP is the treatment of choice for OSA but lack of adherence to CPAP is an ongoing challenge to clinicians. Supportive care, education, and motivational enhancement programs do show promise in improving compliance. Alternatives to CPAP have not been proved as efficacious but may provide some benefit in patients who would otherwise go untreated. In the future, personalized treatment targeting various aspects of OSA, not just the anatomic aspect, may be the best way to approach this condition.

CSA can be seen in patients with heart failure, chronic opioid use, and other medical conditions but is rarely idiopathic. Treatment largely depends on the underlying condition. ASV can be used in patients with central apnea provided these patients do not have heart failure with a low ejection fraction. Oxygen therapy can be used to attenuate Cheyne-Stokes respirations associated with heart failure.

Complex sleep apnea occurs in OSA patients being titrated to CPAP, and the natural course of this condition is to self-resolve. Otherwise, ASV can be used to treat this condition.

Sleep-related hypoventilation occurs commonly in patients with morbid obesity, COPD, and neuromuscular diseases with restrictive chest wall physiology and is characterized by hypercapnia. Treatment involves treating concomitant OSA and the utilization of more advanced modes of noninvasive ventilation such as BiPAP-ST and AVAPS.

The treatment of sleep-related breathing disorders is complex and includes seeking patient input when determining a treatment plan, understanding barriers to treatment, and reevaluating patients after treatment is initiated. Successful treatment of sleep-disordered breathing can lead to improvements in daytime function, quality of life, and overall health.

REFERENCES

1. Young T, Peppard P, Gottlieb D. Epidemiology of obstructive sleep apnea: A population health perspective. *Am J Resp Crit Care Med.* 2002;65:1217–1239.
2. Young T, Palta M, Dempsey J, et al. The occurrence of sleep-disordered breathing among middle-aged adults. *N Engl J Med.* 1993;328(17):1230–1235.
3. Peppard PE, Young T, Barnet JH, et al. Increased prevalence of sleep-disordered breathing in adults. *Am J Epidemiology.* 2013;177(9):1006–1014.
4. Eckert DJ, White DP, Jordan AS, et al. Defining phenotypic causes of obstructive sleep apnea: Identification of novel therapeutic targets. *Am J of Resp Crit Care Med.* 2013;188(8):996–1004.
5. Young T, Finn L, Austin D, et al. Menopausal status and sleep-disordered breathing in the Wisconsin Sleep Cohort Study. *Am J Resp Crit Care Med.* 2003;167:1181–1185.
6. Schwartz AR, Patil SP, Laffan AM, et al. Obesity and obstructive sleep apnea: Pathogenic mechanisms and therapeutic approaches. *Proc Am Thor Soc.* Feb 15 2008;5(2):185–192.
7. Malhotra A, White D. Obstructive sleep apnea. *Lancet.* 2002;360:237–245.
8. Young T, Peppard P, Gottlieb D. Epidemiology of obstructive sleep apnea: A population health perspective. *Am J Resp Crit Care Med.* 2002;165:1217–1239.
9. Tsai W, Remmers J, Brant R, et al. A decision rule for diagnostic testing in obstructive sleep apnea. *Am J Resp Crit Care Med.* 2003;167:1427–1432.
10. Cakirer B, Hans M, Graham G, et al. The relationship between craniofacial morphology and obstructive sleep apnea in whites and in African-Americans. *Am J Resp Crit Care Med.* 2001;163:947–950.
11. Redline S, Sotres-Alvarez D, Loredo J, et al. Sleep-disordered breathing in Hispanic/Latino individuals of diverse backgrounds; The Hispanic Community Health Study/Study of Latinos. *Am J Resp Crit Care Med.* 2014;189(3):335–344.

12. Ip M, Lam B, Lauder I, et al. A community study of sleep-disordered breathing in middle-aged Chinese men in Hong Kong. *Chest.* 2001;119:62–69.

13. Watanabe T, Isono S, Tanaka A, et al. Contribution of body habitus and craniofacial characteristics to segmental closing pressures of the passive pharynx in patients with sleep-disordered breathing. *Am J Resp Crit Care Med.* 2002;165:260–265.

14. Mitler MM, Dawson A, Henriksen SJ, et al. Bedtime ethanol increases resistance of upper airways and produces sleep apneas in asymptomatic snorers. *Alcohol Clin Exp Res.* Dec 1988;12(6):801–805.

15. Nuckton T, Glidden D, Browner W, et al. Physical examination: Mallampati score as an independent predictor of obstructive sleep apnea. *Sleep.* 2006;29:903–908.

16. Kapur VK, Auckley DH, Chowdhuri S, et al. Clinical practice guideline for diagnostic testing for adult obstructive sleep apnea: An American Academy of Sleep medicine clinical practice guideline. *J Clin Sleep Med.* 2017;13(3):479–504.

17. Adult Obstructive Sleep Apnea Task Force of the American Academy of Sleep Medicine. Clinical guideline for the evaluation, management and long-term care of obstructive sleep apnea in adults. *J Clin Sleep Med.* 2009;5(3):263–276.

18. Engleman H, Joffe D. Neuropsychological function in obstructive sleep apnoea. *Sleep Med Rev.* 1999;3(1):59–78.

19. Tregear S, Reston J, Schoelles K, Phillips B. Obstructive sleep apnea and risk of motor vehicle crash: Systematic review and meta-analysis. *J Clin Sleep Med.* 2009;5(10):573–581.

20. Gurubhagavatula I, Sullivan S, Meoli A, et al. Management of obstructive sleep apnea in commercial motor vehicle operators: Recommendations of the AASM Sleep and Transportation Safety Awareness Task Force. *J Clin Sleep Med.* 2017;13(5):745–758.

21. Young T, Finn L, Peppard PE, et al. Sleep-disordered breathing and mortality: Eighteen-year follow-up of the Wisconsin sleep cohort. *Sleep.* 2008;31(8):1071–1078.

22. Wang X, Ouyang Y, Wang Z, et al. Obstructive sleep apnea and risk of cardiovascular disease and all-cause mortality: A meta-analysis of prospective cohort studies. *Int J Cardiol.* 2013;169(3):207–214.

23. Peppard PE, Young T, Palta M, et al. Prospective study of the association between sleep-disordered breathing and hypertension. *N Engl J Med.* 2000;342:1378–1384.

24. Dernaika TA, Kinasewitz GT, Tawk MM. Effects of nocturnal continuous positive airway pressure therapy in patients with resistant hypertension and obstructive sleep apnea. *J Clin Sleep Med.* 2009;5(2):103–107.

25. Marin JM, Carrizo SJ, Vicente E, et al. Long-term cardiovascular outcomes in men with obstructive sleep apnoea-hypopnoea with or without treatment with continuous positive airway pressure: An observational study. *Lancet.* 2005;365(9464):1046–1053.

26. Mehra R, Benjamin EJ, Shahar E, et al. Association of nocturnal arrhythmias with sleep-disordered breathing: The Sleep Heart Health Study. *Am J Respir Crit Care Med.* 2006;173(8):910–916.

27. Abe H, Takahashi M, Yaegashi H. Efficacy of continuous positive airway pressure om arrythmias in obstructive sleep apnea. *Heart Vessels.* 2010;25(1):63–69.

28. Kanagala R, Murali NS, Friendman PA. Obstructive sleep apnea and the recurrence of atrial fibrillation. *Circulation.* 2003;107:2589–2594.

29. Arzt M, Young T, Finn L, Skatrud JB, Bradley TD. Association of sleep-disordered breathing and the occurrence of stroke. *Am J Respir Crit Care Med.* 2005;172(11):1447–1451.

30. Yaggi HK, Concato J, Kernan WN, Lichtman JH, Brass LM, Mohsenin V. Obstructive sleep apnea as a risk factor for stroke and death. *N Engl J Med.* 2005;353(19):2034–2041.

31. Redline S, Yenokyan G, Gottlieb DJ, et al. Obstructive sleep apnea-hypopnea and incident stroke: The Sleep Heart Health Study. *Am J Respir Crit Care Med.* 2010;182(2):269–277.

32. Shalin C, Sandburg O, Gastafson Y. Obstructive sleep apnea is a risk factor for death in patients with stroke: A 10-year follow-up. *Arch Int Med.* 2008;168(3):297–301.

33. Martinez-Garcia MA, Soler-Cataluna JJ, Ejarque-Martinez L, et al. Continuous positive airway pressure treatment reduces mortality in patients with ischemic stroke and obstructive sleep apnea: A 5-year followup study. *Am J Respir Crit Care Med.* 2009;180(1)36–41.

34. Punjabi N, Shahar E, Redline S. Sleep-disordered breathing, glucose intolerance, and insulin resistance: The sleep heart health study. *Am J Epidemiology,* 2004;160(6):521–530.

35. Gross JB, Apfelbaum JL, Caplan RA, et al. Practice guidelines for the perioperative management of patients with obstructive sleep apnea: An updated report by the American Society of Anesthesiologists Task Force on Perioperative Management of Patients with Obstructive Sleep Apnea. *Anesthesiology.* 2014;120:268–286.

36. American Academy of Sleep Medicine. In an Age of Constant Activity, the Solution to Improving the Nation's Health May Lie in Helping It Sleep Better. 2016. http://www.aasmnet.org/sleep-apnea-economic-impact.aspx.

37. Sullivan CE, Issa FG, Berthon-Jones M, et al. Reversal of obstructive sleep apnoea by continuous positive airway pressure applied through the nares. *Lancet.* 1981;1(8225):862–865.

38. Gay P, Weaver T, Loube D, et al. Evaluation of positive airway pressure treatment for sleep related breathing disorders in adults. *Sleep.* 2006;29(3):381–401

39. Giles TL, Lasserson TJ, Smith BJ, et al. Continuous positive airways pressure for obstructive sleep apnoea in adults. *Cochrane Database Syst Rev.* 2006;(3):CD001106.

40. Karimi M, Hedner J, Häbel H, et al. Sleep apnea related risk of motor vehicle accidents is reduced by continuous positive airway pressure: Swedish Traffic Accident Registry Data. *Sleep.* 2015;38(3):341–349.

41. Weaver TE, Mancini C, Maislin G, et al. Continuous positive airway pressure treatment of sleepy patients with milder obstructive sleep apnea: Results of the CPAP Apnea Trial North American Program (CATNAP) randomized clinical trial. *Am J Respir Crit Care Med.* 2012 Oct 1;186(7):677–683.

42. Positive Airway Pressure Titration Task Force of the American Academy of Sleep Medicine. Clinical guidelines for the manual titration of positive airway pressure in patients with obstructive sleep apnea. *J Clin Sleep Med.* 2008;4(2):157–171.

43. Weaver T, Maislin G, Dinges D, et al. Relationship between hours of CPAP use and achieving normal levels of sleepiness and daily functioning. *Sleep.* 2007;30:711–719.

44. Zhao YY, Wang R, Gleason KJ, et al. Effect of continuous positive airway pressure treatment on health-related quality of life and sleepiness in high cardiovascular risk individuals with sleep apnea: Best Apnea Interventions for Research (BestAIR) trial. *Sleep.* 2017;40(4):zsx040. doi:10.1093/sleep/zsx040.

45. Engleman HM, Wild MR. Improving CPAP use by patients with the sleep apnoea/hypopnoea syndrome (SAHS). *Sleep Med Rev.* 2003;7:81–99.

46. Weaver TE, Grunstein RR. Adherence to continuous positive airway pressure therapy: The challenge to effective treatment. *Proc Am Thorac Soc.* 2008 Feb 15;5(2):173–178.

47. Billings ME, Auckley D, Benca R, et al. Race and residential socioeconomics as predictors of CPAP adherence. *Sleep.* 2011 Dec 1;34(12):1653–1658.

48. Sawyer AM, Gooneratne N, Marcus CL, et al. A systematic review of CPAP adherence across age groups: Clinical and empiric insights for developing CPAP adherence interventions. *Sleep Med Rev.* 2011;15(6):343–356. doi:10.1016/j.smrv.2011.01.003.

49. Aloia MS, Arnedt JT, Stanchina M, et al. How early in treatment is PAP adherence established? Revisiting night-to-night variability. *Behav Sleep Med.* 2007;5:229–240.

50. Wozniak DR, Lasserson TJ, Smith I. Educational, supportive and behavioural interventions to improve usage of continuous positive airway pressure machines in adults with obstructive sleep apnoea. *Cochrane Database Syst Rev.* 2014;(1):CD007736. doi:10.1002/14651858.CD007736.pub2.

51. Lai AYK, Fong DYT, Lam JCM, et al. The efficacy of a brief motivational enhancement education program on CPAP adherence in OSA: A Randomized Controlled Trial. *Chest.* 2014;146(3):600–610.

52. Padilla AJ, Katalbas M, Deutsch P, et al. Adaptation of a brief motivational enhancement education program during CPAP initiation to an academic public sleep clinic. 31st Annual Meeting of the Associated Professional Sleep Societies (Abstract Supplement). *Sleep.* 2017;40:Abstract 1192.

53. Bakker JP, Wang R, Weng J, et al. Motivational enhancement for increasing adherence to CPAP: A randomized controlled trial. *Chest.* 2016;150(2):337–345.

54. Mechanick JI, Kushner RF, Sugerman HJ, et al. American Association of Clinical Endocrinologists, The Obesity Society, and American Society for Metabolic & Bariatric Surgery Medical guidelines for clinical practice for the perioperative nutritional, metabolic, and nonsurgical support of the bariatric surgery patient. *Endocr Pract.* 2008;14(Suppl 1):1–83.

55. Phillips CL, Grunstein RR, Darendeliler MA, et al. Health outcomes of continuous positive airway pressure versus oral appliance treatment for obstructive sleep apnea: A randomized controlled trial. *Am J Respir Crit Care Med.* 2013;187:879–887.

56. Boyd SB, Walters AS, Waite P, Harding SM, Song Y. Long-term effectiveness and safety of maxillomandibular advancement for treatment of obstructive sleep apnea. *J Clin Sleep Med.* 2015;11(7):699–708.

57. Strollo PJ, Jr, Soose RJ, Maurer JT, et al. Upper-airway stimulation for obstructive sleep apnea. *N Engl J Med.* 2014;370:139–149.

58. Guimaraes KC, Drager LF, Genta PR, Marcondes BF, Lorenzi-Filho G. Effects of oropharyngeal exercises on patients with moderate obstructive sleep apnea syndrome. *Am J Respir Crit Care Med.* 2009;179:962–966.

59. Camacho M, Certal V, Abdullatif J, et al. Myofunctional therapy to treat obstructive sleep apnea: A systematic review and meta-analysis. *Sleep.* 2015;38(5):669–675. doi:10.5665/sleep.4652.

60. Riaz M, Certal V, Nigam G, et al. Nasal expiratory positive airway pressure devices (Provent) for OSA: A systematic review and meta-analysis. *Sleep Dis.* 2015;2015:734798. doi:10.1155/2015/734798.

61. Prasad B, Radulovacki MG, Carley DW. Proof of concept trial of dronabinol in obstructive sleep apnea. *Front Psychiatry.* 2013;4:1.

62. Carley DW, Prasad B, Reid KJ, et al. Pharmacotherapy of apnea by cannabimimetic enhancement, the PACE Clinical Trial: Effects of dronabinol in obstructive sleep apnea. *Sleep.* 2018;41(1):1–13.

63. Bradley TD, Logan AG, Kimoff RJ. Continuous positive airway pressure for central sleep apnea and heart failure. *N Engl J Med.* 2005;353:2025–2033.

64. Arzt M, Floras JS, Logan AG. Suppression of central sleep apnea by continuous positive airway pressure and transplant free survival in heart failure: A post-hoc analysis of the Canadian Continuous Positive Airway Pressure for patients with Central Sleep Apnea and Heart Failure Trial (CANPAP). *Circulation.* 2007;115(25):3173–3180.

65. Cowie MR, Woehrle H, Wegscheider K. Adaptive servo-ventilation for central sleep apnea in systolic heart failure. *N Engl J Med.* 2015;373:1095–1105.

66. Javaheri S, Smith J, Chung E. The prevalence and natural history of complex sleep apnea. *J Clin Sleep Med.* 2009;5(3):205–211.

67. Morgenthaler TI, Kuzniar TJ, Wolfe LF, et al. The Complex Sleep Apnea Resolution Study: A prospective randomized controlled trial of continuous positive airway pressure versus adaptive servoventilation therapy. *Sleep.* 2014;37(5):927–934. doi:10.5665/sleep.3662.

32

Circadian Sleep Disorders

SHADAB A. RAHMAN AND ELIZABETH B. KLERMAN

Overview

Circadian rhythm sleep wake disorders (CRSWDs) are characterized by sleep occurring at an "inappropriate time." The timing, content, and consolidation of sleep depends on the interaction of at least two physiologic factors[1,2]: (1) the internal circadian clock's influence, and (2) the homeostatic need for sleep, which builds with increasing duration awake and dissipates during sleep (also see Chapter 5). For most people, the physiologically promoted time for sleep initiation is at night at a circadian phase (i.e., time) shortly (~2 hours) after melatonin begins to be secreted and when the homeostatic need for sleep is high. Some CRSWDs may arise if sleep occurs when these two processes are not optimally aligned. Current CRSWD treatment involves ocular light exposure, oral melatonin dosing, sleep scheduling, modifying behavioral choices, and/or meal and exercise timing, rather than the types of interventions used by conventional medicine (e.g., a prescription drug or device or an invasive intervention [e.g., surgery]); most current CRSWD-related interventions are designed to improve the timing of sleep relative to the internal circadian clock.

Circadian Rhythm Sleep Wake Disorders

CRSWDs are diagnosed based on the criteria presented in the *International Classification of Sleep Disorders* (ICSD-3).[3] The ICSD-3 includes seven subtypes: (1) delayed sleep–wake phase disorder (DSWPD), (2) advanced sleep–wake phase disorder (ASWPD), (3) non–24-hour sleep–wake rhythm disorder (N24SWD),

(4) irregular sleep–wake rhythm disorder (ISWRD), (5) shift work disorder (SWD), (6) jet lag disorder (JLD), and (7) circadian sleep–wake disorder not otherwise specified. The ICSD-3 requires 3 months of symptoms except for jet lag disorder. The ICSD-3 applies a general set of criteria to all CRSWDs. These include (1) the sleep–wake rhythm is chronically or recurrently disrupted primarily due to either changes in the endogenous circadian timing system or misalignment between the endogenous circadian rhythm and the desired or required sleep–wake schedule, (2) the sleep–wake disturbance leads to symptoms of insomnia and/or excessive sleepiness, and (3) clinically significant distress or impairment is present. The following sections review the CRSWD subtypes, diagnostics, and treatment options.

Specific Circadian Rhythm Sleep–Wake Disorders

DELAYED SLEEP–WAKE PHASE DISORDER

DSWPD is characterized by bedtimes and wake times that are markedly delayed relative to desired or conventional times.[4] Habitual bedtimes can range between 2 and 4 AM, though some are later than 6 AM, and wake times can be past noon.[5,6] Due to the delayed sleep and wake times, individuals with DSWPD find it difficult to conform to social and/or work schedules that occur earlier in the day; this can precipitate social isolation in some individuals. Multiple studies have documented frequent comorbid psychiatric disorders in patients with DSWPD,[7–10] including depression. Treating patients for DSWPD with melatonin improves depressive symptomatology.[11] When asked to conform to earlier bedtimes, patients with DSWPD face difficulty falling asleep both subjectively and objectively as verified by polysomnography (PSG).[4,12,13]

Patients may also have excessive daytime sleepiness,[14] likely precipitated both by sleep duration being truncated when they must awaken earlier than preferred times and the fact that these awakenings (at earlier than preferred times) occur at circadian phases when subjective sleepiness is high and cognitive performance rhythms are near their nadir.[5] When patients sleep at their preferred times, sleep is of normal quality and duration for age.[5,15] It is common for sleep–wake patterns to differ dramatically between work/school days and non-work/school days in these patients[16] because they can sleep at their preferred times on non-work/school days. Approximately 10% of patients at sleep clinics with complaints of sleep onset insomnia may instead have DSWPD.[4]

DSWPD is one of the more commonly studied CRSWDs, and the estimated prevalence of DSWPD is between 0.2% and 16%,[17,18] with higher rates in younger age groups.

Multiple factors likely contribute to the pathophysiology of DSWPD. People choosing to delay bedtime and stay up later into the evening and early night expose their circadian system to more of the phase-delaying region of the photic phase response curve,[19] causing a circadian phase delay and higher likelihood of staying awake later. Patients with DSWPD may be more sensitive to evening light exposure than are healthy individuals,[4] as evidenced by greater melatonin suppression in DSWPD patients compared to healthy individuals.[20,21] Concurrently, later wake times minimize exposure to phase-advancing light in the morning[19] which would further delay the circadian system.[22] The endogenous circadian phase and sleep can be delayed in healthy individuals without sleep disorders when they live in urban environments with access to nighttime electrical lighting compared to when they are in the wilderness with access to only the natural solar light–dark cycle.[23] Controlled lab-based studies also provide evidence supporting disruptive effects of evening light exposure from personal electronic device usage—pervasive in modern society—on the circadian system and sleep.[24] Since light is the strongest circadian time cue, behavioral choices shaping the light–dark schedule can precipitate a delayed sleep–wake phenotype, especially in vulnerable populations (e.g., those with longer endogenous circadian period or changes in sensitivity to light).

Other potential biological causes of DSWPD include genetics, delayed circadian phase, a long endogenous circadian period, the timing of sleep relative to endogenous circadian phase, and altered dynamics in sleep homeostatic mechanisms. Among the biological factors contributing to the pathophysiology of DSWPD, the most extensively studied is endogenous circadian phase. Several reports show a delayed circadian phase in patients with DSWPD, on average, compared to healthy individuals.[4,13,25,26] However, it is important to note that about 40% of DSPWD patients exhibit a relatively normal circadian phase[13,27]; in a recent study[27] including 103 patients with DSWPD only about 55% of the patients had abnormal circadian phase. Based on these studies, it appears that patients with DSWPD can be further categorized based on their circadian phase as those with and without a delay in their endogenous circadian phase. Even those without a delay in their circadian phase may have an abnormality in their circadian system because the delayed sleep timing, with its associated change in light–dark cycle, would be expected to delay the circadian system, which it does not.

In addition to circadian phase delay, a longer circadian period has been postulated in patients with DSWPD compared to healthy individuals;[25,28] this may contribute to delayed sleep and wake times. Endogenous period is determined by the dynamics in the transcription–translation loops of the molecular circadian clock. The *CRY1* clock gene is part of this molecular clock, and a single report to date has associated a gain of function mutation in the *CRY1* gene in unrelated families with strong heritability of DSWPD.[29] The prevalence rate of this variant, which may play a role in delayed bedtimes, is estimated to be around 0.6% in the general population.[29]

Another biological cause may be altered sleep homeostatic mechanisms, including a slower rate of sleep pressure accumulation across the waking day; this would be expected to be associated with delayed bedtimes. Slower rate of sleep pressure accumulation has been observed in individuals with an evening chronotype.[30] While PSG-based sleep assessments in patients with DSWPD and healthy controls do not suggest differences in sleep architecture (i.e., the duration spent in each stage of sleep) or markers of homeostatic sleep pressure (e.g., sleep latency or amount of slow wave sleep), when DSWPD patients sleep at their habitual bedtimes,[15] DSWPD patients had smaller (compared to a normal cohort) sleep compensatory response following sleep deprivation, suggesting a slower rate of sleep pressure accumulation.[31] Additional studies are required to elucidate the putative role of altered sleep homeostasis in DSWPD patients.

ADVANCED SLEEP–WAKE PHASE DISORDER

In contrast to DSWPD, patients with ASWPD have sleep and wake times that are earlier than desired or conventional.[3] Bedtimes range typically between 6 and 9 PM, and wake times between 2 and 5 AM. Similar to DSWPD, sleep is disrupted when individuals are made to conform to conventional times; when sleep can occur at ASWPD patient's habitual times, then there is minimal deleterious effect on sleep duration or quality.

Prevalence estimates for ASWPD range between 1% and 7% depending on the population studied[32] and are typically higher in men and older individuals. ASWPD may be misdiagnosed as early morning awakening insomnia, which has a prevalence estimate of around 5–8% in the general population[33]; circadian phase has been reported to be 2–4 hours earlier in patients with early morning awakening insomnia as compared to healthy controls,[34] further supporting the possibility of misdiagnosis as insomnia instead of ASWPD. These prevalence estimates for ASWPD also may be lower than the actual prevalence because of underreporting since there are relatively few adverse functional consequences faced by individuals with ASWPD and better accommodation of the early sleep–wake schedules in society. ASWPD is associated with fewer psychiatric comorbidities than DSWPD.

There are strong genetic associations for ASWPD, and several familial cohorts have been identified. The common genetic factor identified is a mutation in either Casein Kinase 1 epsilon (CK1ε) or the phosphorylation site for CK1ε on the human core clock gene Period 2 (hPer2).[35-38] The mutation leads to reduced phosphorylation of the Per2 protein, which in turn reduces its stability and increases the rate of the transcription–translation feedback loop, effectively shortening the period of the circadian cycle. The familial cases are associated with shorter circadian periods,[35,38] which can lead to an abnormal phase of circadian entrainment. It is possible that subtypes within ASWPD have relatively normal circadian phases (as seen in DSWPD); additional studies with objective assessment of circadian phase are required.

NON–24-HOUR SLEEP–WAKE RHYTHM DISORDER

N24SWD, also often referred to as *free-running disorder, non-entrained disorder,* or *hypernychthemeral syndrome,* is characterized by periodic episodes of insomnia and excessive sleepiness.[39] In these patients, sleep timing usually continues to delay, such that sleep may occur over at any clock time over months.[39,40] Since some (but not all) individuals may try to maintain a fixed sleep schedule relatively aligned to the geophysical night to allow them to maintain a normal work and social schedule, some patients with N24SWD may have intervals of debilitating sleep disruption, including sleep onset and maintenance insomnia, fragmentation, and excessive daytime sleepiness with significant impairment of daytime cognitive function.[41] Longitudinal assessment of circadian phase markers such as plasma melatonin or urinary melatonin sulfate rhythms show clear progressive delays or advances cycling across days,[41] demonstrating a lack of entrainment of the circadian system to a 24-hour day. Importantly, while there is a strong correlation between the rate of drift of the circadian phase markers and overt sleep–wake cycles,[42] environmental factors, such as meal and exercise timing, and social cues may modulate the rate of drift, suggesting that additional factors may be affecting the non–24 hour sleep–wake pattern.[42]

N24SWD is most common in totally blind individuals, as expected since their circadian systems cannot respond to the ocular light input stimuli for entrainment.[43,44] Blind individuals without N24SWD may remain entrained to the 24-hour social day through nonphotic cues such as daily meal cycles, exercise, social interaction, and maintaining strict schedules.[45] There are reports of N24SWD in sighted individuals.[46] Large epidemiologic studies to estimate the prevalence of N24SWD in sighted or blind individuals are lacking. Sighted N24SWD appears to be more prevalent in men (~70–80% of the studied population) with a majority of the cases incident between late teens to early 20s.[46]

The underlying pathophysiology of N24SWD in sighted individuals may include weak photic input to the suprachiasmatic nucleus (SCN), altered photic phase response curves for phase resetting, altered light exposure, or long circadian periods.[47] N24SWD and DSWPD may share a common pathology such that persistent delays of the sleep episode (as may occur in chronotherapy for DSWPD[48]) may precipitate N24SWD.[46] Additionally, N24SWD may also follow traumatic brain injury in some cases.[49] Comorbid psychopathology, including major depression and mood disorders, is commonly associated with N24SWD, with evidence supporting comorbid psychopathology preceding or following the development of N24SWD.[46] Social isolation is both a mediator and outcome of N24SWD that can exacerbate both the N24SWD and comorbid psychopathology. It is also important to recognize that social isolation may influence the light–dark cycle experienced by these patients, leading to aberrant or inadequate light exposure that worsens the condition.

IRREGULAR SLEEP–WAKE RHYTHM DISORDER

ISWRD is characterized by a loss of rhythmicity in sleep–wake behavior across the 24-hour day.[50] It typically manifests in children with neurologic developmental disabilities,[51] older adults with neurodegenerative diseases, and patients with schizophrenia.[52] Patients exhibit three or more sleep episodes within a 24-hour interval, although the major sleep episode is typically during the night.[50] The total duration of sleep across the 24-hour day appears to be normal for age but is characterized by a lack of consolidation (into clinically normal nocturnal 6- to 8-hour intervals).[50]

There is evidence suggesting that the circadian system may be disrupted in these patients. In the elderly population, irregular and inverted sleep–wake patterns have been reported in patients with dementia[53] and Alzheimer's disease (AD).[54] In patients with AD, a decrease in the amplitude of the sleep–wake rhythm, primarily due to irregular sleep–wake patterns, was correlated with a decrease in the neuronal population in the SCN in postmortem samples.[55] Circadian core clock gene expression rhythms in postmortem samples of different brain regions from AD patients and control individuals showed significant differences in the phase of these rhythms between the groups, as well as in the relative alignment of these rhythms between the brain regions.[56] Taken together, these results suggest that disruption in the circadian system in these patients may contribute to the irregular sleep–wake patterns observed.

"EXTRINSIC" CIRCADIAN RHYTHM SLEEP WAKE DISORDERS

The CRSWDs just described can be broadly considered as "intrinsic" given their assumed underlying internal biological cause(s) while the patient lives in a regular 24-hour light–dark cycle. In contrast, shift work disorder (SWD) and jet lag disorder (JLD) can be considered as "extrinsic" because their etiology is due to a misalignment between our internal biological time and a shifted external daily light–dark (e.g., remaining awake during solar nighttime and trying to sleep during solar daytime). Shift work can cause 8- to 12-hour shifts in rest–activity schedules and, similarly, jet travel allows shifts in multiple time zones within a few hours. These multihour shifts are too large for within-a-day adjustment by the circadian system. Both SWD and JLD are common in modern society; prevalence rates for JLD are not available and prevalence for SWD is estimated to be about 10% of those who work night and rotating shift work.[58]

Symptoms of JLD include sleep onset and maintenance insomnia, excessive sleepiness, and gastrointestinal disturbance. Similarly, symptoms of SWD include insomnia at home and excessive sleepiness during work. There is considerable interindividual variability in symptom severity, and various factors contribute to these differences including age, gender, and chronotype. Recently, genetic polymorphisms in the core clock gene PER3 have been associated with dichotomizing patients with SWD into those with insomnia and sleepiness versus those with only insomnia.[59,60] PER3 polymorphisms are associated with changes in homeostatic sleep pressure.[61] The adverse health consequences of shift work are well-documented, ranging from depression to diabetes, and are reviewed extensively elsewhere.[62,63] Current studies are systematically investigating the relative contributions of disruptions in the homeostatic and circadian processes associated with jet lag and shift work in mediating these adverse health effects.

Diagnosing Circadian Rhythm Sleep Wake Disorders

As detailed in the ICSD-3,[3] diagnosis starts with a clinical interview and documenting sleep–wake behavior with sleep diaries; objective assessment of sleep–wake patterns using actigraphy is also recommended.[64] The duration for sleep–wake monitoring with sleep diaries and actigraphy should be a minimum of 7 days for most diagnoses and 14 days for N24SWD. Questionnaires that assess an individual's preferred sleep–wake times are also recommended. Optional diagnostic assessment includes measuring endogenous circadian phase, which is currently most reliably estimated by the time at which the secretion of the hormone melatonin begins. This time is termed *dim light melatonin onset* (DLMO) since it must be assessed under dim light conditions to prevent melatonin suppression induced by light exposure. For some CRSWDs (e.g., N24SWD), multiple DLMO assessments several weeks apart are required. DLMO testing is not usually covered by insurance in the United States.

Importantly, the current clinical criteria[3] for diagnosis is purely symptomatic without any guidelines or standards for assessing the underlying pathophysiology. This is problematic because the efficacy of a treatment will likely depend on how well it addresses the underlying pathophysiology.[13,65] As described earlier, sleep is a complex process regulated by at least two interacting physiological processes and then impacted by behavioral choices and external environmental influences. Treatment aimed to change circadian phase will not typically correct problems with sleep homeostasis. Currently, the main diagnostic criterion is a misalignment between a patient's sleep pattern and the patient's *desired* time for sleep by about 2 hours. Therefore, a patient who desires to sleep by 9:00 PM but typically begins sleeping 11:00 PM can be classified as DSWPD, provided they meet other diagnostic criteria related to daytime insomnia, sleepiness, and functional impairment.

Although DLMO assessment is an accurate method of measuring endogenous phase and is beneficial in informing treatment options,[13,65] it is resource-intensive and difficult to implement clinically.[66] Recent studies have tested the feasibility of home saliva collection (rather than in-laboratory blood or saliva collection) for DLMO assessment,[67,68] including in DSWPD patients,[69] with promising results. However, these methods still require individuals to collect sequential salivary samples, typically over 6–8 hours, with strict control over environmental and behavioral conditions. Alternatives may include 24- to 48-hour urine collections to assess rhythmic metabolites such as 6-sulfatoxy melatonin or cortisol, but again, these require careful sample collection procedures and are very sensitive to errors in documentation of the collection sequence. A method to determine circadian phase based on only one or two samples would be ideal, akin to a blood test for assessing fasting glucose levels or lipid profiles. Several candidate approaches are being developed that rely on estimating circadian phase based on the relative levels of several biomarkers present in that one sample[70-72]; validation in clinical populations will be required. Methods to determine circadian phase from non-invasive measures such as actigraphy (i.e., wrist worn devices that measure activity, light, heart rate and/or skin temperature) are being developed and tested.

Treatment of Circadian Rhythm Sleep Wake Disorders

The American Academy of Sleep Medicine (AASM) formed a task force in 2012 to review the practice parameter guidelines for circadian rhythm sleep disorders. Recommendations were provided for the *intrinsic* CRSWDs (i.e., DSWPD, ASWPD, ISWRD, and N24SWD), but not for the *extrinsic* types (i.e., JLD and SWD). Recommendations were classified as "strong" or "weak" and "for" or "against." All recommendations provided were in the weak category, which reflects a "lower degree of certainty in the appropriateness of the patient-care strategy for all patients, and require that the clinician use his or her knowledge and experience, and consider the patient's individual values and preferences, to determine the best course of treatment."

The recommendations[73] supported the use of timed melatonin administration in those with DSWPD, blind adults with N24SWD, and children/adolescents with ISWRD. Light therapy with or without concurrent behavioral interventions was recommended for adults with ASWPD, children/adolescents with DSWPD, and the elderly with dementia and ISWRD. The use of melatonin or hypnotics in demented or elderly patients was strongly recommended against. Provided here is a brief description of and special considerations for each of the main treatment modalities for CRSWDs. Note that the two most common of these—melatonin and light—are complementary/integrative rather than pharmaceutical.

MELATONIN

The hormone melatonin is synthesized and secreted into circulation primarily from the pineal gland; secretion time is tightly regulated by the circadian clock. Melatonin levels are nearly undetectable during the day and start to rise typically 2 hours before bedtime in individuals who are normally entrained and maintain normative sleep–wake schedules[74]; these levels are suppressed by ocular light exposure. Melatonin is the biological signal of darkness (reviewed by Skene and Arendt[75]) and, similar to light exposure, exogenous melatonin can phase shift the endogenous circadian clock in either advance or delay directions. The phase response curve for melatonin is nearly opposite that of light, and the magnitude of the shift is smaller for melatonin than for light.[76]

For a person with clinically normative circadian phase, melatonin treatment in the evening, prior to DLMO, will advance the circadian clock; conversely, administration in the morning will delay the clock. Exogenous melatonin treatment (0.3–5 mg) 5–6 hours before DLMO or 6–8 hours before bedtime has shown consistent effects in advancing the timing of sleep and is a recommended treatment option for DSWPD.[6,77] Exogenous melatonin also has soporific effects, especially when administered at a time when endogenous melatonin levels are low.[78] Therefore, the timing of melatonin administration should be carefully considered when developing treatment plans so that patients are not required to take melatonin at a time when they need to be active and alert, as when driving or operating heavy machinery, for example. This includes not administering melatonin too early in the evening prior to bedtime or at the start of the day.

Ideally, melatonin administration should occur about 1 hour prior to bedtime. However, since DLMO is rarely assessed in the clinics, practitioners rely on the general rule of thumb that DLMO occurs approximately 2 hours before bedtime.[79] While this may be appropriate in young healthy adults without any sleep disorders,[74] such stable timing relationships between DLMO and bedtime may not be present in different populations and in individuals with sleep disorders,[80] especially CRSWDs. For example, there is considerable variability in circadian phase between individuals even when they maintain the same bedtimes and wake times (up to 5 hours in young adults and 9 hours in college students[81,82]); therefore timing melatonin (or light) therapy based on sleep–wake times alone can be ineffective or counterproductive,[83] and the timing of melatonin treatment based solely on bedtime should be avoided. The AASM does not recommend morning administration of melatonin to treat ASWPD.

The phase resetting and soporific effects of melatonin depend on the administration timing, not dosage.[76,78] Given the possible residual sedative effects of melatonin that may continue even after scheduled sleep, the lowest effective dose is always preferred, which typically is approximately 0.3 mg. Moreover, (1) higher doses (≥5 mg) may potentially remain physiologically active for longer and produce phase resetting in the wrong direction and (2) approximately 5 mg of exogenous melatonin impairs glucose tolerance both at night and during the day.[84] Importantly, melatonin is considered a dietary supplement—not a pharmaceutical product—and so is not subject to quality-control regulations. Consequently, there is considerable variability in purity and potency of melatonin formulations, and product labels may not accurately reflect content.[85] Mild side effects including headache, nausea, dizziness, and drowsiness have been reported but typically do not prevent patients from continuing treatment. Rarely, worsening of depressive symptoms, alopecia areata, and impaired glucose tolerance may occur. Moreover, recent work suggests that melatonin concentrations may correlate with uterine contractions in late-term pregnant women[86]; additional research is required to determine the safety of exogenous melatonin during pregnancy. A helpful resource describing the effects of melatonin on human physiology with a special focus on clinical applications and generic treatment plans can be found elsewhere.[79]

LIGHT

Ocular light exposure is the main circadian time cue: it can efficiently advance or delay the circadian clock depending on the circadian (not clock) time of administration.[87] Using only bedtime to determine the timing of light therapy is not advised for the same reasons as detailed in the melatonin section.[83] Additionally, although the phase response curve to light exposure is very well-characterized, it is important to recognize the existence of interindividual variability in phase resetting[87] or sensitivity to light, including some that may be related to the CRSWD itself.[20] Therefore, several attempts to adjust phase with timed light exposure may be necessary before ideal phase resetting is achieved. The most significant concern with light therapy, however, is poor patient compliance due to the burdensome time commitment of at least 30 minutes to 1 hour per treatment session.[73] Minor side effects such as eyestrain, headache, nausea, and agitation have been reported.[73]

It is important to consider the intensity of the light exposure. Typically, higher intensity light (~2,500 lux) is recommended, although under laboratory conditions individuals spending several days in very dim light show maximal phase resetting responses to around 1,000 lux of light. Generally, sensitivity to light is less during the daytime than in the evening, and therefore, brighter intensity light may be necessary to promote phase advances in patients with DSWPD. It is reasonable, therefore, to try to use the highest tolerable intensity of light for inducing maximal phase resetting. Bright light therapy is recommended as a treatment option for ASWPD[73] and can be timed to begin about 2 hours before habitual bedtime to help delay sleep until the desired bedtime is established. Bright light therapy in the morning to advance circadian rhythms in patients with DSWPD has been tried, but the effectiveness is questionable and therefore not recommended.[73] Given the large interindividual variability in response to bright light therapy, however, it may be tried in patients with DSWPD if the intensity and timing are well tolerated. Importantly, light exposure to advance circadian rhythms must occur shortly after the circadian nadir of the core body temperature rhythm, and waking patients up to receive light at this time may not be desirable if that comes at the expense of curtailing sleep, which in turn can increase the risk of higher daytime somnolence and the risk of errors and accidents associated with daytime sleepiness.

Novel research suggests that the human circadian system is exquisitely sensitive to short duration light pulses, as short as a single 15-second pulse or trains of millisecond flashes administered over 60 minutes,[88,89] which suggests that such short-duration exposures may be helpful for designing new treatment strategies that may have better compliance and adherence. Similarly, emergent data suggest that bright light exposure given through the eyelids while an individual is sleeping can potentially reset the circadian clock.[90] This can be another attractive treatment option in the future. However, studies in clinical populations are required to confirm the clinical efficacy and validity of such trials in the home. A helpful resource describing the effects of light on human physiology with a special focus on clinical applications and generic treatment plans can be found elsewhere.[79]

OTHER TREATMENT OPTIONS

Hypnotics are sometimes considered for treating insomnia associated with CRSWDs.[73] There is limited evidence that hypnotics can be beneficial in DSWPD and no evidence that they can be useful in treating ASWPD. Hypnotics can help with insomnia related to JLD and SWD, but carryover sedation and associated increased risk of errors and accidents need to be considered carefully. Currently, only modafinil and armodafinil are approved by the US Food and Drug Administration (FDA) for treating excessive daytime sleepiness associated with SWD; several trials have demonstrated the efficacy of modafinil in reducing sleepiness and increasing alertness during night shifts.[91,92] The US FDA approved the medication tasimelteon for the treatment of N24SWD, the first medication to be approved by the FDA for treatment of any type of CRSWD. In a randomized placebo-controlled clinical trial in 84 blind patients with N24SWD, 20 mg tasimelteon taken one hour before target bedtime promoted circadian entrainment in 20% (8 out of 40) of the patients who received the medication as compared to 3% (1 out of 38) patients who received placebo.[93]

Chronotherapy, which includes gradually delaying an individual's bedtime until the desired bedtime is achieved, was introduced in 1981 as a method to correct sleep timing in patients with delayed sleep phase syndrome.[25] Since patients with DSWPD find it difficult to advance their sleep to their desired bedtime, in chronotherapy, they (counterintuitively) are advised to progressively delay their bedtimes by 2–3 hours each day until they reach their desired bedtime. There are no randomized controlled trials of this approach; most evidence is from case studies with mixed results, and only one case study exists for chronotherapy in treating ASWPD.[93] Related to chronotherapy is *sleep scheduling*, which consists of prescribing sleep–wake times and, in turn, the light–dark schedule that will help entrain circadian rhythms and build homeostatic sleep pressure. Cognitive-behavioral therapy (CBT) may be a beneficial addition to standard CRSWD treatment protocols due to some of the behavioral components of CRSWD symptoms.[94] Combining CBT with bright light therapy in treating DSWPD has shown to be beneficial, but whether CBT improves treatment outcomes beyond light therapy alone is not clear.[95] One of the challenges with CRSWD treatment is that it requires sustained therapy; stopping treatment with melatonin and/or light exposure leads to symptom relapse.[96]

As described earlier, recognizing that behavioral choices can precipitate CRSWDs such as DSWPD is critical for planning effective treatment protocols. *Stimulus control therapy* or CBT, as used in insomnia treatment, may also be a beneficial addition to standard treatment for CRSWDs.[94] For example, the importance of avoiding behaviors that promote wakefulness instead of sleepiness (e.g., consuming coffee or exposure to bright light) before bed need to be emphasized. Conversely, such behavior can be promoted in patients with ASWPD. In shift workers, sleep scheduling combined with optimizing the sleep environment at home (e.g., by using shades or window treatments to darken the room) can significantly improve sleep.[97] Other potentially beneficial interventions include minimizing bright light exposure (e.g., sunlight) when traveling home from work after the night shift, taking melatonin prior to the daytime sleep period, timed napping before and during night shift work, and, as previously mentioned, the use of modafinil/armodafinil prior to the start of the night shift. Minimizing bright light exposure during the commute after the night shift may facilitate circadian adaptation, but it may also reduce alertness, which can be detrimental when driving and therefore likely best limited to shift workers who are not driving after the overnight shift. Likewise, exogenous melatonin prior to daytime sleep should be taken after returning home and not before the commute if the individual will be driving post overnight shift.

Conclusion

CRSWDs were reported in the scientific literature about four decades ago, starting as syndromes and more recently being classified as disorders. Emerging evidence, however, shows that such a classification may be sometimes misleading and/or incomplete. As noted, sleep regulation is profoundly influenced by circadian and sleep physiology, behavioral choices, and external factors; therefore, expanding from a limited view of the underlying pathophysiology that all CRSWDs must have an underlying phase disorder will likely aid diagnosis, treatment, and outcome. Recent advances in estimating circadian phase from single time-point samples or ambulatory methods will aid the diagnosis and classification of CRSWD subtypes. Current treatment modalities rely extensively on integrative medicine approaches, mostly behavioral, melatonin, or light-based used singly or in combination. Randomized controlled trials of treatment modalities using novel interventions or combinations of interventions, with a particular focus on improving patient compliance and sustained adherence, are much needed. To this end, future research trials need to incorporate patient-centered outcomes; trial designs may benefit from incorporating the views of patients and patient advocacy groups. While AASM practice guidelines currently only provide weak support for treatment strategies such as melatonin and light therapy, it is important to recognize that there are considerable interindividual differences in response and that these therapies could be very effective in some individual patients and therefore should not be overlooked. Successful therapy may require sustained engagement between the patient and care provider(s).

CRSWDs cover a broad spectrum of disorders that share numerous phenotypic traits and pathophysiologic mechanisms. These disorders are often undiagnosed but can have significant adverse effects on health and well-being; therefore, early detection and treatment are critical as prevention strategies. Education of physicians and other providers about CRSWDs will be integral to providing effective treatment; documentation of the timing of sleep–wake activity (including its regularity), diurnal preference, and work schedules should to be incorporated into routine clinical assessment of all patients with complaints of poor sleep.

REFERENCES

1. Borbely AA. A two process model of sleep regulation. *Hum Neurobiol.* 1982;1(3):195–204.
2. Dijk DJ, Czeisler CA. Contribution of the circadian pacemaker and the sleep homeostat to sleep propensity, sleep structure, electroencephalographic slow waves, and sleep spindle activity in humans. *J Neurosci.* 1995;15(5 Pt 1):3526–3538.

3. American Academy of Sleep Medicine, ed. *International classification of sleep disorders*, 3rd ed. Darien, IL: American Academy of Sleep Medicine; 2014.

4. Weitzman ED, Czeisler CA, Coleman RM, et al. Delayed sleep phase syndrome. A chronobiological disorder with sleep-onset insomnia. *Arch Gen Psychiatry.* 1981;38(7):737–746.

5. Chang AM, Reid KJ, Gourineni R, Zee PC. Sleep timing and circadian phase in delayed sleep phase syndrome. *J Biol Rhythms.* 2009;24(4):313–321.

6. Mundey K, Benloucif S, Harsanyi K, Dubocovich ML, Zee PC. Phase-dependent treatment of delayed sleep phase syndrome with melatonin. *Sleep.* 2005;28(10):1271–1278.

7. Abe T, Inoue Y, Komada Y, et al. Relation between morningness-eveningness score and depressive symptoms among patients with delayed sleep phase syndrome. *Sleep Med.* 2011;12(7):680–684.

8. Shirayama M, Shirayama Y, Iida H, et al. The psychological aspects of patients with delayed sleep phase syndrome (DSPS). *Sleep Med.* 2003;4(5):427–433.

9. Reid KJ, Jaksa AA, Eisengart JB, et al. Systematic evaluation of Axis-I DSM diagnoses in delayed sleep phase disorder and evening-type circadian preference. *Sleep Med.* 2012;13(9):1171–1177.

10. Dagan Y, Stein D, Steinbock M, Yovel I, Hallis D. Frequency of delayed sleep phase syndrome among hospitalized adolescent psychiatric patients. *J Psychosom Res.* 1998;45(1):15–20.

11. Rahman SA, Kayumov L, Shapiro CM. Antidepressant action of melatonin in the treatment of Delayed Sleep Phase Syndrome. *Sleep Med.* 2010;11(2):131–136.

12. Solheim B, Langsrud K, Kallestad H, Engstrom M, Bjorvatn B, Sand T. Sleep structure and awakening threshold in delayed sleep–wake phase disorder patients compared to healthy sleepers. *Sleep Med.* 2018;46:61–68.

13. Rahman SA, Kayumov L, Tchmoutina EA, Shapiro CM. Clinical efficacy of dim light melatonin onset testing in diagnosing delayed sleep phase syndrome. *Sleep Med.* 2009;10(5):549–555.

14. Wilhelmsen-Langeland A, Saxvig IW, Pallesen S, et al. A randomized controlled trial with bright light and melatonin for the treatment of delayed sleep phase disorder: Effects on subjective and objective sleepiness and cognitive function. *J Biol Rhythms.* 2013;28(5):306–321.

15. Saxvig IW, Wilhelmsen-Langeland A, Pallesen S, et al. Objective measures of sleep and dim light melatonin onset in adolescents and young adults with delayed sleep phase disorder compared to healthy controls. *J Sleep Res.* 2013;22(4):365–372.

16. Crowley SJ, Acebo C, Carskadon MA. Sleep, circadian rhythms, and delayed phase in adolescence. *Sleep Med.* 2007;8(6):602–612.

17. Schrader H, Bovim G, Sand T. The prevalence of delayed and advanced sleep phase syndromes. *J Sleep Res.* 1993;2(1):51–55.

18. Gradisar M, Crowley SJ. Delayed sleep phase disorder in youth. *Curr Opin Psychiatry.* 2013;26(6):580–585.

19. Joo EY, Abbott SM, Reid KJ, et al. Timing of light exposure and activity in adults with delayed sleep–wake phase disorder. *Sleep Med*. 2017;32:259–265.

20. Watson LA, Phillips AJK, Hosken IT, et al. Increased sensitivity of the circadian system to light in delayed sleep–wake phase disorder. *J Physiol*. 2018;596(24):6249–6261.

21. Aoki H, Ozeki Y, Yamada N. Hypersensitivity of melatonin suppression in response to light in patients with delayed sleep phase syndrome. *Chronobiol Int*. 2001;18(2):263–271.

22. Burgess HJ, Eastman CI. Short nights reduce light-induced circadian phase delays in humans. *Sleep*. 2006;29(1):25–30.

23. Wright KP, Jr., McHill AW, Birks BR, Griffin BR, Rusterholz T, Chinoy ED. Entrainment of the human circadian clock to the natural light-dark cycle. *Curr Biol*. 2013;23(16):1554–1558.

24. Chang AM, Aeschbach D, Duffy JF, Czeisler CA. Evening use of light-emitting eReaders negatively affects sleep, circadian timing, and next-morning alertness. *Proc Natl Acad Sci U S A*. 2015;112(4):1232–1237.

25. Czeisler CA, Richardson GS, Coleman RM, et al. Chronotherapy: Resetting the circadian clocks of patients with delayed sleep phase insomnia. *Sleep*. 1981;4(1):1–21.

26. Wyatt JK, Stepanski EJ, Kirkby J. Circadian phase in delayed sleep phase syndrome: Predictors and temporal stability across multiple assessments. *Sleep*. 2006;29(8):1075–1080.

27. Murray JM, Sletten TL, Magee M, et al. Prevalence of circadian misalignment and its association with depressive symptoms in delayed sleep phase disorder. *Sleep*. 2017;40(1). doi:10.1093/sleep/zsw002. PMID: 28364473.

28. Micic G, de Bruyn A, Lovato N, et al. The endogenous circadian temperature period length (tau) in delayed sleep phase disorder compared to good sleepers. *J Sleep Res*. 2013;22(6):617–624.

29. Patke A, Murphy PJ, Onat OE, et al. Mutation of the human circadian clock gene CRY1 in familial delayed sleep phase disorder. *Cell*. 2017;169(2):203–215 e213.

30. Mongrain V, Dumont M. Increased homeostatic response to behavioral sleep fragmentation in morning types compared to evening types. *Sleep*. 2007;30(6):773–780.

31. Uchiyama M, Okawa M, Shibui K, et al. Poor recovery sleep after sleep deprivation in delayed sleep phase syndrome. *Psychiatry Clin Neurosci*. 1999;53(2):195–197.

32. Paine SJ, Fink J, Gander PH, Warman GR. Identifying advanced and delayed sleep phase disorders in the general population: A national survey of New Zealand adults. *Chronobiol Int*. 2014;31(5):627–636.

33. Ohayon MM. Epidemiology of insomnia: What we know and what we still need to learn. *Sleep Med Rev*. 2002;6(2):97–111.

34. Campbell SS, Dawson D, Anderson MW. Alleviation of sleep maintenance insomnia with timed exposure to bright light. *J Am Geriatr Soc*. 1993;41(8):829–836.

35. Jones CR, Campbell SS, Zone SE, et al. Familial advanced sleep-phase syndrome: A short-period circadian rhythm variant in humans. *Nat Med*. 1999;5(9):1062–1065.

36. Toh KL, Jones CR, He Y, et al. An hPer2 phosphorylation site mutation in familial advanced sleep phase syndrome. *Science*. 2001;291(5506):1040–1043.

37. Xu Y, Padiath QS, Shapiro RE, et al. Functional consequences of a CKIdelta mutation causing familial advanced sleep phase syndrome. *Nature*. 2005;434(7033):640–644.

38. Shanware NP, Hutchinson JA, Kim SH, Zhan L, Bowler MJ, Tibbetts RS. Casein kinase 1-dependent phosphorylation of familial advanced sleep phase syndrome-associated residues controls PERIOD 2 stability. *J Biol Chem*. 2011;286(14):12766–12774.

39. Uchiyama M, Lockley SW. Non–24-hour sleep–wake rhythm disorder in sighted and blind patients. *Sleep Med Clin*. 2015;10(4):495–516.

40. Uchiyama M, Shibui K, Hayakawa T, et al. Larger phase angle between sleep propensity and melatonin rhythms in sighted humans with non–24-hour sleep–wake syndrome. *Sleep*. 2002;25(1):83–88.

41. Lockley SW, Dijk DJ, Kosti O, Skene DJ, Arendt J. Alertness, mood and performance rhythm disturbances associated with circadian sleep disorders in the blind. *J Sleep Res*. 2008;17(2):207–216.

42. Emens JS, Laurie AL, Songer JB, Lewy AJ. Non–24-hour disorder in blind individuals revisited: Variability and the influence of environmental time cues. *Sleep*. 2013;36(7):1091–1100.

43. Lockley SW, Arendt J, Skene DJ. Visual impairment and circadian rhythm disorders. *Dialogues Clin Neurosci*. 2007;9(3):301–314.

44. Sack RL, Lewy AJ, Blood ML, Keith LD, Nakagawa H. Circadian rhythm abnormalities in totally blind people: Incidence and clinical significance. *J Clin Endocrinol Metab*. 1992;75(1):127–134.

45. Klerman EB, Rimmer DW, Dijk DJ, Kronauer RE, Rizzo JF, 3rd, Czeisler CA. Nonphotic entrainment of the human circadian pacemaker. *Am J Physiol*. 1998;274(4 Pt 2):R991–996.

46. Hayakawa T, Uchiyama M, Kamei Y, et al. Clinical analyses of sighted patients with non–24-hour sleep–wake syndrome: A study of 57 consecutively diagnosed cases. *Sleep*. 2005;28(8):945–952.

47. Kitamura S, Hida A, Enomoto M, et al. Intrinsic circadian period of sighted patients with circadian rhythm sleep disorder, free-running type. *Biol Psychiatry*. 2013;73(1):63–69.

48. Oren DA, Wehr TA. Hypernyctohemeral syndrome after chronotherapy for delayed sleep phase syndrome. *N Engl J Med*. 1992;327(24):1762.

49. Boivin DB, James FO, Santo JB, Caliyurt O, Chalk C. Non–24-hour sleep–wake syndrome following a car accident. *Neurology*. 2003;60(11):1841–1843.

50. Zee PC, Vitiello MV. Circadian rhythm sleep disorder: Irregular sleep wake rhythm type. *Sleep Med Clin*. 2009;4(2):213–218.

51. MacDuffie KE, Munson J, Greenson J, et al. Sleep problems and trajectories of restricted and repetitive behaviors in children with neurodevelopmental disabilities. *J Autism Dev Disord*. 2020;50(11):3844–3856.

52. Bromundt V, Koster M, Georgiev-Kill A, et al. Sleep–wake cycles and cognitive functioning in schizophrenia. *Br J Psychiatry*. 2011;198(4):269–276.

53. Van Someren EJ. Circadian and sleep disturbances in the elderly. *Exp Gerontol*. 2000;35(9–10):1229–1237.

54. Figueiro MG. Light, sleep and circadian rhythms in older adults with Alzheimer's disease and related dementias. *Neurodegener Dis Manag*. 2017;7(2):119–145.

55. Wang JL, Lim AS, Chiang WY, et al. Suprachiasmatic neuron numbers and rest-activity circadian rhythms in older humans. *Ann Neurol*. 2015;78(2):317–322.

56. Cermakian N, Lamont EW, Boudreau P, Boivin DB. Circadian clock gene expression in brain regions of Alzheimer 's disease patients and control subjects. *J Biol Rhythms*. 2011;26(2):160–170.

57. Martin JL, Webber AP, Alam T, Harker JO, Josephson KR, Alessi CA. Daytime sleeping, sleep disturbance, and circadian rhythms in the nursing home. *Am J Geriatr Psychiatry*. 2006;14(2):121–129.

58. Drake CL, Roehrs T, Richardson G, Walsh JK, Roth T. Shift work sleep disorder: Prevalence and consequences beyond that of symptomatic day workers. *Sleep*. 2004;27(8):1453–1462.

59. Gumenyuk V, Belcher R, Drake CL, Roth T. Differential sleep, sleepiness, and neurophysiology in the insomnia phenotypes of shift work disorder. *Sleep*. 2015;38(1):119–126.

60. Drake CL, Belcher R, Howard R, Roth T, Levin AM, Gumenyuk V. Length polymorphism in the Period 3 gene is associated with sleepiness and maladaptive circadian phase in night-shift workers. *J Sleep Res*. 2015;24(3):254–261.

61. Archer SN, Schmidt C, Vandewalle G, Dijk DJ. Phenotyping of PER3 variants reveals widespread effects on circadian preference, sleep regulation, and health. *Sleep Med Rev*. 2018;40:109–126.

62. Boivin DB, Tremblay GM, James FO. Working on atypical schedules. *Sleep Med*. 2007;8(6):578–589.

63. Chellappa SL, Vujovic N, Williams JS, Scheer F. Impact of circadian disruption on cardiovascular function and disease. *Trends Endocrinol Metab*. 2019;30(10):767–779.

64. Smith MT, McCrae CS, Cheung J, et al. Use of actigraphy for the evaluation of sleep disorders and circadian rhythm sleep–wake disorders: An American Academy of Sleep Medicine systematic review, meta-analysis, and grade assessment. *J Clin Sleep Med*. 2018;14(7):1209–1230.

65. Keijzer H, Smits MG, Duffy JF, Curfs LM. Why the dim light melatonin onset (DLMO) should be measured before treatment of patients with circadian rhythm sleep disorders. *Sleep Med Rev*. 2014;18(4):333–339.

66. Rahman SA. Are we ready to assess circadian phase at home? *Sleep*. 2015;38(6):849–850.

67. Pullman RE, Roepke SE, Duffy JF. Laboratory validation of an in-home method for assessing circadian phase using dim light melatonin onset (DLMO). *Sleep Med*. 2012;13(6):703–706.

68. Burgess HJ, Wyatt JK, Park M, Fogg LF. Home circadian phase assessments with measures of compliance yield accurate dim light melatonin onsets. *Sleep.* 2015;38(6):889–897.

69. Burgess HJ, Park M, Wyatt JK, Fogg LF. Home dim light melatonin onsets with measures of compliance in delayed sleep phase disorder. *J Sleep Res.* 2016;25(3):314–317.

70. Braun R, Kath WL, Iwanaszko M, et al. Universal method for robust detection of circadian state from gene expression. *Proc Natl Acad Sci U S A.* 2018;115(39):E9247–E9256.

71. Wittenbrink N, Ananthasubramaniam B, Munch M, et al. High-accuracy determination of internal circadian time from a single blood sample. *J Clin Invest.* 2018;128(9):3826–3839.

72. Laing EE, Moller-Levet CS, Poh N, Santhi N, Archer SN, Dijk DJ. Blood transcriptome based biomarkers for human circadian phase. *Elife.* 2017;6.

73. Auger RR, Burgess HJ, Emens JS, Deriy LV, Thomas SM, Sharkey KM. Clinical practice guideline for the treatment of intrinsic circadian rhythm sleep–wake disorders: Advanced sleep–wake phase disorder (ASWPD), delayed sleep–wake phase disorder (DSWPD), non–24-hour sleep–wake rhythm disorder (N24SWD), and irregular sleep–wake rhythm disorder (ISWRD). An update for 2015: An American Academy of Sleep Medicine clinical practice guideline. *J Clin Sleep Med.* 2015;11(10):1199–1236.

74. Gooley JJ, Chamberlain K, Smith KA, et al. Exposure to room light before bedtime suppresses melatonin onset and shortens melatonin duration in humans. *J Clin Endocrinol Metab.* 2011;96(3):E463–472.

75. Skene DJ, Arendt J. Human circadian rhythms: Physiological and therapeutic relevance of light and melatonin. *Ann Clin Biochem.* 2006;43(Pt 5):344–353.

76. Burgess HJ, Revell VL, Molina TA, Eastman CI. Human phase response curves to three days of daily melatonin: 0.5 mg versus 3.0 mg. *J Clin Endocrinol Metab.* 2010;95(7):3325–3331.

77. Morgenthaler TI, Lee-Chiong T, Alessi C, et al. Practice parameters for the clinical evaluation and treatment of circadian rhythm sleep disorders. An American Academy of Sleep Medicine report. *Sleep.* 2007;30(11):1445–1459.

78. Wyatt JK, Dijk DJ, Ritz-de Cecco A, Ronda JM, Czeisler CA. Sleep-facilitating effect of exogenous melatonin in healthy young men and women is circadian-phase dependent. *Sleep.* 2006;29(5):609–618.

79. Emens JS, Burgess HJ. Effect of light and melatonin and other melatonin receptor agonists on human circadian physiology. *Sleep Med Clin.* 2015;10(4):435–453.

80. Flynn-Evans EE, Shekleton JA, Miller B, et al. Circadian phase and phase angle disorders in primary insomnia. *Sleep.* 2017;40(12).

81. Wright KP, Jr., Gronfier C, Duffy JF, Czeisler CA. Intrinsic period and light intensity determine the phase relationship between melatonin and sleep in humans. *J Biol Rhythms.* 2005;20(2):168–177.

82. Phillips AJK, Clerx WM, O'Brien CS, et al. Irregular sleep/wake patterns are associated with poorer academic performance and delayed circadian and sleep/wake timing. *Sci Rep.* 2017;7(1):3216.

83. Klerman EB, Rahman SA, St Hilaire MA. What time is it? A tale of three clocks, with implications for personalized medicine. *J Pineal Res.* 2020:e12646.

84. Rubio-Sastre P, Scheer FA, Gomez-Abellan P, Madrid JA, Garaulet M. Acute melatonin administration in humans impairs glucose tolerance in both the morning and evening. *Sleep.* 2014;37(10):1715–1719.

85. Erland LA, Saxena PK. Melatonin natural health products and supplements: Presence of serotonin and significant variability of melatonin content. *J Clin Sleep Med.* 2017;13(2):275–281.

86. Rahman SA, Bibbo C, Olcese J, Czeisler CA, Robinson JN, Klerman EB. Relationship between endogenous melatonin concentrations and uterine contractions in late third trimester of human pregnancy. *J Pineal Res.* 2019;66(4):e12566.

87. St Hilaire MA, Gooley JJ, Khalsa SB, Kronauer RE, Czeisler CA, Lockley SW. Human phase response curve to a 1 h pulse of bright white light. *J Physiol.* 2012;590(13):3035–3045.

88. Rahman SA, St Hilaire MA, Chang AM, et al. Circadian phase resetting by a single short-duration light exposure. *JCI Insight.* 2017;2(7):e89494.

89. Najjar RP, Zeitzer JM. Temporal integration of light flashes by the human circadian system. *J Clin Invest.* 2016;126(3):938–947.

90. Zeitzer JM, Fisicaro RA, Ruby NF, Heller HC. Millisecond flashes of light phase delay the human circadian clock during sleep. *J Biol Rhythms.* 2014;29(5):370–376.

91. Czeisler CA, Walsh JK, Roth T, et al. Modafinil for excessive sleepiness associated with shift-work sleep disorder. *N Engl J Med.* 2005;353(5):476–486.

92. Grady S, Aeschbach D, Wright KP, Jr., Czeisler CA. Effect of modafinil on impairments in neurobehavioral performance and learning associated with extended wakefulness and circadian misalignment. *Neuropsychopharmacology.* 2010;35(9):1910–1920.

93. Lockley SW, Dressman MA, Licamele L, Xiao C, Fisher DM, Flynn-Evans EE, Hull JT, Torres R, Lavedan C, Polymeropoulos MH. Tasimelteon for non-24-hour sleep-wake disorder in totally blind people (SET and RESET): two multicentre, randomised, double-masked, placebo-controlled phase 3 trials. *Lancet.* 2015 Oct 31;386(10005):1754–1764.

93. Moldofsky H, Musisi S, Phillipson EA. Treatment of a case of advanced sleep phase syndrome by phase advance chronotherapy. *Sleep.* 1986;9(1):61–65.

94. Culnan E, McCullough LM, Wyatt JK. Circadian rhythm sleep–wake phase disorders. *Neurol Clin.* 2019;37(3):527–543.

95. Gradisar M, Dohnt H, Gardner G, et al. A randomized controlled trial of cognitive-behavior therapy plus bright light therapy for adolescent delayed sleep phase disorder. *Sleep.* 2011;34(12):1671–1680.

96. Richardson C, Cain N, Bartel K, Micic G, Maddock B, Gradisar M. A randomised controlled trial of bright light therapy and morning activity for adolescents and young adults with delayed sleep–wake phase disorder. *Sleep Med.* 2018;45:114–123.

97. Isherwood CM, Chinoy ED, Murphy AS, Kim JH, Wang W, Duffy JF. Scheduled afternoon-evening sleep leads to better night shift performance in older adults. *Occup Environ Med.* 2020;77(3):179–184.

33

Restless Legs Syndrome and Sleep-Related Movement Disorders

STEPHEN PAUL DUNTLEY

Movement and Sleep

Behavioral quiescence is one of the cardinal features in any definition of sleep. This inactivity is mediated by behavioral disengagement, with reduced awareness of the environment and muscular relaxation which is seen in all stages of sleep. During rapid eye movement (REM) sleep, potent descending inhibition of motor neurons results in a complete paralysis of all muscles except extraocular and respiratory muscles. There are exceptions to this quiescence, and some animals, such as dolphins, are able to maintain swimming behaviors while sleeping; indeed, dolphins and ducks are capable of *unihemispheric sleep* to maintain increased environmental awareness. In most animals, including humans, behavioral quiescence is a requirement for sleep, and maintaining motor activity is the most reliable method of preventing sleep onset.

It is important to remember, however, that even in humans this quiescence is relative. Now that personal sleep tracking devices are nearly ubiquitous, it is essential for us to understand that 8 hours of uninterrupted sleep is not a reasonable expectation and that some arousals, awakenings, and occasional movements are present in normal sleep. Excessive movement during sleep can be seen during arousals from pathological conditions such as sleep apnea, which in severe cases can result in repetitive violent thrashing or the patient bolting upright in the bed. Even more dramatic movements can be seen in parasomnias such as REM sleep behavior disorder, where the muscular paralysis during REM sleep fails and the patient engages in dream enactment behavior.

This chapter deals with conditions that are listed by the *International Classification of Sleep Disorders* (ICSD-3) as "sleep-related movement disorders," which are "primarily characterized by relatively simple, usually stereotyped, movements that disturb sleep or its onset" (American Academy of Sleep Medicine, 2014). The disorders covered in this chapter include restless legs syndrome (RLS) also known as *Willis-Ekbom syndrome*, periodic limb movement disorder (PLMD), sleep-related leg cramps, sleep-related bruxism (SRB), and sleep starts (SS), also known as *hypnic jerks*. Optimal treatment of these disorders requires an integrative approach that involves accurate diagnosis, addressing underlying contributing medical disorders and lifestyle or sleep hygiene issues, instituting nonpharmacological therapy when possible, and prescribing appropriate pharmacotherapy when necessary.

RESTLESS LEGS SYNDROME

RLS is also known as Willis-Ekbom syndrome, named after the two prominent physicians in the Western literature who published early work on the disorder. The first description is generally attributed to Willis, in 1672, who described persons suffering from this disorder as "no more being able to sleep than if they were in the place of greatest torture." Willis noted that opioids were beneficial in treating this disorder (Willis, 1685). The cardinal features of RLS were systematically described by Ekbom in 1945. An earlier description, however, may have been given in Traditional Chinese Medicine (TCM) literature in 1529, and there is an extensive published work on what is likely RLS that unfortunately has not been widely explored by Western medicine (Yan et al., 2012).

RLS is a sensorimotor disorder characterized by a strong, often irresistible urge to move the legs and sometimes arms. Legs are almost always involved first, and, as the disease progresses, arms are often involved. Other body regions are occasionally involved. Initial arm involvement is uncommon. Symptoms are usually bilateral but can fluctuate. Strictly unilateral symptoms should prompt concern for a structural lesion of the nervous system. This urge to move is usually but not always accompanied by sensations that can be variously described as a "a creepy crawly feeling," a tightness, a need to stretch, or a painful sensation. Patients often have difficulty describing the sensation. The ICSD-3 also requires the three following essential features: symptoms must "1. Begin or worsen during periods or rest or inactivity such as lying down or sitting. 2. Be partially or totally relieved by movement such as walking or stretching, at least as long as the activity continues, and 3. Occur exclusively or predominantly in the evening or night rather than during the day" (American Academy of Sleep Medicine, 2014). As the disorder progresses, symptoms may become severe throughout the day and night but are initially worse near bedtime.

Unlike other sleep-related movement disorders characterized by movements that occur at sleep onset or during sleep, the hallmark of RLS is an abnormal conscious sensation with an urge to move which by definition must occur during waking. Unlike the other sleep-related movement disorders, the movements that result from this disorder are typically not simple and usually not particularly stereotyped. These movements consist of walking, stretching, and various other movements or counter-stimulatory activities such as rubbing. RLS is listed among the sleep-related movement disorders because of the prominence of the motor activity, the profound sleep disturbance that it can cause, and the tight link to behaviors that are necessary for normal sleep onset. While mental and physical relaxation and appropriate timing in the evening are essential for normal sleep, these are the very features that precipitate the abnormal sensations and the need to engage in physical activity in RLS patients. Motor activity can be repressed with conscious effort, at least temporarily, but with prolonged duration of immobility the urge to move may become irresistible or truly involuntary movements may occur. Once asleep, more than 80% of patients with RLS develop periodic limb movements (Michaud, Paquet, Lavigne, Desautels, & Montplaisir, 2002), which can cause arousals and awakenings, and these movements are simple and stereotyped. It has recently become clear that RLS is also a disorder of arousal, with patients exhibiting hyperarousal and exhibiting less sleepiness than expected despite often obtaining 4–5 hours or less of sleep a night (Ferre et al., 2017).

RLS is a clinical diagnosis that requires the four essential features just noted and the exclusion of other mimics. No objective diagnostic testing is required for the diagnosis, and no testing exists that can establish the diagnosis with certainty. The presence of periodic limb movements on polysomnography (PSG) and response to dopaminergic agents are considered supporting features but are not required for a diagnosis. The suggested immobilization test (SIT) is sometimes used as a confirmatory test or measure of severity. The patient is monitored for an hour before bedtime, with the subject sitting awake and upright in bed with legs outstretched. Periodic leg movements during waking are counted during this hour. An index of greater than 40 per hour is supportive of a diagnosis of RLS (American Academy of Sleep Medicine, 2014). The International Restless Legs Symptoms (IRLS) rating scale is a 10-item questionnaire with scores ranging from 0 to 40; it is a common clinical tool for assessing severity (Walters et al., 2003).

RLS must be differentiated from akathisia, arthralgia, habitual foot tapping, neuropathic pain, painful leg and moving toes syndrome, peripheral venous insufficiency, and sleep-related leg cramps (SRLC). Estimates of the prevalence vary, partly depending on the symptom threshold chosen. Symptoms can range from a nuisance symptom that is barely noticed to a devastating, life-altering problem that renders sleep and even sitting nearly impossible. By any definition, RLS is a common disorder, and the ICSD-3 estimates it to occur in 5–10% of adults of European or African descent (Allen & Earley, 2001). Clinically significant RLS is estimated to affect about 2.5% of adults (Hening et al., 2004). It is less common in Asian populations. It increases in prevalence with increasing age, but is present in 2–4% of children (Picchietti et al., 2007; Turkdogan, Bekiroglu, & Zaimoglu, 2011), where it is often difficult to diagnose and is often misdiagnosed as attention deficit hyperactivity disorder (ADHD). Onset tends to be earlier in familial cases, and it is about twice as common in women than men.

RLS is classified as either primary, with no known cause, or secondary, in which symptoms are presumably attributable to an underlying medical condition. The secondary conditions with widely accepted causality include pregnancy, iron deficiency, and renal failure. A long list of conditions have been noted to have a looser association, and most involve structural damage to the nervous system, either central or peripheral, or inflammatory conditions. A partial list includes neurological disorders including neuropathy, multiple sclerosis, myelopathy, and stroke; rheumatological disorders including rheumatoid arthritis, lupus, and scleroderma; metabolic disorders including diabetes, hypothyroidism, and acromegaly; pulmonary disorders including sleep apnea, sarcoidosis, and chronic obstructive pulmonary disease (COPD); and gastrointestinal disorders including celiac disease and Crohn's disease (Weinstock, Walters, & Paueksakon, 2012). Vitamin D deficiency has also been linked to RLS (Wali et al., 2018). Medications that may cause or exacerbate RLS include dopamine antagonists, anticholinergic agents, lithium, antidepressants (mirtazapine may be more likely and bupropion least likely to precipitate), ethanol, and methylxanthines, such as caffeine (Patatanian & Claborn, 2018). Theobromine, which is found in chocolate, seems to be particularly likely to precipitate symptoms. Sleep deprivation from any etiology seems to aggravate symptoms.

The pathophysiology of RLS remains uncertain. There is a strong genetic component, and it is estimated that 42.3% of RLS patients have definite hereditary RLS and 12.6% possible hereditary RLS. Many large family cohorts exhibit what appears to be autosomal dominant transmission, with nearly 50% penetrance in families, and genome-wide association studies have identified a number of genes all of which confer a relatively small increased risk. The well-established linkages include *BTBD9*, *MEISI*, *PTPRD*, *MAP2K5*, *SKORI*, and *TOX3*, and at least 13 more risk loci have been identified recently. Most of these genes are associated with regulatory regions and not protein coding, and the strongest risk factor, *MEISI* governs the development of basal ganglia, suggesting that hereditary RLS may be a neurodevelopmental disorder (Spieler et al., 2014).

The genetic studies have yet to yield clear insight into the pathophysiology of RLS. The most robust experimental finding is a brain iron deficiency. The prevalence of RLS in patients with iron deficiency anemia is six times that of the general population and improves with iron supplementation (Allen et al., 2005). While most patients with RLS do not have systemic iron deficiency, the cerebrospinal fluid (CSF) of patients reveals elevated transferrin and reduced ferritin levels, and neuroimaging studies reveal reduced brain iron, especially of the substantia nigra (Allen, Barker, Wehrl, Song, & Earley, 2001; Earley et al., 2000). In animal models, dietary induction of brain iron deficiency leads to a variety of neuro-chemical abnormalities resulting in a hyperdopaminergic, hyperglutamergic, and hypoadenosergic state. Similar abnormalities are found in human RLS patients. It is currently hypothesized that the dopaminergic abnormalities are responsible for the sensorimotor abnormalities of RLS, while the glutamate and adenosine abnor-malities are responsible for the abnormal arousal and sleep found in RLS (Ferre, Garcia-Borreguero, Allen, & Earley, 2019).

The source of brain iron deficiency is poorly understood in patients without a systemic iron deficiency, and genetic studies suggest the need for environmental factors in addition to genetic predisposition. The medical conditions reported to be associated with RLS may give clues to the nature of these environmental factors. A gastroenterologist at my institution noticed that his patients with small intes-tinal bacterial overgrowth (SIBO) had a high incidence of RLS, and the symptoms improved with antibiotic treatment. In a subsequent unblinded trial, patients with SIBO treated with rifaximin 1,200 mg/d for 10 days followed by long-term tegaserod resulted in a greater than 85% improvement in RLS symptoms in 10 of 13 patients. Many of the patients experienced a long-term remission of symptoms. We hypoth-esized that the intestinal inflammation led to systemic (3 patients) and/or brain iron deficiency in these patients, and antibiotic treatment led to a resolution of this deficiency (Weinstock, Fern, & Duntley, 2008). The possible role of inflamma-tion in secondary RLS was then assessed by a literature review of secondary RLS. Thirty-eight medical conditions are reported to have a high association with RLS. Thirty-six of these conditions demonstrate evidence of systemic inflammation or altered immunity, and 14 are associated with systemic iron deficiency (Weinstock et al., 2012). Further evidence for the role of inflammation in RLS is provided by studies finding elevated C-reactive protein in RLS patients, which is also related to periodic limb movement frequency, an elevated neutrophil-to-lymphocyte ratio, and the finding in RLS patients of five unique proteins by gel electrophoresis that are associated with inflammation, immune response, and cardiovascular dis-ease (Varim et al., 2016). It is widely known that inflammation leads to increased hepcidin levels, which reduces GI iron absorption. Recent evidence suggests that increased hepcidin levels also decreases free iron efflux from human endothelial cells into the brain, providing a likely link between systemic inflammation and brain iron deficiency (Chiou et al., 2018).

Whatever the cause of RLS, disturbed sleep, with both sleep onset and mainte-nance difficulty, is the most prominent and usually most distressing aspect of RLS and is seen in 60–90% of patients (Montplaisir et al., 1997). Because of the frequent motor activity, the sleep of a bed partner may also be severely disturbed. Daytime fatigue and less commonly sleepiness may be seen. There is a consistent decre-ment in quality of life indices, such as the SF-36, and this decrement in quality of life is similar to that seen in diseases such as diabetes and depression (Allen et al., 2005). It is important to stress that the impact of symptoms on daily life can be profound and that things we take for granted, such as being able to sit for a movie or on an airplane flight, may be virtually impossible for a person with severe restless legs. Work productivity is impaired. Depression, anxiety, and panic disorder are commonly associated with RLS. Epidemiological studies suggest an increased risk of hypertension and cardiovascular disease in patients with RLS. In a study 2,832 men who had a comprehensive sleep assessment and were then followed for a mean of 8.7 years, a diagnosis of RLS was associated with an incident myocardial infarction hazard ratio of 2.02 even after controlling for other covariates. A recent meta-analysis of nine population-based studies concludes that there is an increased risk of hypertension in RLS patients (Shen et al., 2018) although another recent meta-analysis found no increased risk of cerebrovascular or cardiovascular events when potential cofounding variables were accounted for, thus leading to uncertainty at present regarding the cardiovascular effects of RLS (Katsanos et al., 2018). There is high-quality evidence that pharmacotherapy of RLS results in significant improvement in sleep disturbance, mood disorders, and quality of life indices. There are currently no data that treatment reduces long-term cardiovascular risk. RLS is often difficult to diagnose in children, and it may be misdiagnosed as ADHD.

When a patient presents with RLS symptoms, an integrative approach is necessary. Potential secondary causes of RLS should be sought through a careful history and physical examination, and these should be treated when present. RLS symptoms may improve when the associated condition is effectively treated. Given the likely role of inflammation in the pathophysiology of RLS, it seems prudent to aggressively treat any source of systemic inflammation. Potential aggravating factors such as medications should be assessed and behavioral interventions implemented prior to pharmacotherapy. Pharmacotherapy will be necessary for many patients.

Ferritin, iron, total iron-binding capacity (TIBC), percent saturation, and renal function should be assessed in all patients, and other blood work may be suggested by clinical presentation. A complete blood count (CBC) and hemoglobin measurements alone are inadequate because relative deficits in body iron stores, as reflected in a low ferritin level, can result in aggravation of RLS symptoms before causing anemia. There is recent evidence of an association between vitamin D and RLS, with improvement of RLS after supplemental vitamin D (Wali et al., 2018). Aggressive iron supplementation should be instituted when systemic iron deficiency is found. The IRLS group (Allen et al., 2018) suggests a target ferritin of greater than 75. They recommend oral iron supplementation (ferrous sulfate 325 mg with vitamin C 100 mg) for ferritin levels of less than 75 in adults and less than 50 in children. Intravenous (IV) ferric carboxy maltose 1,000 mg, can be given to patients in whom oral iron is not tolerated or when there is no improvement after

12 weeks of oral iron therapy. Initial use of IV iron is recommended in patients with a ferritin of 75–100, or in patients in whom more rapid symptom relief may be required. IV iron may be effective even in patients without evidence of systemic iron deficiency, but it should not be used if the ferritin level is greater than 300 or the transferrin saturation is more than 45. This recommendation is based on Level A evidence (highly likely to be effective). It may take 4–6 weeks for a full response to IV iron. Pregnancy-induced symptoms usually resolve with delivery. Hemodialysis is notoriously unhelpful for symptoms secondary to uremia, but symptoms may resolve completely with renal transplantation.

The patient's medication list and dietary habits should be assessed for possible aggravating substances. Many patients develop serious sleep hygiene issues. Since symptoms are most severe in the first half of the sleep period, RLS patients often report that they obtain their best sleep late in the sleep period, leading to a tendency to sleep in late when their schedule allows. The resulting delayed sleep phase of their circadian rhythm further contributes to sleep onset difficulties. Many patients do not recognize the contribution of caffeine or ethanol to symptoms, and patients may use ethanol as a hypnotic or increase caffeine consumption to compensate for fatigue from chronic sleep deprivation. These sleep hygiene issues need to be addressed for optimal treatment.

Patients should be assessed for sleep apnea when clinically indicated. In a retrospective study of 56 patients with RLS and obstructive sleep apnea (OSA), treatment of the OSA led to an improvement in symptoms in 20 patients, with 9 patients stopping medications and 8 reducing their dose (Silva, Peralta, & Bentes, 2017). It should also be noted that RLS may result in difficulty tolerating constant positive airway pressure (CPAP), and sometimes treating the RLS leads to improved CPAP compliance.

A number of nonpharmacological treatments have been recommended for RLS symptoms. Although evidence-based data are scarce, there are some data to guide selection. The temporary relief of physical symptoms by movement is one of the essential diagnostic features of RLS so exercise can be used for the relief of symptoms when they occur. There is increasing evidence, however, that regular exercise may play an important role in preventing and treating RLS. In a recent prospective study, 12,812 men and 42,728 women who were free of RLS symptoms at baseline were followed for 4–6 years. Individuals who were physically active, nonsmokers, and alcohol consumption had significantly lower risks of developing RLS (Batool-Anwar et al., 2016).

Most of the clinical trials of exercise regimens for the treatment of RLS have been in hemodialysis patients, where pharmacotherapy can be challenging. A recent meta-analysis of exercise in these patients found 15 randomized controlled trials of acceptable quality (Song, Hu, Diao, Chen, & Jiang, 2018). Exercise regimens were quite variable both in type (cycling, jogging, walking, swimming, calisthenics, resistance exercises), intensity, and timing of exercise, with some

exercise occurring during hemodialysis and some between hemodialysis sessions. One study compared a 6-month exercise regimen to low-dose dopamine
agonist therapy and found similar improvement in uremic patients. Despite this
variability, this analysis found that exercise training was effective in reducing RLS
symptoms in these patients, along with comorbid depression and fatigue. The
American Academy of Neurology (AAN) evidence-based practice guidelines
(Winkelman et al., 2016) consider exercise possibly effective in treating symptoms
(Level C evidence) and improving sleep quality in hemodialysis patients. Several
studies also showed improvement in depression and quality of life measures with
exercise. There is less evidence supporting the use of exercise in primary RLS, but
in one randomized controlled trial patients with primary RLS were prescribed
lower body resistance exercises and treadmill walking for 30 minutes at a pace
resulting in a heart rate of 40–60% the predicted maximum rate three times a
week for 12 weeks. The mean RLS score decreased from 20.6 to 12.1 in the exercise
group, compared to 22.5 to 21.5 in the control group (Aukerman et al., 2006). It
should be noted that, although anecdotal, many patients report that overexertion
on any given day may precipitate significant worsening of RLS, and the regularity
of the exercise program is probably an important component for efficacy. While
work remains to be done to confirm this benefit in primary RLS and to define the
optimal treatment regimen, when coupled with the general health benefits of regular exercise, exercise should be considered one of the most important tools for
preventing and treating RLS.

Yoga is an ancient mind–body discipline that incorporates elements of relaxation training and exercise. It is increasingly accepted in modern medicine as a
useful integrative medicine technique, and although evidence is generally of low to
moderate quality, studies consistently find that yoga improves mood, sleep quality,
and quality of life measures in a variety of medical conditions. While widely
studied in a variety of other neurological disorders, the evidence in RLS is scant.
In one randomized controlled trial, 75 women with RLS were randomly assigned
to receive either an 8-week gentle yoga program designed for older adults or an
educational film program. Classes were held for 90 minutes twice weekly, with 30
minutes of home sessions on non-class days (Innes & Selfe, 2012). Although specific RLS measures were not performed, subjective sleep quality on the Pittsburgh
Sleep Quality Index, mood, perceived stress, and blood pressure all improved in
the treatment group compared to the control group. In a later study, the same
authors conducted a pilot study of 10 women with moderate to severe RLS. Those
who attended an average of 13.4 yoga classes and 4.1 home yoga sessions a week
had a reduction in RLS scores of 21.0 to 10.8, with subjective improvement in sleep
and mood measures (Innes, Selfe, Agarwal, Williams, & Flack, 2013). Although
there are inadequate controlled trials to make evidence-based recommendations
specific for RLS, given the general health benefits of yoga and its possible benefits

in RLS, it is reasonable to consider prescribing yoga for patients with RLS pending further high-quality studies.

Since patients spontaneously develop counter-stimulatory techniques, it is logical to think that the use of devices designed to deliver predictable stimulus should be of some benefit. The AAN practice guidelines (Winkelman et al., 2016) list pneumatic compression devices (PCD) as likely effective in the treatment of primary RLS, and near-infrared spectroscopy (Level B evidence) and repetitive transcranial magnetic stimulation (rTMS) as possibly effective. Pneumatic devices are readily available and also shown to improve sleep quality and quality of life measures, but they are often difficult to use in RLS patients who may need to pace at night. Restiffic, a commercially available device that produces targeted pressure on the abductor halluces and flexor halluces brevis muscles, reduced RLS symptoms in an open label trial. An MM507 foot massager, used alone or combined with a heating pad for 30 minutes before bedtime, resulted in improvement in RLS symptoms in a randomized controlled trial (Park, Ambrogi, & Hade, 2020). Weighted blankets, often used for treatment of insomnia, have been anecdotally reported to reduce RLS symptoms in some patients. Massage of the legs with either glycerin or lavender oil during dialysis was found to be beneficial for hemodialysis patients, and warm or cold water immersion for 10 minutes prior to bedtime was found to be beneficial in pregnant women in randomized controlled trials (Mirbagher Ajorpaz, Rahemi, Aghajani, & Hashemi, 2020; Jafarimenish, Vakilian, & Mobasseri, 2020). Vitamins C (200 mg) and E (400 mg) alone or in combination are likely effective in the treatment of secondary RLS in end-stage renal disease (ESRD) (Sagheb et al., 2012).

In a recent evidence-based review of complementary and alternative treatment for RLS, only 18 studies met inclusion and exclusion criteria, with most already discussed (Xu et al., 2018). One single, blinded, placebo-controlled trial of sham acupuncture revealed an improvement in the IRLS rating scale scores of 5.5 in the acupuncture group compared to 1.4 in the control group (Pan et al., 2015). Magnesium supplementation has been recommended but appears most beneficial in pregnant women (Bartell & Zallek, 2006). Venous insufficiency has been proposed as a secondary cause of RLS, and one unblinded, randomized study revealed significant improvement with sclerotherapy (Hayes, Kingsley, Hamby, & Carlow, 2008). A patient with a spinal cord stimulator implanted for neuropathic pain also reported a significant improvement is his RLS symptoms (Holland et al., 2016). Deep brain stimulators for the treatment of movement disorders have been reported to both improve and worsen RLS. In a small double-blind, placebo-controlled trial, the injection of botulinum toxin resulted in symptom improvement (Mittal, Machado, Richardson, Dubey, & Jabbari, 2018). A variety of other treatments are advocated by RLS patients, such as massage and whirlpool treatment, but evidence supporting their use in the general RLS populations is lacking.

Given the expected lack of side effects from these treatments, including them in treatment options for receptive patients would seem reasonable.

Although differences in definitions, methods of diagnosis and symptom measurement, and often obscure methodologies limit comparisons with Western medical literature, more than 40 herbal formulas are described in TCM literature. A recent review noted 85 studies, with 9 randomized and 3 controlled, dealing with treatments of likely RLS (Yan et al., 2012). Many of these studies suggested effectiveness, and some included medications such as clonazepam and L-dopa in comparison groups. The apparent safety and efficacy of these herbal preparations warrant more rigorous studies. In areas where available, referral to a practitioner of TCM would be reasonable for a patient interested in alternative medicines.

Many patients with severe RLS symptoms will require pharmacotherapy. Medications that have FDA approval for treating RLS symptoms fall into two categories: alpha-2-delta ligands (gabapentin encarbil 300–1,200 mg) and dopamine agonists (pramipexole 0.125 to .75 mg, ropinirole 0.25 to 4 mg; rotigotine1 3 mg). Although not FDA approved, the alpha-2-ligand pregabalin also has evidence supporting efficacy in RLS. Despite the prominence of the response to dopamine agonists, their use is complicated by augmentation (occurrence of symptoms earlier in the day or spread to other body regions) and rebound (the occurrence of symptoms as the medication wears off). These occur in a significant percentage of patients and can result in RLS shifting to other times of the day or a paradoxical worsening of symptoms with increasing doses. Up to 76% of patients on long-term dopaminergic therapy are reported to experience augmentation, and up to 35% exhibit rebound. Stomach upset and headache can sometimes be severe enough to limit use. Other less common but potentially dangerous side effects include abrupt onset of sleepiness, orthostatic hypotension, and impulse control disorder, most commonly presenting as increased gambling or inappropriate sexual activity. Common side effects of gabapentin enacarbil include somnolence, dizziness, and edema. It can worsen mood disorders, which are already common in this population. Pramipexole, rotigotine, and gabapentin encarbil have Level A evidence supporting their use for symptom relief; and ropinirole and pregabalin have Level B evidence supporting their use. Gabapentin encarbil may be more effective than dopamine agonists in treating subjective sleep complaints in RLS patients (Winkelman et al., 2016).

Although lacking FDA approval for treatment of RLS, there is evidence that opioids are effective for refractory cases. One randomized trial of a prolonged-release formulation of oxycodone and naloxone (usual dose 10–30 mg) found an improvement in IRLS scores (Level C evidence), quality of life scores, and improvements in sleep quality (Trenkwalder et al., 2013). Methadone (usual dose 5–20 mg) is supported by only two open label trials, but it may be the most effective opioid, especially in patients requiring 24-hour coverage or long-term treatment.

Guidelines for the appropriate use of opioids have been recently published. Other medications that are sometimes used and for which there is some evidence for effectiveness include benzodiazepines, particularly clonazepam. In small case series, istradefylline and dipyridamole, both of which act on central adenosinergic systems, were effective in reducing RLS symptoms (Garcia-Borreguero et al., 2018; Nuermaimaiti, Oyama, Kasemsuk, & Hattori, 2018). Cannabis is reported to provide total relief in a report of six patients but has not been systematically studied (Megelin & Ghorayeb, 2017).

PERIODIC LIMB MOVEMENT DISORDER

Unlike RLS, PLMD requires objective documentation of periodic limb movements during sleep (PLMS), with current diagnostic criteria requiring PSG. PSG must demonstrate movements more than 5 movements per hour in children and more than 15 per hour in adults. In clinical practice limb movements associated with and without arousals are usually quantified separately, but arousals are not required by the ICSD-3, and the practical importance of distinguishing between movements with and without arousals is not well established. The PLMS must cause clinically significant sleep disturbance or impairment in mental, physical, social, occupational, educational, or other important areas of functioning. According to ICSD-3 criteria, PLMD cannot be diagnosed in the presence of RLS, narcolepsy, or untreated sleep apnea.

PLMS are highly stereotyped movements that occur most commonly in the legs but may affect the arms. The leg movements consist of extension of the big toe and flexion of the foot, knee, and sometimes the hip. Movements typically occur in both legs but the movements may be asynchronous. When associated with a cortical arousal, the arousal may precede, occur concurrently with, or follow the beginning of the limb movement. The movements are associated with autonomic arousals which result in an increase in heart rate and blood pressure. The movements are most frequent in the first half of the night. Similar periodic limb movements can be seen secondary to OSA or secondary to medications. Treatment of the sleep apnea or removal of the causative medication will result in a resolution of the movements.

The prevalence of more than 15 PLMS per hour is reported to be present in 7.6% of 18- to 65-year-olds (American Academy of Sleep Medicine, 2014); however other studies have suggested a much higher prevalence, with the Wisconsin Sleep Cohort finding a periodic limb movement index (PLMI) of greater than 15 in 25.3% of people in this population-based study of adults (Leary et al., 2018). Up to 45% of the elderly may have PLMS. PLMS are more common in Caucasians than African Americans. Unlike RLS, there is no gender difference in PLMS. Although

PLMS are common in adults, the actual prevalence of PLMD is unknown and believed to be uncommon once exclusionary factors are accounted for.

Like RLS, impaired dopamine neurotransmission and CNS iron deficiency appear to be involved in the pathophysiology of PLMS (Ferre et al., 2017). Family members of RLS patients have a higher incidence of PLMS, suggesting a *form fruste* of RLS in these patients. The genetics is similar, with *BTBD9* and *MEIS1* being implicated in genome-wide studies (Winkelman et al., 2015). As in RLS, selective serotonin reuptake inhibitors (SSRIs), tricyclic antidepressants, dopamine antagonists, and lithium can cause or aggravate PLMS.

Insomnia, hypersomnia, and daytime fatigue are the most common reported consequences of PLMS. The sleep of a bed partner may be disturbed as much or more than that of the patient. Occasionally, the limb movements may be violent enough to cause injury to the patient or bed partner. Because other disorders, such as sleep apnea, are felt to be much more common causes of these symptoms, a careful search for other causes is essential before attributing these symptoms to PLMS. Mood disorders, anxiety, and an increased risk of automobile accidents has been reported (Liu, Perez, & Lau, 2018). Attention deficits suggestive of attention deficit disorder (ADD) may be present, especially in children (Silvestri et al., 2009). Leg movements are associated with a surge in sympathetic nervous system activity resulting in increased heart rate and blood pressure and a blunting of the nocturnal dip in blood pressure (Sieminski, Pyrzowski, & Partinen, 2017). Epidemiological studies suggest a link to hypertension and adverse cardiovascular events (Dean et al., 2015; Kendzerska, Kamra, Murray, & Boulos, 2017). Treatment with ropinirole blunts the surge in blood pressure and heart rate, but there is yet no evidence that treatment of PLMS reduces adverse cardiovascular outcomes (Manconi et al., 2011).

Unlike RLS, which is a purely clinical diagnosis, PLMD can be strongly suspected on clinical grounds, but confirmation with PSG is recommended. Evaluation and treatment are otherwise similar, although evidence-based data are relatively scarce compared to RLS and there are little data on the effect of both alternative methods and pharmacotherapy on PLMD. Sleep hygiene should be addressed, and secondary etiologies, especially iron deficiency, should be sought and treated when present. In one trial, acupuncture resulted in an improvement in nighttime motor activity in primary RLS, and exercise reduced waking leg movements during hemodialysis in ESRD patients (Dean et al., 2015; Giannaki et al., 2010). The AAN practice summary concludes that there is strong evidence to support the use of ropinirole in PLMS; moderate evidence for the use of pramipexole, rotigotine, cabergoline, and pregabalin; and weak evidence supporting the use of levodopa (Winkelman et al., 2016). There are little data on gabapentin encarbil or other pharmacological agents.

SLEEP-RELATED LEG CRAMPS

SRLC are defined as a painful sensation in the leg or foot associated with sudden involuntary muscle hardness or tightness, indicating a strong muscle contraction. The muscle contraction occurs during the time in bed but can arise from either wakefulness or sleep. The pain is relieved by forceful stretching of the affected muscle.

The diagnosis is based on clinical criteria. Diagnostic testing such as electromyography and nerve conduction testing, serum creatine kinase (CK), or neuroimaging may be indicated to rule out secondary causes if associated neurological signs or symptoms are present, if the cramps involve areas other than the legs, or if prominent daytime cramping occurs.

The prevalence and frequency of leg cramps increases with age, with an occasional cramp becoming a nearly universal experience. Occasional cramps are seen in 7% of children, in 33% of adults older than 60 (with 6% reporting nightly cramps), and in 50% of adults older than 80 (American Academy of Sleep Medicine, 2014). Gender and ethnic factors are not well established.

Most SRLC are considered idiopathic. Electrophysiological recordings during a cramp begin with a spontaneous firing of lower motor neurons at rates of about 300 Hz (American Academy of Sleep Medicine, 2014). Vigorous physical activity, dehydration, hypokalemia, hypocalcemia, and hypomagnesemia may precipitate cramps. A number of medications may precipitate or aggravate cramps, including oral contraceptives, long-acting beta-agonists, and statins. Leg cramps are common in pregnancy and generally remit after delivery. Secondary leg cramps are seen in myelopathy, amyotrophic lateral sclerosis (ALS), neuropathy, and hypocalcemia.

The most common consequence of leg cramps is insomnia. The pain from the cramp awakens the patient and can prevent return to sleep. In severe cases, the dread of painful cramps can lead to anxiety about falling asleep. Cramping must be distinguished from *dystonia*, where there is a co-contraction of agonist and antagonist muscles that is not relieved by stretching. Nocturnal leg cramps can also be confused with RLS, in which patients may complain of a muscle tightness but where a sustained involuntary muscle contraction does not occur.

As in RLS, an integrative approach includes assessing for secondary etiologies with a careful history and physical examination and removing potential precipitating causes such as medications. Also as in RLS, assessment for and treatment of OSA should be performed if clinically indicated. In one case series, for 3 of 4 patients with both sleep apnea and leg cramps, treatment of the sleep apnea resulted in a resolution of the cramps, and there was a marked improvement in the remaining patient (Westwood, Spector, & Auerbach, 2014). There is some evidence that stretching exercises may be beneficial, with an uncontrolled trial suggesting improvement with calf stretching exercises, although a subsequent randomized trial found no benefit (Coppin, Wicke, & Little, 2005). Quinine at doses of 200–500 mg is effective in reducing the frequency and severity of cramping, but the FDA recommends quinine not be used for the treatment of cramps because of the risk of cardiac arrhythmias. The use of diltiazem (Voon & Sheu, 2001) or magnesium (Roffe, Sills, Crome, & Jones, 2002; Sebo, Cerutti, & Haller, 2014) is supported by some evidence, with the latter being most effective in pregnancy. Gabapentin, carbamazepine, verapamil, and carisoprodol have been suggested as treatment but lack evidence. Botulinum toxin injection was found to be safe and effective in patients with secondary nocturnal leg cramps from lumbar spinal stenosis (Park, Yoon, Yoon, & Kim, 2017).

SLEEP-RELATED BRUXISM

SRB is defined as the presence of regular or frequent tooth grinding noises occurring during sleep, with abnormal tooth wear consistent with tooth grinding, transient morning jaw muscle pain or fatigue, temporal headache, and/or jaw locking upon awakening.

The diagnosis is typically made on clinical grounds. PSG reveals rhythmic masticatory muscle activity with phasic and tonic masseter and temporalis muscle activity associated with grinding noises. Bruxism can arise from any stage of sleep but is most commonly seen in stages 1 and 2 sleep.

The majority of bruxism events occur after an arousal from sleep. Decreased sleep stability appears to be involved but the exact pathophysiology remains unclear. Symptoms may be precipitated or aggravated by anxiety, use of caffeine or tobacco, and dental occlusal defects. SSRIs may precipitate or aggravate bruxism (Melo et al., 2018). Familial factors appear to be present, but the genetics has not been elucidated. A recent study in Japan looked as associations between SRB and personality measures, alcohol, caffeine, tobacco use, past stressful life events, snoring and sleep apnea symptoms, and RLS, along with daytime tooth grinding symptoms. Thirteen polymorphisms in four genes related to serotonergic neurotransmission were studied. Only a single polymorphism was associated with bruxism as measured by 3 nights of electromyographic recording (Abe et al., 2012). A systematic review of the literature found that when considering the results of seven qualifying studies, SRB was associated with drinking more than 8 cups of coffee a day and alcohol and tobacco use (Bertazzo-Silveira et al., 2016). Gastroesophageal reflux also appears to be associated with SRB. SRB must be distinguished from waking bruxism, which is generally considered a separate entity with a distinct pathophysiology.

The prevalence peaks in childhood at 14–17%, decreasing to 12% in young adults and 8% in middle-aged adults (American Academy of Sleep Medicine, 2014). There does not appear to be a gender difference. Characteristic tooth wear is the most frequent consequence. Morning jaw pain and headache are common. Temporomandibular joint (TMJ) disorders may occur, but causality is unclear. As with other sleep-related movement disorders, bruxism may disturb the sleep of the bed partner.

The integrative approach to SRB includes addressing lifestyle issues such as reducing tobacco, caffeine, and alcohol intake. There is some literature suggesting a link between OSA and SRB, but data are inconclusive. PSG studies of SRB found that 85% of bruxism events are associated with limb movements, usually with cortical arousal, suggesting that they are part of a descending volley of motor activity arising from a central generator (Zhang et al., 2017). The primary treatment of bruxism is with dental appliances. A recent meta-analysis found that among the nine studies using objective SRB measurement with PSG, eight revealed an improvement with most types of dental appliances, with a greater improvement seen with devices that provided mandibular advancement (Jokubauskas, Baltrusaityte, & Pileicikiene, 2018). Cognitive-behavioral therapy added to occlusal splint therapy was more effective than splint therapy alone in one study of 22 patients (Trindade, Orestes-Cardoso, & de Siqueira, 2015). Biofeedback has been proposed, but evidence is limited. An unblinded pilot study of rTMS in 12 patients found a reduction in objectively measured bruxing events and jaw soreness with treatment (Zhou et al., 2016). Myofascial trigger point dry needling of patients with SRB resulted in decreased pain and other jaw symptoms both immediately and after 1 week (Blasco-Bonora & Martin-Pintado-Zugasti, 2017). In cases where significant pain or sleep disruption is present, botulinum injections have been demonstrated to be effective in four randomized, placebo-controlled trials (Fernandez-Nunez, Amghar-Maach, & Gay-Escoda, 2019). Clonazepam and clonidine have been proposed for treatment but data are quite limited. A randomized, open label crossover study did not find pramipexole to be beneficial despite its link to PLMS noted earlier (Cahlin, Hedner, & Dahlstrom, 2017).

Sleep Starts

SS, also known as *hypnic jerks*, are a brief sudden contraction of one or multiple body segments that occurs at sleep onset. The movements are sometimes associated with a sensory sensation including falling, a banging noise, or a bright light flash. The sensory phenomenon can be seen without the movement in some individuals. These are usually solitary events and are so common that they are considered a normal variant. Prevalence is estimated at 60–70%, and all ages are affected (American Academy of Sleep Medicine, 2014). The pathophysiology is uncertain, but the transition between sleep and wakefulness is an unstable state for both the sensory and motor systems. A sympathetic autonomic response including tachycardia can accompany the jerks.

In most individuals, these are a sporadic occurrence and do not interfere with sleep. In rare individuals, the SS can become repetitive, leading to sleep onset insomnia. Aggravating lifestyle features should be assessed and addressed and include excessive caffeine consumption, stress, sleep deprivation, and excessive physical exertion. A hypnotic such as clonazepam may occasionally be necessary.

Conclusion

When the normal quiescence of sleep is interrupted by abnormal motor activity, this may be a mere nuisance, or it may result in devastating and life-altering symptoms. Unless integrative medicine is practiced by combining complementary medicine with traditional medical approaches, the practitioner will not be able to deliver optimal care. In the mild RLS patient, in whom lifestyle modification and exercise or yoga may be adequate, pharmacotherapy with a dopamine agonist runs a very real risk of overtreatment, with dosage escalation due to augmentation and rebound resulting in avoidable cost and unnecessary risk. In the most severe RLS patients, even polypharmacy may not provide adequate relief, and complementary medicine may offer real additional benefit. For some disorders, such as SRB and SRLC, traditional medicine provides remarkably few therapeutic options. While evidence-based recommendations are sparse, complementary medicine techniques add real options to otherwise limited treatments. Much work remains to be done to establish the best treatments for these disorders, but with the evidence we have, integrative medicine will deliver the best patient outcomes.

REFERENCES

Abe, Y., Suganuma, T., Ishii, M., Yamamoto, G., Gunji, T., Clark, G. T., . . . Baba, K. (2012). Association of genetic, psychological and behavioral factors with sleep bruxism in a Japanese population. *Journal of Sleep Research, 21*(3), 289–296. doi:10.1111/j.1365-2869.2011.00961.x.

Allen, R. P., Barker, P. B., Wehrl, F. W., Song, H. K., & Earley, C. J. (2001). MRI measurement of brain iron in patients with restless legs syndrome. *Neurology, 56*(2), 263–265. doi:10.1212/wnl.56.2.263.

Allen, R. P., & Earley, C. J. (2001). Restless legs syndrome: A review of clinical and pathophysiologic features. *Journal of Clinical Neurophysiology, 18*(2), 128–147.

Allen, R. P., Picchietti, D. L., Auerbach, M., Cho, Y. W., Connor, J. R., Earley, C. J., . . . Winkelman, J. W. (2018). Evidence-based and consensus clinical practice guidelines for the iron treatment of restless legs syndrome/Willis-Ekbom disease in adults and children: An IRLSSG task force report. *Sleep Medicine, 41*, 27–44. doi:10.1016/j.sleep.2017.11.1126.

Allen, R. P., Walters, A. S., Montplaisir, J., Hening, W., Myers, A., Bell, T. J., & Ferini-Strambi, L. (2005). Restless legs syndrome prevalence and impact: REST general population study. *Archives of Internal Medicine, 165*(11), 1286–1292. doi:10.1001/archinte.165.11.1286.

American Academy of Sleep Medicine. (2014). *The international classification of sleep disorders: Diagnostic & coding manual* (3rd ed.). Westchester, IL: American Academy of Sleep Medicine.

Aukerman, M. M., Aukerman, D., Bayard, M., Tudiver, F., Thorp, L., & Bailey, B. (2006). Exercise and restless legs syndrome: A randomized controlled trial. *Journal of the American Board of Family Medicine, 19*(5), 487–493.

Bartell, S., & Zallek, S. (2006). Intravenous magnesium sulfate may relieve restless legs syndrome in pregnancy. *Journal of Clinical Sleep Medicine, 2*(2), 187–188.

Batool-Anwar, S., Li, Y., De Vito, K., Malhotra, A., Winkelman, J., & Gao, X. (2016). Lifestyle factors and risk of restless legs syndrome: Prospective cohort study. *Journal of Clinical Sleep Medicine, 12*(2), 187–194. doi:10.5664/jcsm.5482.

Bertazzo-Silveira, E., Kruger, C. M., Porto De Toledo, I., Porporatti, A. L., Dick, B., Flores-Mir, C., & De Luca Canto, G. (2016). Association between sleep bruxism and alcohol, caffeine, tobacco, and drug abuse: A systematic review. *Journal of the American Dental Association, 147*(11), 859–866.e4. doi:10.1016/j.adaj.2016.06.014.

Blasco-Bonora, P. M., & Martin-Pintado-Zugasti, A. (2017). Effects of myofascial trigger point dry needling in patients with sleep bruxism and temporomandibular disorders: A prospective case series. *Acupuncture in Medicine, 35*(1), 69–74. doi:10.1136/acupmed-2016-011102.

Cahlin, B. J., Hedner, J., & Dahlstrom, L. (2017). A randomised, open-label, crossover study of the dopamine agonist, pramipexole, in patients with sleep bruxism. *Journal of Sleep Research, 26*(1), 64–72. doi:10.1111/jsr.12440.

Chiou, B., Neal, E. H., Bowman, A. B., Lippmann, E. S., Simpson, I. A., & Connor, J. R. (2018). Endothelial cells are critical regulators of iron transport in a model of the human blood-brain barrier. *Journal of Cerebral Blood Flow and Metabolism*, 271678x18783372. doi:10.1177/0271678x18783372.

Coppin, R. J., Wicke, D. M., & Little, P. S. (2005). Managing nocturnal leg cramps--calf-stretching exercises and cessation of quinine treatment: A factorial randomised controlled trial. *British Journal of General Practice, 55*(512), 186–191.

Dean, D. A., Wang, R., Jacobs, D. R., Duprez, D., Punjabi, N. M., Zee, P. C., . . . Redline, S. (2015). A systematic assessment of the association of polysomnographic indices with blood pressure: The Multi-Ethnic Study of Atherosclerosis (MESA). *Sleep, 38*(4), 587–596. doi:10.5665/sleep.4576.

Earley, C. J., Connor, J. R., Beard, J. L., Malecki, E. A., Epstein, D. K., & Allen, R. P. (2000). Abnormalities in CSF concentrations of ferritin and transferrin in restless legs syndrome. *Neurology, 54*(8), 1698–1700. doi:10.1212/wnl.54.8.1698.

Ekbom, K. A. (1945). Restless legs. Acta Med Scandinavia, 158 (Suppl), 1–123.

Fernandez-Nunez, T., Amghar-Maach, S., & Gay-Escoda, C. (2019). Efficacy of botulinum toxin in the treatment of bruxism: Systematic review. *Medicina Oral, Patología Oral y Cirugía Bucal, 24*(4), e416–e424. doi:10.4317/medoral.22923.

Ferre, S., Garcia-Borreguero, D., Allen, R. P., & Earley, C. J. (2019). New insights into the neurobiology of restless legs syndrome. *Neuroscientist, 25*(2), 113–125. doi:10.1177/1073858418791763.

Ferre, S., Quiroz, C., Guitart, X., Rea, W., Seyedian, A., Moreno, E., . . . Garcia-Borreguero, D. (2017). Pivotal role of adenosine neurotransmission in restless legs syndrome. *Frontiers in Neuroscience, 11*, 722. doi:10.3389/fnins.2017.00722.

Garcia-Borreguero, D., Guitart, X., Garcia Malo, C., Cano-Pumarega, I., Granizo, J. J., & Ferre, S. (2018). Treatment of restless legs syndrome/Willis-Ekbom disease with the non-selective ENT1/ENT2 inhibitor dipyridamole: Testing the adenosine hypothesis. *Sleep Medicine, 45*, 94–97. doi:10.1016/j.sleep.2018.02.002.

Giannaki, C. D., Sakkas, G. K., Hadjigeorgiou, G. M., Karatzaferi, C., Patramani, G., Lavdas, E., . . . Stefanidis, I. (2010). Non-pharmacological management of periodic limb movements during hemodialysis session in patients with uremic restless legs syndrome. *ASAIO Journal, 56*(6), 538–542. doi:10.1097/MAT.0b013e3181f1cc04.

Hayes, C. A., Kingsley, J. R., Hamby, K. R., & Carlow, J. (2008). The effect of endovenous laser ablation on restless legs syndrome. *Phlebology, 23*(3), 112–117. doi:10.1258/phleb.2007.007051.

Hening, W., Walters, A. S., Allen, R. P., Montplaisir, J., Myers, A., & Ferini-Strambi, L. (2004). Impact, diagnosis and treatment of restless legs syndrome (RLS) in a primary care population: The REST (RLS epidemiology, symptoms, and treatment) primary care study. *Sleep Medicine, 5*(3), 237–246. doi:10.1016/j.sleep.2004.03.006.

Holland, M. T., Rettenmaier, L. A., Flouty, O. E., Thomsen, T. R., Jerath, N. U., & Reddy, C. G. (2016). Epidural spinal cord stimulation: A novel therapy in the treatment of restless legs syndrome. *World Neurosurgery, 92*, 582.e515-582.e518. doi:10.1016/j.wneu.2016.05.077.

Innes, K. E., & Selfe, T. K. (2012). The effects of a gentle yoga program on sleep, mood, and blood pressure in older women with restless legs syndrome (RLS): A preliminary randomized controlled trial. *Evidence-Based Complementary and Alternative Medicine, 2012*, 294058. doi:10.1155/2012/294058.

Innes, K. E., Selfe, T. K., Agarwal, P., Williams, K., & Flack, K. L. (2013). Efficacy of an eight-week yoga intervention on symptoms of restless legs syndrome (RLS): A pilot study. *Journal of Alternative and Complementary Medicine, 19*(6), 527–535. doi:10.1089/acm.2012.0330.

Hornyak M, Feige B, Riemann D, Voderholzer U. Periodic leg movements in sleep and periodic limb movement disorder: prevalence, clinical significance and treatment. *Sleep Med Rev.* 2006 Jun;10(3):169–177. doi:10.1016/j.smrv.2005.12.003. PMID: 16762807.

Jafarimanesh, H., Vakilian, K., & Mobasseri, S. (2020). Thermo-therapy and cryotherapy to decrease the symptoms of restless leg syndrome during the pregnancy: A randomized clinical trial. *Complementary Therapy Medicine, 50*, 102409. doi:10.1016/j.ctim.2020.102409.

Jokubauskas, L., Baltrusaityte, A., & Pileicikiene, G. (2018). Oral appliances for managing sleep bruxism in adults: A systematic review from 2007 to 2017. *Journal of Oral Rehabilitation, 45*(1), 81–95. doi:10.1111/joor.12558.

Katsanos, A. H., Kosmidou, M., Konitsiotis, S., Tsivgoulis, G., Fiolaki, A., Kyritsis, A. P., & Giannopoulos, S. (2018). Restless legs syndrome and cerebrovascular/cardiovascular events: Systematic review and meta-analysis. *Acta Neurologica Scandinavica, 137*(1), 142–148. doi:10.1111/ane.12848.

Kendzerska, T., Kamra, M., Murray, B. J., & Boulos, M. I. (2017). Incident cardiovascular events and death in individuals with restless legs syndrome or periodic limb movements in sleep: A systematic review. *Sleep, 40*(3). doi:10.1093/sleep/zsx013.

Leary, E. B., Moore, H. E. t., Schneider, L. D., Finn, L. A., Peppard, P. E., & Mignot, E. (2018). Periodic limb movements in sleep: Prevalence and associated sleepiness in the Wisconsin Sleep Cohort. *Clinical Neurophysiology, 129*(11), 2306–2314. doi:10.1016/j.clinph.2018.08.022.

Liu, S. Y., Perez, M. A., & Lau, N. (2018). The impact of sleep disorders on driving safety-findings from the Second Strategic Highway Research Program naturalistic driving study. *Sleep, 41*(4). doi:10.1093/sleep/zsy023.

Manconi, M., Ferri, R., Zucconi, M., Clemens, S., Rundo, F., Oldani, A., & Ferini-Strambi, L. (2011). Effects of acute dopamine-agonist treatment in restless legs syndrome on heart rate variability during sleep. *Sleep Medicine, 12*(1), 47–55. doi:10.1016/j.sleep.2010.03.019.

Megelin, T., & Ghorayeb, I. (2017). Cannabis for restless legs syndrome: A report of six patients. *Sleep Medicine, 36*, 182–183. doi:10.1016/j.sleep.2017.04.019.

Melo, G., Dutra, K. L., Rodrigues Filho, R., Ortega, A. O. L., Porporatti, A. L., Dick, B., . . . De Luca Canto, G. (2018). Association between psychotropic medications and presence of sleep bruxism: A systematic review. *Journal of Oral Rehabilitation, 45*(7), 545–554. doi:10.1111/joor.12633.

Michaud, M., Paquet, J., Lavigne, G., Desautels, A., & Montplaisir, J. (2002). Sleep laboratory diagnosis of restless legs syndrome. *European Neurology, 48*(2), 108–113. doi:10.1159/000062996.

Mirbagher Ajorpaz, N., Rahemi, Z., Aghajani, M., & Hashemi, S. H. (2020). Effects of glycerin oil and lavender oil massages on hemodialysis patients' restless legs syndrome. *Journal of Bodywork and Movement Therapy, 24*(1), 88–92. doi:10.1016/j.jbmt.2019.06.012.

Mittal, S. O., Machado, D., Richardson, D., Dubey, D., & Jabbari, B. (2018). Botulinum toxin in restless legs syndrome: A randomized double-blind placebo-controlled crossover study. *Toxins, 10*(10). doi:10.3390/toxins10100401.

Montplaisir, J., Boucher, S., Poirier, G., Lavigne, G., Lapierre, O., & Lesperance, P. (1997). Clinical, polysomnographic, and genetic characteristics of restless legs syndrome: A study of 133 patients diagnosed with new standard criteria. *Movement Disorders, 12*(1), 61–65. doi:10.1002/mds.870120111.

Nuermaimaiti, M., Oyama, G., Kasemsuk, C., & Hattori, N. (2018). Istradefylline for restless legs syndrome associated with Parkinson's disease. *Tremor and Other Hyperkinetic Movements (New York, N.Y.), 8*, 521. doi:10.7916/d86h5r1h.

Pan, W., Wang, M., Li, M., Wang, Q., Kwak, S., Jiang, W., & Yamamoto, Y. (2015). Actigraph evaluation of acupuncture for treating restless legs syndrome. *Evidence-Based Complementary and Alternative Medicine, 2015,* 343201. doi:10.1155/2015/343201.

Park, A., Ambrogi, K., & Hade, E. M. (2020). Randomized pilot trial for the efficacy of the MMF07 foot massager and heat therapy for restless legs syndrome. *PLoS One, 15*(4), e0230951. doi:10.1371/journal.pone.0230951.

Park, S. J., Yoon, K. B., Yoon, D. M., & Kim, S. H. (2017). Botulinum toxin treatment for nocturnal calf cramps in patients with lumbar spinal stenosis: A randomized clinical trial. *Archives of Physical Medicine and Rehabilitation, 98*(5), 957–963. doi:10.1016/j.apmr.2017.01.017.

Patatanian, E., & Claborn, M. K. (2018). Drug-induced restless legs syndrome. *Annals of Pharmacotherapy, 52*(7), 662–672. doi:10.1177/1060028018760296.

Picchietti, D., Allen, R. P., Walters, A. S., Davidson, J. E., Myers, A., & Ferini-Strambi, L. (2007). Restless legs syndrome: Prevalence and impact in children and adolescents: The Peds REST study. *Pediatrics, 120*(2), 253–266. doi:10.1542/peds.2006-2767.

Roffe, C., Sills, S., Crome, P., & Jones, P. (2002). Randomised, cross-over, placebo controlled trial of magnesium citrate in the treatment of chronic persistent leg cramps. *Medical Science Monitor, 8*(5), Cr326–330.

Sagheb, M. M., Dormanesh, B., Fallahzadeh, M. K., Akbari, H., Sohrabi Nazari, S., Heydari, S. T., & Behzadi, S. (2012). Efficacy of vitamins C, E, and their combination for treatment of restless legs syndrome in hemodialysis patients: A randomized, double-blind, placebo-controlled trial. *Sleep Medicine, 13*(5), 542–545. doi:10.1016/j.sleep.2011.11.010.

Sebo, P., Cerutti, B., & Haller, D. M. (2014). Effect of magnesium therapy on nocturnal leg cramps: A systematic review of randomized controlled trials with meta-analysis using simulations. *Family Practice, 31*(1), 7–19. doi:10.1093/fampra/cmt065.

Shen, Y., Liu, H., Dai, T., Guan, Y., Tu, J., & Nie, H. (2018). Association between restless legs syndrome and hypertension: A meta-analysis of nine population-based studies. *Neurological Sciences, 39*(2), 235–242. doi:10.1007/s10072-017-3182-4.

Sieminski, M., Pyrzowski, J., & Partinen, M. (2017). Periodic limb movements in sleep are followed by increases in EEG activity, blood pressure, and heart rate during sleep. *Sleep Breath, 21*(2), 497–503. doi:10.1007/s11325-017-1476-7.

Silva, C., Peralta, A. R., & Bentes, C. (2017). The urge to move and breathe: The impact of obstructive sleep apnea syndrome treatment in patients with previously diagnosed, clinically significant restless legs syndrome. *Sleep Medicine, 38,* 17–20. doi:10.1016/j.sleep.2017.06.023.

Silvestri, R., Gagliano, A., Arico, I., Calarese, T., Cedro, C., Bruni, O., . . . Bramanti, P. (2009). Sleep disorders in children with attention-deficit/hyperactivity disorder (ADHD) recorded overnight by video-polysomnography. *Sleep Medicine, 10*(10), 1132–1138. doi:10.1016/j.sleep.2009.04.003.

Song, Y. Y., Hu, R. J., Diao, Y. S., Chen, L., & Jiang, X. L. (2018). Effects of exercise training on restless legs syndrome, depression, sleep quality, and fatigue among hemodialysis patients: A systematic review and meta-analysis. *Journal of Pain and Symptom Management, 55*(4), 1184–1195. doi:10.1016/j.jpainsymman.2017.12.472.

Spieler, D., Kaffe, M., Knauf, F., Bessa, J., Tena, J. J., Giesert, F., . . . Winkelmann, J. (2014). Restless legs syndrome-associated intronic common variant in Meis1 alters enhancer function in the developing telencephalon. *Genome Research, 24*(4), 592–603. doi:10.1101/gr.166751.113.

Trenkwalder, C., Benes, H., Grote, L., Garcia-Borreguero, D., Hogl, B., Hopp, M., . . . Kohnen, R. (2013). Prolonged release oxycodone-naloxone for treatment of severe restless legs syndrome after failure of previous treatment: A double-blind, randomised, placebo-controlled trial with an open-label extension. *Lancet Neurology, 12*(12), 1141–1150. doi:10.1016/s1474-4422(13)70239-4.

Trindade, M., Orestes-Cardoso, S., & de Siqueira, T. C. (2015). Interdisciplinary treatment of bruxism with an occlusal splint and cognitive behavioral therapy. *General Dentistry, 63*(5), e1–4.

Turkdogan, D., Bekiroglu, N., & Zaimoglu, S. (2011). A prevalence study of restless legs syndrome in Turkish children and adolescents. *Sleep Medicine, 12*–4), 315–321. doi:10.1016/j.sleep.2010.08.013.

Varim, C., Acar, B. A., Uyanik, M. S., Acar, T., Alagoz, N., Nalbant, A., . . . Ergenc, H. (2016). Association between the neutrophil-to-lymphocyte ratio, a new marker of systemic inflammation, and restless legs syndrome. *Singapore Medical Journal, 57*(9), 514–516. doi:10.11622/smedj.2016154.

Voon, W. C., & Sheu, S. H. (2001). Diltiazem for nocturnal leg cramps. *Age and Ageing, 30*(1), 91–92. doi:10.1093/ageing/30.1.91.

Wali, S., Alsafadi, S., Abaalkhail, B., Ramadan, I., Abulhamail, B., Kousa, M., . . . Hamed, M. (2018). The association between vitamin D level and restless legs syndrome: A population-based case-control study. *Journal of Clinical Sleep Medicine, 14*(4), 557–564. doi:10.5664/jcsm.7044.

Walters, A. S., LeBrocq, C., Dhar, A., Hening, W., Rosen, R., Allen, R. P., & Trenkwalder, C. (2003). Validation of the International Restless Legs Syndrome Study Group rating scale for restless legs syndrome. *Sleep Medicine, 4*(2), 121–132.

Weinstock, L. B., Fern, S. E., & Duntley, S. P. (2008). Restless legs syndrome in patients with irritable bowel syndrome: Response to small intestinal bacterial overgrowth therapy. *Digestive Diseases and Sciences, 53*(5), 1252–1256. doi:10.1007/s10620-007-0021-0.

Weinstock, L. B., Walters, A. S., & Paueksakon, P. (2012). Restless legs syndrome: Theoretical roles of inflammatory and immune mechanisms. *Sleep Medicine Reviews, 16*(4), 341–354. doi:10.1016/j.smrv.2011.09.003.

Westwood, A. J., Spector, A. R., & Auerbach, S. H. (2014). CPAP treats muscle cramps in patients with obstructive sleep apnea. *Journal of Clinical Sleep Medicine, 10*(6), 691–692. doi:10.5664/jcsm.3806.

Willis, T. (1685). *The London Practice of Physic.* London: Bassett and Crooke.

Winkelman, J. W., Armstrong, M. J., Allen, R. P., Chaudhuri, K. R., Ondo, W., Trenkwalder, C., . . . Zesiewicz, T. (2016). Practice guideline summary: Treatment of restless legs syndrome in adults: Report of the Guideline Development, Dissemination, and Implementation Subcommittee of the American Academy of Neurology. *Neurology, 87*(24), 2585–2593. doi:10.1212/wnl.0000000000003388.

Winkelman, J. W., Blackwell, T., Stone, K., Ancoli-Israel, S., Tranah, G. J., & Redline, S. (2015). Genetic associations of periodic limb movements of sleep in the elderly for the MrOS sleep study. *Sleep Medicine, 16*(11), 1360–1365. doi:10.1016/j.sleep.2015.07.017.

Xu, X. M., Liu, Y., Jia, S. Y., Dong, M. X., Cao, D., & Wei, Y. D. (2018). Complementary and alternative therapies for restless legs syndrome: An evidence-based systematic review. *Sleep Medicine Reviews, 38*, 158–167. doi:10.1016/j.smrv.2017.06.003.

Yan, X., Wang, W. D., Walters, A. S., Wang, Q., Liu, Y. J., & Chu, F. Y. (2012). Traditional Chinese medicine herbal preparations in restless legs syndrome (RLS) treatment: A review and probable first description of RLS in 1529. *Sleep Medicine Reviews, 16*(6), 509–518. doi:10.1016/j.smrv.2012.01.003.

Zhang, Y., Lu, J., Wang, Z., Zhong, Z., Xu, M., Zou, X., . . . Yao, D. (2017). Companion of oral movements with limb movements in patients with sleep bruxism: Preliminary findings. *Sleep Medicine, 36*, 156–164. doi:10.1016/j.sleep.2017.05.015.

Zhou, W. N., Fu, H. Y., Du, Y. F., Sun, J. H., Zhang, J. L., Wang, C., . . . Wang, K. L. (2016). Short-term effects of repetitive transcranial magnetic stimulation on sleep bruxism: A pilot study. *International Journal of Oral Science, 8*(1), 61–65. doi:10.1038/ijos.2015.35.

34

Sleep-Related Parasomnias

JACLYN L. LEWIS-CROSWELL AND JOSÉ COLÓN

Parasomnias are sleep disorders that occur during rapid eye movement (REM) sleep or arousals from non–REM (NREM) sleep. Parasomnias occur in specific stages of sleep or during the transition from sleep to wakefulness or wakefulness to sleep. They result in undesirable verbal or physical behaviors such as sleeptalking or sleepwalking and often disrupt the bed partner as well as the patient. In this chapter, parasomnias are categorized as NREM parasomnias and REM parasomnias.[1] The NREM parasomnias include sleepwalking, sleep terrors, and confusional arousals, while REM parasomnias include REM sleep behavior disorder (RBD), recurrent isolated sleep paralysis, and nightmare disorder. The use of integrative approaches for treatment of parasomnias from sleepwalking to nightmares dates back to before recorded literature, and these are still found to be effective. Integrative modalities such as herbal supplements, hypnosis, and psychotherapy offer advantages over medications as they have a safer side-effect profile when compared to medications. For many parasomnias, medications are infrequently used.

NREM Parasomnias

NREM parasomnias are depicted in early literature; witness the sleepwalking scene from William Shakespeare's tragedy *Macbeth*, written in 1607. The twentieth-century Disney cartoon from 1947 "Sleepy Time Donald" shows how a sleepwalking Donald Duck created headaches for Daisy Duck, thus demonstrating how parasomnias can negatively impact others.

The NREM parasomnias include somnambulism (sleepwalking), sleep terrors also known as night terrors (*pavor nocturnus*), and confusional arousals. The stage of sleep in which NREM parasomnias usually occur is slow wave sleep (SWS) or while coming out of SWS.[1] These disorders are more common in childhood because children have a greater percentage of SWS. Although they can occur at any time of the night, it is far more common for these parasomnias to occur in the first third of the night because people tend to spend more time in SWS in the earlier part of the night. These parasomnias are considered to have a genetic component, and people with disorders of arousal often have family members with one of these parasomnias. Circumstances that increase the likelihood of experiencing an NREM parasomnias include fever, certain medications, being overly tired, or being sleep deprived as these can result in increased SWS. Some sleep disturbances can be elucidated secondary to periodic limb movement disorders (PLMD) or sleep apnea, as these can cause cortical arousals during SWS which can lead to awakenings that result in a parasomnia. Children tend to "outgrow" these parasomnias in early adulthood, when they experience less SWS, a normal change in sleep architecture.[2]

Confusional arousals are an NREM parasomnia characterized by confusion, disorientation, or slow mentation during arousal from NREM sleep. These occur during incomplete or slow awakenings from stage N3 sleep or SWS. The patient may begin to vocalize and occasionally have complex motor movement or behaviors. A hallmark of confusional arousals is to have poor to no recall of the event the following day. This often predictable parasomnia usually occurs in the first third of the night and generally at the same time every night.

INTEGRATIVE TREATMENT OF DISORDERS OF AROUSAL, NREM PARASOMNIAS

Ruling out easily remedied causes of the arousal disorders includes reviewing prescribed medications that are known to trigger the episodes just noted. Additionally, a comprehensive history from the patient or family member should be obtained and evaluated for triggers of the disorder of arousal, such as intense physical activity, sleep deprivation, poor sleep hygiene, and other medical conditions such as hyperthyroidism.[2]

The initial treatment of these disorders should include providing education and reassurance to patients and family members. The family should be informed about how to help console the patient and gently help the patient back to sleep. It is paramount to discuss safety parameters, especially for sleepwalkers.[3] During a sleepwalking episode, for children as well as adults, it is helpful to provide comfort to the sleepwalker and gently redirect him or her back to bed; confrontation or awakening the patient during events can lengthen the parasomnia and lead to confusion, resistance, or agitation.[2,4]

Other primary sleep disorders should be identified and treated, including sleep apnea, restless leg syndrome, narcolepsy, sleep-related epilepsy, parasomnia overlap syndrome, insomnia, nocturnal eating, and gastroesophageal reflux. It can be advantageous to avoid medications or substances such as alcohol, antipsychotics, antidepressants, antihistamines, sedative-hypnotics, and benzodiazepines.[1]

For sleepwalkers, safety is of the utmost concern and an immediate focus of treatment. Initial steps include removing anything that may be hazardous or harmful (candles, knives, fire arms). If the home is a two-story house, it is important to secure the sleepwalker away from stairs and place gates at the top and bottom of stairs. If possible, the sleepwalker should sleep on the ground floor to decrease risk of falling down stairs or over railings. Also, windows and doors should be locked and monitored by an alarm system.

For all parasomnias, it can be helpful to teach the patient and family good sleep hygiene and sleep behaviors to ensure that the patient is not experiencing sleep deprivation. Interventions include eliminating and learning how to manage stress, regulating the sleep cycle by keeping the same wake time and bedtime daily and nightly, and having a calming bedtime ritual such as a warm bath, reading time, and a meditation/relaxation routine to help manage stress before bedtime.[2,4]

Given the emphasis on safety, there are times when a patient may benefit from medical management. When the use of medication is indicated, benzodiazepines such as diazepam, lorazepam, and clonazepam have been shown to be helpful to decrease sleepwalking episodes, but, as noted earlier, they have the potential to cause daytime fatigue. As an integrative/alternative medicine treatment option, boiled onions have been reported to reduce sleepwalking although there are no clinical studies to substantiate these patient reports.[5-7] Melatonin has been documented to decrease night terror episodes.[8]

Scheduled awakenings are an integrative approach to improve sleep hygiene, as consistent bed and rise times are beneficial for solidifying sleep cycles. Initially, a patient's sleep pattern needs to be monitored over the course of a week to determine the typical time of the arousal episode. The optimal time to awaken the patient is approximately 15–30 minutes before the usual time of the partial arousal episode. The patient should be awakened by a light touch or verbal prompt; once the patient is aroused, he or she can be allowed to return to sleep. The patient should acknowledge that they are awake, verbally or with eye opening. This should be continued for 1 full week, and, if there are no further episodes of sleepwalking or night terrors after 1 week, then treatment tapering can begin. If there are additional episodes of partial arousals, then the treatment needs to continue until an entire week passes without episodes. Treatment tapering occurs initially by not waking the patient up on 1 out of 7 nights. If there are no episodes during that week, then each subsequent week an additional night without a scheduled awakening is added on.[9]

HYPNOSIS FOR NREM PARASOMNIAS

Hypnosis has long been embraced in integrative medicine. According to the Society of Psychological Hypnosis (Division 30 of the American Psychology Association), "hypnosis is a procedure involving cognitive processes (like imagination) in which a subject is guided by a hypnotist to respond to suggestions for changes in sensations, perceptions, thoughts, feelings, and behaviors." Patients can be trained to guide themselves through a hypnotic procedure, coined "self-hypnosis." Hypnosis can create a state of deep relaxation which helps the mind to concentrate intensely on a specific thought, memory, feeling, or sensation without distraction, thus increasing the ability to be open to suggestions that can be used to change certain thoughts or behaviors.[10,11] Hypnosis is known to cause a state of consciousness involving focused attention and reduced peripheral awareness characterized by an enhanced capacity for response to suggestion. This shift in consciousness enables us to tap into many of our natural abilities and allows us to make change more quickly.[12-14]

Hypnosis is used integratively to treat many conditions, but, with regard to sleep disorders, hypnosis has been successfully used to treat sleepwalking, night terrors, parasomnia overlap disorder, nocturnal enuresis, bruxism, sleep paralysis, and nightmares, as well as posttraumatic stress disorder (PTSD)-associated nightmares.[15] In one study, 27 adult sleepwalkers and sleep terror patients were treated with hypnosis. The results of this study found that 6 (22%) of the patients reported "very much improvement," 14 (52%) reported "much improvement," and none reported minimal improvement, whereas 7 (26%) reported that the symptoms were unchanged. None of the study participants reported worsened symptoms after treatment with hypnosis.[16]

A study treating sleepwalkers found that subjects who were provided hypnosis sessions with suggestions such as "you will wake when your feet are on the ground" and "you do not need the sleep eating, that time has passed; leave it behind" was repeated 6 times over 3 weeks. Every subject in the active treatment group improved on all parameters by the end of the 3 weeks and were symptom-free at a 1-year follow-up.[17] In another study, 12 men in the military facing discharge secondary to sleepwalking were treated with hypnosis. Six of the patients engaged in hypnosis and four reported total alleviation of the sleepwalking.[18] A 5-year follow-up study on hypnosis-treated sleepwalking, night terrors, nightmares, epic dreaming, and sleep eating was published in 2007. Of 36 patients, 40.5% were symptom-free or much improved at the end of 5 years.[15]

Hypnosis has been successfully used to treat patients with primary parasomnias including nightmares, sleepwalking, and sleep terrors. Hypnotic suggestion given to decrease the frequency of nightmares or to alter nightmare content was found to be effective. Relaxation induced from hypnosis is partially helpful in improving sleep and decreasing parasomnias.[19]

REM Parasomnias

REM parasomnias are sleep disorders occurring during the REM stage of sleep. These include nightmare disorder, recurrent isolated sleep paralysis, and RBD, which is dream enactment during REM sleep. Frequently, RBD patients present for treatment due to self-injury or secondary to a bed partner complaint.[20] These parasomnias are only similar in that they occur during the REM stage of sleep.

RECURRENT ISOLATED SLEEP PARALYSIS

Fuseli's 1781 painting *The Nightmare* depicts an incubus-like image that has been associated with sleep paralysis. Sleep paralysis episodes account for early depictions of ancient demon attacks and, in more modern times, alien abductions.

Recurrent isolated sleep paralysis also known as *sleep paralysis* (SP) occurs when REM-based atonia persists into wakefulness.[20] During episodes of sleep paralysis, the sufferer awakens to atonia combined with conscious awareness. This is usually a frightening event often accompanied by vivid, waking dreams (i.e., hallucinations). When sleep paralysis occurs independently of narcolepsy and other medical conditions, it may be termed "recurrent isolated sleep paralysis" and is a recognized sleep–wake disorder.[21]

In understanding SP, there is some core basic science about REM sleep that must be understood. REM sleep is an active brain time and is associated with autonomic fluctuations. In REM sleep, body atonia occurs, believed to be protective so that the sleeper does not act out dreams. For several reasons, but primarily related to decreased muscle tone, there can be increased apnea in REM sleep. Memory consolidation occurs during various stages throughout sleep, but the memory consolidation associated with emotions is thought to occur during REM sleep. Physiologically, there is increased blood flow to organs, including sexual organs (males can have erections and females can have clitoral engorgement during REM sleep). It is not difficult to see how waking up during REM in the setting of SP along with an increased heart rate, possible apnea, and an emotional cognitive state could be terrifying to an individual.

SP is surprisingly common; however, patients are reluctant to discuss these issues with healthcare providers because they find the sensations embarrassing. Patients who find SP episodes to be terrifying may simply report that they had a nightmare without further elaboration. A systematic review of the literature found that 7.6% of the general population have experienced at least one SP episode over the course of their lifetimes.[22] Medical conditions associated with sleep paralysis include hypertension, idiopathic hypersomnia, narcolepsy, sleep apnea, alcohol use, and Wilson's disease, but the most common condition associated with SP is insufficient sleep syndrome.[21]

Integrative Treatments for Sleep Paralysis

There are no medications formally approved by the US Food and Drug Administration (FDA) for SP. Much of the information regarding pharmaceutical treatment of SP is extrapolated from the treatment of narcolepsy, including reports of benefit from antidepressants and sodium oxybate.[21] The efficacy of antidepressants in reducing SP may be due to their REM-suppressing properties and/or their reduction of anxiety.

Integrative treatments for SP include performing a root cause analysis. Given that sleep deprivation is the most common trigger, measures such as sleep hygiene and counseling to avoid the use of alcohol or caffeine before bed may serve as preventive measures.[23] A behavioral approach using cognitive-behavioral therapy (CBT) for sleep paralysis has been shown to be effective.[24] Also, psychoeducation and reassurance are the most basic therapy a clinician can provide,[21] especially considering the high rates of anxiety associated with SP.[25] Another potential treatment for SP may be lucid dreaming. Episodes of sleep paralysis and lucid dreaming are related but different experiences of REM sleep. While sleep paralysis is related primarily to issues of sleep quality and well-being, lucid dreaming may reflect a continuation of greater imaginative capacity and positive imagery in waking states.[26] There are no formal studies using lucid dream therapy to treat SP; however, the use of lucid dream therapy for the treatment of nightmares is outlined later in this chapter. There are people who have used their awareness of being in a state of SP to allow them to enter a lucid dream upon returning to sleep.

REM SLEEP BEHAVIOR DISORDER

RBD was first noted as a sleep disorder in the 1980s; however, REM sleep disorders were described long before that. The 1950 animated feature *Cinderella* features a cartoon dog, Bruno, having nightmares with dream enactment. The dog's behavior resembled RBD, a REM parasomnia.

RBD is manifested by vivid, often frightening dreams associated with simple or complex motor behavior during REM sleep.[27] RBD is characterized by loss of normal skeletal muscle atonia during REM sleep, accompanied by prominent motor activity and dreaming.[28] The polysomnographic (PSG) features of RBD include dream enactment behavior with increased electromyographic tone.[27] While a patient may not have an episode of RBD during PSG, REM sleep without atonia

(RSWA) can still be identified in the absence of an event. RBD often occurs concomitantly with the alpha-synucleinopathy family of neurodegenerative disorders, which includes idiopathic Parkinson disease, Lewy body dementia, and multiple system atrophy.[29] RBD may predate the development of neurodegenerative disorders by years, and patients should be counseled regarding the potential development of neurologic symptoms and neurodegenerative diseases.

The age of RBD onset is typically 40–70 years, and there is a male gender predominance.[27] When RBD is seen in younger adults it may be associated with narcolepsy, parasomnia overlap disorder, antidepressants, and possibly autoimmune disorders such as multiple sclerosis.[30]

The timing of RBD episodes reflects when the patient is in REM sleep, and, since the majority of REM sleep occurs during the latter half of the sleep period (particularly the latter third of the sleep period, which for most individuals is after 3 AM), RBD tends to be exhibited in the few hours prior to wake onset. Unlike most pleasant dreams and nightmares, which are typically vividly recalled on awakening but rapidly forgotten afterward, those with RBD can often recall vivid details of the dream for days, and sometimes for weeks or years.[27]

Differential diagnosis of RBD may include NREM parasomnias, nocturnal panic attacks, nocturnal seizures, nightmares, nocturnal wandering associated with dementia, and obstructive sleep apnea (OSA).[27] The presence of OSA causing disruption of REM sleep leading to symptoms of RBD is called "pseudo-RBD," which requires PSG to differentiate.[31] However, it should be noted that pseudo-RBD can coexist with true RBD.[32]

Integrative Treatments for RBD

One simple measure for management of RBD is assessing the environment. The American Academy of Sleep Medicine (AASM) best practice guidelines recommend modifying the sleep environment for patients who have had sleep-related injury.[33] Suggested modifications can include placing bed rails to prevent falls, bringing the mattress to floor level to minimize the height of a potential fall, and placing pillows or cushions on the floor. Other measures may include padding corners of furniture, window protection, and removing potentially dangerous objects such as glass lamps, guns, or sharp objects from the bedroom. Additionally, for the safety of the bed partner, it may be recommended that he or she sleep in a different room until the RBD symptoms are controlled.

Given that injury can occur, some cases of RBD may warrant management with supplements or medications. Medication management recommendations per AASM best practice guidelines suggest clonazepam and a few other medications with limited data. Clonazepam, though suggested for the treatment of RBD, should be used with caution in patients with dementia, gait disorders, or concomitant

OSA. There are limited data for the use of other medications, but other options may include pramipexole, zopiclone, benzodiazepines other than clonazepam, desipramine, clozapine, carbamazepine, sodium oxybate, ramelteon, gabapentin, and pregabalin.[33,34] The use of sodium oxybate is based on one case report and is not FDA approved for RBD. It is typically used for treatment of narcolepsy.[33]

An important factor in the approach to RBD is to look for underlying causes. Subjects taking serotonergic antidepressants have more electromyelographic (EMG) activity in the submental lead during REM sleep than do controls. Individuals taking such medications may be at increased risk of developing RBD, particularly with increasing age.[35] RBD has been noted to have a high incidence of comorbidity with PTSD,[36] and RBD can mimic PTSD-related nightmares. In PTSD, an accurate diagnosis of sleep disturbance using PSG is relevant for treatment and prognostic evaluation.[37]

Other integrative approaches to RBD may include nonpharmacologic approaches. Melatonin can be considered a possible sole or add-on therapy with clonazepam in select patients with RBD.[38] Yi-gan san, a traditional herbal mixture, has been widely used for the management of neurodegenerative disorders in traditional East Asian medicine because it has neuroprotective effects and rescues dopaminergic neurons.[39] It is proposed that the efficacy demonstrated by yi-gan san may reflect the gamma-aminobutyric acid (GABA)-ergic and serotonergic (5-HT2) properties of angelicae radix (angelica root; *Angelica sinensi*), which is one of its constituents.[40]

Another proposed recommendation for the management of RBD is to decrease the unpleasant dreams, thereby reducing the anticipatory concerns about nightmares that sometimes results in overt "sleep phobia."[27] Recommendations for treatment of nightmares later in this chapter may be applied.

NIGHTMARE DISORDER

Dreams were rediscovered in the modern era by Dr. Sigmund Freud. He started an entire branch of psychology devoted to unlocking his patients' "unconscious" minds through the interpretation of dreams. Dr. Carl Jung was a student of Freud. He felt that dreams show us what we are striving to achieve as well as what stands in our way. Jung refers to nightmares as "shadow elements," and he believed that they are missing parts of ourselves.

Nightmares consist of dream imagery that is often elaborate and lengthy and may elicit anxiety, fear, or other dysphoric emotions. The content of the nightmares often focuses on avoidance of imminent danger or may evoke other negative emotions such as fear, guilt, or anger. Nightmares can occur during any stage of sleep but most frequently occur during REM sleep.[41] The *International Classification of Sleep Disorders* (ICSD-3) has classified nightmare disorder as a parasomnia usually associated with REM sleep, including recurrent episodes of awakenings from sleep with recall of intensely disturbing dreams. Nightmares usually involve fear or anxiety but also anger, sadness, disgust, and other dysphoric emotions. The nightmare episode may cause delayed return to sleep, and the nightmare episodes are more likely to occur in the latter half of the typical sleep period, which is when REM sleep episodes are of greater duration.[20] Most nightmares are "idiopathic," indicating they have no clear cause. Nightmare disorder is common, affecting about 2–6% of the adult population, with a higher proportion of children and adolescents affected.[1,4] Nightmares are more likely to occur in children if they experience significant life psychosocial stress, and, in those cases, they generally do not resolve on their own. These children would likely benefit from interventions noted later in this chapter. For adults, nightmares are reported to be monthly in 6% of the population but in the severe range (nightly) in only 1–2% of the population.[41] The presence of nightmare disorder can impair quality of life, resulting in sleep avoidance and sleep deprivation, with a consequent increase in the intensity of the nightmares.[1,2,4,10,20] Unfortunately nightmare disorder can lead to other consequences such as a predisposition to insomnia, daytime sleepiness, and fatigue. It may also cause or exacerbate underlying psychiatric distress and illness. Once nightmares are successfully treated, patients usually report feeling more rested upon awakening and report less daytime fatigue and sleepiness.[1,2,4,10,20]

Integrative Treatments for Nightmare Disorder

Treatment of nightmares is required for severe, recurrent nightmares as well as for children or even adults who report distress. It can be useful to limit television exposure prior to going to sleep. Also, life stressors or anxiety triggers need to be identified and managed along with engagement in good sleep skills, such as regular bedtime and rise time, avoiding caffeine 8 hours prior to bed time, and avoiding alcohol before bed.[1,10] Various prescription drug classes can increase the rate of nightmares or bizarre dreams, and these include catecholaminergic agents, some antidepressants (e.g., bupropion), barbiturates, alcohol, and beta-blockers. Drugs of abuse known to cause nightmares included cocaine, marijuana, and alcohol, and alcohol withdrawal also increases nightmare prevalence.[1]

Chamomile can be used to treatment nightmares. Chamomile is one of the most ancient medicinal herbs known. The dried flowers of chamomile contain many terpenoids and flavonoids that contribute to its medicinal properties.[42] Chamomile in the form of an aqueous extract (tea) has been frequently used as a mild sedative to calm nerves and reduce anxiety, and it has also been used to treat hysteria, insomnia, and nightmares.[43] Valerian root has long been associated with sleep and has been found to be as effective as diazepam in reducing anxiety.[44]

However, in patients with nightmare disorder, caution should be used because there have been reports of developing nightmares as a side effect.[45]

Given that nightmares may be associated with distress and poor sleep quality, there are times when medication management may be appropriate. Prazosin is the drug with the most robust data for treatment of nightmares associated with PTSD; it is an alpha-adrenergic antagonist originally used for the treatment of high blood pressure. This medication has been found to reduce nightmares and improve sleep in patients with PTSD.[10,46,47]

Image rehearsal therapy (IRT) is a modified CBT technique that treats nightmare disorder by altering the nightmare's content. IRT involves recalling the nightmare, writing it down, and changing the theme, story, and ending as well as any negative dream content to create a more positive dream. The patient is asked to write down the nightmare, replace unwanted content, and shift cognitively to more positive endings. The patient should rehearse the new dream content for 10–20 minutes daily prior to going to sleep.[10,48,49] IRT has been found to be effective for the treatment of nightmare disorder in patients with PTSD. In one study, 114 patients with PTSD and nightmares were treated with IRT and found at 3- or 6-month follow-up to have improvements in nightmares, sleep, and PTSD severity.[50]

Exposure, relaxation, and rescripting therapy (ERRT) is similar to IRT in many ways and has been shown to be effective for treating nightmares with onset after trauma exposure. The treatment involves psychoeducation, sleep hygiene, and progressive muscle relaxation training. Homework is assigned in this treatment modality and is practiced at home. This is similar to IRT, except that the exposure utilized is slightly different. Exposure procedures such as writing out and rescripting the nightmares, homework assignments, problem-solving, and coping strategies are intended to help deal with the nightmares.[10,51]

Other integrative approaches to nightmares include behavioral interventions. *Systematic desensitization and progressive deep muscle relaxation* (PDMR) training are suggested for treatment of idiopathic nightmares. This technique has also been called *graduated exposure therapy*. In this treatment, the patient is gradually exposed to his fears. The patient is taught to cope with and manage stress by learning relaxation strategies prior to being exposed to the feared object or situation.

PDMR training alone has been suggested as an effective treatment for idiopathic nightmares. The technique involves learning to tense and relax muscles, one body part at a time, to elicit relaxation.[10,50]

Hypnosis is another integrative approach that has been found to be an effective treatment for nightmares. In a small case series of 10 patients with nightmares treated with hypnosis, 71% had improvement or were symptom-free at 18 months, and 67% were symptom-free at 5-year follow-up.[15] Another study with 3 subjects showed that brief hypnotic therapy of 1 to 5 sessions was beneficial for repetitive nightmares.[12] Research has shown that hypnosis can be effective in treating nightmares related to trauma or nontraumatic or imagined experiences. Transformation of the nightmares can occur while the patient is reliving or replaying it under hypnosis. In a study by Eichelman, two combat veterans with PTSD and nightmares were able to obtain cessation of nightmares with dream substitutions and rehearsal during hypnotic trance.[52] In another study from 1998, Gorton worked with a woman with depression, anxiety, insomnia, and chronic nightmares. He was able to eliminate nightmares through the use of hypnosis.[53]

As early as 1959, Milton Erikson talked about the use of hypnosis with patients who have nightmares, not to alter the actual memory of the traumatic event but instead to add elements that could help the patient cope with the frightening content of the nightmare. During hypnotic sessions, the practitioner has the patient go through the nightmare, and, with repeated exposure, the patient is able to develop more control over the nightmare. Another hypnotic technique is to have the patient imagine running the nightmare on a movie or television screen with a remote control; the remote control can slow down or stop the movie as it plays on the screen. In some interventions, the patient may learn to stop the movie prior to the "bad part" or the patient may learn to "change the ending" of the nightmare to a more pleasant scene. One study treating recurrent nightmares in 11 children demonstrated that hypnosis-enhanced dream review is effective in greatly reducing the frequency of or resolving nightmares.[54]

Other exciting integrative approaches to reduce or defuse nightmares involve the use of *lucid dreaming* and *dream incubation*. Once again, the use of these techniques is perhaps prehistoric. In the ancient Greek religion, Hypnos presided over sleep, and his son, Morpheus, ruled dreams. Scattered across the Mediterranean, the Greeks built hundreds of shrines to serve as dream temples. Dreams were embraced by these early cultures. The ancient Egyptians piggybacked the use dream temples and practiced dream incubation. While ancient Egyptians and Greeks knew the power of dreams, the Tibetan Buddhists used dream yoga and were pioneers of lucid dreaming, a technique used today that helps defuse nightmares.

Lucid dreaming was discovered in 1975, by researcher Keith Hearne. By monitoring a sleeping subject during PSG, he was able to validate the concept of lucid dreaming, which is that one can have awareness within dreams. Prior to the PSG, he had collaborated with his subject to create essentially a Morse code of eye movements. Through this, his subject provided confirmation of his awareness while the PSG confirmed that he was still asleep. Three years later, Stephen LaBerge conducted a similar test at Stanford University. He had no knowledge of Hearne's experiments but successfully used the same eye signaling technique to confirm one could be conscious during dreams. This technique would later be called signal-verified lucid dreaming (SVLD).[55]

Lucid dream therapy (LDT) is a variant of IRT. The cognitive restructuring technique of LDT allows an individual to alter the nightmare storyline during the nightmare itself by realizing that one is dreaming, or being "lucid" during the nightmare. Data show that lucid dreaming constitutes a hybrid state of consciousness with definable and measurable differences from waking and from REM sleep, particularly in the frontal areas.[56] The prevalence of this sleep phenomenon may be more common than one may assume. In a representative sample of German adults ($N = 919$), 51% of the participants reported that they had experienced a lucid dream at least once.[57]

There are several ways to achieve lucid dreaming, but for brevity they can be divided into *dream-induced lucid dreaming* (DILD) and *wake-induced lucid dreaming* (WILD). In the more common case, subjects report having been in the midst of a dream when a bizarre occurrence causes sufficient reflection to lead to the realization that they are dreaming (DILD). In the other less frequent case, subjects report briefly awakening from a dream and then falling back asleep and entering directly into the dream with no (or very little) break in consciousness (WILD). Research by LaBerge in the confirmation of lucid dreaming through SVLDs showed that 72% of the confirmed lucid dreams were classified as DILDs and the remaining 28% as WILDs.[55] Lucid dreams are reported to occur more frequently late in the sleep cycle.[58] Hence, encouraging patients to engage in LDT encourages them to catch their last REM cycle, thus promoting a full night of sleep.

Dream recall is perhaps the simplest technique that can induce lucid dreaming. The technique does not require much more effort than merely trying to remember the dream. Stephen LaBerge tells of one such event in his book, *Exploring the World of Lucid Dreaming*.[59] His 7-year-old niece told LaBerge that she had a bad dream. In her dream she was swimming in a local reservoir when she noticed a shark. LaBerge told his niece that the next time she saw a shark, she would know that she was inside a dream. He also suggested that she make friends with the shark. Later, when she had another dream with a shark, she told him she decided to ride on the back of the shark.

Dream incubation is another way to achieve lucid dreams. Dream incubation actually has many broad applications, and it has been found to be practical and effective, as demonstrated by a 1993 study at Harvard. Seventy-six college students were asked to incubate dreams as part of a class on dreaming. For 1 week, the subjects went to sleep trying to incubate a dream that would solve a particular problem. One half of the students reported a dream that related to their problems. Seventy percent of these believed that their dream contained a solution to the problem. The students' dream journals were rated by judges who agreed with most of the students' conclusions as to whether the dreams addressed or solved their problems.[60]

Conclusion

From alien abductions to healing powers of dreams, parasomnia tales may be as old as sleep itself. The first accounts of hospitals were in fact dream temples. The Temple of Asclepias at Epidaurus was built in the early fourth century BCE. Aesculapius would walk around the temple with his rod, alongside slithering non-venomous snakes, and this is where the sick and injured traveled to seek healing. In these first accounts of hospitals, patients did not travel there for medications, but rather for sleep.

While dream temples no longer exist, parasomnias are still commonly seen sleep disorders. Some parasomnias may be benign and self-limited, while others may be a sign of an underlying neurological disorder, as in RBD. Proper identification of parasomnias is necessary to determine the appropriate approach to therapy, and integrative treatment modalities are often effective treatment options.

REFERENCES

1. Kothare SV, Ivanenko A. *Parasomnias.* New York: Springer; 2013.
2. Morin CM, Espie CA. *The Oxford handbook of sleep and sleep disorders.* New York: Oxford University Press; 2012.
3. Broughton RJ. Sleep disorders: Disorders of arousal? *Science.* 1968;159:1070–1078.
4. Thorpy MJ, Plazzi G. *The parasomnias and other sleep-related movement disorders.* New York: Cambridge University Press; 2010.
5. Broughton RJ. NREM arousal parasomnias. In Kryger MH, Roth T, Dement WC, eds. *Principles and practice of sleep medicine.* Philadelphia: Saunders; 2005: 693–706.
6. Schenck CH, Mahowald MW. Long-term, nightly benzodiazepine treatment of injurious parasomnias and other disorders of disrupted nocturnal sleep in 170 adults. *Am J Med.* 1996;100(3):333–337.
7. Schenck CH, Mahowald MW. Parasomnias: Managing bizarre sleep-related behavior disorders. *Postgrad Med.* 2000;107(3):145–156.
8. Jan JE, Freeman RD, Wasdell MB, Bomben MM. A child with severe night terrors and sleep-walking responds to melatonin therapy. *Dev Med Child Neurol.* 2004 Nov;46(11):789.
9. Perlis M, Aloia M, Kuhn B. *Behavioral treatments for sleep disorders: A comprehensive primer of behavioral sleep medicine interventions.* London: Elsevier Press; 2011.
10. Aurora RN, Zak RS, Auerbach SH, et al. Best practice guide for the treatment of nightmare disorder in adults. *J Clin Sleep Med.* 2010;6(4):389–401.
11. Hammond DC. *Hypnotic induction and suggestion.* Bloomington, IL: American Society of Clinical Hypnosis; 1998.
12. Kohler WC, Kurz PJ. *Hypnosis in the management of sleep disorders.* Abingdon, UK: Routledge; July 13, 2017.

13. Definition and Description of Hypnosis. APA division 30. 2014; https://www.apadivisions.org/division-30/about.

14. Eric Spiegel, Ph.D., Hypnosis and You: An Introduction to Professionals and the Public. ASCH.NET 7/5/2017; https://www.asch.net/Public/HypnosisandYou-AnIntroduction.aspx.

15. Hauri PJ, Silber MH, Boeve BF. The treatment of parasomnias with hypnosis: A 5-year follow-up study. *J Clin Sleep Med.* 2007;3(4):369–373.

16. Hurwitz TD, Mahowald MW, Schenck CH, Schluter JL, Bundlie SR. A retrospective outcome study and review of hypnosis as treatment of adults with sleepwalking and sleep terror. *J Nerv Ment Dis.* 1991;179(4):228–233.

17. Reid WH, Ahmed I, Levie CA. Treatment of sleepwalking: A controlled study. *Am J Psychother.* 1981 Jan;35(1):27–37.

18. Reid WH. Treatment of somnambulism in military trainees. *Am J Psychother.* 1975;29(1):101–106.

19. Kennedy G. A review of hypnosis in the treatment of parasomnias: Nightmare, sleepwalking, and sleep terror disorders. *Austral J Clin Exp Hypnosis.* 2002;30(2), 99–155.

20. American Academy of Sleep Medicine. *International classification of sleep disorders: Diagnostic and coding manual.* 3 ed. Darien, IL: American Academy of Sleep Medicine; 2014.

21. Sharpless BA. A clinician's guide to recurrent isolated sleep paralysis. *Neuropsychiatr Dis Treatm.* 2016;12:1761–1767.

22. Sharpless BA, Barber JP. Lifetime prevalence rates of sleep paralysis: A systematic review. *Sleep Med Rev.* 2011;15(5):311–315.

23. Edinger JD, Carney CE. *Overcoming insomnia: A cognitive-behavioral therapy approach.* New York: Oxford University Press; 2008.

24. Sharpless BA, Doghramji K. *Sleep paralysis: Historical, psychological, and medical perspectives.* New York: Oxford University Press; 2015.

25. Otto MW, Simon NM, Powers M, Hinton D, Zalta AK, Pollack MH. Rates of isolated sleep paralysis in outpatients with anxiety disorders. *J Anxiety Disord.* 2006;20(5):687–693.

26. Denis D, Poerio GL. Terror and bliss? Commonalities and distinctions between sleep paralysis, lucid dreaming, and their associations with waking life experiences. *J Sleep Res.* 2017 Feb;26(1):38–47.

27. Boeve BF. REM sleep behavior disorder: Updated review of the core features, the RBD-Neurodegenerative Disease Association, evolving concepts, controversies, and future directions. *Ann NY Acad Sci.* 2010;1184:15–54.

28. Boeve B, Silber M, Saper C, et al. Pathophysiology of REM sleep behaviour disorder and relevance to neurodegenerative disease. *Brain.* 2007;130:2770–2788.

29. McCarter SJ, St Louis EK, Boeve BF. REM sleep behavior disorder and REM sleep without atonia as an early manifestation of degenerative neurological disease. *Curr Neurol Neurosci Rep.* 2012;12(2):182–192.

30. Ju Y-ES. Rapid eye movement sleep behavior disorder in adults younger than 50 years of age. *Sleep Med.* 2013;14(8):768–774.

31. Neikrug AB, Ancoli-Israel S. Diagnostic tools for REM sleep behavior disorder. *Sleep Med Rev.* 2012;16(5):415–429.

32. Schenck CH. Expanded insights into idiopathic REM sleep behavior disorder. *Sleep.* 2016;39(1):7–9.

33. Aurora RN, Zak RS, Maganti RK, et al. Best practice guide for the treatment of REM sleep behavior disorder (RBD). *J Clin Sleep Med* 2010;6(1):85–95.

34. Esaki Y, Kitajima T, Koike S, et al. An open-labeled trial of ramelteon in idiopathic rapid eye movement sleep behavior disorder. *J Clin Sleep Med* 2016;12(5):689–693.

35. Winkelman JW, James L. Serotonergic antidepressants are associated with REM sleep without atonia. *Sleep.* 2004;27(2):317–321.

36. Husain AM, Miller PP, Carwile ST. REM sleep behavior disorder: Potential relationship to post-traumatic stress disorder. *J Clin Neurophysiol.* 2001 Mar;18(2):148–157.

37. Roepke S, Hansen M-L, Peter A, Merkl A, Palafox C, Danker-Hopfe H. Nightmares that mislead to diagnosis of reactivation of PTSD. *Eur J Psychotraumatol.* 2013;4:10.3402/ejpt.v4io.18714. doi:10.3402/ejpt.v4io.18714.

38. Boeve BF, Silber MH, Ferman TJ. Melatonin for treatment of REM sleep behavior disorder in neurologic disorders: Results in 14 patients. *Sleep Med.* 2003 Jul;4(4):281–284.

39. Doo AR, Kim SN, Park JY, et al. Neuroprotective effects of an herbal medicine, Yi-Gan San on MPP+/MPTP-induced cytotoxicity in vitro and in vivo. *J Ethnopharmacol.* 2010 Sep 15;131(2):433–42. doi:10.1016/j.jep.2010.07.008.

40. Shinno H, Kamei M, Nakamura Y, Inami Y, Horiguchi J. Successful treatment with Yi-Gan San for rapid eye movement sleep behavior disorder. *Prog Neuropsychoparmacol Biol Psychiatry* 2008;32:1749–1751.

41. American Psychiatric Association. *Diagnostic and statistical manual of mental disorders,* 5th ed. (DSM-V). Washington, DC: American Psychiatric Association; 2013.

42. Srivastava JK, Shankar E, Gupta S. Chamomile: A herbal medicine of the past with bright future. *Mol Med Rep.* 2010;3(6):895–901. doi:10.3892/mmr.2010.377.

43. Alramadhan E, Hanna MS, Hanna MS, Goldstein TA, Avila SM, Weeks BS. Dietary and botanical anxiolytics. *Med Sci Monit.* 2012;18(4):RA40–RA48.

44. Gurley BJ, Gardner SF, Hubbard MA, et al. In vivo effects of goldenseal, kava kava, black cohosh, and valerian on human cytochrome P450 1A2, 2D6, 2E1, and 3A4 phenotypes. *Clin Pharmacol Ther.* 2005;77(5):415–426.

45. Laberge S, Levitan L, Dement WC. Lucid dreaming: Physiological correlates of consciousness during REM sleep. *J Mind Behav.* 1986;7:251–258.

46. Raskind MA, Peskind ER, Hoff DJ, Hart KL, Holmes HA, Warren D, McFall M. A parallel group placebo controlled study of prazosin for trauma nightmares and sleep disturbance in combat Veterans with post-traumatic stress disorders. *Biol Psychiatry.* 2007;61:928–934.

47. Raskind MA, Peterson K, Williams T, Hoff D, Hart K, Holmes H, Peskind ER. A trial of prazosin for combat trauma PTSD with nightmares in active-duty soldiers returned from Iraq and Afghanistan. *Am J Psychiatry.* 2013;170:1003–1010.

48. Krakow V, Hollifield M, Johnston L, et al. Imagery rehearsal therapy for chronic nightmares in sexual assault survivors with posttraumatic stress disorder: A randomized controlled trial. *JAMA*. 2001;286:584–588.

49. Krakow B, Hollifield M, Johnston L, Koss M, Schrader R, Warner T. Imagery rehearsal therapy for chronic nightmares in sexual assault survivors with posttraumatic stress disorder: A randomized controlled trial. *JAMA*. 2001; 286(5):537–545

50. Miller WR, DiPilato M. Treatment of nightmares via relaxation and desensitization: A controlled evaluation. *J Consult Clin Psychol* 1983;51:870–877.

51. Davis JL, Wright DC. Case series utilizing exposure, relaxation, and rescripting therapy: Impact on nightmares, sleep quality and psychological distress. *Behav Sleep Med* 2005;3:151–157

52. Eichelman B. Hypnotic change in combat dreams of two veterans with posttraumatic stress disorder. *Am J Psychiatry*. 1985;142(1):112–114.

53. Gorton GE. Life-long nightmares: An eclectic treatment approach. *Am J Psychother*. 1988 Oct;42(4):610–618.

54. Linden JH, Bhardwaj A, Anbar RD. Hypnotically enhanced dreaming to achieve symptom reduction: A case study of 11 children and adolescents. *Am J Clin Hypnosis*. 2006 Apr;48:4.

55. Voss U, Holzmann R, Tuin I, Hobson A. Lucid dreaming: A state of consciousness with features of both waking and non-lucid dreaming. *Sleep*. 2009;32(9):1191–1200.

56. Schredl M, Erlacher D. Frequency of lucid dreaming in a representative German sample. *Percept Mot Skills*. 2011 Feb;112(1):104–108.

57. Stumbrys T, Erlacher D, Johnson M, Schredl M. The phenomenology of lucid dreaming: An online survey. *Am J Psychol*. 2014 Summer;127(2):191–204.

58. LaBerge S. Lucid dreaming: Psychophysiological studies of consciousness during REM sleep. In Bootsen RR, Kihlstrom JF, Schacter DL, eds., *Sleep and cognition*. Washington, DC: APA Press; 1990: 109–126.

59. LaBerge S, Rheingold H. *Exploring the World of Lucid Dreaming*. New York: Ballantine Books; 1990.

60. Barrett D. The Committee of Sleep: A study of dream incubation for problem solving. *Dreaming*. 1993;3(2):115–122.

35

Treatment of Pediatric Sleep Disorders

CHANA CHIN AND IRIS A. PEREZ

Pediatric Sleep Issues from Infancy to Childhood

Sleep problems are common in the pediatric population and may include poor sleep habits, delayed or inappropriate timing of sleep, prolonged night waking, and fragmented sleep. These sleep disturbances may emanate from infancy and are harbingers of sleep disorders in adulthood. They are associated with mortality and significant morbidities that negatively impact both the patient and family. Thus, prevention and appropriate treatment that are initiated early are essential.

Treatment of sleep disorders in childhood is focused on addressing the etiology and the predisposing, precipitating, and persisting factors, as well as parental and family concerns. In this chapter, we review current recommendations for safe infant sleep, promotion of sleep hygiene strategies in childhood (see table 35.1), and treatment options of representative pediatric sleep disorders.

Sleep in the Infant

SAFE INFANT SLEEP: AAP RECOMMENDATIONS

According to the US Centers for Disease Control and Prevention (CDC) 2016 Data and Statistics, approximately 3,600 infants die annually in the United States from sleep-related deaths, including sudden infant death syndrome (SIDS), accidental suffocation, and strangulation in bed.[1] With the adoption of the "Safe to Sleep" campaign, there has been a dramatic decline in SIDS.[2] However, infant

Table 35.1 Strategies for sleep hygiene in young infants and children

Place infant or child in crib or bed drowsy but awake	• Encourage sleeping alone without intervention from parents/caregivers • Avoid making the child sleep while being held or sleep other than his/her bed/room • Avoid bottle feeding/breastfeeding to sleep
Use transitional object to help baby/child fall asleep	
Establish a regular bedtime routine that is appropriate and helps child sleep on his/her own	• <6 months: Feeding or rocking then laying down in crib drowsy but awake • ≥6 months and toddlers: Brief, ≤30–45 minutes, of quiet relaxing activities (warm bath, reading stories, lullabies)
Maintain sleep conducive environment	• Cool, comfortable, calm, quiet, dark • No televisions or electronic devices
Appropriate sleep schedule	• Regular bedtimes and wake times • Appropriately timed naps geared to age and development at
Consistent sleep schedule	• Similar on weekdays and weekends
Promote good daytime behavior	• Bright light in the morning • Exercise/physical activity during the day • Avoid stimulating activity and foods (sugar, caffeine) near bedtime
Don't use bed or room for punishment ("time out")	
Avoid electronics/media viewing before bed or placing them in the bedroom	

deaths remain high,[2,3] and a recent report indicates an increasing mortality rate for unintentional suffocation and strangulation in bed among infants.[1]

Sudden unexpected infant death (SUID) refers to sudden and unexpected death, whether explained or unexplained (including SIDS) occurring in infancy.[4] SIDS is a subcategory of SUIDS and refers to infant deaths that cannot be explained after a thorough investigation, including autopsy, scene investigation, and review of clinical history.[2] There are striking risk factor similarities for SUID and SIDS. To reduce all sleep-related infant deaths, the American Academy of Pediatrics (AAP) published in 2016 an updated recommendation focused on safe sleeping environment for infants up to 1 year of age.[2,5] These include supine sleep positioning, use of a firm sleep surface, room sharing without bedsharing, and avoidance of soft bedding and overheating.[2]

All infants, including those who are hospitalized and preterm (at least from 32 weeks postmenstrual age [PMA]) should be placed wholly on the back for every sleep opportunity until they reach 1 year of age.[2] Prone sleeping is associated with reduced cerebral oxygenation,[6] increased risk of rebreathing expired gases resulting in hypercapnia and hypoxemia, overheating (by decreasing the rate of heat loss),[7] altered autonomic control of the cardiovascular system,[8] and decreased arousability.[9,10] Side sleeping is inherently unstable, predisposing an infant to rolling to the prone position, and thus must be avoided.[11] Elevating the head of the infant's crib is not recommended as it may result in the infant sliding to the foot of the crib and into a position that may compromise respiration.[2] Around 4–6 months of age, infants learn to roll over. Once the infant can roll from supine to prone and from prone to supine, the infant may remain in the sleep position that he or she assumes.[2]

Infants should be placed on a firm, tight-fitting crib mattress covered by a fitted sheet. Use of soft bedding such as mattress toppers, blankets, pillows, quilts, comforters, bumper pads, and bed positioners should not be used because they create overheating, rebreathing, and suffocation risk.

A crib that conforms to consumer Product Safety Commission (CPSC) is the safest place for an infant to sleep. Portable cribs, play yards, and bassinets that meet safety standards are adequate alternatives. Sofas have been found to be hazardous to sleeping infants.[12] Currently, there is no AAP recommendation for or against the use of bedside sleepers attached to the side of the parental bed. Sitting devices such as car seats, strollers, swings, infant carriers, and infant slings are not safe for routine sleep in young infants because they have poor head control, thus increasing the risk of upper airway obstruction and oxygen desaturation.[13,14] When an infant falls asleep in sitting device, he or she should be moved to a crib or other appropriate safe surface as soon as safe and practical.

Co-sleeping refers to parent and infant sleeping in close proximity (on the same surface or different surfaces) whereas *bedsharing* refers to parent(s) and infant sleeping together on any surface (bed, couch, chair). Because, the term "co-sleeping" is confusing and often misconstrued, the AAP recommends using the terms "bedsharing" and "room sharing" (when infant sleeps in the parents' room but on a separate sleep surface close to the parents' bed). In one study as many as 60% of mothers of infants from birth to 12 months admit to bedsharing at least once.[15] This practice may be due to cultural, personal, and economic influences. Although bedsharing facilitates breastfeeding, a known protective factor against SIDS, it is recommended that room sharing without bedsharing is the safest sleeping arrangement to reduce the risk of SIDS. SIDS risk while bedsharing is highest in very young infants; when mother smoked during pregnancy; when parents smoke, ingest alcohol, or arousal-altering medications; when bedsharing occurs on the sofa or couch; when there is soft bedding; or when the infant bedshares the whole night.[16]

Swaddling or wrapping the infant in a light blanket may calm infants, promote sleep, and encourage supine sleep position. When swaddled, infants should be placed wholly in supine position, and swaddling should be discontinued when the child exhibits signs of attempting to roll. Velcro and other fasteners should be securely attached when wearable blankets (infant bags) and swaddle wraps (wearable blankets with bands of fabric that can be wrapped around the infant) are used.[17] Correct swaddling application avoids hip dysplasia, overheating, head covering, and strangulation.[18–20]

Breastfeeding or giving expressed milk to an infant to any extent or duration is protective against SIDS[2,21] particularly when used exclusively; thus, breastfeeding should be encouraged as soon as and as long as possible. Use of a pacifier is also protective, especially when used at sleep onset, even if the pacifier falls from the mouth when the infant falls asleep. A pacifier can be introduced to formula-fed infants right away, and when breastfeeding is well-established.[21,22]

In summary, observing safe infant sleep practices is essential to decreasing the risk of SIDS and other sleep-related infant deaths. The mnemonic SAFE (Supine, Alone, Firm mattress, and Empty) is a good guide in maintaining a safe sleeping environment for any infant up to 1 year of age. Other essential practices to safe infant sleep include breastfeeding; use of a pacifier; the avoidance of overheating and exposure to smoke, alcohol, and illicit drugs; and routine immunization.[2,5]

INFANT SLEEP-DISORDERED BREATHING: CENTRAL SLEEP APNEA

Infants are at risk for sleep-disordered breathing predominated by central sleep apnea (CSA) or obstructive sleep apnea (OSA) due to immature respiratory control, high loop gain, impaired arousal threshold, laryngeal reflexes with a prominent cardiorespiratory depressant effect, adverse chest wall properties impairing load compensation, pulmonary mechanics favoring lower resting functional residual capacity (FRC) and lung compliance, highly compliant upper airway, and the predominance of rapid eye movement (REM) sleep.[23–25] Central apneas are common in infants, with a prevalence of 5%[26]; incidence is inversely proportional to age and gestational age. In one study, apneas were present in almost all infants born at 28 weeks of gestation or less, in 20% of infants born at 34 weeks of gestation, and it disappeared in all infants by 40 weeks PMA,[27] indicating that apneas resolve as infants mature. Prolonged recurrent central apneas in children less than 37 weeks conceptional age is termed *apnea of prematurity,* while those occurring in infants of at least 37 weeks conceptual age are termed *apnea of infancy.* Periodic breathing is common and is seen in almost all preterm infants with birth weights of less than 1,000 grams and in up to 80% of term infants.[28,29] It typically appears at 2–4 weeks of age then declines in frequency such that they are rarely present by 6 months of age.[28–30]

Central apneas and periodic breathing may be signs of a pathologic condition such as congenital central hypoventilation syndrome, Chiari malformation with myelomeningocele, Prader-Willi syndrome (PWS), or achondroplasia. Short central apneas associated with oxygen desaturation suggest decreased pulmonary reserve rather than a central nervous system (CNS) abnormality. Periodic breathing for 5% or more of sleep time in term infants[31] and 10% of sleep time in preterm infants[30] is considered abnormal and can reflect respiratory control or CNS abnormality, illness, or physiologic stressors.[30,31]

The approach to treatment of central apneas is focused on stabilization of irregular breathing and relief of hypoxemia with supplemental oxygen with or without ventilatory support and the use of respiratory stimulants (caffeine and theophylline) for apnea of prematurity. When hypoventilation is a concern, noninvasive positive pressure ventilation, continuous positive airway pressure (CPAP), or a high-flow nasal cannula can be used to provide respiratory support in apnea of prematurity while the infant is in the hospital.[32]

Xanthines (caffeine and theophylline) are primarily used for the treatment of apnea of prematurity (infants born between 29 and 32 weeks) and should be considered in symptomatic infants of 34 weeks of gestation or older.[32] Xanthines improve minute ventilation and carbon dioxide sensitivity and cause decreases in periodic breathing and hypoxic depression of breathing. Their primary mechanism of action is thought to be blockade of inhibitory adenosine A_1 receptors, with resultant excitation of respiratory neural output, as well as blockade of excitatory adenosine A_{2A} receptors located on gamma-aminobutyric acidergic neurons. However, they are associated with adverse effects including tachycardia, emesis, and jitteriness, limiting their use. Caffeine citrate is preferred because it has longer half-life, higher therapeutic index, and does not require drug-level monitoring. The standard dosing of caffeine citrate includes a loading dose of 20 mg/kg followed by maintenance of 5 mg/kg per day up to 10 mg/kg per day for persistent apnea. The optimal time to start caffeine in premature infants is not known but generally initiated when apnea occurs in infants of greater than 28 weeks of gestation. A trial off caffeine may be considered when an infant has been free of clinically significant apnea/bradycardia events, off positive pressure for 5–7 days, or at 33–34 weeks PMA. Infants with an unusually prolonged course of recurrent, extreme apnea or bradycardia may be discharged with home cardiorespiratory monitoring.[32] When prescribing a home apnea monitor, caregiver training addressing appropriate responses to the alarms and reiterating that the home apnea monitor does not prevent SIDS cannot be overemphasized.

Brief, isolated bradycardic episodes that spontaneously resolve and feeding-related events that resolve with interruption of feeding are common and should not delay weaning off caffeine. "Extreme events" (apnea >30 seconds and/or heart rate <60 beats per minute for >10 seconds) have been found to decrease dramatically after 43 weeks PMA. Current evidence suggests that caffeine and elective home monitoring can be discontinued in most infants after 43 weeks PMA unless otherwise clinically indicated.[32]

SLEEP-DISORDERED BREATHING: OBSTRUCTIVE SLEEP APNEA

Infants are predisposed to OSA due to their upper airway anatomy, obligate nasal breathing, and REM sleep predominance. OSA is more common in infants with a history of prematurity, bronchopulmonary dysplasia, obesity, and being born to a mother with a history of prenatal smoking.[23] Craniofacial malformations are the most common causes of infant OSA. Other causes of infant OSA are listed in Box 35.1.

The diagnosis of OSA may be delayed in an infant because of lack of symptoms or decreased recognition of symptoms.[33,34] For example, infants with Robin sequence and OSA may not snore.[35] Parents may underestimate the presence and severity of OSA in children with Down syndrome.[36] Thus, the AAP recommends screening for OSA at least once during the first 6 months of life as part of anticipatory guidance of infants with Down syndrome.[37]

Overnight in-lab polysomnography (PSG) remains the gold standard in establishing the diagnosis of OSA.[38,39] Infants diagnosed with OSA need to undergo airway endoscopy to identify the sites of obstruction and assess associated conditions. Other tests to consider include (1) lateral neck x-ray to assess the presence of adenotonsillar hypertrophy, (2) chest x-ray to assess for cardiopulmonary disease which may explain the severity of associated hypoxemia, (3) blood gas to assess for daytime hypoventilation, and (4) echocardiogram to assess for the presence of pulmonary hypertension.

Infants with mild OSA and whose conditions are likely to resolve may benefit from positional therapy, supplemental oxygen, nasopharyngeal tube, and treatment of associated conditions like gastroesophageal reflux disease (GERD). Noninvasive positive pressure ventilation with CPAP or bilevel positive airway pressure (BiPAP) delivered via nasal mask, prongs, or oronasal mask can successfully reverse OSA.[40] It is safe and effective, but success can be hindered by adherence; availability of an appropriate and proper fitting PAP interface, particularly in the very young; and family buy-in for the treatment.[41] In addition, prolonged use of CPAP or BiPAP can predispose to midface hypoplasia and malocclusion due to pressure of the tight fitting mask on the growing face. Therefore, family training and regular follow-up cannot be overemphasized. High-flow nasal cannula therapy (HFNC) has been reported to be successful in an infant with severe OSA, hypotonia, and craniofacial anomalies for whom CPAP therapy was not possible.[42] It has been used as a form of noninvasive respiratory support for preterm

> **Box 35.1 Predisposing factors and medical conditions associated with infant obstructive sleep apnea (OSA)**
>
> **Craniofacial abnormalities**
>
> Maxillary hypoplasia: Craniosynostosis, achondroplasia, Down syndrome, Treacher-Collins
>
> Micrognathia: Robin sequence, hemifacial microsomia
>
> Macroglossia: Beckwith Wiedemann syndrome, Down syndrome
>
> **Airway abnormalities**
>
> Laryngomalacia, subglottic stenosis, choanal atresia, cleft palate
>
> Adenotonsillar hypertrophy
>
> Obesity
>
> Neurologic disorders
>
> Cerebral palsy
>
> Chiari malformation
>
> Neuromuscular weakness
>
> Prader-Willi syndrome
>
> Gastroesophageal reflux
>
> Maternal smoking exposure
>
> Respiratory infection
>
> Post pharyngeal flap surgery

infants[43] and in the acute management of bronchiolitis in infants and children.[42,44] For infants with OSA, vigilant monitoring of symptoms, development of failure to thrive, or pulmonary hypertension is critical. A repeat PSG is key to document resolution of OSA, optimal oxygen requirement for relief of hypoxemia, or CPAP/ BiPAP titration to achieve the best setting to relieve OSA and hypoventilation.

Supratoglottoplasty is the first line of treatment for severe laryngomalacia. It is indicated in infants with worsening airway symptoms, feeding difficulties, and failure to thrive.[45] It is effective in reversing abnormal respiratory parameters in patients with moderate to severe OSA.[46] Infants with Down syndrome and laryngomalacia may benefit from supratoglottoplasty, but many would still require additional procedures.[47]

Adenotonsillectomy is indicated in infants with enlarged tonsils and adenoids. The risk for postoperative complications is high (up to 28% in one series), thus infants should be admitted for careful monitoring after the surgery.[48] Parents need to be counseled on the potential for adenoidal regrowth and thus to screen for recurrence of symptoms.[48] When symptoms recur, a repeat overnight PSG is indicated.

Mandibular distraction osteogenesis (MDO) is indicated in infants with micrognathia where the tongue abuts the posterior pharyngeal wall. The procedure involves osteotomies on the mandible bilaterally, stabilizing it in a rigid fixator, and gradually lengthening the mandible using the principle of distraction osteogenesis until the distractors are fully extended (30 mm distraction in one center).[49] MDO is highly successful in preventing tracheostomy in infants with isolated Robin sequence.[49,50] Infants with other sites of obstruction, such as laryngomalacia, subglottic stenosis, or significant tracheomalacia, or with significant untreatable central apnea have high failure rates with MDO and should be considered for tracheostomy.[51] Complications of MDO include nerve injuries, facial scarring, tooth injury, and temporomandibular joint dysfunction.[52] Other interventions include tongue-lip adhesion for infants with Robin sequence and significant glossoptosis[51] and tongue reduction for infants with Beckwith-Wiedemann syndrome.[53]

When infants have multiple sites of obstruction or are expected to require multiple surgeries, tracheostomy placement should be highly considered.[51] Complications of tracheostomy include suprastomal collapse, tracheal wall granuloma, laryngotracheal stenosis, tracheal wall erosion, catastrophic bleeding, recurrent infections, fistulas, tracheomalacia, and accidental decannulation.[54]

INFANT SLEEP AND COLIC

Colic presents as crying for more than 3 hours per day for more than 3 days a week, most often in the late afternoon or early evening in an otherwise healthy infant. Colic first presents during the second week of life, decreases significantly by 8–9 weeks, and is rare in infants older than 9 weeks.[55,56] There are no proven treatments for colic. Management includes parental reassurance that the condition is benign, behavioral interventions to soothe the infant, and evaluation for organic causes.[57] Behavior interventions may include swaddling, gentle rocking, decreased stimulation, calming sounds (such as white noise machines), vibration, and use of a pacifier. Organic causes may include constipation, GERD, infections, feeding disorders, acute abdominal pain, and occult fracture; maternal drug effects should be addressed.[58] Dietary modification, such as lactase supplementation, diet change in breastfeeding mothers, and a change to a hydrolysate formula are of unclear efficacy.[59] Soy milk is not recommended for infants younger than 6 months. Simethicone and proton pump inhibitors are ineffective, and dicyclomine, an anticholinergic drug, is contraindicated because it can cause apnea and seizures.[60,61] Other therapies, such as manipulative therapies, massage, acupuncture, herbal supplements,[62] and "gripe water" (dill seed oil, bicarbonate, and hydrogenated glucose) are contraindicated or lack sufficient evidence to support their routine use.[60,62,63]

Sleep in the Child

NORMAL SLEEP IN A CHILD

Adequate sleep duration for age on a regular basis leads to improved attention, behavior, learning, memory, emotional regulation, quality of life, and mental and physical health. The AAP has issued a Statement of Endorsement supporting the American Academy of Sleep Medicine (AASM) guidelines outlining recommended sleep duration for children from infants to teens. To promote optimal health, the recommended sleep hours, including naps, are listed in Table 35.2.[64,65]

Table 35.2 Recommended sleep duration

Child's age	Sleep duration
Infants 4 months–12 months	12–16 hours per 24 hours (including naps)
Children 1–2 years of age	11–14 hours per 24 hours (including naps)
Children 3–5 years of age	10–13 hours per 24 hours (including naps)
Children 6–12 years of age	9–12 hours per 24 hours
Teenagers 13–18 years of age	8–10 hours per 24 hours

COMMON CONCERNS THAT INTERRUPT A CHILD'S NORMAL NIGHT OF SLEEP: BEHAVIORAL INSOMNIA

Insomnia is the most common sleep problem in childhood, with a prevalence of up to 30% in infants, toddlers, and preschoolers.[66,67] Infants do not usually sleep through the night for the first 3–6 postnatal months, therefore the diagnosis of insomnia is usually not made before 6 months of age. Sleep problems can manifest as difficulty in initiating sleep without caregiver's intervention, in maintaining sleep (frequent night waking and difficulty returning to sleep without a caregiver's intervention), and waking up earlier than usual, with inability returning to sleep. There are generally two types of behavioral insomnia in children: sleep onset association disorder and limit setting disorder.[66–68]

In behavioral insomnia of childhood, *sleep onset association type*, infants and children become dependent on specific sleep onset associations (e.g., rocking, feeding, parental presence) to fall asleep at bedtime and to return to sleep during the night. This type of insomnia tends to improve by 3–4 years of age.[66,68]

In behavioral insomnia of childhood, *limit-setting type*, parents have difficulties in adequately enforcing bedtime limits. The child exhibits bedtime refusal (e.g., verbal protests, crying, getting out of bed, attention-seeking behaviors, "curtain calls"). This disorder typically presents after 2 years of age, when children are sleeping in a bed or are capable of climbing out of the crib. It is present in up to 10–30% of toddlers and in up to 15% of school-age children, and it may coexist with nighttime awakenings. In toddlers, it may manifest as increased nighttime awakenings and may reflect a manifestation of separation anxiety.[66,68]

Management of pediatric insomnia includes establishing optimal sleep hygiene, behavioral therapies, and rarely, pharmacotherapy.[66,67,69–73] The AASM recommends behavioral interventions in the treatment of bedtime problems and night waking in young children. The main objectives of behavioral therapy are to eliminate negative associations that lead to insomnia. The behavioral approaches include (1) unmodified extinction (extinction with parental presence and preventive parent education) and (2) graduated extinction, bedtime fading/positive routines, and scheduled awakenings. At present, there is insufficient evidence to recommend standardized bedtime routines and positive reinforcement as single therapies.[66,67,74]

Unmodified extinction involves the parents putting the child to bed at a designated bedtime and then ignoring the child until morning, although parents continue to monitor for issues such as safety and illness. This can be performed with parental presence in the child's bedroom. However, the parents do not interact with the child until the predetermined time.

Graduated extinction helps the infant or child learn to fall asleep independently by slowly increasing the amount of time the infant cries until he or she learns to "self-soothe." An infant is allowed to cry only a few minutes (1–2 minutes) before being soothed. The time to intervention is slowly increased until the infant learns to calm him- or herself. For older children, graduated extinction consists of putting the child to sleep safely and the parents ignoring bedtime crying and tantrums for predetermined periods before briefly checking on the child. A progressive checking schedule (e.g., 5 minutes, then 10 minutes) or fixed checking schedule (e.g., every 5 minutes) may be used. The goal is to reduce undesired behaviors (e.g., crying, screaming) by eliminating parental attention and enable the child to develop self-soothing skills and return to sleep alone. This intervention is often referred to as "sleep training." Parental acceptance of graduated extinction techniques tends to be greater than that of unmodified extinction. Parents should also be prepared for the "extinction burst," which is a worsening of the behavior, usually occurring on the second night.

Delayed bedtime with removal from bed/positive bedtime routines involves temporarily delaying the child's bedtime in order to more closely approximate the actual sleep onset time. The parent is also to remove the child from bed for a specific time period if sleep onset is not achieved within a prescribed time (15–30 minutes); this allows them to perform some calming activity to induce sleepiness. The child should be put to bed drowsy but awake. Once the time when the child goes to bed spontaneously is established, put the child to bed 15–30 minutes earlier every day until the appropriate time is established. Positive bedtime routines involve the institution of a set sequence of pleasurable and calming activities preceding bedtime in order to establish a behavioral chain leading up to sleep onset. Both of these treatments are based on stimulus control techniques and are targeted toward reducing affective and physiologic arousal at bedtime.

Scheduled awakenings consist of documentation of the pattern of night waking, followed by the institution of preemptive waking of the child 15–30 minutes prior to the expected time of spontaneous awakenings and subsequent fading out of the awakenings over time. Providing the "usual" responses (e.g., feeding, rocking, soothing) as if child had awakened spontaneously can also be supplemented during the preemptive awakening. Studies suggest that this technique may have less utility in very young children.

"Fading" of the adult intervention involves gradually decreasing parental involvement in the child's falling asleep. This involves an "exit plan" in which the parents institute a regular bedtime and sleep schedule and then gradually decrease direct contact with the child as he or she falls asleep. The goal for the plan is for the parent to "exit" the room and allow the child to fall asleep independently.

Approach to behavioral insomnia of childhood, sleep onset type is through gradual extinction of association stimulus. For the limit setting type, behavioral techniques and parent involvement are key. It is essential for parents to establish the limits and rules and maintain them firmly.

COMMON CONCERNS THAT INTERRUPT A CHILD'S NORMAL NIGHT OF SLEEP: NOCTURNAL ENURESIS

Sleep enuresis refers to recurrent involuntary voiding during sleep, occurring at least twice per week for at least 3 months in a patient older than 5 years of age. In primary enuresis, the patient has never been consistently dry during sleep. With secondary enuresis, there is recurrence of bedwetting in a patient who has previously been consistently dry during sleep for at least 6 months.[68,75]

The etiology of sleep enuresis is complex but may be due to three interrelated factors: large nocturnal urine volume production, nocturnal bladder hyperactivity, and difficulty arousing from sleep. It is suggested that difficulty arousing from sleep is important in primary enuresis, and poor bladder instability/overactivity is more important in secondary enuresis.[68,76,77]

Treatment of nocturnal enuresis (NE) involves evaluation of conditions such as sleep-disordered breathing, heart abnormalities, metabolic conditions, constipation, psychologic stressors, and/or excess nocturnal fluid and solute intake as well as small bladder capacities. Bladder capacity can be determined by using the voiding diary and maximum voided volume to look for a pattern of frequent small-volume voids during the day.[75,78–80]

All children with NE should attempt to limit their fluid consumption during the evening, empty their bladder before going to sleep, and void again whenever they wake up at night as well. First-line treatments for NE include bed alarms and desmopressin.[75] The bedwetting alarm (vibratory and/or auditory) is focused on altering the sleep arousal associated with voiding[75,79,80]

Desmopressin is a vasopressin analogue that reduces the amount of urine produced at night and can result in dryness in up to 30% and partial response in up to 40% of patients. However, relapse rate is high particularly with the nasal spray preparation. There is a risk of hyponatremia and water intoxication requiring limiting fluid intake to 200 mL starting 1 hour before the medication intake and until the child wakes the next morning. To assess continued need, desmopressin can be withdrawn every 3 months.[79–81]

Anticholinergics (oxybutynin and tolterodine) and imipramine are an effective adjunctive therapy in children with overactive bladders and small bladder capacity. However, the relapse rate is high. Constipation is a common side effect.[75,82] Imipramine increases the risk of QT prolongation in children, and a family history of sudden cardiac death should raise concern for QT prolongation. At present, use of imipramine is limited to specialty centers with extensive experience in treating NE.[75]

Hypnosis and acupuncture are alternative treatments that can be incorporated in children with refractory NE. They are not recommended as first-line therapy.[83]

COMMON CONCERNS THAT INTERRUPT A CHILD'S NORMAL NIGHT OF SLEEP: PARASOMNIA

Parasomnias are disorders of sleep that comprise complex behaviors that occur during non–REM sleep, REM sleep, or during transitions to and from sleep. Disorders of arousal (sleepwalking, sleep terror, and confusional arousals) consist of complex behaviors that are usually initiated during partial arousal from slow wave N3 sleep. Most episodes are brief, but they may last as long as 30–40 minutes. Most episodes emerge in the first third or half of typical sleep but can occur during the daytime nap. They are triggered by sleep deprivation, stress, medical illness (fever), noise, or medications such as antihistamines and stimulants. Disorders of arousals typically resolve by puberty but infrequently persist or arise in adolescence or adulthood.[68] PSG is not routinely indicated, although it is indicated when there is uncommon age of onset for presenting symptoms, the diagnosis is unclear, there are medical or legal consequences, with the risk injury to self or others, a high frequency of episodes, suspicion of other sleep disorders (OSA, periodic limb movement disorder [PLMD], or nocturnal epilepsy), and safety risks (e.g., leaving the house).

Sleep terrors differ from other disorders of arousal in that they are associated with autonomic nervous system and behavioral manifestations of intense fear. During a sleep terror, parents should remain calm because the episode is often more frightening for the parent than for the child. Attempts to awaken a child fully during a sleep terror may increase the child's agitation. The parent should not try to wake the child but make sure the child cannot hurt himself or herself by keeping the child in bed and safe. After the episode, the parent can focus on improving sleep debt to minimize sleep deprivation. Scheduled awakening may be considered for a child who is having nightly episodes. Using this approach, parents identify the time of the episodes and wake the child to the point of arousal 15–30 minutes before that time. This can be done for 2–4 weeks, until the episodes stop occurring, and can be repeated if the episodes recur. The rare child with frequent severe or violent episodes that place him or her at high risk of injury can be treated with benzodiazepines (clonazepam). Treatment can be considered for 3–6 months, until the episodes cease completely. Benzodiazepines (clonazepam) should be slowly tapered because abrupt discontinuation results in slow wave sleep rebound and a return of the nocturnal episodes. Low doses should be used initially, with upward titration as needed; patients should be monitored for daytime sedation due to the drug's long half-life. Medications should be given at least 90 minutes before bedtime to achieve effective drug levels in the first part of the night. L-5-hydroxytryptophan, a precursor of serotonin, has been found efficacious in the treatment of sleep terrors.

During a sleepwalking episode, the parent should not try to wake the child up but instead gently guide the child back to bed. The parent should focus on ensuring the child is safe during these episodes. Safety measures may include securing doors and windows, alarms such as bells placed on the doorknob, placing mattresses on the floor, using sleeping bags, and blocking access to stairs and kitchen. Parent should optimize good sleep hygiene with a regular sleep–wake schedule. Very rarely, in a child whose nightly events result in injury, benzodiazepines (clonazepam) may be given. Most episodes resolve by puberty, with the age-related decrease in slow wave sleep. OSA and other sleep-related respiratory events are increasingly recognized precipitants of disorders of arousal in children. Thus, treatment of these may reduce or eliminate the recurrence of sleepwalking.

Nightmares are very common in children. They typically occur in the last third of the night. They result in complete awakening, after which the child can often provide a detailed description of the frightening scenario. Post awakening anxiety and difficulty returning to sleep may be present and can lead to sleep avoidance and sleep deprivation. *Nightmare disorder* occurs when the dream experience or the sleep disturbance causes clinically significant distress or impairment. Nightmare disorder in children is most likely to occur in those exposed to severe psychosocial stressors, in physically or sexually abused children, and in those suffering from posttraumatic stress disorder (PTSD). Because childhood nightmares often resolve spontaneously, the diagnosis of nightmare disorder should be given only if there is persistent distress or impairment. Emotions are characteristically negative and most frequently involve anxiety, fear, or terror but may also involve anger, rage, embarrassment, and disgust. Nightmare content most often focuses on imminent physical danger to the individual, and the child has the ability to detail the nightmare contents upon awakening. Traumatic trauma-related nightmares are the most consistent problem reported by patients with PTSD. Although approximately 50% of PTSD cases resolve within 3 months, posttraumatic nightmares may persist throughout life.[84]

Parents should focus on maintaining good sleep hygiene and limiting exposure to frightening or overstimulating television shows and movies before bedtime. Some children may respond well to parental reassurance or the use of security objects such as blankets. A developmental-behavioral pediatrician or psychologist referral may be needed because some children may respond to relaxation strategies or systemic desensitization. For pediatric PTSD-associated nightmares, prazosin improved nightmares and sleep.[85]

REM behavior disorder (RBD) in children is rare and virtually never idiopathic. It is usually associated with narcolepsy,[86] brainstem tumors, antidepressants, medications (selective serotonin reuptake inhibitors [SSRIs]), neurodevelopmental disorders (autism, Smith-Magennis, Moebius syndrome),[87,88] Tourette syndrome,[89] and various rare conditions. Safety remains key in management. RBD in childhood seems to respond to clonazepam and melatonin.[87,88]

COMMON CONCERNS THAT INTERRUPT A CHILD'S NORMAL NIGHT OF SLEEP: SLEEP-RELATED MOVEMENT DISORDERS

Restless legs syndrome (RLS), PLMD, bruxism, and rhythmic movement disorder (RMD) can occur and interrupt sleep.

RLS is an increasingly recognized sleep disorder in children characterized by an urge to move accompanied by a disagreeable sensation in the legs that commonly occurs in the evening prior to sleep onset. Periodic limb movements in sleep (PLMS) are characterized by periodic episodes of repetitive and highly stereotypic limb movements during sleep. PLMD is defined by the presence of PLMS associated with symptoms of insomnia or excessive daytime sleepiness. RLS and PLMD are closely related conditions especially in children and adolescents. RLS is associated with attention deficit hyperactivity disorder (ADHD), migraine, and chronic kidney disease. The diagnosis of RLS must meet the four essential features seen in adults. In addition, the child must be able to describe the symptoms in his or her own words. Because it is often difficult for children to provide a reliable history, other features can help in establishing the diagnosis, including a Periodic Limb Movement Index score of 5 or more per hour of sleep, a family history of RLS *and*

PLMD in first-degree relatives, and a family history of periodic limb movements in sleep. For a diagnosis of periodic limb movements in sleep, an overnight PSG is required (PLM index ≥5).[68]

The best initial form of treatment is to reduce factors or conditions that may worsen or precipitate RLS. These include enforcing good sleep hygiene with a regular sleep–wake schedule; avoiding heavy meals, fluids, or exercise within a few hours of bedtime; and discouraging non–sleep-inducing activities such as watching television or playing games near bedtime. Iron deficiency should be considered in a child with RLS so measuring serum ferritin is recommended, but it should not be tested in ill children because it can be falsely elevated. The first line of therapy in children is iron supplementation.[90–92] Consensus guidelinefor treating iron deficiency in children with RLS, suggests initiation of treatment for fasting ferritin levels less than 50 mcg/l with titration of iron until the ferritin level is greater than ≥50 mcg/l–.[93] It may take weeks or months of treatment with iron supplementation to detect improvements in RLS symptoms.

Medications such as SSRIs and tricyclic antidepressants (TCAs) can precipitate RLS or PLMD in predisposed individuals, and switching to another class of antidepressant is recommended. Caffeine, sedating antihistamines, and dopamine antagonists such as compazine and metoclopramide may also worsen RLS.

Currently, there no approved medications for RLS in children. Certain medications have been tried in children with RLS, including levodopa/carbidopa, dopamine agonists (e.g., ropinirole, pramipexole), benzodiazepines (e.g., clonazepam), and alpha-adrenergic (e.g., clonidine). The long-term risks of treating children for RLS or PLMD with the existing medications are unknown. Clonidine and clonazepam have been fairly well-tolerated in children. However, clonazepam should be used with caution in children suspected of sleep-disordered breathing because it can relax the upper airway muscles, thereby increasing risk of upper airway collapse. Dopaminergic medications may be considered in children with severe cases of RLS, although the long-term effects are unknown. They are generally well-tolerated in children; however, up to 20% of children taking carbidopa/levodopa may develop nausea. Several case studies demonstrate good efficacy and tolerance of carbidopa/levodopa and ropinirole in children with ADHD and RLS. Although there is emerging literature supporting medical therapy in children with RLS and PLMD, the overall experiences with these medications in children are still limited. Regular follow-up is important to assess clinical improvement and to modify medication regimen. Further studies are needed to evaluate the safety and efficacy of pharmacologic therapy on RLS and PLMD in children.[94]

Rhythmic movement disorder (RMD) is repetitive, stereotyped, rhythmic motor behaviors that occur predominantly during sleep onset but may occur in all sleep stages, particularly N2. It may include headbanging, head rolling, or body rolling. It is typically seen in infants and children and frequency decreases by 5 years of age. If persistent, it may be an indication of mental retardation, autism, or other pathologies. RMD most often relies on parental report. PSG with video monitoring may aid in diagnosis by allowing direct visualization of whole-body movements.[95]

Treatment is focused on reducing injury risk by ensuring that the child's bed is stable, using bedrails, moving the bed away from the wall, and, when necessary, installing padding. Behavioral approaches, including teaching replacement behaviors, cognitive behavioral treatments, reward systems, and aversion therapy, have been reported in a small number of small studies and case reports, but no two studies have replicated a consistent treatment protocol.

There are no randomized controlled trials of pharmacological treatments for RMD, and current knowledge is based on limited case studies. Benzodiazepines (clonazepam, flurazepam, and oxazepam) have been reported to have partial success in eliminating RMD but rapid development of tolerance has also been reported. TCAs (imipramine) and dopamine antagonists (haloperidol and pimozide) have also been reported in case studies.[95]

SLEEP-DISORDERED BREATHING IN THE CHILD: SLEEP APNEA

Pediatric OSA is common with a prevalence of 1.2 -5.7 % in general pediatric population. The prevalence is higher due to the pediatric obesity epidemic. The prevalence peaks between 2 and 8 years of age in association with adenotonsillar hypertrophy. There is equal prevalence in prepubertal boys and girls; higher in adolescent males, African American children, and those of lower socioeconomic status.[38]

All children should be screened for OSA, and those with symptoms of snoring and signs and symptoms of OSA should undergo an overnight PSG.[38] The gold standard test is an overnight, attended, in-laboratory PSG/sleep study[38] with non-invasive tests involving the measurement of a number of physiologic functions, typically including electroencephalogram (EEG), pulse oximetry, oronasal airflow, abdominal and chest wall movements, partial pressure of carbon dioxide (PCO_2), and video recording.[96] Specific pediatric scoring criteria should be used. Obstructive apnea is defined as cessation of airflow ($\geq$90% decrease in apnea sensor excursions from baseline) of a minimum duration of 2 missed breaths. Obstructive hypopnea is defined as a 30% or greater drop in flow for 2 or more breaths in association with 3% or greater oxygen desaturation or an arousal. Hypoventilation is defined as arterial PCO_2 (or surrogate) of greater than 50 mm Hg for more than 25% of total sleep time.[96] When adult diagnostic criteria is used, the presence and severity of OSA may be underestimated.

An obstructive apnea hypopnea index (AHI) of 1.5 or more episodes per hour but less than 5 per hour is considered mild; an AHI of 5 or more per hour but less than 10 per hour is considered moderate; and an AHI of 10 or more per hour is considered severe. Currently, the AASM does not recommend home sleep apnea testing (HSAT) in children.[97] If PSG is not available, then clinicians may order alternative diagnostic tests, such as nocturnal video recording, nocturnal oximetry, daytime nap PSG, or ambulatory PSG.[38] Although PSG is the gold standard for diagnosis of OSA, the availability of sleep laboratories with pediatric expertise is limited and may not be readily available in certain regions of the country. If an alternative test fails to demonstrate OSA in a patient with a high pretest probability, full PSG should be sought.

The goals of treatment of a child with OSA include achieving normal respiratory pattern, gas exchange, and sleep architecture during sleep and resolution of associated complications. Adenotonsillectomy is the first line of treatment in a child with adenotonsillar hypertrophy who does not have a contraindication to surgery.[38] Adenotonsillectomy is safe and is associated with a low incidence of postoperative complications.[98] High-risk patients undergoing adenotonsillectomy should be performed as inpatients and observed postoperatively for respiratory complications such as worsening of OSA or pulmonary edema in the immediate postoperative period. Death attributable to respiratory complications in the immediate postoperative period has been reported in patients with severe OSA. Risk factors for postoperative respiratory complications include young age (<3 years), severe OSA, asthma, sickle cell disease, failure to thrive, morbid obesity, craniofacial anomalies, Down syndrome, neuromuscular disorders, and pulmonary hypertension.[38] Children with an acute respiratory infection on the day of surgery, as documented by fever, cough, and/or wheezing, are at increased risk of postoperative complications and therefore should be rescheduled or monitored closely postoperatively. Adenotonsillectomy results in significant improvement in 70% of children. However, those who older (> 7 years of age), obese, have severe OSA, or have asthma warrant repeat overnight PSG as they are at risk for residual OSA.[99] Patients who remain symptomatic should undergo reevaluation with PSG.

Weight loss should be recommended in addition to other therapy in a child who is overweight or obese. Weight loss has been shown to improve OSA, although the degree of weight loss required has not been determined. Intranasal corticosteroids[100] and montelukast[101,102] are effective in the treatment of children with mild OSAS.[100] Children with a lower AHI, smaller waist circumference, higher positioned soft palate, smaller neck circumference, and of non-black race may have spontaneous resolution of their OSA and thus may benefit with watchful waiting.[103] Rapid maxillary expansion can be effective in children with isolated maxillary narrowing.[104,105]

CPAP is recommended if adenotonsillectomy is not performed or for persistent OSA.[38] Success of CPAP therapy depends on adequate education, including hands-on demonstration, careful mask fitting, and acclimatization prior to initiation of therapy. This can include videos, brochures, or educational sessions. Acclimatization can include providing masks for parents to take home for practice as part of the bedtime routine, age-appropriate explanations for the child, and behavioral modification techniques. Providers should take a calm, consistent, committed, and confident approach to reassure parents and patients that they can succeed with an explanation of how therapy works and its goals and benefits. A child life specialist can incorporate play therapy, especially in the hospitalized child, and a psychologist can provide desensitization therapies effective in specially selected patients.

There is increasing use of auto-titrating CPAP in children.[106] Reports indicate that it is safe and effective, and the mean pressures are found to be below those obtained from sleep studies.[106]

PAP therapy in children can be challenging. Despite significant improvement of PAP interfaces, finding appropriately sized interfaces and headgear remains difficult. Specific interfaces also have weight requirements for pediatric population. It is imperative to partner with a reliable home vendor that can supply the appropriate tubing, filters, interfaces, and headgear and be available for troubleshooting.

Adherence poses a challenge to successful PAP therapy. Despite advances in the device and interfaces, adherence is generally poor in the pediatric population.[107,108] Predictors of low adherence include low maternal education, race (African American), poor family social support, and being a teenager.[109] Adherence may be enhanced by education, peer support, developmentally targeted and individualized support strategies,[110] and improving caregiver CPAP-specific self-efficacy.[111]

Once initiated PAP therapy must be closely monitored by the prescriber. Periodic re-titration to account for changes related to growth and development, surgical interventions, change in body mass index (BMI), and increased adherence is also indicated for children. Despite all the methods trialed to improve pediatric adherence, this continues to be low. Multidisciplinary approaches may be taken at specialized pediatric sleep centers.

For children with mild to moderate OSA intolerant to CPAP, HFNC has been tried and found to be effective.[42,112] However, its use in the home setting remains sparse.

Adolescent Sleep and Special Pediatric Cases

NORMAL ADOLESCENT SLEEP

Adolescents experience a natural delay in their circadian rhythm compounded by unhealthy sleep behaviors, poor sleep hygiene, irregular sleep–wake patterns, electronic media use in the bedroom, and excessive caffeine use.[113] Thus, the average adolescent in the United States is chronically sleep-deprived and pathologically sleepy and regularly experiences sleepiness rated as highly as those with narcolepsy.

ADOLESCENT CIRCADIAN RHYTHM DISORDERS

Delayed sleep phase syndrome (DSPS) is a common disorder among adolescents.[114] The condition is characterized by habitual sleep–wake patterns that are delayed relative to conventional sleep times by 2 hours or more. Adolescents have a natural predisposition to a phase delay, but those with this disorder complain of sleep onset insomnia and extreme difficulty waking in the morning. Almost all report themselves to be evening types, with optimal functioning during afternoon, evening, and late evening. They make up for the short nighttime sleep period by taking afternoon naps or by extending sleep time on weekends. A positive family history is found in up to 40% of patients, along with polymorphisms in the clock gene *per3*.

The aim of treatment in DSPS is to realign the sleep schedule to a more conventional and socially acceptable pattern. Treatment involves improving sleep hygiene by avoiding naps and caffeinated beverages and decreasing bright light exposure (from TV, computers, or phones) in the evening. Weekend oversleep time should not extend more than 2 hours beyond the desired wake time.

Management of DSPS in children and adolescents includes strategically timed light therapy post awakening and strategically timed melatonin.[115] In one study, optimal results were obtained with a melatonin dose of 0.15 mg/kg, taken 1.5–2.0 hours prior to habitual bedtime. Melatonin 10 mg taken daily (higher than typical chronobiotic doses) should be used with caution in children due to its effect on growth hormone regulation. Adverse effects include headaches, somnolence, hypotension, hypertension, gastrointestinal upset, and exacerbation of alopecia areata. Side effects of light therapy include hypomania in patients with seasonal depression. Other commonly described side effects include eyestrain, nausea, agitation, and treatment-emergent headaches, albeit with predominantly spontaneous remission.[115]

ADOLESCENT INSOMNIA

Insomnia is the most prevalent sleep disorder in adolescence, particularly in late adolescence and in girls. Insomnia in adolescents is associated with mood disorders and suicidality. Adolescents are predisposed to insomnia and sleep hygiene problems due to a biological tendency to sleep later, increased school demands, participation in sports and other enrichment activities, after-school and evening jobs, and unhealthy sleep-related behaviors such as social and peer interactions including use of social media at bed and nighttime and high caffeine intake. During adolescence, there is also less parental control of bedtimes.[113]

Management focuses on adequate sleep routine, behavioral therapy, and use of melatonin in selected cases.[116] Cognitive-behavioral therapy for insomnia (CBT-I) is an effective intervention for insomnia in adolescents that includes stimulus control (adopt regular schedules, consolidate sleep to nighttime, and improve bed–sleep association), arousal reduction (quieting pre-bedtime activities and relaxation-imagery), cognitive therapy, and improving sleep hygiene practices (increase behaviors and environmental conditions that promote improved sleep quality). Sleep restriction (temporarily limit hours in bed to increase sleep efficiency) is typically not considered appropriate in adolescents because they already experience restricted sleep schedules (e.g., due to later bedtimes and early school start times) and thus this approach may exacerbate the consequences of insomnia disorder. CBT-I has demonstrated longer lasting improvement than pharmacological treatment. Internet-based CBT-I is a cost-effective option to group therapy.[117,118] There is also a Cochrane Review examining the use of hypnosis[119] and acupuncture[120] for the treatment of chronic insomnia, and these modalities are currently not recommended.

Melatonin is a hormone synthesized by the pineal gland and secreted by the suprachiasmatic nucleus of the hypothalamus, reaching peak levels between 2 and 4 AM. It is efficacious in children with ADHD and autism spectrum disorder. The recommended dose is 0.5–3 mg in children given 1–2 hours before dim light melatonin onset or at bedtime. In one study, melatonin significantly advanced sleep onset and dim-light melatonin onset by approximately 1 hour and decreased sleep onset latency by 35 minutes when given at least 1 hour prior to bedtime.

There are no drugs currently FDA approved for treatment of insomnia in childhood and adolescence. For most adolescents, sleep disorders improve using the sleep hygiene approach and behavioral intervention. When pharmacological therapy is required, the medication should act on the target symptom and should be appropriate for age and neurodevelopmental level, always weighing the benefits against the risks. Drugs that have been prescribed for pediatric insomnia include melatonin, antihistaminic agents, alpha-agonist (clonidine), L5-hydroxytryptophan, benzodiazepines, and TCAss. [121]

Antihistamines (diphenhydramine, hydroxyzine, promethazine) promote sedation via H_1-receptor blocking properties, with minimal effects on sleep architecture. Diphenhydramine reaches blood and tissue levels 2 hours after ingestion; it has a duration of 4–6 hours and plasma levels of 30 ng/mL induces drowsiness. Doses of diphenhydramine in children are 0.5 mg/kg up to 25 mg, while hydroxyzine is effective at a dose of 0.5 mg/kg in children. Side effects include daytime sedation, dizziness, or paradoxical hyperactivity.[121]

The alpha-agonist (clonidine) has a duration of action of 3 hours and half-life of 6–12 hours. Side effects of clonidine include anticholinergic effects, hypotension, and REM suppression. With abrupt discontinuation, there can be hypertension and REM rebound. Clonidine has a narrow therapeutic index, and overdose has been associated with cardiotoxicity and death. There is no recommended starting dose, but 0.05–0.1 mg has been suggested.[121]

Benzodiazepines are considered in children with neurological/and or psychiatric problems but are contraindicated in suspected sleep-disordered breathing.

L-5 hydroxytryptophan is a serotonin precursor that acts as a sleep stabilizing factor and thus can be used in those with multiple nocturnal awakenings or those who awaken in the middle of the night and have difficulty returning to sleep. It has been shown to be effective in those with night terrors at a dose of 1–2 mg/kg per day at bedtime.[121]

The safety and efficacy of herbal supplements such as valerian root have not been tested in children. Herbal preparations containing lemon balm, chamomile, and passion flower have not been found to be effective Kava-kava is associated with necrotizing hepatitis, while tryptophan has been associated with eosinophilic myalgia. Lavender aromatherapy has been suggested to reduce nighttime arousals but this has not been tested in children.

ADOLESCENT HYPERSOMNIA

Providers usually investigate an organic etiology for hypersomnia with a clinical history targeted toward symptoms consistent with sleep apnea, limb movement disorder, insufficient sleep, psychiatric disorders, medications, or circadian rhythm disorder. Providers may also inquire about symptoms consistent with narcolepsy, such as cataplexy, sleep paralysis, and hypnagogic and hypnopompic hallucinations. A PSG (with at least 6 hours sleep) and multiple sleep latency test (MSLT) may be indicated for these patients who present with possible hypersomnia narcolepsy as well as other diagnoses leading to excessive sleepiness. [122, 123] MSLT in adolescents may need to be interpreted with caution because sleep onset REM periods (SOREMPs) are fairly common in adolescents, as demonstrated by one study of normal adolescents that reported 48% of subjects had at least one SOREMP.

Treatment objectives should include control of daytime sleepiness to improve function at work, at school, at home, and socially and to control cataplexy, hypnagogic hallucinations, and sleep paralysis in narcolepsy. As previously recommended for narcolepsy, a healthcare provider should consider the risk-benefit ratio of medication. Modafinil is effective for treatment of daytime sleepiness due to narcolepsy and even idiopathic hypersomnia. Treatment of hypersomnias of central origin with methylphenidate or modafinil in children between the ages of 6 and 15 appears to be relatively safe. There is one study of modafinil in children with narcolepsy or idiopathic hypersomnolence that indicated it was safe and well-tolerated in children who did not have other preexisting neurologic or psychiatric conditions. Sodium oxybate is effective for treatment of cataplexy, daytime sleepiness, and disrupted sleep due to narcolepsy and may be effective for treatment of hypnagogic hallucinations and sleep paralysis; it is now FDA approved for patients 7 years and older. Amphetamine, methamphetamine, dextroamphetamine, and methylphenidate are effective for treatment of daytime sleepiness due to narcolepsy. An electrocardiogram (ECG) should be considered prior to initiation, especially in the patient who presents with concern for arrythmias, such as a family history of sudden cardiac death. It is important to expand the history to include specific cardiac symptoms, Wolf-Parkinson-White syndrome, sudden death in the family, hypertrophic cardiomyopathy, and long QT syndrome. TCAs, SSRIs, venlafaxine, and reboxetine may also be effective treatments for cataplexy.[122–124]

Scheduled naps can be beneficial to combat sleepiness but seldom suffice as primary therapy for narcolepsy. The combination of regular bedtimes and two 15-minute, regularly scheduled naps reduced unscheduled daytime sleep episodes and sleepiness when compared to stimulant therapy alone.[122–124]

Regular follow-up of patients with hypersomnia of central origin is necessary to monitor response to treatment, respond to potential medication side effects, and enhance the patient's adaptation to the disorder. The patients should be seen at least once every 6 months, to assess the development of medication side effects, including sleep disturbances, mood changes, and cardiovascular or metabolic abnormalities. Patients with severe sleepiness should be advised to avoid potentially dangerous activities at home, school, or work and should not operate a motor vehicle until sleepiness is appropriately controlled by stimulant medications.[124]

Sleep in Patients with Special Diagnoses

COMMON MEDICAL DISORDERS IN CHILDREN AND ADOLESCENTS THAT EFFECT SLEEP: ATTENTION-DEFICIT HYPERACTIVITY DISORDER

ADHD is the most common neurobehavioral disorder of childhood. ADHD has been estimated to affect approximately 5.3% of children and adolescents worldwide and to persist into adulthood in approximately two-thirds of patients.[125] Among recommendations, a clinician should include assessment for other conditions that might coexist with ADHD such as sleep apnea.[126,127] Objective measures (PSG, actigraphy, and MSLT) and subjective measures such and parent self-rated questionnaires and diaries/logs are used to assess sleep in patients with ADHD.[126]

The relationships of ADHD with sleep problems, psychiatric comorbidities, and medications are complex and multidirectional. Hypopnea/apnea and peripheral limb movements in sleep or nocturnal motricity in PSG studies; increased sleep onset latency and shorter sleep time in actigraphic studies; and bedtime resistance, difficulty with morning awakenings, sleep onset difficulties, sleep-disordered breathing, night awakenings, and daytime sleepiness in subjective studies have been reported. Significant PSG findings in children with ADHD include lower sleep efficiency, higher AHI scores, a larger number of sleep stage shifts per hour, and increased limb movements. ADHD is also frequently coincident with sleep disorders (OSA, PLMD, RLS, and circadian rhythm sleep disorders). Problems with sleep can, however, also lead to the development of ADHD or ADHD-like symptoms, potentially resulting in misdiagnosis. Psychostimulant medications are associated with disrupted or disturbed sleep but also can paradoxically calm some patients with ADHD for sleep by alleviating their symptoms. Long-acting formulations may have insufficient duration of action, leading to symptom rebound at bedtime. Thus, current US and European guidelines recommend assessment of sleep disturbances during evaluation of ADHD and before initiation of pharmacotherapy, with healthy sleep practices as the first-line option for addressing sleep problems. Psychiatric illnesses such as bipolar disorder, autism, PTSD, and obsessive-compulsive disorder often occur coincidently with ADHD and are also associated with sleep problems. The interactions of comorbid disorders and associated medications with ADHD and sleep disturbances are therefore important to consider when managing patients.[127,128]

ADHD is associated with bedtime resistance, difficulty with morning awakenings, sleep onset difficulties, sleep-disordered breathing, night awakenings, and daytime sleepiness. Other sleep problems seen in children with ADHD include parasomnias, nightmares, delayed sleep phase, short sleep time, and anxiety around bedtime.[126,127]

Behavior therapy is the first line of treatment. Behavior therapy usually is implemented by training parents in specific techniques that improve their abilities to modify and shape their child's behavior and improve the child's ability to regulate his or her own behavior. The training involves techniques to more effectively provide rewards when their child demonstrates the desired behavior via positive reinforcement and learn what behaviors can be reduced or eliminated by using planned ignoring as an active strategy or to provide appropriate consequences or punishments when their child fails to meet goals. To shape behaviors, there is a need to consistently apply rewards and consequences as tasks are achieved and then to gradually increase the expectations for each task as they are mastered.[129,130]

Similarly, sleep hygiene and routines are encouraged. Implementing healthy sleep practices is the recommended first-line option for addressing problems with sleep in both medicated and unmedicated patients with ADHD. In a study of children with ADHD and initial insomnia receiving stimulants, implementing sleep hygiene reduced sleep onset delay to below 60 minutes in about 20% of patients.[131]

Ball blankets are blankets that are filled with loose balls to stimulate sensory receptors in the skin, muscles, and joints that transmit inhibitory signals to the CNS. In a study of children with ADHD, the use of ball blankets was found to reduce sleep onset latency, the number of awakenings, and intraindividual variability in sleep parameters.[132]

Data on sleep medication use in patients with ADHD are scarce. The immediate -release form of clonidine has been suggested as a treatment option for stimulant-associated sleep onset delay in patients with ADHD Hypnotic agents, including zolpidem, mirtazapine, trazodone, and antihistamines, have been used off-label in the treatment of insomnia in children with ADHD.[126]

The incidence of organic sleep disorders such as OSA and RLS appear to be elevated in patients with ADHD. A recent systematic review indicated that the prevalence of OSA in patients with ADHD (25–30%) is higher than in the general population (~3%). The US guidelines recommend that children undergoing evaluation for ADHD be assessed for sleep apnea. In children with diagnoses of ADHD and OSA, significant improvements in ADHD symptoms, including hyperactivity,occurred following adenotonsillectomy or PAP. Therapy. A complex interaction of propensity for obesity and ADHD has also been reported.[126]

While 2% of typically developing children and adolescents (aged 8–17 years) are reported to meet the diagnostic criteria for RLS, up to 44% of children with ADHD have symptoms of RLS, and 26% of children with RLS have symptoms of ADHD. The impact of RLS or PLMD on sleep can lead not only to the diurnal manifestation of ADHD-like symptoms but also manifest as bedtime resistance and be mistaken for opposition or defiance due to the unpleasant symptoms.[134]

COMMON MEDICAL DISORDERS IN CHILDREN AND ADOLESCENTS THAT EFFECT SLEEP: AUTISM SPECTRUM DISORDER

Autism spectrum disorder (ASD) is common, with a prevalence of 1 in 59 children. As high as 80% of children with ASD have possible sleep disorders. Children with ASD are described as poor sleepers with difficulties initiating and maintaining sleep, short sleep duration, early morning awakening, and parasomnias. These sleep problems predispose to insufficient sleep, resulting in exacerbation of severity of the core symptoms of ASD and maladaptive behaviors. Therefore, it is critical to evaluate for the presence of sleep disorders in these patients.[135-138]

Several factors contribute to sleep disruption in ASD and include epilepsy, gastroesophageal reflux, constipation, anxiety, and/or depression. Children with ASD have decreased awareness of social cues, resulting in impaired synchronization of circadian rhythms. Medications that are prescribed to treat ASD symptoms and comorbid psychiatric conditions may cause insomnia or hypersomnolence. For example, the atypical antipsychotics risperidone, used for treating aggressive or self-injurious behavior, severe mood swings, tantrums, and irritability, causes daytime sleepiness but insomnia may also occur. The primary action of risperidone is serotonin 5-HT2 receptor blockade, but it is also a potent dopamine D_2 receptor antagonist. SSRIs used for treating repetitive behaviors in ASD have also been shown to have negative effects on sleep, including insomnia.[135–138]

Promoting sleep hygiene is important for patients with ASD. A good sleep environment with a dark, cool, and quiet bedroom is recommended as children with ASD may be particularly sensitive to noises and/or have sensory issue. Bedtime routines are essential as transitioning can be difficult for ASD patients. The routine should be relatively short (20–30 minutes) and include relaxing activities such as reading or listening to quiet music and avoiding the use of electronics close to bedtime. Additional recommendations for caretakers and providers are available via the organization Autism Speaks.[135–138]

Behavioral modifications including graduated extinction and faded bedtime (delaying the child's bedtime until he or she is ready for sleep) are useful strategies. Melatonin supplementation has been shown to be effective at improving sleep initiation with minimal reports of adverse events. Melatonin is primarily used as a sedative at low doses (1–3 mg) given approximately 30 minutes prior to bedtime. Given that the half-life of melatonin is rather short (<1 hour), the controlled-release melatonin preparations are sometimes effective when night awakening is present.[135]

A few psychotropic medications have been evaluated for treating insomnia in children with ASD.[139] These include clonidine, mirtazapine, and gabapentin. Risperidone has been shown to improve sleep latency but not sleep duration.

COMMON MEDICAL DISORDERS IN CHILDREN AND ADOLESCENTS THAT EFFECT SLEEP: DOWN SYNDROME

Per current AAP guidelines, clinicians should screen for symptoms of OSA, including heavy breathing, snoring, restless sleep, uncommon sleep positions, frequent night awakening, daytime sleepiness, apneic pauses, and behavior problems at each well-child visit. Parental perception of the presence and severity of OSA is poor in patients with Down syndrome. Therefore, a sleep study for all children with Down syndrome by 4 years of age is recommended, along with referral to a pediatric sleep specialist if OSA is present. [36,37] First-line treatment is adenotonsillectomy. Persistent or recurrent OSA occurs in up to 50% of patients due to relative macroglossia, glossoptosis, regrowth of adenoid and tonsillar tissue, enlarged lingual tonsils, and hypopharyngeal collapse. Those with residual OSA may require CPAP/BiPAP, or additional airway surgery such as lingual tonsillectomy, tongue base reduction, mandibular distraction, rapid maxillary expansion, and hypoglossal nerve stimulation. Patients with Down syndrome undergo thyroid function screening every 6 months until 1 year of age, then annually; for those with OSA, it is important to verify normal thyroid function.[140–142] Those who are intolerant to CPAP may be tried on HFNC.[143]

COMMON MEDICAL DISORDERS IN CHILDREN AND ADOLESCENTS THAT EFFECT SLEEP: PRADER-WILLI SYNDROME

PWS is a genetic disorder estimated to affect between 1 in 10,000 and 1 in 30,000 live births. PWS is caused by loss of imprinted gene expression from the paternal copy of chromosome 15q11.2-q13. Sleep problems occur frequently among individuals with PWS and include sleep-related breathing disorder and excessive daytime sleepiness. Narcolepsy has also been associated with PWS. Children with PWS progress from failure to thrive during infancy to hyperphagia and morbid obesity during later childhood and onward.[144] CSA predominates in infants and children with PWS who are less than 2 years old, while OSA is the most common finding in those older than 2 years. The phenotype of sleep-disordered breathing in PWS patients also evolves over time from predominantly CSA in infancy to OSA in older children. Behavioral difficulties are common and may make establishing effective therapy with CPAP more challenging when OSA persists after adenotonsillectomy. Excessive daytime sleepiness is also common in patients with PWS and may continue after OSA is effectively treated. Altered ventilatory control, obesity, airway hypotonia, micrognathia, narrowing of the upper airway, and respiratory muscle weakness all make individuals with PWS vulnerable to OSA, which can be severe. Some patients have associated hypothyroidism, which also contributes to the risk for OSA.[144]

Children 2 years and younger with CSA can be treated with supplemental oxygen. Those with OSA should be treated with adenotonsillectomy if adenotonsillar hypertrophy is present. For PWS patients with residual OSA after airway surgery, treatment with CPAP is recommended. Supplemental oxygen may be needed as oxygen desaturation is often severe even when OSA is mild. Weight loss may also be helpful, traditionally approached through diet and behavioral modifications. More recently, some patients have undergone laparoscopic sleeve gastrectomy. Residual excessive daytime sleepiness can be treated with stimulant medication (methylphenidate or dextroamphetamine derivatives) and/or modafinil (Provigil). By 3 months of age, PWS children should be screened for hypothyroidism.[140,144,145]

The development of OSA during growth hormone (GH) therapy is of particular concern due to several reports of sudden death in individuals with PWS undergoing GH therapy. In PWS patients receiving GH therapy, most fatal events occurred during the first 9 months of therapy. It is important to note that sudden death in PWS deaths occurred in both untreated patients and those on GH therapy and were often associated with respiratory insufficiency or respiratory infection.[144–146]

Current recommendations include PSG (sleep study) before and 6–10 weeks after beginning GH treatment and at 1 year, regardless of age, to assess for central and obstructive apneas. When present, delaying (or stopping) GH treatment until PSG results improve with treatment may be considered. It is also recommended that GH therapy not be initiated during an acute respiratory illness. A repeat PSG at any time there are new or worsening symptoms is suggested.[146-147] First line of treatment is adenotonsillectomy. If OSA or sleep disordered breathing persists, then CPAP or BiPAP therapy is recommended.[140]

REFERENCES

1. Centers for Disease Control (CDC). Data and statistics - SIDS and SUID. https://www.cdc.gov/sids/data.htm

2. American Academy of Pediatrics. Task Force on Sudden Infant Death Syndrome. AAP policy statement: SIDS and other sleep-related infant deaths: Updated 2016 recommendations for a safe infant sleeping environment. *Pediatrics*. 2016 Nov;138(5):e20162938 doi:10.1542/peds.2016–2938.

3. Centers for Disease Control (CDC). FastStats–Infant Health. https://www.cdc.gov/nchs/fastats/infant-health.htm

4. Tieder JS, Bonkowsky JL, Etzel RA, et al. Brief resolved unexplained events (formerly apparent life-threatening events) and evaluation of lower-risk infants. *Pediatrics*. 2016;137(5):e20160590–e20160590. doi:10.1542/peds.2016–0590.

5. Carlin RF, Moon RY. Risk factors, protective factors, and current recommendations to reduce sudden infant death syndrome. *JAMA Pediatr*. 2017;171(2):175. doi:10.1001/jamapediatrics.2016.3345.

6. Wong FY, Witcombe NB, Yiallourou SR, et al. Cerebral oxygenation is depressed during sleep in healthy term infants when they sleep prone. *Pediatrics*. 2011;127(3):e558–65. doi:10.1542/peds.2010–2724.

7. Tuffnell CS, Petersen SA, Wailoo MP. Prone sleeping infants have a reduced ability to lose heat. *Early Hum Dev*. 1995;43(2):109–116. http://www.ncbi.nlm.nih.gov/pubmed/8903756

8. Wong F, Yiallourou SR, Odoi A, Browne P, Walker AM, Horne RSC. Cerebrovascular control is altered in healthy term infants when they sleep prone. *Sleep*. 2013;36(12):1911–1918. doi:10.5665/sleep.3228.

9. Horne RS, Ferens D, Watts AM, et al. The prone sleeping position impairs arousability in term infants. *J Pediatr*. 2001;138(6):811–816. doi:10.1067/mpd.2001.114475.

10. Richardson HL, Horne RSC. Arousal from sleep pathways are affected by the prone sleeping position and preterm birth: Preterm birth, prone sleeping and arousal from sleep. *Early Hum Dev*. 2013. doi:10.1016/j.earlhumdev.2013.05.001.

11. Li D-K, Petitti DB, Willinger M, et al. Infant sleeping position and the risk of sudden infant death syndrome in California, 1997–2000. *Am J Epidemiol*. 2003;157(5):446–455. http://www.ncbi.nlm.nih.gov/pubmed/12615609

12. Rechtman LR, Colvin JD, Blair PS, Moon RY. Sofas and infant mortality. *Pediatrics*. 2014;134(5):e1293–300. doi:10.1542/peds.2014-1543.

13. Bergounioux J, Madre C, Crucis-Armengaud A, et al. Sudden deaths in adult-worn baby carriers: 19 cases. *Eur J Pediatr*. 2015;174(12):1665–1670. doi:10.1007/s00431-015-2593-6.

14. Batra EK, Midgett JD, Moon RY. Hazards associated with sitting and carrying devices for children two years and younger. *J Pediatr*. 2015;167(1):183–187. doi:10.1016/j.jpeds.2015.03.044.

15. Hauck FR, Signore C, Fein SB, Raju TNK. Infant sleeping arrangements and practices during the first year of life. *Pediatrics*. 2008;122(Suppl 2):S113–120. doi:10.1542/peds.2008-13150.

16. Vennemann MM, Hense H-W, Bajanowski T, et al. Bed sharing and the risk of sudden infant death syndrome: Can we resolve the debate? *J Pediatr*. 2012;160(1):44–8.e2. doi:10.1016/j.jpeds.2011.06.052.

17. Varghese S, Gasalberti D, Ahern K, Chang JC. An analysis of attitude toward infant sleep safety and SIDS risk reduction behavior among caregivers of newborns and infants. *J Perinatol*. 2015;35(11):970–973. doi:10.1038/jp.2015.111.

18. Pease AS, Fleming PJ, Hauck FR, et al. Swaddling and the risk of sudden infant death syndrome: A meta-analysis. *Pediatrics*. 2016;137(6):e20153275–e20153275. doi:10.1542/peds.2015-3275.

19. McDonnell E, Moon RY. Infant deaths and injuries associated with wearable blankets, swaddle wraps, and swaddling. *J Pediatr*. 2014;164(5):1152–1156. doi:10.1016/j.jpeds.2013.12.045.

20. Kelly BA, Irigoyen MM, Sherry PC, Pomerantz C, Mondesir M, Isaza-Brando N. Swaddling and infant sleeping practices. *J Community Health*. 2017;42:10–14. doi:10.1007/s10900-016-0219-1.

21. Alm B, Wennergren G, Möllborg P, Lagercrantz H. Breastfeeding and dummy use have a protective effect on sudden infant death syndrome. *Acta Paediatr*. 2016;105(1):31–38. doi:10.1111/apa.13124.

22. Eidelman AI. Breastfeeding and the use of human milk: An analysis of the American Academy of Pediatrics 2012 Breastfeeding Policy Statement. *Breastfeed Med*. 2012;7(5):323–324. doi:10.1089/bfm.2012.0067.

23. Katz ES, Mitchell RB, D'Ambrosio CM. Obstructive sleep apnea in infants. *Am J Respir Crit Care Med*. 2012;185(8):805–816. doi:10.1164/rccm.201108-1455CI.

24. Horne RSC, Parslow PM, Harding R. Respiratory control and arousal in sleeping infants. *Paediatr Respir Rev*. 2004;5(3):190–198. doi:10.1016/j.prrv.2004.04.011.

25. Carroll JL, Agarwal A. Development of ventilatory control in infants. *Paediatr Respir Rev*. 2010;11(4):199–207. doi:https://doi.org/10.1016/j.prrv.2010.06.002.

26. Kritzinger FE, Al-Saleh S, Narang I. Descriptive analysis of central sleep apnea in childhood at a single center. *Pediatr Pulmonol*. 2011;46(10):1023–1030. doi:10.1002/ppul.21469.

27. Henderson-Smart DJ. The effect of gestational age on the incidence and duration of recurrent apnoea in newborn babies. *Aust Paediatr J*. 1981;17(4):273–276. http://www.ncbi.nlm.nih.gov/pubmed/7347216

28. Glotzbach SF, Baldwin RB, Lederer NE, Tansey PA, Ariagno RL. Periodic breathing in preterm infants: Incidence and characteristics. *Pediatrics.* 1989;84(5):785–792. http://www.ncbi.nlm.nih.gov/pubmed/2797974

29. Fenner A, Schalk U, Hoenicke H, Wendenburg A, Roehling T. Periodic breathing in premature and neonatal babies: Incidence, breathing pattern, respiratory gas tensions, response to changes in the composition of ambient air. *Pediatr Res.* 1973. doi:10.1203/00006450-197304000-00020.

30. Patel M, Mohr M, Lake D, et al. Clinical associations with immature breathing in preterm infants: Part 2-periodic breathing. *Pediatr Res.* 2016. doi:10.1038/pr.2016.58.

31. Sateia MJ. International classification of sleep disorders-third edition highlights and modifications. *Chest.* 2014. doi:10.1378/chest.14-0970.

32. Eichenwald EC. Apnea of prematurity. *Pediatrics.* 2016;137(1):e20153757. doi:10.1542/peds.2015-3757.

33. Ward SL, Marcus CL. Obstructive sleep apnea in infants and young children. *J Clin Neurophysiol.* 1996;13(3):198–207. doi:10.1097/00004691-199605000-00003.

34. Leiberman A, Tal A, Brama I, Sofer S. Obstructive sleep apnea in young infants. *Int J Pediatr Otorhinolaryngol.* 1988;16(1):39–44. doi:10.1016/0165-5876(88)90098-5.

35. Anderson ICW, Sedaghat AR, McGinley BM, Redett RJ, Boss EF, Ishman SL. Prevalence and severity of obstructive sleep apnea and snoring in infants with Pierre Robin sequence. *Cleft Palate-Craniofacial J.* 2011;48(5):614–618. doi:10.1597/10-100.

36. Rosen D, Lombardo A, Skotko B, Davidson EJ. Parental perceptions of sleep disturbances and sleep-disordered breathing in children with Down syndrome. *Clin Pediatr (Phila).* 2011;50(2):121–125. doi:10.1177/0009922810384260.

37. Bull MJ. Committee on Genetics. Health supervision for children with Down syndrome. *Pediatrics.* 2011;128(2):393–406. doi:10.1542/peds.2011-1605.

38. Marcus CL, Brooks LJ, Draper KA, et al. Diagnosis and management of childhood obstructive sleep apnea syndrome. *Pediatrics.* 2012;130(3):576–584. doi:10.1542/peds.2012-1671.

39. Ramgopal S, Kothare S V., Rana M, Singh K, Khatwa U. Obstructive sleep apnea in infancy: A 7-year experience at a pediatric sleep center. *Pediatr Pulmonol.* 2014. doi:10.1002/ppul.22867.

40. Leonardis RL, Robison JG, Otteson TD. Evaluating the management of obstructive sleep apnea in neonates and infants. *JAMA Otolaryngol Head Neck Surg.* 2013;139(2):139–146. doi:10.1001/jamaoto.2013.1331.

41. Adeleye A, Ho A, Nettel-Aguirre A, Buchhalter J, Kirk V. Noninvasive positive airway pressure treatment in children less than 12 months of age. *Can Respir J.* 2016;2016:7654631. doi:10.1155/2016/7654631.

42. Joseph L, Goldberg S, Shitrit M, Picard E. High-flow nasal cannula therapy for obstructive sleep apnea in children. *J Clin Sleep Med.* 2015;11(9):1007–1010. doi:10.5664/jcsm.5014.

43. Wilkinson D, Andersen C, O'Donnell CPF, De Paoli AG, Manley BJ. High flow nasal cannula for respiratory support in preterm infants. *Cochrane Database Syst Rev.* 2016;2:CD006405. doi:10.1002/14651858.CD006405.pub3.

44. Goh CT, Kirby LJ, Schell DN, Egan JR. Humidified high-flow nasal cannula oxygen in bronchiolitis reduces need for invasive ventilation but not intensive care admission. *J Paediatr Child Health.* 2017;53(9):897–902. doi:10.1111/jpc.13564.

45. Ramprasad VH, Ryan MA, Farjat AE, Eapen RJ, Raynor EM. Practice patterns in supraglottoplasty and perioperative care. *Int J Pediatr Otorhinolaryngol.* 2016;86:118–123. doi:10.1016/j.ijporl.2016.04.039.

46. O'Connor TE, Bumbak P, Vijayasekaran S. Objective assessment of supraglottoplasty outcomes using polysomnography. *Int J Pediatr Otorhinolaryngol.* 2009;73(9):1211–1216. doi:10.1016/j.ijporl.2009.05.007.

47. Cockerill CC, Frisch CD, Rein SE, Orvidas LJ. Supraglottoplasty outcomes in children with Down syndrome. *Int J Pediatr Otorhinolaryngol.* 2016;87:87–90. doi:10.1016/j.ijporl.2016.05.022.

48. Cheng J, Elden L. Outcomes in children under 12 months of age undergoing adenotonsillectomy for sleep-disordered breathing. *Laryngoscope.* 2013;123(9):2281–2284. doi:10.1002/lary.23796.

49. Hammoudeh J, Bindingnavele VK, Davis B, et al. Neonatal and infant mandibular distraction as an alternative to tracheostomy in severe obstructive sleep apnea. *Cleft Palate Craniofac J.* 2012;49(1):32–38. doi:10.1597/10-069.

50. Breik O, Tivey D, Umapathysivam K, Anderson P. Mandibular distraction osteogenesis for the management of upper airway obstruction in children with micrognathia: A systematic review. *Int J Oral Maxillofac Surg.* 2016;45(6):769–782. doi:10.1016/j.ijom.2016.01.009.

51. Khansa I, Hall C, Madhoun LL, et al. Airway and feeding outcomes of mandibular distraction, tongue-lip adhesion, and conservative management in Pierre Robin sequence. *Plast Reconstr Surg.* 2017;139(4):975e–983e. doi:10.1097/PRS.0000000000003167.

52. Master DL, Hanson PR, Gosain AK. Complications of mandibular distraction osteogenesis. *J Craniofac Surg.* 2010;21(5):1565–1570. doi:10.1097/SCS.0b013e3181ecc6e5.

53. Cielo CM, Duffy KA, Vyas A, Taylor JA, Kalish JM. Obstructive sleep apnoea and the role of tongue reduction surgery in children with Beckwith-Wiedemann syndrome. *Paediatr Respir Rev.* February 2017. doi:10.1016/j.prrv.2017.02.003.

54. Sherman JM, Davis S, Albamonte-Petrick S, et al. Care of the child with a chronic tracheostomy. This official statement of the American Thoracic Society was adopted by the ATS Board of Directors, July 1999. *Am J Respir Crit Care Med.* 2000;161(1):297–308. doi:10.1164/ajrccm.161.1.ats1-00.

55. Wessel MA, Cobb JC, Jackson EB, Harris GS, Detwiler AC. Paroxysmal fussing in infancy, sometimes called colic. *Pediatrics.* 1954;14(5):421–435. http://www.ncbi.nlm.nih.gov/pubmed/13214956

56. Wolke D, Bilgin A, Samara M. Systematic review and meta-analysis: Fussing and crying durations and prevalence of colic in infants. *J Pediatr.* 2017;185:55–61.e4. doi:10.1016/j.jpeds.2017.02.020.

57. Bell G, Hiscock H, Tobin S, Cook F, Sung V. Behavioral outcomes of infant colic in toddlerhood: A longitudinal study. *J Pediatr.* 2018;201:154–159. doi:10.1016/j.jpeds.2018.05.010.

58. Barr RG. Colic and crying syndromes in infants. *Pediatrics.* 1998;102(5 Suppl E):1282–1286. http://www.ncbi.nlm.nih.gov/pubmed/9794970

59. Gordon M, Biagioli E, Sorrenti M, et al. Dietary modifications for infantile colic. *Cochrane Database Syst Rev.* October 2018. doi:10.1002/14651858.CD011029.pub2.

60. Johnson JD, Cocker K, Chang E. Infantile colic: Recognition and treatment. *Am Fam Physician.* 2015;92(7):577–582. http://www.ncbi.nlm.nih.gov/pubmed/26447441

61. Williams J, Watkins-Jones R. Dicyclomine: Worrying symptoms associated with its use in some small babies. *Br Med J (Clin Res Ed).* 1984;288(6421):901. http://www.ncbi.nlm.nih.gov/pubmed/6423135

62. Pace CA. Infantile colic: What to know for the primary care setting. *Clin Pediatr (Phila).* 2017;56(7):616–618. doi:10.1177/0009922816664062.

63. Sarasu JM, Narang M, Shah D. Infantile colic: An update. *Indian Pediatr.* 2018;55(11):979–987. http://www.ncbi.nlm.nih.gov/pubmed/29941700

64. Paruthi S, Brooks LJ, D'Ambrosio C, et al. Recommended amount of sleep for pediatric populations: A consensus statement of the American Academy of Sleep Medicine. *J Clin Sleep Med.* 2016;12(6):785–786. doi:10.5664/jcsm.5866.

65. Paruthi S, Brooks LJ, D'Ambrosio C, et al. Recommended amount of sleep for pediatric populations. *Pediatrics.* 2016;138(2):e20161601. doi:10.1542/peds.2016-1601.

66. Owens JA, Moore M. Insomnia in infants and young children. *Pediatr Ann.* 2017;46(9):e321–e326. doi:10.3928/19382359-20170816-02.

67. Morgenthaler TI, Owens J, Alessi C, et al. Practice parameters for behavioral treatment of bedtime problems and night wakings in infants and young children. *Sleep.* 2006;29(10):1277–1281. http://www.ncbi.nlm.nih.gov/pubmed/17068980

68. American Academy of Sleep Medicine. *International Classification of Sleep Disorders.* 3rd ed. Darien, IL: Author; 2014.

69. Meltzer LJ. Clinical management of behavioral insomnia of childhood: Treatment of bedtime problems and night wakings in young children. *Behav Sleep Med.* 2010;8(3):172–189. doi:10.1080/15402002.2010.487464.

70. Mindell JA, Li AM, Sadeh A, Kwon R, Goh DYT. Bedtime routines for young children: A dose-dependent association with sleep outcomes. *Sleep.* 2015;38(5):717–722. doi:10.5665/sleep.4662.

71. Honaker SM, Meltzer LJ. Bedtime problems and night wakings in young children: An update of the evidence. *Paediatr Respir Rev.* 2014;15(4):333–339. doi:10.1016/j.prrv.2014.04.011.

72. Owens JA, Moturi S. Pharmacologic treatment of pediatric insomnia. *Child Adolesc Psychiatr Clin N Am.* 2009;18(4):1001–1016. doi:10.1016/j.chc.2009.04.009.

73. Mindell JA, Kuhn B, Lewin DS, Meltzer LJ, Sadeh A, American Academy of Sleep Medicine. Behavioral treatment of bedtime problems and night wakings in infants and young children. *Sleep.* 2006;29(10):1263–1276. http://www.ncbi.nlm.nih.gov/pubmed/17068979

74. Meltzer LJ, Mindell JA. Systematic review and meta-analysis of behavioral interventions for pediatric insomnia. *J Pediatr Psychol.* 2014;39(8):932–948. doi:10.1093/jpepsy/jsu041.

75. Bayne AP, Skoog SJ. Nocturnal enuresis: An approach to assessment and treatment. *Pediatr Rev.* 2014;35(8):327–335. doi:10.1542/pir.35-8-327.

76. Robson WLM, Leung AKC, Van Howe R. Primary and secondary nocturnal enuresis: Similarities in presentation. *Pediatrics.* 2005;115(4):956–959. doi:10.1542/peds.2004-1402.

77. Nevéus T. Pathogenesis of enuresis: Towards a new understanding. *Int J Urol.* 2017;24(3):174–182. doi:10.1111/iju.13310.

78. Haid B, Tekgül S. Primary and secondary enuresis: Pathophysiology, diagnosis, and treatment. *Eur Urol Focus.* 2017;3(2–3):198–206. doi:10.1016/j.euf.2017.08.010.

79. Vande Walle J, Rittig S, Bauer S, Eggert P, Marschall-Kehrel D, Tekgul S. Practical consensus guidelines for the management of enuresis. *Eur J Pediatr.* 2012;171(6):971–983. doi:10.1007/s00431-012-1687-7.

80. Robson WLM. Evaluation and management of enuresis. *N Engl J Med.* 2009;360(14):1429–1436. doi:10.1056/NEJMcp0808009.

81. Glazener CM, Evans JH. Desmopressin for nocturnal enuresis in children. *Cochrane Database Syst Rev.* 2002;(3):CD002112. doi:10.1002/14651858.CD002112.

82. Neveus T, Eggert P, Evans J, et al. Evaluation of and treatment for monosymptomatic enuresis: A standardization document from the international Children's Continence Society. *J Urol.* 2010;183(2):441–447. doi:10.1016/j.juro.2009.10.043.

83. Glazener CMA, Evans JHC, Cheuk DKL. Complementary and miscellaneous interventions for nocturnal enuresis in children. *Cochrane Database Syst Rev.* 2005;(2):CD005230. doi:10.1002/14651858.CD005230.

84. Kovachy B, O'Hara R, Hawkins N, et al. Sleep disturbance in pediatric PTSD: Current findings and future directions. *J Clin Sleep Med.* 2013;9(5):501–510. doi:10.5664/jcsm.2678.

85. Keeshin BR, Ding Q, Presson AP, Berkowitz SJ, Strawn JR. Use of prazosin for pediatric PTSD-associated nightmares and sleep disturbances: A retrospective chart review. *Neurol Ther.* 2017;6(2):247–257. doi:10.1007/s40120-017-0078-4.

86. Nevsimalova S, Prihodova I, Kemlink D, Lin L, Mignot E. REM behavior disorder (RBD) can be one of the first symptoms of childhood narcolepsy. *Sleep Med.* 2007;8(7-8):784–786. doi:10.1016/j.sleep.2006.11.018.

87. Lloyd R, Tippmann-Peikert M, Slocumb N, Kotagal S. Characteristics of REM sleep behavior disorder in childhood. *J Clin Sleep Med.* 2012;8(2):127–131. doi:10.5664/jcsm.1760.

88. Kotagal S. Rapid eye movement sleep behavior disorder during childhood. *Sleep Med Clin.* 2015;10(2):163–167. doi:10.1016/j.jsmc.2015.02.004.

89. Trajanovic NN, Voloh I, Shapiro CM, Sandor P. REM sleep behaviour disorder in a child with Tourette's syndrome. *Can J Neurol Sci.* 2004;31(4):572–575. http://www.ncbi.nlm.nih.gov/pubmed/15595270

90. Munzer T, Felt B. The role of iron in pediatric restless legs syndrome and periodic limb movements in sleep. *Semin Neurol.* 2017;37(4):439–445. doi:10.1055/s-0037-1605342.

91. Allen RP, Picchietti DL, Garcia-Borreguero D, et al. Restless legs syndrome/Willis-Ekbom disease diagnostic criteria: Updated International Restless Legs Syndrome Study Group (IRLSSG) consensus criteria: History, rationale, description, and significance. *Sleep Med.* 2014;15(8):860–873. doi:10.1016/j.sleep.2014.03.025.

92. Amos LB, Grekowicz ML, Kuhn EM, et al. Treatment of pediatric restless legs syndrome. *Clin Pediatr (Phila).* 2014;53(4):331–336. doi:10.1177/0009922813507997.

93. Allen RP, Picchietti DL, Auerbach M, Cho YW, Connor JR, Earley CJ, Garcia-Borreguero D, Kotagal S, Manconi M, Ondo W, Ulfberg J, Winkelman JW; International Restless Legs Syndrome Study Group (IRLSSG). Evidence-based and consensus clinical practice guidelines for the iron treatment of restless legs syndrome/Willis-Ekbom disease in adults and children: an IRLSSG task force report. *Sleep Med.* 2018 Jan;41:27–44. doi:10.1016/j.sleep.2017.11.1126. Epub 2017 Nov 24. PMID: 29425576.

94. Rulong G, Dye T, Simakajornboon N. Pharmacological management of restless legs syndrome and periodic limb movement disorder in children. *Pediatr Drugs.* 2018;20(1):9–17. doi:10.1007/s40272-017-0262-0.

95. Gwyther ARM, Walters AS, Hill CM. Rhythmic movement disorder in childhood: An integrative review. *Sleep Med Rev.* 2017;35:62–75. doi:10.1016/j.smrv.2016.08.003.

96. Berry RB, Brooks R, Gamaldo Charlene E, et al., for the AASM. *The AASM Manual for the scoring of sleep and associated events: Rules, terminology and technical specifications.* Version 2. Darien, IL: American Academy of Sleep Medicine; 2017.

97. Kirk V, Baughn J, D'Andrea L, et al. American Academy of Sleep Medicine position paper for the use of a home sleep apnea test for the diagnosis of OSA in children. *J Clin Sleep Med.* August 2017. http://www.ncbi.nlm.nih.gov/pubmed/28877820

98. Konstantinopoulou S, Gallagher P, Elden L, et al. Complications of adenotonsillectomy for obstructive sleep apnea in school-aged children. *Int J Pediatr Otorhinolaryngol.* 2015;79(2):240–245. doi:10.1016/j.ijporl.2014.12.018.

99. Bhattacharjee R, Kheirandish-Gozal L, Spruyt K, et al. Adenotonsillectomy outcomes in treatment of obstructive sleep apnea in children: A multicenter retrospective study. *Am J Respir Crit Care Med.* 2010;182(5):676–683. doi:10.1164/rccm.200912-1930OC.

100. Chan CCK, Au CT, Lam HS, Lee DLY, Wing YK, Li AM. Intranasal corticosteroids for mild childhood obstructive sleep apnea: A randomized, placebo-controlled study. *Sleep Med.* 2015;16(3):358–363. doi:10.1016/j.sleep.2014.10.015.

101. Goldbart AD, Greenberg-Dotan S, Tal A. Montelukast for children with obstructive sleep apnea: A double-blind, placebo-controlled study. *Pediatrics.* 2012;130(3):e575–80. doi:10.1542/peds.2012-0310.

102. Kheirandish-Gozal L, Bandla HPR, Gozal D. Montelukast for children with obstructive sleep apnea: Results of a double-blind, randomized, placebo-controlled trial. *Ann Am Thorac Soc.* 2016;13(10):1736–1741. doi:10.1513/AnnalsATS.201606-432OC.

103. Chervin RD, Ellenberg SS, Hou X, et al. Prognosis for spontaneous resolution of OSA in children. *Chest.* 2015;148(5):1204–1213. doi:10.1378/chest.14-2873.

104. Machado-Júnior A-J, Zancanella E, Crespo A-N. Rapid maxillary expansion and obstructive sleep apnea: A review and meta-analysis. *Med Oral Patol Oral Cir Bucal.* 2016;21(4):e465–469. http://www.ncbi.nlm.nih.gov/pubmed/27031063

105. Pirelli P, Saponara M, Guilleminault C. Rapid maxillary expansion (RME) for pediatric obstructive sleep apnea: A 12-year follow-up. *Sleep Med.* 2015;16(8):933–935. doi:10.1016/j.sleep.2015.04.012.

106. Mihai R, Vandeleur M, Pecoraro S, Davey MJ, Nixon GM. Autotitrating CPAP as a tool for CPAP initiation for children. *J Clin Sleep Med.* 2017;13(5):713–719. doi:10.5664/jcsm.6590.

107. Marcus CL, Rosen G, Ward SLD, et al. Adherence to and effectiveness of positive airway pressure therapy in children with obstructive sleep apnea. *Pediatrics.* 2006;117(3):e442–51. doi:10.1542/peds.2005-1634.

108. Hawkins SMM, Jensen EL, Simon SL, Friedman NR. Correlates of pediatric CPAP adherence. *J Clin Sleep Med.* 2016;12(6):879–884. doi:10.5664/jcsm.5892.

109. DiFeo N, Meltzer LJ, Beck SE, et al. Predictors of positive airway pressure therapy adherence in children: A prospective study. *J Clin Sleep Med.* 2012;8(3):279–286. doi:10.5664/jcsm.1914.

110. Prashad PS, Marcus CL, Maggs J, et al. Investigating reasons for CPAP adherence in adolescents: A qualitative approach. *J Clin Sleep Med.* 2013;9(12):1303–1313. doi:10.5664/jcsm.3276.

111. Xanthopoulos MS, Kim JY, Blechner M, et al. Self-efficacy and short-term adherence to continuous positive airway pressure treatment in children. *Sleep.* 2017;40(7). doi:10.1093/sleep/zsx096.

112. Hawkins S, Huston S, Campbell K, Halbower A. High-flow, heated, humidified air via nasal cannula treats CPAP-intolerant children with obstructive sleep apnea. *J Clin Sleep Med.* 2017;13(8):981–989. doi:10.5664/jcsm.6700.

113. Owens J. Insufficient sleep in adolescents and young adults: An update on causes and consequences. *Pediatrics.* 2014;134(3):e921–32. doi:10.1542/peds.2014-1696.

114. Sivertsen B, Pallesen S, Stormark KM, Bøe T, Lundervold AJ, Hysing M. Delayed sleep phase syndrome in adolescents: Prevalence and correlates in a large population based study. *BMC Public Health.* 2013;13(1):1163. doi:10.1186/1471-2458-13-1163.

115. Auger RR, Burgess HJ, Emens JS, Deriy L V, Thomas SM, Sharkey KM. Clinical practice guideline for the treatment of intrinsic circadian rhythm sleep-wake disorders: Advanced sleep-wake phase disorder (ASWPD), delayed sleep-wake phase disorder (DSWPD), non-24-hour sleep-wake rhythm disorder (N24SWD), and irregular sleep-wake rhythm disorder (ISWRD). An Update for 2015: An American Academy of Sleep Medicine clinical practice guideline. *J Clin Sleep Med.* 2015;11(10):1199–1236. doi:10.5664/jcsm.5100.

116. Riemann D, Baglioni C, Bassetti C, et al. European guideline for the diagnosis and treatment of insomnia. *J Sleep Res.* 2017;26(6):675–700. doi:10.1111/jsr.12594.

117. Blake MJ, Sheeber LB, Youssef GJ, Raniti MB, Allen NB. Systematic review and meta-analysis of adolescent cognitive-behavioral sleep interventions. *Clin Child Fam Psychol Rev.* 2017;20(3):227–249. doi:10.1007/s10567-017-0234-5.

118. de Zambotti M, Goldstone A, Colrain IM, Baker FC. Insomnia disorder in adolescence: Diagnosis, impact, and treatment. *Sleep Med Rev.* 2018;39:12–24. doi:10.1016/j.smrv.2017.06.009.

119. Zhou ES, Gardiner P, Bertisch SM. Integrative medicine for insomnia. *Med Clin North Am.* 2017;101(5):865–879. doi:10.1016/j.mcna.2017.04.005.

120. Cheuk DK, Yeung W-F, Chung K, Wong V. Acupuncture for insomnia. *Cochrane Database Syst Rev.* September 2012. doi:10.1002/14651858.CD005472.pub3. doi:10.1183/13993003.01090-2016.

121. Owens JA, Babcock D, Blumer J, Chervin R, Ferber R, Goetting M, Glaze D, Ivanenko A, Mindell J, Rappley M, Rosen C, Sheldon S. The use of pharmacotherapy in the treatment of pediatric insomnia in primary care: rational approaches. A consensus meeting summary. *J Clin Sleep Med.* 2005 Jan 15;1(1):49–59. PMID: 17561616.

122. Merdad RA, Akil H, Wali SO. Sleepiness in Adolescents. *Sleep Med Clin.* 2017 Sep;12(3):415–428. doi:10.1016/j.jsmc.2017.03.014. Epub 2017 Jun 9. PMID: 28778239.

123. Owens JA, Babcock D, Weiss M. Evaluation and Treatment of Children and Adolescents With Excessive Daytime Sleepiness. *Clin Pediatr (Phila).* 2020 May;59(4–5):340–351. doi:10.1177/0009922820903434. Epub 2020 Mar 13. PMID: 32167377; PMCID: PMC7160754.

124. Kotagal S. Treatment of narcolepsy and other organic hypersomnias in children. *Paediatr Respir Rev.* 2018 Jan;25:19–24. doi:10.1016/j.prrv.2017.06.012. Epub 2017 Jun 20. PMID: 28735675.

125. Polanczyk G, de Lima MS, Horta BL, Biederman J, Rohde LA. The worldwide prevalence of ADHD: a systematic review and metaregression analysis. *Am J Psychiatry.* 2007 Jun;164(6):942–948. doi:10.1176/ajp.2007.164.6.942. PMID: 17541055.

126. Hvolby A. Associations of sleep disturbance with ADHD: implications for treatment. *Atten Defic Hyperact Disord.* 2015 Mar;7(1):1–18. doi:10.1007/s12402-014-0151-0. Epub 2014 Aug 17. PMID: 25127644; PMCID: PMC4340974.

127. Wolraich ML, Hagan JF Jr, Allan C, Chan E, Davison D, Earls M, Evans SW, Flinn SK, Froehlich T, Frost J, Holbrook JR, Lehmann CU, Lessin HR, Okechukwu K, Pierce KL, Winner JD, Zurhellen W; Subcommittee on children and adolescents with attention-Deficit/Hyperactive disorder. Clinical Practice Guideline for the Diagnosis, Evaluation, and Treatment of Attention-Deficit/Hyperactivity Disorder in Children and Adolescents. *Pediatrics.* 2019 Oct;144(4):e20192528. doi: 10.1542/peds.2019-2528. Erratum in: Pediatrics. 2020 Mar;145(3): PMID: 31570648; PMCID: PMC7067282.

128. Graham J, Banaschewski T, Buitelaar J, Coghill D, Danckaerts M, Dittmann RW, Döpfner M, Hamilton R, Hollis C, Holtmann M, Hulpke-Wette M, Lecendreux M, Rosenthal E, Rothenberger A, Santosh P, Sergeant J, Simonoff E, Sonuga-Barke E, Wong IC, Zuddas A, Steinhausen HC, Taylor E; European Guidelines Group. European guidelines on managing adverse effects of medication for ADHD. *Eur Child Adolesc Psychiatry.* 2011 Jan;20(1):17–37. doi: 10.1007/s00787-010-0140-6. Epub 2010 Nov 3. PMID: 21042924; PMCID: PMC3012210.

129. Cortese S, Holtmann M, Banaschewski T, Buitelaar J, Coghill D, Danckaerts M, Dittmann RW, Graham J, Taylor E, Sergeant J; European ADHD Guidelines Group. Practitioner review: current best practice in the management of adverse events during treatment with ADHD medications in children and adolescents. *J Child Psychol Psychiatry.* 2013 Mar;54(3):227–246. doi: 10.1111/jcpp.12036. Epub 2013 Jan 7. PMID: 23294014.

130. Yoon SY, Jain U, Shapiro C. Sleep in attention-deficit/hyperactivity disorder in children and adults: past, present, and future. *Sleep Med Rev.* 2012 Aug;16(4):371–388. doi:10.1016/j.smrv.2011.07.001. Epub 2011 Oct 26. PMID: 22033171.

131. Weiss MD, Wasdell MB, Bomben MM, Rea KJ, Freeman RD. Sleep hygiene and melatonin treatment for children and adolescents with ADHD and initial insomnia. *J Am Acad Child Adolesc Psychiatry.* 2006 May;45(5):512–519. PMID: 16670647.

132. Hvolby A, Bilenberg N. Use of Ball Blanket in attention-deficit/hyperactivity disorder sleeping problems. *Nord J Psychiatry.* 2011 Apr;65(2):89–94. doi: 10.3109/08039488.2010.501868. Epub 2010 Jul 22. PMID: 20662681.

133. Efron D, Lycett K, Sciberras E. Use of sleep medication in children with ADHD. *Sleep Med.* 2014 Apr;15(4):472–475. doi:10.1016/j.sleep.2013.10.018. Epub 2014 Feb 7. PMID: 24684977.

134. Cortese S, Konofal E, Lecendreux M, Arnulf I, Mouren MC, Darra F, Dalla Bernardina B. Restless legs syndrome and attention-deficit/hyperactivity disorder: a review of the literature. Sleep. 2005 Aug 1;28(8):1007–1013.

135. Williams Buckley A, Hirtz D, Oskoui M, Armstrong MJ, Batra A, Bridgemohan C, Coury D, Dawson G, Donley D, Findling RL, Gaughan T, Gloss D, Gronseth G, Kessler R, Merillat S, Michelson D, Owens J, Pringsheim T, Sikich L, Stahmer A, Thurm A, Tuchman R, Warren Z, Wetherby A, Wiznitzer M, Ashwal S. Practice guideline: Treatment for insomnia and disrupted sleep behavior in children and adolescents with autism spectrum disorder: Report of the Guideline Development, Dissemination, and Implementation Subcommittee of the American Academy of Neurology. *Neurology.* 2020 Mar 3;94(9):392–404. doi: 10.1212/WNL.0000000000009033. Epub 2020 Feb 12. PMID: 32051244; PMCID: PMC7238942.

136. Reynolds AM, Malow BA. Sleep and autism spectrum disorders. *Pediatr Clin North Am.* 2011 Jun;58(3):685–698. doi:10.1016/j.pcl.2011.03.009. PMID: 21600349.

137. Souders MC, Zavodny S, Eriksen W, Sinko R, Connell J, Kerns C, Schaaf R, Pinto-Martin J. Sleep in Children with Autism Spectrum Disorder. *Curr Psychiatry*

Rep. 2017 Jun;19(6):34. doi:10.1007/s11920-017-0782-x. PMID: 28502070; PMCID: PMC5846201.

138. Malow BA, Byars K, Johnson K, Weiss S, Bernal P, Goldman SE, Panzer R, Coury DL, Glaze DG; Sleep Committee of the Autism Treatment Network. A practice pathway for the identification, evaluation, and management of insomnia in children and adolescents with autism spectrum disorders. *Pediatrics.* 2012 Nov;130 Suppl 2:S106–S124. doi: 10.1542/peds.2012-0900I. PMID: 23118242.093/sleep/28.8.1007. PMID: 16218085.

139. Blackmer AB, Feinstein JA. Management of Sleep Disorders in Children With Neurodevelopmental Disorders: A Review. *Pharmacotherapy,* 2016;36:84–98. https://doi.org/10.1002/phar.1686

140. Kaditis AG, Alonso Alvarez ML, Boudewyns A, Alexopoulos EI, Ersu R, Joosten K, Larramona H, Miano S, Narang I, Trang H, Tsaoussoglou M, Vandenbussche N, Villa MP, Van Waardenburg D, Weber S, Verhulst S. Obstructive sleep disordered breathing in 2- to 18-year-old children: diagnosis and management. *Eur Respir J.* 2016 Jan;47(1):69–94. doi: 10.1183/13993003.00385-2015. Epub 2015 Nov 5. PMID: 26541535.

141. Nehme Bsc J, Laberge R, Pothos M, et al. Treatment and persistence/recurrence of sleep-disordered breathing in children with Down syndrome. *Pediatr Pulmonol.* 2019;54:1291–1296. doi:10.1002/ppul.24380

142. Rosen D. Severe hypothyroidism presenting as obstructive sleep apnea. *Clin Pediatr (Phila).* 2010;49(4):381–383. doi:10.1177/0009922809351093

143. Hawkins S, Huston S, Campbell K, Halbower A. High-Flow, Heated, Humidified Air Via Nasal Cannula Treats CPAP-Intolerant Children With Obstructive Sleep Apnea. *J Clin Sleep Med.* 2017 Aug 15;13(8):981–989. doi: 10.5664/jcsm.6700. PMID: 28728621; PMCID: PMC5529135.

144. Gillett ES, Perez IA. Disorders of Sleep and Ventilatory Control in Prader-Willi Syndrome. *Diseases.* 2016 Jul 8;4(3):23. doi:10.3390/diseases4030023. PMID: 28933403; PMCID: PMC5456282.

145. Duis J, van Wattum PJ, Scheimann A, Salehi P, Brokamp E, Fairbrother L, Childers A, Shelton AR, Bingham NC, Shoemaker AH, Miller JL. A multidisciplinary approach to the clinical management of Prader-Willi syndrome. *Mol Genet Genomic Med.* 2019 Mar;7(3):e514. doi: 10.1002/mgg3.514. Epub 2019 Jan 29. PMID: 30697974; PMCID: PMC6418440.

146. McCandless SE; Committee on Genetics. Clinical report—health supervision for children with Prader-Willi syndrome. *Pediatrics.* 2011 Jan;127(1):195–204. doi: 10.1542/peds.2010-2820. Epub 2010 Dec 27. PMID: 21187304.

147. Deal CL, Tony M, Höybye C, Allen DB, Tauber M, Christiansen JS; 2011 Growth Hormone in Prader-Willi Syndrome Clinical Care Guidelines Workshop Participants. GrowthHormone Research Society workshop summary: consensus guidelines for recombinant human growth hormone therapy in Prader-Willi syndrome. *J Clin Endocrinol Metab.* 2013 Jun;98(6):E1072–87. doi:10.1210/jc.2012-3888. Epub 2013 Mar 29. PMID: 23543664; PMCID: PMC3789886.

36

Technology and Sleep: Wearable Sleep Devices, Apps, and Consumer Products

DIANA GRIGSBY-TOUSSAINT, KAUSTUBH VIJAY PARAB, AND
JONG CHEOL SHIN

Introduction

The proliferation of various forms of technology has made defining, measuring, and evaluating sleep both exciting and daunting at the same time. In this chapter, we summarize both old and new technology used to study sleep, and we highlight its clinical implications.

WHITE NOISE MACHINES

White noise machines are used as nonpharmacological interventions for sleep. They are based on white noise principles that aid sensory integration,[1] and the sound is delivered in the range of human hearing (i.e., 20–20,000 Hz). White noise is hypothesized to work through recurrent exposure, which is thought to lead to sleep as a habitual response.

Intrauterine sounds such as maternal blood flow are considered natural sources of white noise. As such, white noise machines have been used quite extensively to calm babies.[2-5] A recent systematic review[1] focusing on sleep problems among children (0–18 years) found that white noise exposure resulted in favorable sleep outcomes across several studies using various designs. Interestingly, exposure to white noise seems to settle babies after a feed[6] and may be an effective intervention against gas pain.[7] Compared to swinging, which stimulates endorphin secretion, white noise has been found to be more effective for decreasing daily crying duration among colicky babies.[8]

Among healthy adults, exposure to white noise has not demonstrated consistent benefits for sleep architecture.[8-10] While some studies have found that exposure to white noise does not influence total sleep time (TST),[8] others have found a reduction in wake after sleep onset (WASO).[9] Consequently, additional studies on white noise machines are needed to fully evaluate their impact on night arousals and sleep stages, particularly among adults. Among children, specifically babies, white noise machines seem to be an effective nonpharmacological intervention for sleep.

BLUE LIGHT–BLOCKING GLASSES (BLUE BLOCKERS)

Blue blocker lenses, which are yellow-tinged lenses that filter short-wavelength blue light, have received increased attention for attenuating the impact of artificial light exposure on sleep.[11,12] For example, Ostrin et al. demonstrated that adults who wore blue blockers for approximately 4 hours before bedtime for 2 weeks had improved melatonin levels and sleep duration.[12] Van der Lely et al. found that the use of a blue blocker lens lessened the suppression of melatonin by light-emitting diode (LED) computer screens and increased self-reported sleepiness suppressed, in comparison to clear lens users, on the Karolinska Sleepiness Scale (KSS).[11]

Currently, blue blocker technology also is being ~~been~~ tried in intraocular lenses as well as eyeglasses.[13] Blue blocker lenses in eyeglasses are ubiquitously used to reduce eye strain due to long-term exposure to computer screens—so-called *computer vision syndrome*,[14] which is a group of vision-related problems arising from the increasing use of electronic devices. Although blue blockers are encouraged for full-time wear in eyeglasses, their long-term effects on melatonin, circadian patterns, and eye growth in children have not been clarified. However, there have been studies assessing the association between blue-blocking intraocular lenses and sleep quality, melatonin, and mood.[15,16] In subjects receiving neutral versus blue-blocking intraocular lenses, at 3 weeks after surgery, no difference was found in sleep quality and melatonin levels.[17] On the other hand, after 1 year, those receiving blue blocker intraocular lenses had a 50% lower peak in melatonin levels compared to those receiving neutral intraocular lenses.[16] Since the intraocular lenses are fixed surgically inside the eye, this effect can be justified by the fact that the blue light was blocked both during night and day. When subjective sleep quality was assessed in other studies 6 months after implantation of clear, blue-blocking, or UV-blocking intraocular lenses, no adverse impact was found.

A major practical implication of blue blockers is their suggested use for night shift workers to prevent the resynchronization effect of morning sunlight on the way back home.[18,19] In terms of visual comfort, research participants reported that the environment appeared significantly darker (n = 13; F(1,12) = 17.70; p = .001) although less glaring (F(1,12) = 17.66; p = .001) through blue blockers.[11] Importantly, blue blockers have been shown to impair chromatic perception.[20] Thus, distinguishing traffic signals could be difficult while wearing blue blockers, and thus wear might not be recommended while driving. Notwithstanding, blue blocker use in the evening during LED bright light exposure inside the home could be recommended for better sleep.

SLEEP AND TEMPERATURE

Temperature is one of the most significant environmental determinants of both falling asleep and staying asleep. Body temperature usually follows a 24-hour clock or circadian rhythm, which is associated with the human wake–sleep cycle.[21,22] Several studies have shown that skin and body temperature are high around sleep onset but low during sleep and periods right before wakefulness.[21,23] This occurs because blood vessels in the skin dilate to expedite heat loss when preparing for sleep, resulting in a reduction of core body temperature. The lowered body temperature is maintained during sleep but increases before one wakes up.

Ambient temperature is able to interrupt regular sleep patterns by altering circadian thermoregulation.[24] Obradovich et al. examined the relationship between anomalous nighttime temperature and sleep quality in the US population.[25] The research team linked data from 765,000 survey respondents and nighttime temperature data from 2002 to 2011, and then predicted the future incidence of insufficient sleep from nighttime heat in 2050 and 2099 while accounting for seasonal effects. Findings from the study showed anomalous nighttime temperature significantly increased insufficient sleep in all age groups, especially among the elderly, low-income groups, and during the summer months. Specifically, a 1°C warming in nighttime temperatures resulted in 0.28 days of insufficient sleep per month (β = 0.028, p = 0.014).[25] The change in ambient temperature also affects skin temperature and is consequently related to sleep propensity.[26,27] Raymann et al. found that distal skin warming is helpful to reduce the difference between core body and distal temperatures and also contributes to shorter sleep latency and better sleep quality.[28] For example, sleep onset latency (SOL), which is the length of time to transition from full wakefulness to sleep, was shortened by a 1°C warming of proximal (0.23 minutes) and distal (0.40 minutes) skin temperatures.[26,27] On the other hand, a sleep environment that provides a reduced core temperature (i.e., neck and back cooling system) results in better sleep efficiency (11.12%), shorter SOL (17.28 minutes) and WASO (36.57 minutes), and a smaller number of awakenings (7.62).[29]

Since thermoregulation influences both sleep quality and quantity, controlling body temperature is considered one way to improve sleep. Richardson et al.

suggest avoiding moderate- to high-intensity evening exercise[30] as it may delay core body temperature rhythms and increase the risk of delayed sleep–wake phase disorder (DSWPD), ultimately increasing difficulty of sleep onset. Reducing core body temperature also promotes better sleep. Ebb, which is a forehead cooling device, was developed to reduce metabolic activity in the frontal cortex of the brain during sleep. According to a randomized clinical trial of 2 days of treatment, Ebb used in adults with insomnia shortened light sleep (stage 1 non–rapid eye movement [NREM] sleep latency, 12.4 minutes and stage 2 NREM sleep latency, 11.5 minutes) compared to a control group.[31] Moreover, another study showed that veterans with chronic insomnia disorder and comorbid medical and psychiatric conditions experienced shortened SOL (29.9 minutes) and WASO (19.7 minutes) and increased sleep quality score after 4 weeks of treatment with Ebb.[32]

Notwithstanding these benefits of distal skin temperature regulation, the evidence remains equivocal.[23] Raymann et al. found warm (hyperthermic) foot baths before bedtime were excellent to prevent heat dissipation and improve sleep.[28] In contrast, recent studies have argued that warm foot baths before bedtime did not significantly reduce sleep latency.[33,34] Moreover, Liao et al. have indicated that some studies examining temperature control and sleep did not adequately account for the differences in thermoregulation in individuals with good compared to poor sleep. Therefore, additional studies are needed to further explore the role of distal skin thermoregulation in sleep outcomes.

SENSORY INTEGRATION AND WEIGHTED BLANKETS

Weighted blankets are a relatively new therapeutic tool in the field of occupational therapy and sleep clinics. Muller et al. evaluated the safety and effectiveness of weighted blankets with 32 adults who constituted a convenience sample.[35] Results showed that all vital sign metrics such as blood pressure, pulse rate, and pulse oximetry supported the evidence of weighted blanket safety, and those using weighted blankets also showed better sleep effectiveness in terms of lower electrodermal activity (EDA) and lower anxiety. The blankets were preferred by users as a calming modality.[35] Weighted blankets have been thought to improve the quality of sleep in children, especially children with autism spectrum disorder (ASD), sensory overresponsivity, and sleep disorders.[36,37] Specifically, several case studies have shown that weighted blankets support better sleep quality by aiding sensory integration and easing chronic pain. Some researchers, however, have cast doubt on the evidence of the positive influences of the weighted blanket on sleep.[38] One recent randomized controlled trial with 67 participants indicated no evidence to support the effectiveness of weighted blankets to improve sleep for children with ASD.[39] Additional studies are needed to fully understand the impact of weighted blankets on sleep across various demographic groups.

SLEEP TRACKERS

Sleep trackers are very popular, and the market is growing fast. A report by Future Market Insights states that the size of the wearable sleep tracker market was approximately US$1,388.3 million in 2017 and is anticipated to reach US$3,072 million by the end of 2028.[40] According to the Worldwide Quarterly Wearable Device Tracker by International Data Corporation (IDC), by market share of wearable trackers from first-quarter sales in 2015, the top five vendors were Apple (16.1%), Xiaomi (14.8%), Fitbit (8.7%), Huawei (5.2%), and Garmin (5%).[41] Sleep trackers are actively developing in terms of functions and features. For example, the most recent Fitbit provides specific information not only about sleep duration but also about quantifiable sleep stages. Also, the auto-sleep detection function on trackers is becoming more accurate. Sleep trackers are available as headbands, wristbands, neckbands, or rings. The Oura ring, which is the most recently developed ring sleep tracker, consists of a three-axis accelerometer and skin temperature sensors.[42] These sensors help to measure physiological signals such as movement during sleep, heart rate, and patterns of heartbeat and then estimate sleep quantity and sleep stages.

Because sleep trackers are personal electronic devices for sleep monitoring, recording, and evaluation they can be used to objectively, accurately, and reliably measure sleep, compared to traditional sleep diaries that are based on memory recall. Although such trackers were initially used primarily for physical activity research,[43,44] they have been developed so that consumers and healthcare providers can monitor and measure sleep. Tracking sleep can help identify what actually happens during sleep. For example, information about deep sleep versus light sleep via motion detection can give feedback on how to address potential issues and risks related to sleep problems. Eventually, sleep experts may use sleep trackers to provide timely sleep counseling via accurate sleep information and intervene by providing personalized suggestions for individuals to improve their sleep quality.

Sleep trackers operate using various embedded sensors. According to a review in 2017, sleep trackers can be either on the body (wearable) or near the body (nearable).[44] Most trackers use eight types of sensors, typically located on two parts of the body. Wearable sleep trackers include sensors for accelerometry, a heart rate (HR) monitor, an electroencephalogram (EEG), galvanic skin response (GSR), an electrocardiogram (ECG), and respiratory rate (RR) sensors (airflow measurement). Nearable sleep trackers include a ballistocardiogram (BCG), RR sensors, and movement/motion sensors. All sensors monitor and record physiological changes during sleep in real time.

This combination of hardware and software lays the foundation to facilitate the gathering of Big Data that will allow the optimization of personalized sleep solutions. To optimize solutions, of course, sensors in the device must be calibrated to obtain accurate sleep measurements. Polysomnography (PSG), which uses EEG, ECG, and respiration sensors, is considered the gold standard sleep measurement tool in the field of sleep research. Because PSG provides a high accuracy of sleep measurements that can determine sleep stages, PSG has been used to calibrate the reliability and validity of sleep trackers in several studies. Zambotti et al. compared sleep outcomes in 32 healthy adolescents using Fitbit, a wearable sleep tracker with accelerometer and HR monitor, to PSG and ECG.[45] Fitbit provided TST, SOL, WASO, and sleep efficiency in addition to a sleep score calculated by summing scores for sleep duration, sleep quality, and restoration. In terms of sleep detection, accelerometers showed high accuracy (90.9 ±4.7%; 95% confidence interval [CI]: 89.1, 92.7%), high sensitivity (97.1 ±2.3%; 95% CI: 96.2, 97.9%), and high predictive value (92.9 ±4.7%; 95% CI: 91.1, 94.6) with PSG. Average HR in the tracker (59.3 ±7.5 bpm) was significantly different from the ECG HR (60.2 ±7.6 bpm; p <0.001), but the difference of 0.88 bpm (±0.43 bpm) may be negligible from a clinical perspective. Tal et al. collected 63 participants' sleep records using EarlySense, a nearable sleep tracker, to compare PSG and tracker parameters (i.e., HR, RR, and body movement).[46] Compared with PSG, the measurement accuracy of HR and RR was 96.1% and 93.3%, respectively, and the sleep detection sensitivity, specificity, and accuracy of the sleep tracker were 92.5%, 80.4%, and 90.5%, respectively. Both wearable and nearable sleep trackers showed good capability to detect sleep stages and measure sleep patterns. Fitbit has validated their sleep stages with PSG data and defines light sleep as stages 1 and 2, while deep sleep is defined as stage 3.[45] Consequently, improved device validity and reliability will improve the relevance of these devices for clinical applications as well. The Oura ring has also been calibrated and validated with PSG.[47] Results of the validation study showed that the Oura ring produced results similar to PSG regarding TST, SOL, and WASO, and also had high sensitivity (96%) for sleep detection. However, it had lower sensitivity for sleep stage detection (65% for light sleep, 51% for deep sleep, and 61% for REM sleep), a 20-minute underestimation of deep sleep, and an 18-minute overestimation of REM sleep.

SLEEP APPLICATIONS (APPS)

A report by Research2Guidance (R2G) indicated that approximately $5.4 billion was invested globally into digital health start-ups in 2016, with continued growth projections based on estimates of market potential.[48] Health apps are one of the major areas of advancement in the digital health area. In addition to more than 84,000 app publishers in the medical and health and fitness market, 325,000 health apps were available in 2017, and 78,000 new health apps were added to Apple App Stores and Google Play Store from 2016 to 2017. This represents a doubling in growth compared to 2015, based on an IMS report (n = 165,169).[49] The sleep app market is also growing significantly, but its growth is relatively slower compared to the growth of the entire health market.

Smartphone applications were developed with various functions to monitor and improve sleep quality. Functions available in current sleep apps include sleep tracking, sleep education, sleep meditation (e.g., lullaby, white noise, light control), and a sleep alarm. With a user-friendly interface and easy use, apps can be used to control external devices such as a smart lightbulbs, smart thermostats, and speakers that enhance the environment for sleep. Regarding the function of sleep tracking, some apps use only an embedded sensor like an accelerometer or self-reported sleep questionnaire, while others use external sleep trackers such as a Fitbit or Oura ring. One of the few studies to examine the effectiveness of sleep apps was conducted by Shin et al., where mobile phone apps used for interventions, sleep disorders, and sleep quality were examined.[50] Findings from the study showed that smartphone apps for interventions typically included functions for tracking, sleep advice for behavioral change, and optimized alarms. All studies in the review indicated that sleep apps improved sleep quality and addressed issues associated with sleep disorders.

Grigsby-Toussaint et al. evaluated commercially available sleep apps to examine the psychological components that can impact sleep behavior.[51] From 330 unique sleep apps available on iOS and Android platforms at the time, a total of 35 apps that were not meditation apps were selected. The results indicated that the most popular apps tend to be well-designed to encourage healthy sleep hygiene. The top three behavioral constructs incorporated were for realistic goal setting ($n = 30$, 86%), time management ($n = 27$, 77%), and self-monitoring ($n = 23$, 66%). Some challenges identified with the use of apps include the constantly changing nature of the availability of apps,[51] as well as high user attrition, high data entry burden, loss of interest, and hidden costs.[52] Therefore, automated or effortless data entry that addresses behavioral change components will be one area of improvement for future sleep app development.

SLEEP AND VIRTUAL REALITY

Virtual reality (VR), defined as a computer-generated three-dimensional replicated environment, permits interactions using various types of equipment, usually a combination of sensors, gloves, and headsets.[53] With recent advances in technology, VR environments have become more immersive, providing stronger sensory and more "real-life" experiences for people.[54] Since well-established VR simulations can repetitively provide a situation that may be hard to confront or duplicate in reality, they can be used to intervene or evaluate the progress of interventions objectively. Despite the prevalence of sleep problems in the general population, however, few sleep studies have utilized VR. Studies that have utilized VR for sleep research have focused on road-crossing tests to assess the adverse effects of sleep disorders[54] or used games as an exercise intervention to reduce stress and improve sleep quality in the elderly.[55] A VR game intervention study involved random assignment of a 30-minute game twice per week for 3 months. The treatment group did improve their sleep score compared to the control group (F = 4.74, p <0.05), suggesting some evidence for future effective sleep interventions using VR.

Of note, the limited use of VR in sleep research may be due to the recent development of commercially available VR devices. VR products such as Kortex[56] or mindZense Sleep[57] have recently become available for sleep management, but there is scant scientific evidence to support their effectiveness using rigorous study designs.

SMART BEDS

Smart beds are rapidly becoming essential components of the new wave of "smart homes." Smart beds have been defined in two ways: (1) as a generic term for new sleep equipment such as a smart mattress, smart pillow, or smart bedframe or (2) to describe innovative technology that optimizes the sleep environment through individual preferences for improving sleep quality and sleep disorders. Two statements support these definitions: "The bed in the master bedroom has special equipment to monitor occupants' sleep patterns and keep track of sleepless nights"[58] and "The unique system can be programmed to remember your preferred sound, smell, light and temperature settings to gently wake up all your senses and give you a good start to every morning."[59] Conceptually, smart beds should address the entire sleep environment, including pillows and blankets, but the majority of smart bed research seems to focus on smart mattresses. And, although some commercial smart beds also include thermostats for temperature control during sleep time, most of the smart bed research focuses on the calibration and validation of the bed's nearable sleep tracker. No clinical studies examining the impact of the smart bed on sleep could be found.[60–62]

PHILIPS SMARTSLEEP DEEP SLEEP HEADBAND

The Philips SmartSleep Deep Sleep Headband is a soft wearable headband designed for 18- to 50-year-olds who do not have trouble with sleep onset but cannot seem to get more than 7 hours of rest. The headband detects stages of slow wave sleep (SWS) by measuring the electrical activity of the brain and intervening with an audio tone that improves the duration and depth of SWS. This generation of the customized audio tone is based on Philips' proprietary advanced sleep analysis algorithms.[63] The SmartSleep device is accompanied by an app that records sleep improvements over a period of time and provides tips for getting the best possible night's sleep. At the Consumer Electronics Show (CES) in 2018, Philips announced the addition to the SmartSleep device of a validated digital analysis tool useful for detecting sleep challenges and solutions.[64] There is an ongoing nonrandomized, unblended, uncontrolled case series study by Philips Respironics to validate the SmartSleep product.[65] The study has a target sample of approximately 50 healthy adults (21–50 years) who self-report shortened sleep due to their lifestyle. The primary outcome measure is the effect of auditory stimulation from the SmartSleep device on short sleep as measured by changes in cumulative or average slow wave activity (CSWA). Secondary outcome measures (e.g., Matrix Reasoning task, Psychomotor Vigilance testing, and a G7-point scale for sleepiness) are also included. Because the results of this ongoing validation study are publicly unavailable, no conclusions can be drawn regarding the SmartSleep device's application to sleep.

Conclusion

Although white noise machines have been well-established as nonpharmacological interventions for sleep, advances in technology have led to the proliferation of other tools that can be used to track and evaluate sleep. For population-based studies that make the use of PSG challenging in community-based settings, sleep apps and trackers hold some promise as tools to measure and assess sleep in addition to serving as a platform by which to educate people about sleep hygiene on a large scale. For the increased evening use of light-emitting devices, particularly among adolescents and young adults, blue blocker glasses may attenuate the impact of artificial light on circadian misalignment. More recent commercial products such as smart beds, deep sleep headbands, and VR games need additional studies to fully assess their impact on sleep outcomes. Notwithstanding, these old and new technologies provide excellent starting points as tools for addressing sleep quality and quantity.

REFERENCES

1. France KG, McLay LK, Hunter JE, France MLS. Empirical research evaluating the effects of non-traditional approaches to enhancing sleep in typical and clinical children and young people. *Sleep Med Rev.* 2018;39:69–81.

2. Standley JM. Music therapy for the neonate. *Newborn Infant Nurs Rev.* 2001;1(4):211–216.

3. Kucukoglu S, Aytekin A, Celebioglu A, Celebi A, Caner I, Maden R. Effect of white noise in relieving vaccination pain in premature infants. *Pain Manag Nurs.* 2016;17(6):392–400.

4. Karakoç A, Türker F. Effects of white noise and holding on pain perception in newborns. *Pain Manag Nurs.* 2014;15(4):864–870.

5. Murooka H, Araki T, Sasaki T, Iwasa Y, Nakamura M, Suda N. Induction of rest and sleep on the neonates by the rhythm of the maternal blood flow. *J Nippon Med Sch.* 1975;42(3):245–247.

6. Spencer JA, Moran DJ, Lee A, Talbert D. White noise and sleep induction. *Arch Dis Child.* 1990;65(1):135–137.

7. Sezici E, Yigit D. Comparison between swinging and playing of white noise among colicky babies: A paired randomised controlled trial. *J Clin Nurs.* 2018;27(3–4):593–600.

8. Stanchina ML, Abu-Hijleh M, Chaudhry BK, Carlisle CC, Millman RP. The influence of white noise on sleep in subjects exposed to ICU noise. *Sleep Med.* 2005;6(5):423–428.

9. Shrivastava D, Jung S, Saadat M, Sirohi R, Crewson K. How to interpret the results of a sleep study. *J Comm Hosp Intern Med Perspect.* 2014;4(5):24983.

10. Ebben MR, Degrazia MQ, Krieger AC. The effect of white noise on individuals complaining of poor quality sleep in a high noise environment in New York City. *Sleep,* 2018;41:A145–A145.

11. Van der Lely S, Frey S, Garbazza C, et al. Blue blocker glasses as a countermeasure for alerting effects of evening light-emitting diode screen exposure in male teenagers. *J Adolesc Heal.* 2015;56(1):113–119.

12. Ostrin LA, Abbott KS, Queener HM. Attenuation of short wavelengths alters sleep and the ip RGC pupil response. *Ophthalmic Physiol Opt.* 2017;37(4):440–450.

13. Davison JA, Patel AS, Cunha JP, Schwiegerling J, Muftuoglu O. Recent studies provide an updated clinical perspective on blue light-filtering IOLs. *Graefe's Arch Clin Exp Ophthalmol.* 2011;249(7):957–968.

14. Ostrin LA. Ocular and systemic melatonin and the influence of light exposure. *Clin Exp Optom.* 2018;102(2), 99–108.

15. Alexander I, Cuthbertson FM, Ratnarajan G, et al. Impact of cataract surgery on sleep in patients receiving either ultraviolet-blocking or blue-filtering intraocular lens implants. *Invest Ophthalmol Vis Sci.* 2014;55(8):4999–5004.

16. Brøndsted AE, Haargaard B, Sander B, Lund-Andersen H, Jennum P, Kessel L. The effect of blue-blocking and neutral intraocular lenses on circadian photoentrainment and sleep one year after cataract surgery. *Acta Ophthalmol.* 2017;95(4):344–351.

17. Brøndsted AE, Sander B, Haargaard B, et al. The effect of cataract surgery on circadian photoentrainment: A randomized trial of blue-blocking versus neutral intraocular lenses. *Ophthalmology.* 2015;122(10):2115–2124.

18. Sasseville A, Benhaberou-Brun D, Fontaine C, Charon M-C, Hebert M. Wearing blue-blockers in the morning could improve sleep of workers on a permanent night schedule: A pilot study. *Chronobiol Int.* 2009;26(5):913–925.

19. Sasseville A, Hébert M. Using blue-green light at night and blue-blockers during the day to improves adaptation to night work: A pilot study. *Prog Neuro-Psychopharmacology Biol Psychiatry.* 2010;34(7):1236–1242.

20. Sasseville A, Martin JS, Houle J, Hébert M. Investigating the contribution of short wavelengths in the alerting effect of bright light. *Physiol Behav.* 2015;151:81–87.

21. Hasselberg MJ, McMahon J, Parker K, Wansing H. The validity, reliability, and utility of the iButton® for measurement of body temperature circadian rhythms in sleep/wake research. *Sleep Med.* 2013;14(1):5–11. doi:10.1016/j.sleep.2010.12.011.

22. Yadlapalli S, Jiang C, Bahle A, Reddy P, Meyhofer E, Shafer OT. Circadian clock neurons constantly monitor environmental temperature to set sleep timing. *Nature.* 2018;555(7694):98–102. doi:10.1038/nature25740.

23. Sarabia JA, Rol MA, Mendiola P, Madrid JA. Circadian rhythm of wrist temperature in normal-living subjects: A candidate of new index of the circadian system. *Physiol Behav.* 2008;95(4):570–580.

24. Okamoto-Mizuno K, Mizuno K, Michie S, Maeda A, Lizuka S. Effects of humid heat exposure on human sleep stages and body temperature. *Sleep.* 1999;22(6):767–773. doi:10.1093/sleep/22.6.767.

25. Obradovich N, Migliorini R, Mednick SC, Fowler JH. Nighttime temperature and human sleep loss in a changing climate. *Sci Adv.* 2017;3(5):1–7. doi:10.1126/sciadv.1601555.

26. Fronczek R, Raymann RJEM, Romeijn N, et al. Manipulation of core body and skin temperature improves vigilance and maintenance of wakefulness in narcolepsy. *Sleep.* 2008;31(2):233–240. doi:10.1093/sleep/31.2.233.

27. Raymann RJEM. Cutaneous warming promotes sleep onset. *AJP Regul Integr Comp Physiol.* 2005;288(6):R1589–R1597. doi:10.1152/ajpregu.00492.2004.

28. Raymann RJEM, Swaab DF, Van Someren EJW. Skin temperature and sleep-onset latency: Changes with age and insomnia. *Physiol Behav.* 2007;90(2–3):257–266. doi:10.1016/j.physbeh.2006.09.008.

29. Lan L, Qian XL, Lian ZW, Lin YB. Local body cooling to improve sleep quality and thermal comfort in a hot environment. *Indoor Air.* 2018;28(1):135–145. doi:10.1111/ina.12428.

30. Richardson CE, Gradisar M, Short MA, Lang C. Can exercise regulate the circadian system of adolescents? Novel implications for the treatment of delayed sleep-wake phase disorder. *Sleep Med Rev.* 2017;34:122–129. doi:10.1016/j.smrv.2016.06.010.

31. Roth T, Mayleben D, Feldman N, Lankford A, Grant T, Nofzinger E. A novel forehead temperature-regulating device for insomnia: A randomized clinical trial. *Sleep.* 2018;41(5):1–11. doi:10.1093/sleep/zsy045.

32. Mysliwiec V, Neylan TC, Chiappetta L, Nofzinger EA. Effects of a forehead cooling device in veterans with chronic insomnia disorder and co-morbid

medical and psychiatric conditions: A pilot study. *Sleep Breath.* 2020. doi:10.1007/s11325-020-02126-w.

33. Naumann J, Grebe J, Kaifel S, Weinert T, Sadaghiani C, Huber R. Effects of hyperthermic baths on depression, sleep and heart rate variability in patients with depressive disorder: A randomized clinical pilot trial. *BMC Complement Altern Med.* 2017;17(1):1–9. doi:10.1186/s12906-017-1676-5.

34. Liao WC, Wang L, Kuo CP, Lo C, Chiu MJ, Ting H. Effect of a warm footbath before bedtime on body temperature and sleep in older adults with good and poor sleep: An experimental crossover trial. *Int J Nurs Stud.* 2013;50(12):1607–1616. doi:10.1016/j.ijnurstu.2013.04.006.

35. Mullen B, Champagne T, Krishnamurty S, Dickson D, Gao RX. Exploring the safety and therapeutic effects of deep pressure stimulation using a weighted blanket. *Occup Ther Ment Heal.* 2008;24(1):65–89.

36. Stephenson J, Carter M. The use of weighted vests with children with autism spectrum disorders and other disabilities. *J Autism Dev Disord.* 2009;39(1):105–114. doi:10.1007/s10803-008-0605-3.

37. Gee BM, Peterson TG, Buck A, Lloyd K. Improving sleep quality using weighted blankets among young children with an autism spectrum disorder. *Int J Ther Rehabil.* 2016;23(4):173–181.

38. Creasey N, Finlay F. Question 2: Do weighted blankets improve sleep in children with an autistic spectrum disorder? *Arch Dis Child.* 2013;98(11):919–920.

39. Gringras P, Green D, Wright B, et al. Weighted blankets and sleep in autistic children—a randomized controlled trial. *Pediatrics.* 2014;134(2):298–306.

40. Future Market Insight. Wearable sleep trackers market: Online distribution channel segment to augment revenue growth during the forecast period: Global industry analysis 2013–2017 and opportunity assessment 2018–2028. 2018. https://www.futuremarketinsights.com/reports/wearable-sleep-trackers-market

41. IDC. Worldwide Quarterly Wearable Device Tracker. 2018. https://www.idc.com/getdoc.jsp?containerId=prUS43900918

42. Oura Health. 2018. https://ouraring.com/

43. Bellone GJ, Plano SA, Cardinali DP, Chada DP, Vigo DE, Golombek DA. Comparative analysis of actigraphy performance in healthy young subjects. *Sleep Sci.* 2016;9(4):272–279. doi:10.1016/j.slsci.2016.05.004.

44. Bianchi MT. Sleep devices: Wearables and nearables, informational and interventional, consumer and clinical. *Metabolism.* 2018;84:99–108. doi:10.1016/j.metabol.2017.10.008.

45. de Zambotti M, Baker FC, Willoughby AR, et al. Measures of sleep and cardiac functioning during sleep using a multi-sensory commercially-available wristband in adolescents. *Physiol Behav.* 2016;158:143–149. doi:10.1016/j.physbeh.2016.03.006.

46. Tal A, Shinar Z, Shaki D, Codish S, Goldbart A. Validation of contact-free sleep monitoring device with comparison to polysomnography. *J Clin Sleep Med.* 2017;13(3):517–522. doi:10.5664/jcsm.6514.

47. de Zambotti M, Rosas L, Colrain IM, Baker FC. The sleep of the ring: Comparison of the ŌURA sleep tracker against polysomnography. *Behav Sleep Med.* 2019;17(2):124–136. doi:10.1177/0333102415576222.Is.

48. Research2guidance. R2G mHealth App Economics 2017 – Current Status and Future Trends in Mobile Health. 2018;(November 2017). https://research2guidance.com/product/mhealth-economics-2017-current-status-and-future-trends-in-mobile-health/

49. Aitken M, Lyle J. Patient adoption of MHealth. 2015. www.theimsinstitute.org

50. Shin JC, Kim J, Grigsby-Toussaint D. Mobile phone interventions for sleep disorders and sleep quality: Systematic review. *JMIR mHealth uHealth.* 2017;5(9):e131. doi:10.2196/mhealth.7244.

51. Grigsby-Toussaint DS, Shin JC, Reeves DM, Beattie A, Auguste E, Jean-Louis G. Sleep apps and behavioral constructs: A content analysis. *Prev Med Reports.* 2017;6:126–129. doi:10.1016/j.pmedr.2017.02.018.

52. Krebs P, Duncan DT. Health app use among us mobile phone owners: A national survey. *JMIR mHealth uHealth.* 2015;3(4):e101. doi:10.2196/mhealth.4924.

53. Virtual Reality Society. What is virtual reality. 2018. https://www.vrs.org.uk/virtual-reality/what-is-virtual-reality.html

54. Freeman D, Reeve S, Robinson A, et al. Virtual reality in the assessment, understanding, and treatment of mental health disorders. *Psychol Med.* 2017;47(14):2393–2400. doi:10.1017/S003329171700040X.

55. Chang LC, Wang CYI, Yu P. Virtual reality improves sleep quality amongst older adults with disabilities. *Int J Geriatr Psychiatry.* 2014;29(12):1312–1313. doi:10.1002/gps.4172.

56. Fisher Wallace Laboratories. Kortex. 2018. https://kortex.health/

57. Minditorium IVS. mindZense Sleep. 2018. https://www.oculus.com/experiences/go/1471880979518893/

58. King J, Jansen E, Helal S, et al. The gator tech smart house: A programmable pervasive space. *Computer (Long Beach Calif).* 2005;38(3):50–60. doi:10.1109/MC.2005.107.

59. Park SH, Won SH, Lee JB, Kim SW. Smart home: Digitally engineered domestic life. *Pers Ubiquitous Comput.* 2003;7(3–4):189–196. doi:10.1007/s00779-003-0228-9.

60. Hart A, Tallevi K, Wickland D, Kearney RE, Cafazzo JA. A contact-free respiration monitor for smart bed and ambulatory monitoring applications. *2010 Annu Int Conf IEEE Eng Med Biol Soc EMBC'10.* 2010:927–930. doi:10.1109/IEMBS.2010.5627525.

61. Kim Y, Yoo S, Han C, Kim S, Shin J, Choi J. Evaluation of unconstrained monitoring technology used in the smart bed for u-health environment. *Telemed e-Health.* 2011;17(6):435–441. doi:10.1089/tmj.2010.0211.

62. Sivanantham A. Measurement of heartbeat, respiration and movements detection using Smart Bed. *2015 IEEE Recent Adv Intell Comput Syst RAICS 2015.* 2016;(December):105–109. doi:10.1109/RAICS.2015.7488397.

63. Royal Philips. Philips Personal Health Solutions at CES 2018 connect people, technology and data. *Bus Wire*. September 2018. http://search.ebscohost.com/login.aspx?direct=true&db=bwh&AN=bizwire.c82506559

64. Philips news center United states. June 2018. Extracted from: https://www.usa.philips.com/a-w/about/news/archive/standard/news/press/2018/20180620-philips-named-best-overall-medtech-company-for-best-sleep-monitoring-solution-with-philips-smartsleep.html

65. Philips Respironics. Smart sleep in-home validation extension study: Full text view. ClinicalTrials.gov. 2019. https://clinicaltrials.gov/ct2/show/study/NCT03665844?cond=Smart+sleep&rank=1

37

The Future of Sleep (and Dream) Medicine

RUBIN NAIMAN

Every man takes the limits of his own field of vision for the limits of the world.

—Arthur Schopenhauer

Notwithstanding the significant progress made in the treatment of sleep disorders reviewed in this text, much remains to be done. Despite the dramatic growth of sleep medicine, related research, and public health initiatives over recent decades, insufficient sleep and sleep disorders, especially insomnia and obstructive sleep apnea (OSA), remain endemic. And the resulting personal suffering as well as social and economic costs are staggering. An integrative revisioning of sleep medicine may help us better understand and more effectively address these concerns in the future.

Based on extensive clinical and teaching experience in integrative approaches to sleep and dreams, this chapter sketches the author's vision of the future of sleep medicine. To do so, we must begin with an examination of our presumptions about sleep itself and the limitations they impose on sleep medicine. Toward this end, our discussion will emphasize insomnia, the most prevalent sleep disorder. How we approach insomnia is illustrative of how we relate to sleep in general and has ramifications for how we manage other sleep disorders. As we will see, the core tenets of integrative medicine provide a foundation for reimagining sleep medicine based on a radically transformed sense of sleep.

Presumptions and Limitations of Conventional Sleep Medicine

Our contemporary sense of sleep has been shaped by three dynamic sociocultural forces: denaturation, industrialization, and medicalization. *Denaturation* refers to the gradual segregation of sleep from the natural environment in which it evolved and on which it depends. It is the nocturnal equivalent of "nature deficit disorder." Most obviously, denaturation is associated with chronic and significant disentrainment from nature's circadian zeitgebers, especially the rhythms of light and darkness and ambient temperatures. Natural sleep was characterized by an intimate dance between the sleeper and the environment. We slept *with* the world around us—in close proximity to and in time with the people and places that comprised our world. Modern sleep, however, is decontextualized, less social and relational, more individual, private, and dysrhythmic. Additionally, the places we sleep, our bedrooms, have become significantly less permeable to the natural nocturnal environment and more polluted with daytime stimulation, especially artificial light,[1] synthetic chemicals,[2] and the rapidly escalating occurrence of electromagnetic fields (EMFs).[3]

The Industrial Revolution further damaged sleep by devaluing it and disrupting circadian rhythms. *Industrialization* transfigured our age-old dance with the environment into a race through it. Beyond its socioeconomic impact, industrialization endorses a mindset that overvalues productivity and undervalues rest. A web search for antonyms of *industrious* reveals numerous pejorative terms like lazy, inactive, sluggish, indolent, dull, lackadaisical, idle, lethargic, and unproductive, alongside a dearth of positive terms. By substantially lengthening the waking day with artificial light at night, industrialization gradually effected a subtle but pernicious constriction of human consciousness that I have previously described as *wake-centrism*. Wake-centrism refers to waking that is runaway—insufficiently modulated by sleep and dreaming. It is amplified and accelerated at the expense of sleep and dreams, which are relegated to secondary and subservient states of consciousness. Wake-centrism establishes waking as the primary or gold standard for consciousness, resulting in a subtle but pernicious psychological "addiction" to it.[4]

Wake-centric waking lies at the root of psychophysiological hyperarousal, the primary cause of insomnia disorder. It is not surprising that speeding is a common infraction of the law and that *crashing* is a common euphemism for getting to sleep. Neither is our extensive reliance on substances and sedative-hypnotics as chemical emergency brakes a surprise. As we will see, the failure to recognize the fundamental conceptual constraints imposed by wake-centrism limits our understanding and management of insomnia.

Our contemporary sense of sleep is also *medicalized*. Historically, sleep was a *personal, subjective experience*—a state of consciousness of equal interest to poets, priests, and ordinary people as it was to physicians. But as concerns about sleep disorders skyrocketed over recent decades, sleep medicine reconceptualized sleep as a *biomedical, objective process*. Today, for health professionals and consumers alike, most conversations about sleep are cast in medical terms.[5] Sleep is about neurophysiology, polysomnography, hypnotics, therapeutic mattresses, and tracking devices. This reconceptualization has spawned a powerful sleep-medical-industrial complex that reinforces medicalization with profits from sleep pharmaceuticals, supplements, gadgetry, and other products.[6]

Sleep medicine has further obscured our understanding of, and therefore our relationship with, sleep by defining it negatively—that is, in terms of what it is not. In much the same way that health is presumed to be the absence of disease, sleep is presumed to be the absence of waking, or awareness, or consciousness. In his classic volume, *The Promise of Sleep*, William Dement states, "It is impossible to have conscious, experiential knowledge of non-dreaming sleep; indeed, one of sleep's defining aspects is that we don't know that we are sleeping while we are doing it."[7] The presumption that sleep is unconscious has significant ramifications for how we relate to sleep as well as dreams. And it is mistaken.

Historically, sleep specialists have dismissed anecdotal reports of awareness of sleep by conceptualizing them as "sleep state misperception." However, it might be more accurate to view these as sleep state perception. A recent opinion piece in *Trends in Cognitive Science* concludes "there are good empirical and theoretical reasons for saying that a range of different types of sleep experience, some of which are distinct from dreaming, can occur in all stages of sleep."[8] This echoes a time-honored perspective that has recently been gaining scientific support. Tibetan Buddhist sleep and dream yogas,[9] Hindu Vedantic scriptures,[10] and Western philosophies like anthroposophy[11] all view sleep as a state of consciousness that can be directly experienced. More recently, studies of yoga nidra[12] and mindfulness meditation confirm the human capacity to cultivate awareness during non–rapid eye movement (NREM) sleep.[13]

Rooted in wake-centrism, the presumption that sleep is unconscious may be sleep medicine's greatest misstep. Medicalization devalues the subjective experience of sleep by obscuring it with biomedical complexities. Scientific attempts to define sleep are largely descriptions of neurophysiological correlates of the subjective experience of sleep. As a result, conventional sleep medicine (CSM) *depersonalizes* sleep. It loses sight of the sleeper, of the patient's experience of sleep, of the importance of *sleep phenomenology.*

A recent manifesto by a coalition of prominent global scientists has raised concerns about philosophical materialism, an ideology that dismisses the value of phenomenology in science and medicine. They assert, "Faith in this ideology, as an exclusive explanatory framework for reality, has compelled scientists to neglect the subjective dimension of human experience. This has led to a severely distorted and impoverished understanding of ourselves and our place in nature."[14]

Dismissing sleep phenomenology discourages us from opening to a more direct experience of and relationship with sleep. It limits our sense of responsibility for our own sleep, erodes sleep self-efficacy, and sets sleep specialists up as gatekeepers. It also encourages overreliance on hypnotics that mimic sleep by inducing states of unconsciousness. Fortunately, recent studies are beginning to acknowledge the value of subjective self-reports in the evaluation and treatment of insomnia.[15]

The most obvious consequences of the depersonalization of sleep lie in CSM's dismissive posture toward the phenomenology of dreaming. Dreaming is commonly viewed as a subset of sleep that is personally meaningless and largely irrelevant to health. Despite the fact that we cannot prove a negative, the prominent activation-synthesis model of REM/dreaming presumes that dreams have no inherent personal meaning.[16] Studies of sleep loss commonly fail to discriminate actual sleep loss from REM sleep or dream loss. As a result, CSM has long been in denial about the existence and ramifications of a silent epidemic of REM sleep loss.[17]

In practice, REM sleep and dreams have been of interest to sleep clinicians only when they might be suggestive of pathology as in REM behavior disorder (RBD) or nightmare disorder. However, mounting evidence confirms that REM sleep and dreaming play a critical role in the pathophysiology of insomnia.[18] More specifically, much of what is designated *wake after sleep onset* (WASO) might more accurately be described as WADO—*wake after dream onset.*

It can be argued that behavioral sleep medicine (BSM) evolved in large part to address the shortcomings associated with the medicalization and depersonalization of sleep, especially in the treatment of insomnia. In contrast to CSM's symptom-suppressive approach that relies primarily on sedative-hypnotics, BSM has adapted and integrated established behavioral and psychotherapeutic techniques to create cognitive-behavioral therapy for insomnia (CBT-I). But this attempt at restoring regard for the sleeper has fallen short.

Although meta-analyses support CBT-I as a first-line treatment for insomnia, as many as 25–40% of patients continue to be symptomatic after treatment,[19] and improvements in quality of life measures are often small.[20] More severe insomnia has, additionally, been found to be significantly less responsive to CBT-I.[21] And although sleep hygiene appears to be useful in supporting healthy sleep, it is of questionable effectiveness as a monotherapy for insomnia.[22]

As its name suggests, behavioral sleep *medicine* is also medicalized, relying on biomedical conceptualizations of sleep that presume it to be unconscious. CBT-I focuses on thoughts and behaviors about sleep, but, like CSM, it largely neglects the phenomenology or experience of sleep. As a result, CBT-I may be more effective at addressing thoughts and behaviors that impede sleep and less effective at directly facilitating sleep induction. And because BSM presumes sleep is unconscious, even relaxation practices that can deliver patients to the shoreline of sleep typically fail to teach them how to swim. Likewise, although BSM may address REM sleep-related pathologies such as nightmares and sleep paralysis, it fails to meaningfully address dreaming. Given clinical psychology's historic roots in phenomenology and dreamwork, BSM's limited regard for dreaming, especially the phenomenology of dreams, is striking.

Sleep medicine has carefully mapped and measured the complex neurophysiology of sleep. But we need to heed Gregory Bateson's admonition that *the map is not the territory and the name is not the thing.* And neither is the number. By confusing the clinical conceptualizations and measurements of sleep with actual sleep, sleep medicine has overshadowed our common sense and sentiments about sleep. Certainly, sleep disorders are medical issues, but sleep, per se, is not. The brain and body do not sleep; people do.

An Integrative Approach to Sleep and Sleep Health

To summarize, our sleep is (1) denatured—disentrained from natural environmental and rhythmic influences, (2) industrialized—damaged by wake-centrism and hyperarousal, and (3) medicalized—depersonalized and dismissive of sleep and dream phenomenology. The basic tenets of integrative medicine that inform this text provide a viable foundation for effectively addressing these challenges and reshaping the future of sleep health. More specifically, the tenets of integrative medicine provide a rationale for naturalizing, deindustrializing, and personalizing sleep. Integrative medicine emphasizes (1) lifestyle factors, (2) natural and less-invasive interventions, (3) the therapeutic relationship (e.g., viewing patients as partners), (4) the critical role of mind, (5) the body's innate healing capacity, and (6) health promotion and prevention.

NATURALIZING SLEEP

Naturalizing sleep requires a fundamental shift in our relationship with nature that acknowledges our profound interdependence. Because sleep is as much an environmental issue as it is a physiological process, greater emphasis needs to be placed on this broader, more comprehensive context of sleep. Naturalizing sleep is about healing our relationship with nature—with night and natural rhythms as well as with human nature. In the future, sleep disorders may be understood as environmental illnesses as much as medical conditions.

In contrast to a culture driven by linear time, the natural world is structured by rhythmic timing. The future of sleep will need to offer greater regard for the role of timing—of rhythmic processes in life as well as in medicine. The *power of when*—that is, the powerful influence of natural rhythmic processes including circadian as well as infradian and ultradian rhythms—needs to be better understood and more thoroughly considered. The critical role of circadian rhythms will be particularly important in making medical, vocational, social, and personal decisions such as timing in the administration of medicines, school start times, and work schedules. The timing of sleep, both nightly sleep and daytime napping, must also receive greater regard in the future. Sleep phases that are aligned with natural night have, for example, long been endorsed by non-Western medical systems such as Ayurveda and Traditional Chinese Medicine (TCM).[23]

Increased recognition and regard for the critical role of timing in health, disease, and treatment should drive greater interdisciplinary interest in the field of circadian medicine.[24] More specifically, attention to the critical role of respiration in sleep health and sleep disorders could open new avenues for treatment. Early in the evolution of integrative medicine, Andrew Weil called attention to the significance of respiration in general health in his audiobook, *Breathing: the Master Key to Self-Healing*.[25] Alternative approaches to respiration in health ranging from classic Ayurvedic *pranayama* practices[26] to more recent Buteyko methods[27] offer creative options for research and management of snoring and apnea.

Barry Krakow's investigation of the relationship between chronic insomnia and sleep-disordered breathing likewise opens new and promising vistas for prevention and treatment. His model draws attention to the critical interaction of body (respiratory) and mind (cognitive) factors in the pathophysiology of insomnia. It suggests that insomnia, posttraumatic stress disorder (PTSD), depression, and anxiety disorders can cause initial sleep fragmentation, which over time results in sleep-disordered breathing that is obscured by insomnia. Krakow reports significant success in treating these patients with adapt-servo ventilation.[28]

In addition to the widely accepted need to sleep in cool, dark, safe, and quiet places, our understanding of a healthy sleep environment should expand to include sensitivity to more subtle environmental factors including toxic chemicals and non-ionizing radiation. Recent advances in biophilic architecture and design emphasize the health as well as aesthetic value of creating greater permeability between interior spaces and the natural world.[29]

Sleep retreats of the future could provide carefully designed healing environments, as are currently seen in exclusive spas around the globe. Or they might involve camping excursions to unspoiled environments sans electronic devices.[30] Reminiscent of the nineteenth-century "rest cure" (without the austerity), home-based personalized sleep retreats might also serve to promote sleep and dream health.

DEINDUSTRIALIZING SLEEP

Deindustrializing sleep is about managing hyperarousal-driven insomnia by modulating runaway waking consciousness with rest and sleep. If we choose to reduce our reliance on hypnotics, managing hyperarousal becomes a psychological and behavioral challenge that falls squarely on the shoulders of BSM. Historically, BSM has responded to this challenge with CBT-I, including sleep hygiene recommendations and cognitive therapy. These are certainly useful interventions, especially for decreasing stimulation, activity, and mentation, but, as previously discussed, they are insufficient.

The limitations of CBT-I are rooted in wake-centrism. That is, CBT-I focuses entirely on behavior and mentation associated with waking consciousness. And, waking is sticky. Believing waking consciousness can be leveraged into sleep keeps us stuck in waking. Although we can effectively utilize waking to take us to the edge of sleep, we cannot think or behave our way directly into sleep. Getting to sleep requires a shift of consciousness—*transcending waking and surrendering to sleep and dreams.*[31]

The future of BSM might witness the evolution of CBT-I from *cognitive-behavioral therapy* to *consciousness*-behavioral therapy. The current cognitive model could be enhanced by drawing from a range of therapies that support transcendence into non-waking states of consciousness. This is already under way, with growing interest in the role of mindfulness in sleep, [32] and will likely continue with the incorporation of interventions from diverse arenas including dreamwork, yoga nidra, and psychedelic therapies.

Because it is rooted in wake-centrism and reinforced by social expectations, it may prove useful to conceptualize hyperarousal-driven insomnia as an "addiction" to waking. Building on emerging support for group approaches,[33] the 12-step recovery model might prove useful in this regard because it is widely accessible, personalized, non-medicalized, focused on surrender, and provides extensive sponsor support at virtually no cost.[34]

PERSONALIZING SLEEP

Understanding and supporting the role of transcendence in sleep requires addressing problems arising from its depersonalization. As the future unfolds, sleep will no longer be viewed as unconsciousness, but as another kind of consciousness. Such a positive redefinition will accommodate phenomenology and counter the limitations of a negative, medicalized definition. A binocular view of sleep that integrates biomedical findings and phenomenological experience will provide a more comprehensive picture of sleep that is consistent with integrative medicine's body–mind approach. In short, this begins by complementing medical assessment with attention to individuals' personal sleep stories.

The prospect of re-personalizing sleep suggests that people are potentially capable of directly experiencing aspects of it. Beyond dreaming, which will be addressed shortly, the common belief that NREM sleep is unconscious can spark negative, anxiety-provoking appraisals of any awareness during sleep, which in turn can trigger wakefulness and insomnia. Awareness of sleep has inadvertently been pathologized by sleep medicine and may deter people from trusting their own experience. As discussed previously, recent evidence of the potential for awareness even during delta states in meditation and yoga nidra practices are consistent with ancient Buddhist and Hindu writings. This author's informal polling of thousands of people during public sleep presentations around the globe routinely found a clear majority of them acknowledged having experienced awareness of their sleep.

More readily captured by poets and mystics (see the works of Mary Oliver, Rudolph Steiner, David Whyte, Rumi, and Sri Auribindo) sleep is difficult to define positively because it cannot be readily translated it into ordinary waking world concepts or terminology. Experientially, sleep might be redefined as a state of serenity with both psychophysiological and phenomenological correlates. It can, furthermore, be understood as a kind of default consciousness. Like the potential for silence in a loud room, sleep is the potential for serenity beneath the din of waking consciousness. It is always present and revealed by surrendering the stimulation of waking consciousness. Recognizing one's potential to become aware of sleep is not to suggest that it is necessary to do so. But it does open the door to a new and richer relationship with sleep and dreams.

All of this suggests the potential benefit of incorporating spiritual or consciousness-expanding practices into sleep health promotion and treatment approaches. Yoga nidra, various forms of meditation, mindfulness-based stress reduction, and other techniques that open the mind can be useful in this regard.

Re-personalizing sleep requires deepening the partnership between practitioners and patients. It requires practitioners to actively elicit and empathically attend to patients' sleep stories. This includes exploring patient experiences with, in, and around the edges of sleep. It calls for a closer examination of common subjective experiences around sleep onset, sleep offset, WASO, napping, dreaming, and daytime sleepiness. Such a professional posture encourages patients to develop more personal and meaningful relationships with their sleep, which can, in turn, increase treatment adherence and improve self-efficacy.[35]

Reconsidering and Restoring Dreaming

Because dreaming is the most accessible direct experience of sleep, it is a practical avenue for reinstating regard for phenomenology. Given that, it is interesting to consider how much dreaming has been marginalized in both general and sleep medicine (see Chapter 13, "Dream Medicine"). This marginalization is even more striking when we acknowledge dreaming's key role in both sleep and mental health. To summarize, REM sleep and dreaming play critical roles in the consolidation of procedural memory and the regulation of emotions and mood.[36] Dreams, even bad ones, appear to represent a kind of endogenous psychotherapy and may be useful in both preventing and healing PTSD.[37]

Given that hypnagogic and hypnopompic dreams, respectively, carry us into and out of sleep, dreaming serves as the bridge between waking and sleep consciousness. Not surprisingly then, dreaming plays a complex role in the path-ophysiology of insomnia disorder (ID). Given that dreaming is a highly aroused state, individuals with persistent hyperarousal are more prone to experience REM sleep–triggered sleep disruptions. Insomnia patients are, in fact, more likely than good sleepers to report REM sleep as waking.[18] Since much WASO may more accurately be characterized as WADO, evaluating and addressing REM/dreaming should be a routine part of managing ID. And, given that significant REM/dream disruptions are also characteristic of OSA, narcolepsy, many parasomnias, and nightmare disorders, clinicians should routinely query all sleep patients about their dreams.

The extent of our marginalization of dreaming is reflected in the silence shrouding the evidence of an epidemic of REM sleep/dream loss. What is particularly salient is practitioners' typical indifference to the fact that many general, sleep, and psychiatric medications interfere with REM sleep. Freud's "royal road to the unconscious" is being washed out by a flood of REM sleep–suppressant drugs as well as excessive dependence on alcohol and cannabis.[17] The impact of dream loss on health, mental health, the quality of life, and daytime functioning warrants more serious research. Excessive daytime sleepiness resulting from actual sleep loss, for example, might differ from the daytime effects dream loss. It would be beneficial to investigate the concept of excessive daytime dreaminess.

Restoring regard for dreaming in general, mental, and sleep health will require all healthcare professionals, especially sleep and BSM practitioners, to obtain fundamental training in REM sleep, dreaming, and dreamwork.

In Closing

Current estimates suggest that more than 60 million Americans suffer from sleep disorders. Given that there are approximately 7,500 board-certified sleep specialists in the United States, the ratio of prospective patients to sleep specialists is about 43,000:1.[38] Certainly we need to increase these numbers. But we also need to train other health specialists to better evaluate and address basic sleep concerns. The future of sleep medicine will need interdisciplinary healthcare teams that are structured around patient needs, not professional identities or boundaries. Primary care providers as well as psychotherapists should, as a matter of course, receive practical training in supporting sleep health and treating insomnia.

The future will, hopefully, emphasize sleep health promotion and prevention beginning with attention to sleep and dreams in primary school. Rest and napping will no longer be seen as time out from waking activities, but as *time in*—into sleep and dreams, into spaces of serenity and imagination. There will be a greater recognition that we cannot separate what we need to do for healthy sleep from what supports our general health. Sleep will be recognized as a touchstone of health and well-being and offered the same regard as exercise, nutrition, and stress management practices.

The future of sleep medicine will be integrative in the broadest sense of the term. Beyond the integration of conventional with complementary and alternative medicine, it will likely encourage a richer integration of objectivity and phenomenology, the individual and the natural world, as well as waking consciousness with sleep and dreams.

The future of sleep medicine may, in fact, be the future of integrative sleep and dream medicine.

REFERENCES

1. Raap T, Pinxten R, Eens M. Light pollution disrupts sleep in free-living animals. *Sci Rep.* 2015;5:13557. https://doi.org/10.1038/srep13557
2. Bader W. *Sleep safe in a toxic world: Your guide to identifying and removing hidden toxins from your bedroom.* Los Angeles: SCB Distributors; 2012.
3. Pall ML. Microwave frequency electromagnetic fields (EMFs) produce widespread neuropsychiatric effects including depression. *J Chem Neuroanatomy.* 2016 Sep;75(Pt B):43–51. doi:10.1016/j.jchemneu.2015.08.001.
4. Naiman R. *Falling for sleep.* London: Aeon; 2016.
5. Moloney ME, Konrad TR, Zimmer CR. The medicalization of sleeplessness: A public health concern. *Am J Public Health.* 2011;101(8):1429–1433.
6. Barbee H, Moloney ME, Konrad TR. Selling slumber: American neoliberalism and the medicalization of sleeplessness. *Sociol Compass.* 2018;12(10):e12622.
7. Dement WC, Vaughan C. *The promise of sleep: A pioneer in sleep medicine explores the vital connection between health, happiness, and a good night's sleep.* New York: Dell; 1999.
8. Windt JM, Nielsen T, Thompson E. Does consciousness disappear in dreamless sleep?. *Trends Cogn Sci.* 2016;20(12):871–882.
9. Rinpoche TW. *The Tibetan yogas of dream and sleep.* New Delhi: Motilal Banarsidass Publisher; 2004.
10. Alexander C. A conceptual and phenomenological analysis of pure consciousness during sleep. *Lucidity Letter.* 1988;7(2):1–7.
11. Lipson M. *Sleep and dreams: A bridge to the spirit.* Hudson, NY: Steiner Books; 2003.
12. Miller R. *Yoga nidra: Awaken to unqualified presence through traditional mind-body practices.* Louisville, CO: Sounds True; 2010.
13. Visser F. *Ken Wilber: Thought as passion.* Albany, NY: SUNY Press; 2012.
14. Beauregard M, Schwartz GE, Miller L, et al. Manifesto for a post- materialist science. *Explore.* 2014;10(5):272–274.
15. Grandner MA, Perlis ML. Pharmacotherapy for insomnia disorder in older adults. *JAMA Network Open.* 2019;2(12):e1918214–e1918214.

16. Hobson JA, McCarley RW. The brain as a dream state generator: An activation-synthesis hypothesis of the dream process. *Am J Psychiatry.* 1977;134(12):1335–1348.

17. Naiman R. Dreamless: The silent epidemic of REM sleep loss. *Ann NY Acad Sci.* 2017;1406(1):77–85.

18. Riemann D, Spiegelhalder K, Nissen C, et al. REM sleep instability–a new pathway for insomnia? Pharmacopsychiatry. 2012;45(5):167–176.

19. Baron KG, Hooker S. Next Steps for patients who fail to respond to cognitive behavioral therapy for insomnia (CBT-I): The perspective from behavioral sleep medicine psychologists. *Curr Sleep Med Rep.* 2017;3(4):327–332.

20. Kyle SD, Morgan K, Espie CA. Insomnia and health-related quality of life. *Sleep Med Rev.* 2010;14:69–82.

21. Bathgate CJ, Edinger JD, Krystal AD. Insomnia patients with objective short sleep duration have a blunted response to cognitive behavioral therapy for insomnia. *Sleep.* 2017;40(1):zsw012.

22. Irish LA, Kline CE, Gunn HE, et al. The role of sleep hygiene in promoting public health: A review of empirical evidence. *Sleep Med Rev.* 2015;22:23–36.

23. Shea B. *Handbook of Chinese Medicine and Ayurveda: An integrated practice of ancient healing traditions.* New York: Simon and Schuster; 2018.

24. Panda S. The arrival of circadian medicine. *Nat Rev Endocrinol.* 2019;15(2):67–69.

25. Weil AT. *Breathing: The master key to self-healing.* Audio CD. Louisville, CO: Sounds True; 2000.

26. Manjunath NK, Telles S. Influence of yoga ayurveda on self-rated sleep in a geriatric population. *Indian J Med Res.* 2005;121(5):683.

27. Courtney R, Cohen M. Investigating the claims of Konstantin Buteyko M.D, PhD: The relationship of breath holding time to end tidal CO_2 and other proposed measures of dysfunctional breathing. *J Alt Compl Med.* 2008;14(2):115–123

28. Krakow B, McIver ND, Ulibarri VA, Krakow J, Schrader RM. Prospective randomized controlled trial on the efficacy of continuous positive airway pressure and adaptive servo-ventilation in the treatment of chronic complex insomnia. *EClinicalMedicine.* 2019;13::57–73.

29. Bolten B, Barbiero G. Biophilic design: How to enhance physical and psychological health and wellbeing in our built environments. *Visions for Sustainability.* 2020;13:1–4.

30. Stothard ER, McHill AW, Depner CM, et al. Circadian entrainment to the natural light-dark cycle across seasons and the weekend. *Curr Biol.* 2017;27(4):508–513.

31. Naiman RR. *Healing night: The science and spirit of sleeping, dreaming, and awakening.* Minneapolis, MN: Syren Book Company; 2006.

32. Ong JC, Moore C. What do we really know about mindfulness and sleep health?. *Curr Opin Psychol.* 2020;34:18–22.

33. Castronovo V, Galbiati A, Sforza M, et al. Long-term clinical effect of group cognitive behavioral therapy for insomnia: A case series study. *Sleep Med.* 2018;47:54–59.

34. Naiman RR. Insomniacs anonymous: Do we need a 12-step program for sleep? Huffington Post. 2011 June. www.huffingtonpost.com/rubin-naiman-phd/

35. Meichenbaum D, Turk DC. *Facilitating treatment adherence: A practitioner's guidebook*. New York: Plenum Press; 1987.
36. Cartwright R. *The 24-hour mind: The role of sleep and dreaming in our emotional lives*. New York: Oxford University Press; 2010.
37. Repantis D, Wermuth K, Tsamitros N, et al. REM sleep in acutely traumatized individuals and interventions for the secondary prevention of post-traumatic stress disorder. *Eur J Psychotraumatol.* 2020;11(1):1740492.
38. Watson NF, Rosen IM, Chervin RD. The past is prologue: The future of sleep medicine. *J Clin Sleep Med.* 2017;13(1):127–135.

INDEX

For the benefit of digital users, indexed terms that span two pages (e.g., 52–53) may, on occasion, appear on only one of those pages.

Tables, figures and boxes are indicated by *t, f* and *b* following the page number

NMDA receptors, 157
nocturnal enuresis, 597–98
non-entrained disorder. *See* non–24-hour
    sleep–wake rhythm disorder
non–24-hour sleep–wake rhythm disorder,
    54–55, 137–38, 529–30, 533–34,
    535, 536–37
NREM sleep
    adulthood/aging, 50–51, 51*f*
    in children, 35, 39, 40–41, 42
    dreaming, 214
    homeostasis biomarkers, 68–69
    lavender induction of, 333
    memory role, 216
    napping and, 93–94
    parasomnias (*see* parasomnias)
    physiology of, 212
    resistance exercise effects, 130
    vitamin A deficiency, 160
N24SWD. *See* non–24-hour sleep–wake
    rhythm disorder
Nurses' Health Study, 472
nutrition. *See* diet/nutrition

obesity
    circadian disruption effects, 79–80
    hypoventilation syndrome, 351, 522–23
    short sleep and, 18–19, 21, 87–88
    sleep deprivation and, 113
Obradovich, N., 627
obsessive-compulsive disorder (OCD), 454
obstructive sleep apnea (OSA)
    ADHD comorbid, 608–10
    adjunctive treatment, 518–20
    antioxidants, 158–59
    background, 509–11
    cannabis, 264–65, 520
    in children, 602–4
    clonazepam, 577–78
    consequences of, 513–14
    CPAP, 6–7, 134, 152, 440, 512–13, 514–20
    CPAP adherence, 515–17
    CPAP alternatives, 518–20
    diagnosis, 512–13
    evaluation of, 511–12
    exercise effects, 134*f*, 134–35
    functional medicine, 347
    GI tract relationship to, 152
    historically, 6–7
    in infants, 590–94, 593*t*

insomnia comorbid, 515
integrative sleep medicine, 439–40
pathophysiology, 510–11
pharmacotherapy, 520
prevalence, 509–10
race/ethnicity, 511, 515
restless legs syndrome relationship
    to, 555
risk factors, 510–11
screening for, 435
structural integrity in functional
    medicine, 351–52
treatment, 512–13, 514–20
vitamin A deficiency, 160
vitamin D deficiency, 160–61
in women, 474, 475–76, 478, 510–11
occupational accidents, 22–23
O'Connor, K., 424
olanzapine, 389–90
older adults. *See* adulthood/aging
oleic acid/oleamide, 159
olibanum, 336
omega-3-fatty acids, 159
operant conditioning, 404
opioids
    drug interactions, 377
    limiting, in OSA, 518
    restless legs syndrome, 558–59
optimism intervention, 205*t*
oral appliances, in OSA, 518–19
orange oil, 339*t*
orexin (hypocretin), 34–35, 489–90,
    491, 493
orexin antagonists, 8–9
Ornish, D., 353
osteopathy, 306–7, 309–10
Ostrin, L. A., 626
Oura ring, 629, 631
oxybutynin, in children, 598
oxytocin, pregnancy effects on, 474–75

Padilla, A. J., 517
Page, A. T., 461
pain, chronic
    cannabis use in, 267
    case study, 436, 442
    energy medicine,
        contraindications, 323–24
    herbs for, 442
    hypnosis, 367